Stress Management for Life

A RESEARCH-BASED, EXPERIENTIAL APPROACH

Second Edition

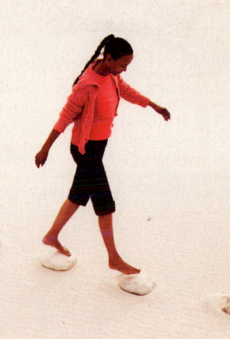

Michael Olpin
Weber State University

Margie Hesson
South Dakota State University

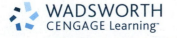

WADSWORTH
CENGAGE Learning™

Australia • Brazil • Japan • Korea • Mexico • Singapore • Spain • United Kingdom • United States

WADSWORTH
CENGAGE Learning

Stress Management for Life: A Research-Based, Experiential Approach, Second Edition
Michael Olpin, Margie Hesson

Publisher: Yolanda Cossio

Health Editor: Laura Pople

Developmental Editor: Anna Lustig

Assistant Editor: Samantha Arvin

Editorial Assistant: Jenny Hoang

Media Editor: Lauren Tarson

Marketing Manager: Laura McGinn

Marketing Assistant: Elizabeth Wong

Marketing Communications Manager:
Belinda Krohmer

Content Project Manager: Trudy Brown

Creative Director: Rob Hugel

Art Director: John Walker

Print Buyer: Linda Hsu

Rights Acquisitions Account Manager, Text:
Bob Kauser

Rights Acquisitions Account Manager, Image:
Leitha Etheridge-Sims

Production Service: Elm Street Publishing
Services

Text Designer: Tani Hasegawa

Photo Researcher: Bill Smith Group

Cover Designer: Jeanne Calabrese

Cover Image: Martin Barraud/Getty Images

Compositor: Integra Software Services Pvt. Ltd.

For product information and technology assistance, contact us at
Cengage Learning Customer & Sales Support, 1-800-354-9706.

For permission to use material from this text or product,
submit all requests online at **www.cengage.com/permissions.**
Further permissions questions can be e-mailed to
permissionrequest@cengage.com.

Library of Congress Control Number: 2009922080

ISBN-13: 978-0-324-59943-5
ISBN-10: 0-324-59943-9

Wadsworth
10 Davis Drive
Belmont, CA 94002-3098
USA

Cengage Learning is a leading provider of customized learning solutions with office locations around the globe, including Singapore, the United Kingdom, Australia, Mexico, Brazil, and Japan. Locate your local office at **www.cengage.com/global.**

Cengage Learning products are represented in Canada by Nelson Education, Ltd.

To learn more about Wadsworth, visit **www.cengage.com/wadsworth.**
Purchase any of our products at your local college store or at our preferred online store **www.ichapters.com.**

Printed in the United States of America
1 2 3 4 5 6 7 13 12 11 10 09

155,9042
O52

Brief Contents

Contents

Part III
Stress-Prevention Strategies

Contents

Preface

A little knowledge that acts is worth infinitely
more than much knowledge that is idle.

—*Kahlil Gibran*

Stress Management for Life is more than just another book about stress. It is an experience. This book will teach you what you need to know about stress—and it doesn't stop there. You will find a toolbox of skills for immediate application and for immediate benefits to prevent and manage stress in your life. You will learn about stress; you will learn and practice specific techniques; and you will be inspired to continue a life-long program of stress management. *Stress Management for Life* provides information, inspiration, and application—a powerful approach to a healthy, balanced life.

Listen to what this student says about *Stress Management for Life:*

> This book really helped me to get in touch with myself and the way I view a variety of things in my life. What I learned will help me well into my future and the book should be required reading for every student. The book was very inspirational in motivating me to take action to live a better, stress-free life. The materials and activities were beyond good. With all the perceived stress we experience in our daily lives, on top of the rigorous academic studies, it is easy to let things get to us. This book would help everyone put things into perspective. The book opened my eyes to the variety of stress-relieving exercises I can use throughout my daily life. The things I learned will last a lifetime.

You too can learn to replace stress and tension with life-enhancing energy. The best news is that it's up to you! You are in charge of the choices you make every day. Through reading, thinking, learning, and actually practicing the many strategies presented in *Stress Management for Life*, you will be on the path to a healthier, more balanced, and more productive life. The real power of this book will be found in the action you take. You will learn to experience the benefits of energizing relaxation immediately. And you will be prepared to develop a lifetime plan to assure that these benefits will continue long after your class is over.

Stress Management for Life is:

- a practical guide for incorporating stress management into your daily life.
- a holistic approach to prevent and manage unhealthy stress.
- a "how to" book with clear instructions on stress management techniques that work.
- a book that will change your life, enhance your health, and improve your quality of life.

> You have complete control over three things in your life: what you think, what you say, and how you behave. To make a change in your life, you must recognize that these gifts are the most powerful tools you possess in shaping the form of your life.
>
> —*Sonya Friedman*

Overview of *Stress Management for Life*

Part I: Getting Started In this introduction to stress management, you will begin thinking about stress in today's world. You will personalize the information by completing a variety of stress self-assessments that will help you understand your own unique stressors and how you handle them.

Part II: Understanding Stress Part II explores the physical and psychological implications of stress—how the body and mind communicate. Have you ever heard of psychoneuroimmunology? Learn about this and other exciting research on the connection between mind and body.

Part III: Stress-Prevention Strategies Part III offers some concrete and effective tools that you can incorporate into your life with immediate results to *prevent* stress In the first place. You will receive some proven tips for eliminating stress by managing time and organizing your schedule. You will read about how to control emotions including anger, fear, and worry. Values clarification, spirituality and stress, financial management, and a healing environment are just a few of the interesting topics covered here.

Part IV: Stress-Reduction Techniques Despite your best efforts to prevent stress, we know that stress happens. In Part IV you will learn a wide variety of techniques designed specifically to help you reduce stress. You will be amazed to find that simple techniques such as the Power Nap, meditation, autogenics, and yoga can leave you feeling relaxed and energized. You will learn about massage, guided imagery, the latest in complementary/alternative approaches, and other powerful stress-reduction techniques.

One of the selling points for *Stress Management for Life* is that you will benefit from the information while you are reading the book and also will be preparing to reap the benefits for a lifetime. You will be able to incorporate the techniques that work best for you and that fit your lifestyle, values, and goals into a plan for life.

New in the Second Edition

Each chapter has been revised to keep you current on the latest in stress-management advancements. New stats from the annual College Student Assessment and data from Healthy People 2010 help you stay abreast on current stress-related issues. New research is reported including research on:

- the relationship between altruism, stress, and academic performance.
- how pets help college students cope with stress.
- intimacy and how close relationships improve psychological health.
- brain changes that occur during meditation.
- weight gain in college and the connection to stress eating.

You will also find new content in this edition including:

- Stress Vulnerability Assessment.
- hardiness and how hardy characteristics relate to stress.
- happiness and gratitude.
- expanded coverage of biofeedback.
- strategies to improve stress-related performance for athletes.

Two new features have been added to the already comprehensive array of engaging features including:

- Stress Busting Behavior boxes for a quick interactive opportunity to personalize what you are reading.
- Stress Management Labs at the end of each chapter to help you review and apply important chapter information.

Features

Stress Management for Life is written in a *clear and easy-to-understand* style. The reading level and content are geared for university students like you. This book doesn't try to cover everything about stress. Instead, it covers everything that matters to successfully prevent and manage stress in your life.

Who said a textbook has to be boring? The authors of *Stress Management for Life* teach stress-management courses to university students every semester. They have taught stress management to thousands of students, and they know from experience that the best learning happens in an *interesting, challenging, positive* environment. This book has many features to make this a positive and interesting experience for you including:

- **chapter quotes** for inspiration and insight.
- **Student Objectives** to clearly guide you in your learning.
- **key words,** bolded in the chapter and tied to definitions in the Glossary.

- **Frequently Asked Questions** to capture your interest about things on your mind to which you want answers.
- **Real People, Real Stories,** beginning each chapter with true stories that bring the information to life.
- **Author Anecdotes** scattered throughout the chapters, which describe the authors' own experiences to help you better understand and relate to the content.
- **Research Highlights** throughout the book to keep you informed on the latest and most interesting research on topics involving stress and stress management.
- **FYI** (For Your Information) tidbits of motivational and interesting information scattered throughout the chapters.
- **Stress Busting Behavior** checklists for quick, interactive application of content.
- **Culture Connections** that will open your mind and increase your awareness of stress topics from divergent cultures around the world.
- **key points and a list of key terms** at the end of each chapter to reinforce the chapter's most important content and terminology.
- **Stress Management Labs** at the end of each chapter to provide you with an opportunity to review and apply important learning.

As an added bonus, *Stress Management for Life* comes with an access code for the book's Premium Website, which includes several resources to help you develop your stress-management skills:

- Inside the Stress Relief audio files, you will find relaxation exercises that go along with Part IV of your textbook. A narrator will guide you through each technique. So not only will you read in the chapters about how to deeply relax, but you will also get to practice as you experience each stress-management technique. Each audio file relaxation technique is in MP3 format so you can download it to your computer and then transfer it to an MP3 device, such as an iPod or MP3 player.
- Also on the Website, the Student Activities Manual provides you with engaging activities, handouts, stress assessments, chapter outlines, and other resources to help you achieve the benefits of stress management.

To the Instructor

The authors of *Stress Management for Life* are full-time professors who teach stress-management courses every semester, both face to face and online, to hundreds of students. Over their many years of teaching stress management to students across the country, they searched high and low for just the right book for their students. They wanted a book that would:

- emphasize experiential learning by clearly explaining the "how to" of stress management and prevention.
- cover the important aspects of stress management without going into so much depth that students get lost and lose interest.
- capture students' interest by presenting the information in a clear, interesting style with a variety of attention-grabbing features throughout the book.
- include topics that are sources of stress for college students today—financial and time management, relationships, spiritual stress, and many others.
- provide motivation and inspiration along with the facts.
- build on a strong foundation of well-researched information.
- provide opportunities for students to practice relaxation techniques while they are learning the content.
- be teacher-friendly and include a comprehensive *Instructor's Manual* and test bank.

The authors wrote *Stress Management for Life* to meet these needs.

Stress Management for Life is written so the chapters can be assigned in the order that works best for you and your students. Combining an activity chapter from Part IV with a chapter from Parts I, II, or III is an especially effective teaching strategy. Students get to start practicing relaxation techniques immediately. You will find a sample 15-week semester schedule in the *Instructor's Manual* to get you thinking about scheduling options.

Ancillaries A deliberate goal of *Stress Management for Life* and the accompanying ancillaries is to provide you with a ready-to-go package to make your job easier. The authors are teachers, just like you, who know what makes the job easier.

Premium Website

Audio Files: Stress-Relief Exercises The unique collection of Audio Relaxation Exercises included on the book's Premium Website provides helpful demonstrations of many stress-management techniques presented in Part IV of the book. Techniques available on the Website include the Power Nap, autogenics, progressive relaxation, restful breathing, a mindful relaxation, and three guided imageries. This collection of Relaxation Exercises was developed specifically to supplement the content in *Stress Management for Life*. The students will be able to read about the methods and also will have the opportunity to practice the techniques for optimal results.

Guided practice creates powerful experiential learning for effective relaxation. Students who have practiced the relaxation exercises often comment that the exercises became one of the most helpful and useful tools in their stress-management course, enabling them to achieve effective relaxation at home. Many instructors use the Stress Relief Audio Files in the classroom to assist them in teaching these methods for relieving stress.

Student Activities Manual Also located on the Premium Website, the *Stress Management for Life Student Activities Manual* guides students through activities that will help them apply what they are learning. Students will find a variety of activities, handouts, worksheets, chapter outlines, assessments, and more to help them integrate what they are learning.

Critical Thinking/Discussion Questions The Premium Website also contains critical thinking/discussion questions to get your students really thinking and to engage them in lively classroom discussion. These questions also make great journaling assignments.

Online *Instructor's Manual* The *Stress Management for Life Instructor's Manual* is chockfull of activities, information, suggestions, and tips that you can adapt for your specific needs. Included in the Instructor's Manual are:

- learning objectives for each chapter
- chapter outlines
- discussion questions
- a sample syllabus
- reproducible handouts
- class activities
- everything you need to teach an interesting and successful class

Ebank Test Bank A complete test bank, containing multiple choice, true/false, and short answer questions for each chapter.

Teaching stress management does not have to be stressful!

About the Authors

Michael Olpin is a professor in the Department of Health Promotion and Human Performance at Weber State University in Ogden, Utah, where he regularly teaches the Stress Management course along with a variety of other courses in Health Promotion. His background includes instruction in stress management at four institutions of higher education and more than 25 years studying the subject. He has presented a large number of workshops and papers on stress management both in his home state and around the country. He consults privately for individuals and corporations in stress management, along with other areas of health and high-level wellness.

Margie Hesson is a Registered Nurse and an instructor in the College of Nursing at South Dakota State University, where her teaching focus areas are stress management, public health, epidemiology, health promotion, and complementary/alternative health care. She is endorsed by the American Holistic Nurses Association as a Certified Holistic Stress Management Instructor. She is the author of two general-audience books on stress and healthy living and is a contributing author to numerous textbooks. In addition to more than 30 years' experience as a nurse and a teacher, she has been director of corporate health promotion and is active as a health ministry consultant to churches. She is a frequent presenter on stress management and health-promotion topics at the state, national, and international levels.

Acknowledgments

This second edition couldn't have happened without the help and support of many.

Thanks to all the top-notch professionals associated with Cengage Learning for their valuable contributions: Anna Lustig, Trudy Brown, and Samantha Arvin; Kristin Jobe, Elm Street Publishing Services; Jennifer Lim, the Bill Smith Group; and many others behind the scenes who helped bring this work together. It has been a great pleasure working with them.

We extend heartfelt appreciation to our contributing author, Dr. James Hesson, for his many insights and especially for his contributions to the chapters addressing time and money management. His expertise on exercise was invaluable in explaining the connections between exercise and stress. As an experienced author, his suggestions and guidance helped shape the book and we learned greatly from him.

Dr. Mark Schwartz went above and beyond the role of reviewer to provide excellent suggestions based on his expertise in stress management and biofeedback, and we thank him.

Thanks, too, to those who served as reviewers: Robert Alman, Indiana Univesity of Pennsylvania; Mary Brown, Utah Valley University; Arlene Lacome, Saint Joseph's University; Dan Mykins, SUNY—Brockport; Christopher J. Rasmussen, Baylor University; Mark Stephen Schwartz, University of North Florida; and Nanette Tummers, Eastern Connecticut State University. We appreciate their time and energy, which helped us make this second edition even better. Their suggestions and wise advice enhanced the quality of this book immeasurably.

Michael's Acknowledgments There are many people who helped make this second edition come together, and I would like to personally thank each of them. Clearly, working with my co-author, Margie Hesson, has been the best gift of all for me. She is thorough, organized, and very clear on the direction we wanted to go this time around.

I'm also grateful to the fine folks at Cengage who made all the parts come together to produce this final product. I was always impressed by the coordinated effort this has been, like many parts to a well-oiled, humming engine.

I'm also deeply grateful to my loving wife, Shanyn, and our four beautiful kids, Analise, Erica, Adam, and our newest addition, little Ben. Their patience with me as I had to spend my nights and weekends writing instead of playing with them has been tremendous. Their ongoing support, as well as all the yummy food they brought to me, allowed me to keep focused to see this through to its end.

I thought the first edition was a really good book. This second edition is far better. This has happened because of the hard work and dedication of many fantastic people.

Margie's Acknowledgments Thanks to my co-author, Dr. Mike Olpin, for his expertise in stress management, positive attitude, and work ethic. His years of teaching stress management have resulted in a keen understanding of how to help others manage stress.

Thanks go to my colleagues and students at South Dakota State University College of Nursing. I greatly appreciate their support and encouragement. Many of my students contributed personal stress stories (I hope I wasn't the cause of too much of that stress!) in an effort to help other students learn about stress management.

Photographer Jenny Evans of Candy Apple Photography provided expert consultation on the photos. Thanks to Jenny and Rich for sharing their pictures and their expertise.

My family continues to be a source of inspiration to me, and I feel very blessed to have them in my life. Thanks to our children, David Hesson and Jenny and Rich Evans. Most of all, I am grateful for my #1 stress-reliever—my husband, Jim. He is my greatest supporter, and I can't thank him enough for encouraging me to set goals and embrace new opportunities. I have felt his support every step of the way.

1 Stress in Today's World

■ Is stress always bad? ■ Stress seems to be everywhere. Can I really do anything about it, or is it just an inevitable demand of living in today's world? ■ Was I born with a certain capacity to handle stress? Is successful stress management a result of heredity or environment?

Study of this chapter will enable you to:

1. Define the terms *stress* and *stressor*.
2. Define and explain the difference between eustress and distress.
3. Differentiate between acute, acute episodic, and chronic stress.
4. Relate stress to the five dimensions of holistic health—physical, intellectual (also referred to as mental), emotional, spiritual, and social.
5. Discuss some of the most common stressors affecting college students today.

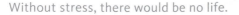

Without stress, there would be no life.

— *Hans Selye*

© Rudi Von Briel/PhotoEdit

2

Nicole's Story Nicole was about to graduate, but reflecting on her first year of college still brought some painful memories. Here is Nicole's story.

* * *

My first year of nursing school proved to be more stressful and more challenging than I had bargained for. In addition to my 18 credits that first semester, I had 6 lab hours each week. It wasn't just the academics that had me floundering. I was also working 20–30 hours per week at a local grocery store and trying to maintain a social life.

Early in the semester I began to feel the stress. I soon began cutting back on my social life because I needed to study or work. Day after day I kept reminding myself that this situation was "just for this semester," and "I can get through this."

My stress started affecting me physically. By the first week in October, I had lost 10 pounds and was starting to have stomach cramps nearly every day. My weight loss and stomach cramps were caused mainly by my not eating. I would get stressed out and skip a meal, which would turn into skipping two meals or, at the worst, three meals. My sleep patterns started changing, too. I needed to sleep more and more to be able to function. Some days I slept 14 to 16 hours but still felt tired. Other days I couldn't sleep at all. By Thanksgiving break I had lost 15 pounds and was taking prescribed muscle relaxants and ulcer medications.

My emotions started changing, too. I cried at the drop of a hat, sometimes over nothing. I took long, hot showers so my roommates wouldn't see me crying. I also angered easily. I couldn't seem to get happy about anything. I quit caring about my appearance, so I stopped wearing makeup and fixing my hair.

School was the main stressor, and my grades began to show it. As my grades initially began to slip, I became even more stressed out. I was worried that I would fail a class and be out of the nursing program, so I spent more and more time studying.

I tried so hard to conceal my problems because I didn't want to admit I couldn't handle things. I didn't want people to think I was stressed out and such a mess. How could I ever be a good nurse and help other people if I couldn't even help myself?

It was really difficult for me to do, but I finally told my family and friends what I was going through. With their help, I made several changes in my life. The first major change came with the end of my busy, class-loaded semester. When registering for classes the next semester, I cut back my class load. I also found a new job that paid more per hour so I could work less. My parents helped me out financially as much as they could. My boyfriend maintained a 24-hour, 7-days-a-week "hotline" for me, and he encouraged me to call him whenever I felt stressed. I started riding my bicycle and doing yoga to "de-stress." I also set aside time each day just for myself, when I could do anything I wanted.

I'm still learning how to handle my stress, but my first year in nursing school taught me a lot about myself and how I handle stress. I learned what my limits are and what can happen if I don't deal with my stress appropriately. I'll graduate in a month, and I know I'll still have stress, but now I know how to deal with stress in a healthier way.

Percentage of College Students Who Felt Frequently Overwhelmed How often do you feel overwhelmed by all you have to do? Do you think men or women are more likely to report feeling overwhelmed? Here are some thought-provoking findings:

Stress levels among college freshmen appear to be increasing with 36% of first-year students reporting they felt overwhelmed nine or more times within the past school year.* It isn't just freshmen that are feeling overwhelmed. The National College Health Assessment surveyed over 20,000 students from 39 colleges and universities and found that 64.5% reported feeling overwhelmed between 1-10 times within the last 12 months. Women were more likely than men to indicate that they frequently felt overwhelmed by all they had to do. Thirty-one percent of the females reported feeling overwhelmed 11 or more times in the last 12 months compared to 19.9% of males.**

Sources: *Pryor, J., Hurtado, S., Saenz, V., Korn, J., Santos, J., & Korn, W. (2006). *The American Freshman: National Norms for Fall 2006.* Los Angeles: Higher Education Research Institute, UCLA.
**American College Health Association–National College Health Assessment: Reference Group Executive Summary Fall 2007. Baltimore: American College Health Association; 2008.

Stress in Today's World

"It was the best of times, it was the worst of times," Charles Dickens wrote of 18th-century France in his masterpiece, *A Tale of Two Cities*. Could the same be said for you, today's college student? Never before have college students been faced with such vast opportunities, such freedom of choice, and such an array of information. Yet these opportunities, the numerous choices, and the information overload can leave you feeling overwhelmed and stressed.

Will this be the best of times or the worst of times for you? With the proper skills and the right information, you will be in control of your destiny. *Stress Management for Life* is packed with information that will help you do more than merely survive your college years. These can be the best of times for you. The decision is yours.

Stress: What Is It?

Stress, stressors, eustress, distress, good stress, bad stress. What is stress all about? Hans Selye, the noted stress researcher, once said: "Stress is a scientific concept which has suffered from the mixed blessing of being too well known and too little understood."

Coming up with an accepted definition of stress is not easy. Nurses and physicians, psychologists, biologists, engineers, and students may each have a different meaning in mind when they talk about stress. One useful definition is: **Stress** is a demand made upon the adaptive capacities of the mind and body.[1] This definition helps us understand three important aspects of stress:

1. How you experience stress depends on your personal view of the stressor, and it can be both a positive and a negative factor in your life.
2. Your *reaction* to the events in life, rather than the actual event, is what will determine whether the outcome will be positive or negative.
3. Stress is a demand upon the body's *capacity*. When your capacity for handling stress is strong and healthy, the outcome is positive. When you lack the ability to handle the demands, the outcome is negative.

We can relate managing stress to building muscle. To build bigger biceps, you faithfully perform arm curls with gradually increasing weight. Over time, your muscles respond to the overload and become bigger, stronger biceps. The key is in finding the proper balance. Too little weight will not produce the desired results, and too much weight may result in fatigue and injury and will not produce the desired results. You need to overload the muscle just enough to make it stronger. So it is with stress: Too little stress leads to boredom and lethargy, and too much stress leads to physical and emotional breakdown. The right balance leads to a productive, healthy life.

Although we often think of stress as negative, we should keep in mind that stress can be stimulating and helpful. Think of how boring life would be without some changes and challenges to push you along, to provide opportunities to learn and grow, and to provide the impetus for accomplishing your goals in life (see Figure 1.1)!

Yerkes–Dodson Principle

Harvard physicians Robert Yerkes and John Dodson first described the relationship between stress and performance in 1908.[2] The **Yerkes–Dodson Principle** implies that to a certain point, a specific amount of stress is healthy, useful, and even beneficial. In addition to enhanced performance, this usefulness can be translated into one's health and well-being.

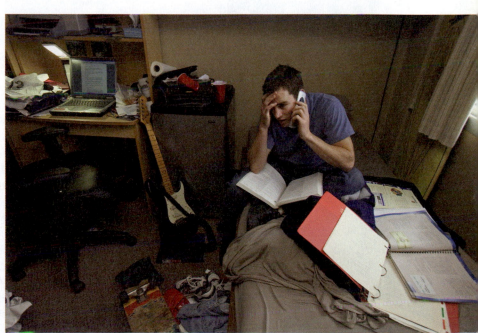

© Bill Varie/CORBIS

College students are faced with many stressors. What is your #1 stressor?

FIGURE 1.1 You Want a Little Stress... Not Too Much

Source: "You Want A Little Stress... Not Too Much," *Wellness Guidelines for a Healthy Lifestyle*, 3rd ed., by W.K. Hoeger, L. Turner, and B. Hafen. From Hope Publications, Kalamazoo, MI.

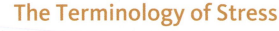

Distress	Stress	Distress
	With the right	
With too little	**amount of**	**With too much**
stress we are:	**stress we are:**	**stress we are:**

1	2	3	4	5	6	7	8	9

bored	productive	burned out
tired	energetic	exhausted
unhappy	happy	overweight
restless	creative	irritable
prone to illness	healthy	prone to illness

Reprinted with permission, Hope Publications, Kalamazoo, Michigan (616) 343-0770.

The stimulus of the stress response is often essential for success. We see this in situations such as sporting events, academic pursuits, and even in creative and social activities. As stress levels increase, so does performance. This relationship between increased stress and increased performance, however, does not continue indefinitely. Stress or arousal can increase performance but when stress exceeds one's ability to cope, this overload contributes to diminished performance, inefficiency, and even health problems.

A good image to remind us that we each have an ideal amount of stress is the tension in the strings of a guitar. When a guitar is strung too tightly (too much tension), the string will sound a note higher than desirable. The guitar string, when tightened to its maximum, is likely to snap. The same string, if not tightened sufficiently, will play a note that is lower than is desirable. If it is strung without any tension, no sound at all will come from it. The proper tension results in the desirable note. The same image can be used to depict how healthy one's body is with too much or too little stress.

The Terminology of Stress

Stress can be good or bad, acute or chronic. These and other variances of stress are explained in the following definitions.

Good and Bad Stress A **stressor** is any event or situation that an individual perceives as a threat that causes him or her to either adapt or initiate the stress response. (The stress response will be explained in detail in Chapter 3.) Therefore, a stressor is a stimulus, and stress is a response. To think of it another way, the stressor is the cause and stress is the effect.

Hans Selye, one of the first to study the effects of stress, coined the term **eustress** to explain the positive, desirable stress that keeps life interesting and helps to motivate and inspire. Events such as going off to college, getting married, starting a new job, or having a baby can be happy, joyous, *and* stress-producing. Eustress also involves managing stress successfully even when dealing with a negative stressor. Notice in Figure 1.2 that eustress is represented on the curve where stress level and health and performance increase simultaneously. Eustress implies that a certain amount of stress is useful, beneficial, and even good for our health, much like the perfectly strung guitar string.

Distress refers to the negative effects of stress that drain us of energy and surpass our capacity to cope. Often when we are talking about stress, we are referring to distress. Notice the place on Figure 1.2 where stress continues to increase yet performance and health begins to decline. This downward curve represents distress. For optimal performance and well-being, you want to stay on top of the curve.

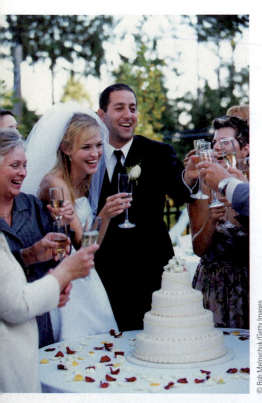

Getting married is an example of a positive stressor, also known as eustress.

© Rob Melnychuk/Getty Images

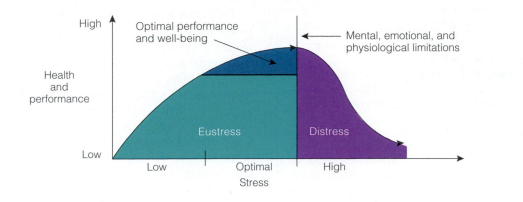

High

Optimal performance
and well-being

Mental, emotional, and
physiological limitations

Health
and
performance

Eustress

Distress

Low

Low

Optimal
Stress

High

FIGURE 1.2 Relationship between Stress and Health and Performance

Source: "Relationship between Stress and Health and Performance," Figure 12.1 from *Lifetime Physical Fitness and Wellness*, 10th ed., by W. K. Hoeger and S. A. Hoeger (Belmont, CA: Wadsworth/Cengage Learning, 2009, p. 381). Used by permission.

Acute and Chronic Stress Stress can be acute or chronic. **Acute stress** results from a short-term stressor. It appears suddenly, is usually quite intense, and then disappears quickly. Imagine being out for a leisurely evening stroll when suddenly, from out of nowhere, a large, mangy dog leaps from the bushes, growling, with teeth bared. Your response would fit the definition of acute stress.

Have you ever been cruising down the highway, relaxing to your favorite tunes when you glanced in your rearview mirror to see the flashing lights of a police car bearing down from behind? If so, chances are you experienced acute stress at that time.

If you have ever parachuted or participated in other exhilarating activities, you will understand that when you manage acute stress well, it can help you think clearly and perform optimally. Acute stress can be exciting and invigorating in small doses—but too much is exhausting.

People experiencing **episodic acute stress** seem to be perpetually in the clutches of acute stress. These are the people who elicit your response "What now?!" when you see them racing toward you. They seem to be always in a rush—but usually late. If something can go wrong, it will. They can't seem to get their act together or organize the many self-inflicted demands and pressures that clamor for their attention. They often blame their problems on other people and external events.

People who have frequent episodes of acute stress tend to be over-aroused, short-tempered, irritable, anxious, and tense. They may describe themselves as having "a lot of nervous energy." As you can imagine, the symptoms of episodic acute stress are the symptoms of extended over-arousal including persistent tension headaches, migraines, digestive problems, hypertension, chest pain, and heart disease.[3]

Chronic stress is long-term stress resulting from those nagging problems that just don't seem to go away. This is the grinding stress that can wear you down day after day, year after year. Chronic stress can result from credit card debt that keeps growing, from long-term health problems, from emotionally draining relationships, or from staying in an unfulfilling, energy-draining job. Chronic stress can be a result of unrelenting demands and pressures that go on for an interminable time.

Author Anecdote **High Stress** The soothing sound of the engine hummed in my ears as the small Cessna airplane slowly climbed to 3,000 feet over Lincoln, Nebraska. I was about to make my first parachute jump—and I was feeling anything but soothed. I have a list of "Things to Do Before I Die," and parachuting was on the list. At this moment I couldn't remember why.

My heart was racing, my jaws were clenched, and I was having trouble thinking clearly. Suddenly the small door flew open and a blast of noisy, cold air brought me to my senses. I knew what to do. Rather awkwardly I maneuvered my parachute-laden body so I was sitting in the doorway with my legs dangling in the wind. I tried not to think about the fact that 3,000 feet separated my dangling boots and the earth below. I eased forward slowly to balance precariously on the extremely small step and held on for dear life to the bar attached under the wing of the airplane.

Every cell in my body was shouting, "Whatever you do, don't let go of this airplane!" Somewhere in the distance I heard my jumpmaster, Gary, shout over the tremendous wind, "Margie, let go!"

There it was—the moment of decision. With a deep breath I released my grip, pushed off, arched my back, spread my arms and legs, and began to fall.

Seconds later my parachute popped open and there I was, floating in the sky. It was exhilarating! I have never felt more alive. My stress response was fully engaged. The powerful stress hormones were surging through my body. As I touched down, my knees shaking, I fully understood the feeling of an adrenaline high. My body had served me well in this experience of acute stress.

—MH

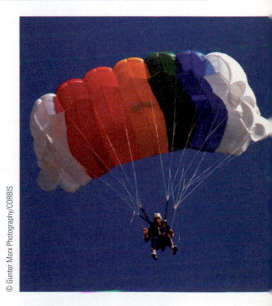

© Gunter Marx Photography/CORBIS

Acute stress can be exhilarating!

Put the Glass Down

A professor is presenting a lecture on stress management. He raises a glass of water and asks the class, "How heavy do you think this glass of water is?" The students guess about 6 ounces.

"It doesn't matter what the absolute weight is," the professor replies. "It depends on how long you hold it. If I hold it for a minute, it is okay. If I hold it for an hour, my arm will start to ache. If I hold it for a day, you will have to call an ambulance. It is the exact same weight, but the longer I hold it, the heavier it becomes."

If you continue to carry your burdens all the time, sooner or later you will not be able to carry on. The burden will be too heavy. You will have to put the glass down and rest a while before you hold it up again. You will have to put your burdens down from time to time so you can be refreshed and able to carry on. Whatever burden you are carrying on your shoulders, let it down. Take a rest. If you must, you can pick it up again later when you have rested. Take time to rest and relax.

—Source unknown

The danger of chronic stress is that people get used to it, lose hope, and gi searching for solutions. As their ph and mental resources are depleted are overcome by feelings of apathy, lessness, and fear. Chronic stress can ally kill—through suicide, heart atta violence. You will learn in later ch that this chronic, long-term stress i results in stress-related disease and re the quality of life.

Holistic Health

Understanding Health To stand how stress affects you and to how to increase your capacity for handling the demands of life, you will have to l stand the relationship between health and stress. Two important points about heal

1. *Health is more than just the absence of disease.* The focus of this book is on mor just controlling stress to prevent disease and the other negative consequen stress. The focus is on increasing your capacity for dealing with stress so you can optimal health and well-being. The text also focuses on promoting good heal improving the quality of life today and in the years to come.

2. *Health is more than just physical.* **Holistic health** encompasses the physical lectual, emotional, spiritual, and social dimensions. An imbalance in any o dimensions will affect your health. Even broader definitions of health includ pational and environmental dimensions. In later chapters we will discuss th two dimensions and how they relate to stress. The important message here is holistically healthy person functions as a total, balanced person.

Dimensions of Health

Figure 1.3 depicts the five dimensions of health—physical, intellectual, emotio tual, and social.

Following is a brief description of each of the dimensions of health and an ex of how stress relates to that dimension. Understanding each of these dimension you plan a more balanced approach to managing stress.

Physical Health When the cells, tissues, organs, and systems that function form your body are in working order, you can claim to be in good **physical heal** able to minimize disease and injury and function optimally. Physical qualities in weight, visual acuity, skin integrity, and level of endurance, among others. promoting health in the physical dimension are taking care of your body by e foods, exercising, getting adequate sleep, avoiding alcohol and drugs, and g health screenings.

Physical health and stress are closely related. Stress is a risk factor for m ous health problems that plague us today. Stress has been shown to weake system, resulting in increased susceptibility to a variety of health prob healthy body is better able to resist many of the damaging physiological c erwise might result from excessive stress. It works both ways: Stress can c illness, and disease and illness can cause stress.

Intellectual Health **Intellectual health,** also called mental health, ity to think and learn from experiences, the ability to assess and question and the openness to new learning. Your mind—how and what you th ful impact on your health and well-being. In this text you will learn research that sheds light on the connection between the body and the

Learning about stress is an important first step in preventing and managing stress. Intellectual understanding of the physical and psychological aspects of stress and wise decision-making skills will allow you to process the information you learn and apply this information to a plan that will improve your health and well-being. In this book you will learn a variety of stress prevention and stress-management techniques. Through critical thinking and informed choice, you will decide on the tools and techniques that work best for you. Your ability to process and act on this information will strengthen the intellectual dimension of your health.

Emotional Health In contrast to mental health, which encompasses thoughts and the mind, **emotional health** pertains to feelings. It involves experiencing and appreciating a wide range of feelings and the ability to express these feelings and emotions in a healthy manner. An indication of emotional wellness is the ability to remain flexible in coping with the ups and downs of life.

Stress and emotional health are strongly related. Everyone is affected by feelings such as anger, fear, happiness, worry, love, guilt, and loneliness. Emotionally healthy people use healthy coping skills to keep from becoming overwhelmed by these feelings. Dealing successfully with stress means taking control of your emotions rather than letting your emotions take control of you.

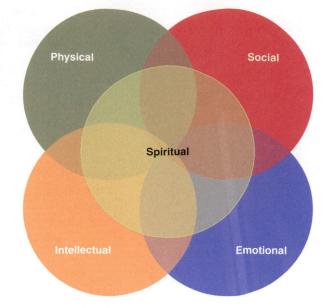

FIGURE 1.3 Dimensions of Health

Spiritual Health **Spiritual health** relates to the principles and values that guide a person and give meaning, direction, and purpose to life. A conviction that life is meaningful and a belief that your life is guided by a reality greater than yourself are indications of spiritual health. Spiritually healthy people believe that their life has value and that they are here for a reason. The spiritual dimension may be the foundation for all other dimensions of health.

Stress, especially chronic stress, often arises from a sense of aimlessness or lack of purpose. Much of the stress in today's society relates to being out of touch with our values and beliefs. Making choices that are not consistent with your core values can be stressful. For example, if you highly value family and find that the demands of work and school leave little time for family, you likely will experience distress. In later chapters you will learn how techniques such as values clarification can contribute to spiritual peace.

Nurturing your spiritual dimension through religion, volunteer work, nature, art, music, or other avenues above and beyond your own immediate needs will most certainly reduce stress and promote health. Spirituality as a key component in stress management will be discussed further in Chapter 10.

Social Health **Social health** refers to the ability to relate to others and express care and concern for others. The ability to interact effectively with others, to develop satisfying interpersonal relationships, and to fulfill social roles is important for social health. Relationships with others, particularly family and friends, affect social well-being. When you are socially healthy, you feel accepted by others and see yourself as an important part of your world.

A strong social support system increases the capacity for handling the demands of life. As you will learn in

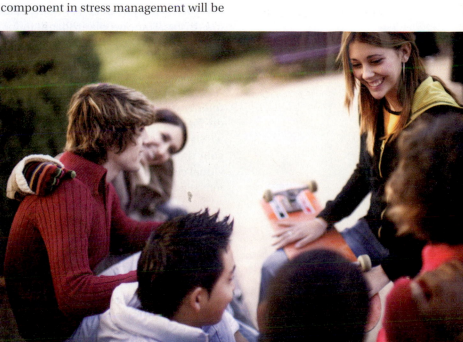

The support of family and friends is vital for health in the social dimension.

© Randy Faris/CORBIS

TABLE 1.1 Negative Effects of Stress on Each Dimension of Holistic Health

Physical	Intellectual	Emotional	Spiritual	Social
Muscle tension	Forgetfulness	Anxiety	Lack of meaning	Isolation
Headaches	Poor concentration	Frustration	Lack of purpose	Lashing out
Teeth grinding	Low productivity	Nervousness	Loneliness	Clamming up
Fatigue	Negative attitude	Worrying	Depression	Lowered sex drive
Insomnia	Confusion	Tension	Low self-esteem	Nagging
Backaches	No new ideas	Mood swings	Loss of self-worth	Fewer friends
Stomach problems	Lethargy	Easily discouraged	Feeling abandoned	Using people
Colds	Boredom	Crying spells	Inability to love	
Neck aches		Irritability		
Shoulder pains				
Drug use				

Chapter 13, study after study shows that people who have the support of friends and family are better able to deal with the ups and downs in life.

Holistic Health: Putting It All Together Upon reviewing Nicole's story in the opening vignette, you will readily see that stress affected every dimension of her health. Physically, she had trouble eating and sleeping. She developed ulcers and required medication for muscle tension. Intellectually, as she became more overwhelmed by all the demands, her grades began to fall. Emotionally, she was overwhelmed by all the pressure, depressed, and felt like a failure. Spiritually, she began to question her purpose and meaning in life. She doubted her value as a person, saying to herself, "How can I ever be a good nurse and help other people if I can't even help myself?" Nicole initially withdrew from her friends and family, cutting back on her social life to study and work. She had difficulty admitting that she needed help and support from others. Table 1.1 is a summary of how stress negatively affects every dimension of health.

You will find in this book a toolbox of various techniques and strategies for managing stress, and you will determine what works best for you. Understanding the holistic model of health will guide you in assessing all dimensions of health.

Nature or Nurture

Everyone is unique. Genetic variations may partly explain the differences in how we react to stressors. Some people are naturally laid-back, while others react strongly at the slightest hint of stress. Life experiences also may increase your sensitivity to stress. Strong stress reactions sometimes can be traced to early environmental factors. People who were exposed to extreme stress as children tend to be particularly vulnerable to stress as adults.[4]

Your unique genetic makeup, your unique experiences in life, and your unique environment as you were growing and developing all play a part in your individual reactions to the inevitable stressors of life.

Many factors affect our experience with stress. The important point is to remember your uniqueness. Stress affects each person differently. Getting in touch with your individual circumstances will help you determine the stress management techniques that are most effective for you.

Sources of Stress

Nobody has to tell you that the college years can be years of high stress. Even though the sources and causes of stress are unique for each person, many college students will face some common stressors. Each of these potential stressors will be dealt with more fully in later chapters, but here are some of the most common sources of stress. See if any of these apply to you.

Time Management Do you have too much to do? No matter how hard you work, do you feel like you never get caught up? If you are like many people, the answer is "yes." You

Stress and the Developing Brain

We know, from a plethora of research, that the early months and years of life are crucial for brain development. Still, the question remains: How do early influences act on the brain to promote or challenge the developmental process? Researchers have suggested that positive and negative experiences, chronic stressors, and various other environmental factors may affect a young child's developing brain. Now, studies involving animals reveal in more detail how this may happen.

One important line of research has focused on brain systems that control stress hormones such as cortisol. Cortisol and other stress hormones play an important role in emergencies: They help make energy available to enable effective responses, temporarily suppress the immune response, and sharpen attention. Excess cortisol may cause shrinkage of the hippocampus, a brain structure required for the formation of certain kinds of memory.

In experiments with animals, scientists have shown that a well-defined period of early postnatal development may be an important determinant of the capacity to handle stress throughout life. In one set of studies, rat pups were removed each day from their mothers as briefly as 15 minutes, and then returned. The natural maternal response of intensively licking and grooming the returned pup was shown to alter the brain chemistry of the pup in a positive way, making the animal less reactive to stressful stimuli. Although these pups are able to mount an appropriate stress response in the face of threat, their response does not become excessive or inappropriate.

Striking differences were seen in rat pups that were removed from their mothers for 3 hours a day—a model of maternal neglect, compared to pups that were not separated. After 3 hours, the mother rats tended to ignore the pups, at least initially, upon their return. In sharp contrast to the pups that were greeted attentively by their mothers after a short absence, the "neglected" pups showed a more profound and excessive stress response in subsequent tests. This response appeared to last into adulthood.

Another study reported that infant monkeys raised by mothers who experienced unpredictable conditions in obtaining food showed markedly high levels of corticotrophin releasing factor (CRF) in their cerebrospinal fluid and, as adults, abnormally low levels of cerebrospinal

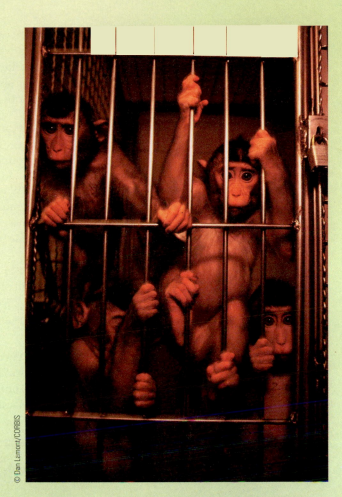

Monkeys deprived of love and support as babies become less social and more anxious as adults.

fluid cortisol. This is a pattern often seen in humans with post-traumatic stress disorder and depression. The distressed monkey mothers, uncertain about finding food, behaved inconsistently and sometimes neglectfully toward their offspring. The affected young monkeys were abnormally anxious when confronted with separations or new environments. They also were less social and more subordinate as adult animals.

It is too early to draw firm conclusions from these animal studies about the extent to which early life experience produces a long-lived or permanent set point for stress responses. Nevertheless, animal models that show the interactive effect of stress and brain development deserve serious consideration and continued study.

Source: National Institute of Health, *Stress and the Developing Brain* (NIH Publication No. 01-4603) (Bethesda, MD: NIH, 2001).

---

will learn in Chapter 11 (on time management) that we don't so much need to manage our time as we need help to manage ourselves!

Personal Expectations Are you your greatest stressor? Do you put demands on yourself that may be unrealistic? Do you have feelings of low self-esteem or feelings that your life is out of control? Do you take on more than you should? Would you be better off if you could learn to say "no" more often?

Family Expectations and Family Life "So what are you going to do for the rest of your life?" Do you find well-intentioned family members about to drive you crazy with their desire to help you find direction in your life? Family life stressors can include, among many others, health problems, substance abuse, strong disagreements, loss of family members, difficulties with stepparents, homesickness, and divorce.

Employment Decisions and Finances Do you work more so you can pay your tuition, or go even deeper in debt so you have more time to study? In Chapter 12 you will learn how to manage your finances to help reduce stress caused by money (or lack of it).

School Pressures Where to begin? Deciding on a major, teachers who expect too much, and failing a test are just the start of a list of school pressures. Do the demands and pressures of school leave you feeling overwhelmed? Figure 1.4 shows that stress is the top impediment to academic performance.

Living Arrangements What do you do with the "roommate from hell"? Would you be better off moving out of the dorm and into an apartment? Maybe you should consider a fraternity or a sorority. How do you find some quiet time for yourself when you are surrounded by people constantly?

Relationships You get a "Dear John" letter from your girlfriend back home. Your best friend meets another best friend. You are left behind when the gang goes out for an evening of fun. University counseling services report that relationship problems are one of the top reasons that students seek professional help.

Physical Health Issues Just a few of the physical challenges facing college students are a lack of sleep, poor nutrition, hormonal fluctuations, and no time to exercise. Is it any wonder that colds and flu plague students, especially during finals? And what about more serious health problems such as sexually transmitted infections; drug, tobacco, and alcohol abuse; anorexia; depression? And the list goes on....

Environmental Stressors You live with environmental stressors including noise, crowding, traffic, weather, pollution, and violence. As a sign of the times, terrorism has been added to the list of things that students most fear. Chapter 14 will teach you how you can create a more healing environment.

Information Overload Never before in history have we had access to such tremendous amounts of information. Surrounded by technology and computers, you have

FIGURE 1.4 Top 10 Reported Impediments to Students' Academic Performance

Source: American College Health Association. National College Health Assessment: Reference Group Executive Summary Fall 2007. Baltimore: American College Health Association, 2008.

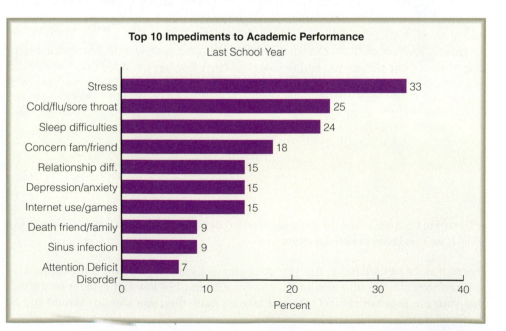

Life Out of Balance Ko.yaa.nis.qatsi,

n. 1. Crazy life. 2. Life in turmoil. 3. Life disintegrating. 4. Life out of balance. 5. A state of life that calls for another way of living.

Does this sound like your life? *Koyaanisqatsi* (Ko-YAWN-is-SCOTS-ee) is a Hopi Indian word that may have meaning for your life today. Consider how another way of living can improve your well-being. Throughout *Stress Management for Life* you will find Culture Connections to offer you different perspectives on stress. Use these opportunities to step out of your box and think about things in a new way.

We become so accustomed to our way of seeing things that we easily may come to believe that everyone thinks the same way we do. Sometimes, if we pause and reflect with an open mind, we may perceive a better way. If *koyaanisqatsi* describes your life, maybe it's time to investigate a different way of living.

Source: Retrieved February 18, 2005, from http://www.philipglass.com/html/filmskoyaanisqatsi.html

---

more information available than you could have imagined two decades ago. One computer search for information on "stress in college students" yielded 357,405 results. And don't forget cell phones, pagers, palm pilots, e-mail. You have information coming at you 24/7. All this information has had such an impact on stress that it has been given a name: **technostress.** In Chapter 14 you will learn more about technostress and how you can control it.

Choices The world of today's college student is filled with choice, much of it consequential. This explosion of choice in the university reflects a pervasive social trend. Americans are overwhelmed with choices in virtually every area of life—from what products to buy (300 kinds of cereal, 50 different cell phones, thousands of mutual funds) to where to go for spring break and how to pay for that vacation (credit card, debit card, check, loan, or even cash).[5]

Daily Hassles Finally, we cannot forget those hundreds of small but significant hassles that can creep into your day and absolutely put you over the edge. Lazarus[6] described **hassles** as the irritating, frustrating, or distressing incidents that occur in our everyday transactions with the environment. His research supports the premise that the petty annoyances, frustrations, and unpleasant surprises that plague us every day may add up to more grief than life's major stressful events.

Hassles can take the form of a flat tire, dead cell phone, computer crash, toothache, the dog who ate your homework, and the list goes on. A wise person once said, "Sometimes it is not the mountain in front of you, but the grain of sand in your shoe that brings you to your knees."[7]

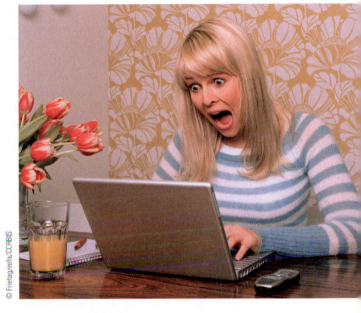

Daily hassles can exceed our ability to cope. Do you know the feeling?

Stress Busting Behavior: Your Sources of Stress

Check those items that are major sources of stress for you. Circle the biggest source of stress.

- ☑ Time Management
- ☑ Personal Expectations
- ☑ Family Expectations and Family Life
- ☑ Employment Decisions and Finances
- ☑ School Pressures
- ☐ Living Arrangements

- ☐ Relationships
- ☐ Physical Health Issues
- ☐ Environmental Stressors
- ☐ Information Overload
- ☐ ~~Choices~~
- ☐ Daily Hassles

Identifying the causes of your stress can be an important first step in developing a plan to reduce or eliminate stress. Throughout the chapters of this book, you will find helpful information and proven strategies to help you deal with many of these common sources of stress.

Conclusion

The key lesson to be derived from this chapter is to strive for balance in your life. Even though stress can be challenging and useful at times, it also can become chronic and excessive to the point where you no longer are able to adapt to and cope with the pressures. An optimal level of stress is characterized by high energy, mental alertness, high motivation, calm under pressure, thorough analysis of problems, improved memory and recall, sharp perception, and a generally optimistic outlook.[8]

In *Stress Management for Life* you will learn that you can prevent and manage stress through three basic approaches:

1. *Eliminate the stressor.* By confronting the problems that are causing you stress, you sometimes can change or eliminate their source.
2. *Change your thinking.* At times you cannot eliminate the cause of your stress, but you do have the power to change your interpretation of the situation and the way you think about it.
3. *Manage the stress.* Sometimes the best you can do is to manage the stress through skills that will help you cope most successfully. When you can't prevent stress, relaxation techniques will help you manage the resulting effects of stress.

You are about to embark on an exciting journey of discovery. You will learn about stress in your life. What factors are causing negative stress for you? You will learn how stress affects you physically, emotionally, intellectually, spiritually, and socially. Most important, though, you will learn how to increase your *capacity* for handling the demands of today's world. You will learn how to prevent stress. You will learn how to manage and cope successfully with the stresses you can't prevent. So what will it be for you? Will these be the best of times, or the worst of times? The decision is yours. Let the journey begin.

LAB

1.1 Dimensions of Health

DIRECTIONS Write a paper including your response to the following statements. You can also complete this Lab activity online at the Premium Website.

Review: Review each of the five dimensions of health. Think about how each dimension relates specifically to your stress. List two specific things you currently do in each dimension to help manage and control stress. If you have trouble coming up with anything, you might consider focusing on that dimension of your health.

1. Physical – What two things in the physical dimension of health have you found effective in managing and controlling stress?

2. Intellectual – What two things in the intellectual dimension of health have you found effective in managing and controlling stress?

3. Emotional – What two things in the emotional dimension of health have you found effective in managing and controlling stress?

4. Spiritual – What two things in the spiritual dimension of health have you found effective in managing and controlling stress?

5. Social – What two things in the social dimension of health have you found effective in managing and controlling stress?

Respond: Select one dimension of health. Plan and implement a specific action to improve your stress in that dimension. For example:

- Physical – Get up early Saturday morning for a long walk in nature.
- Spiritual – Spend 30 minutes in quiet prayer.
- Social – Write a letter of appreciation to someone special in your life.
- Emotional – Do something for no other reason than the fun of it – pack a picnic, watch a funny movie, dance along to an oldies CD,…

You get to decide what would most benefit you. The important thing is that you **do** something.

1. What dimension of health did you select?

2. What was your specific action for improving your health in that dimension?

Reflect: When you have completed your response, reflect on how you felt. Did you feel different after you carried out your activity? If so, how? Reflect on how you can make more stress-busting moments in your life.

Key Points

- Stress is a demand upon the adaptive capacities of the mind and body.
- Eustress is the positive, desirable stress that keeps life interesting and helps to motivate and inspire.
- Distress is the negative, energy-draining form of stress.
- Stress can be acute, episodic acute, or chronic. The effects on health vary with each type of stress.
- A stressor is any event or situation that causes us to adapt or initiates the stress response. A stressor is a stimulus, and stress is a response.
- Health is more than the absence of disease. Health has a direct relationship to stress.

- Holistic health encompasses physical, intellectual, emotional, spiritual, and social dimensions. Imbalance in any of these dimensions affects overall health, and stress affects all dimensions of health.
- Although each of us has different and unique sources of stress, some stressors are common for today's college students.
- *Stress Management for Life* will provide you with tools to increase your capacity to deal more effectively with the stressors of life.
- Your college years can be the best of times. The choice is yours.

Key Terms

stress
Yerkes–Dodson Principle
stressor
eustress
distress
acute stress

episodic acute stress
chronic stress
holistic health
physical health
intellectual health
emotional health

spiritual health
social health
Koyaanisqatsi
technostress
hassles

Discussion Time For Critical Thinking/Discussion Questions, please visit this book's Premium Website.

Notes

1. *Managing Stress,* by D. Fontana (London, England: British Psychology Society and Routledge, Ltd., 1989).

2. "The Relation of Strength of Stimulus to Rapidity of Habit-Formation," by R. M. Yerkes and J. D. Dodson, *Journal of Comparative Neurology and Psychology, 18* (1908): 459–484.

3. "Psychology at Work: The Different Kinds of Stress." American Psychological Association. Retrieved January 30, 2004, from http://helping.apa.org.

4. "Stress: Why You Have It and How It Hurts Your Health." Mayo Clinic staff. Retrieved Sept. 17, 2004, from www.mayoclinic.com.

5. "The Tyranny of Choice," by B. Schwartz, *Chronicle of Higher Education*, Jan. 23, 2004.

6. "Puzzles in the Study of Daily Hassles," by R. Lazarus, *Journal of Behavioral Medicine* 7 (1984): 375–389.

7. "Risk Factors Leading to Chronic Stress-Related Symptoms," by I. Wickramasekera, *Advances* 4(1) (1987): 21.

8. *Corporate Stress*, by R. Forbes (Garden City, NJ: Doubleday, 1979).

2 Self-Assessment

■ I know I feel stressed, but how can I measure my stress? ■ How do I rate my stress level compared to the stress level of others? ■ I often have headaches and tight shoulders, but I am not sure why. Could this be due to stress? ■ When I feel stressed, is it more because of what is happening in my life or because of how I react or think about what is happening?

Study of this chapter will enable you to:

1. Assess your current level of stress from a variety of perspectives.
2. Explain physiological and psychological indicators of stress.
3. Evaluate the impact of stress on the quality of your life.

Normally we do not so much look at things as overlook them.

—Alan Watts

Stress Happens The Stress Management 101 class was about to begin. Today's topic was to be "Assessing Your Stress." Angie sat quietly in the back of the classroom.

"Okay class, let's start by checking our resting heart rate," the teacher announced. Angie's pulse was 105 beats per minute.

"Next, check the number of breaths you take per minute." Angie counted 30 breaths.

"How long does it usually take you to fall asleep once you lie down at night?" Angie said she usually takes at least an hour.

"How much of the time do you feel high levels of stress?" Angie said she feels that way almost all the time.

"Doesn't it feel unpleasant to always feel so stressed?" the teacher questioned. Angie's reply, common among college students, was, "I didn't know there was another way to feel. I assumed that this was the way college life was supposed to be and that everyone feels this way."

Self-Assessment

Several years ago author Richard Carlson created a catchy title for his best-selling book, *Don't Sweat the Small Stuff … and It's All Small Stuff*. He offered some important advice for our over-stressed society: We need to step back and relax. The problem is that not all stuff is small stuff. Some things are worth sweating over. The tricky part is to determine what is really important and worthy of your energy and what constitutes the small stuff that causes needless worry and diminishes the quality of your life.

One of the looming challenges for successful stress management is to determine what causes you stress. A certain level of stress can energize and motivate you to deal with the important issues in your life. You will want to focus your energy on the things in your life that are truly important. How do you determine what factors cause you unnecessary stress? How does your stress level compare to others? We will help you answer these questions in this chapter.

Where Are You Now Stress-Wise?

How is stress measured? This chapter presents a variety of tools to help assess your stress. Some of these tools are simple and fun, and others are more scientific and complex. Each was selected to help you understand the stress in your life and to provide information you can use to develop a stress management plan that works for you.

The first step in developing a plan is assessment. As Alan Watts stated in the beginning quote, "Normally we do not so much look at things as overlook them." You may be so busy living your life that you don't take time to stop and evaluate. You just keep doing what you are doing.

To assess stress, no one best tool will suffice, in part because reactions to events vary from person to person. What distresses one person excites and challenges another. Research increasingly supports the idea that the amount of stress is not what matters but, instead, the individual's ability to control the stressful situation. Often, external events are not what cause stress. How we perceive and cope with stressful events is the determining factor.

Therefore, you should use the information in this chapter in a way that seems relevant to you and your life. These assessments and surveys are not intended to be diagnostic but only to guide you in better understanding yourself. Taken together, the results of these assessments will produce an overall picture of your current stress status and help you decide where you want to go and how you can get there. Starting with a comprehensive assessment is so important that we have devoted this entire chapter to helping you get the picture of your current stress status.

Assess Your Stress Using Figure 2.1, fill in your personal results based on the instructions.

Resting Heart Rate Check your resting heart rate (pulse) after you have been sitting or relaxing for at least 30 minutes. You will need a watch or clock with a second hand

FIGURE 2.1 "Assess Your Stress" Form

Resting Heart Rate	_____ Beats per minute
Breathing Pattern	_____ Abdomen _____ Chest _____ Both
Respiration Rate	_____ Breaths per minute
Stress-o-Meter	1 2 3 4 5 6 7 8 9 10

(or digital seconds). First, find your pulse. You can find your **radial pulse** on the thumb side of your wrist, or your **carotid pulse** on your neck just under the jaw. For 60 seconds count the number of beats you feel. Place this number in the first line of Figure 2.1.

Breathing Pattern Now find a chair with a back. Sit in the chair so your back is primarily straight up and down against the back of the chair. Place one hand on your abdomen with your palm covering your navel. Place your other hand on the upper part of your chest with the palm of that hand just above your heart. For a minute or two, become aware of your breathing. While sitting straight up, notice your breath as it goes in and comes back out. Become aware of your hands as you breathe in and out. Which hand seems to move more—the hand on your abdomen or the one on your chest? Or do your hands both seem to move equally?

Try this second technique to see if you get the same results: First breathe out and empty your lungs. Count to three as you inhale deeply. Now hold it. Did your shoulders go up? Did you feel like the air filled the upper part of your lungs? If so, you probably lean toward what we call chest breathing. By contrast, if you are a diaphragmatic breather, you will feel your abdominal area expand, your belt tighten, and fullness in the lower part of your lungs and chest. Record your results on Figure 2.1 by putting an X by the mode that best describes how you breathe.

Respiration Rate For about a minute, become aware of your breathing again. This time, count how many natural, effortless breaths you take in a minute. Be sure to breathe as normally and naturally as possible. Each inhalation and exhalation cycle is considered one breath. The number of breaths you take in one minute is called your **respiration rate.** On Figure 2.1, record the number of breaths you take per minute.

Stress-o-Meter Think back over the last month of your life, including all of your waking moments. Give yourself a rating on the "Stress-o-Meter" along a continuum in which:

"1" means that you feel your life has been relatively stress-free during that period. You have felt blissful and calm most of the time. Everything seemed to go your way.

"10" means that you felt very high anxiety most of the time and that this was a month packed with high levels of stress. You felt totally overwhelmed, like your life was out of control, and like you were unable to cope.

Considering the last month as a single period of time, you most likely would rank yourself somewhere between these two extremes. To average out the month (we all have highs and lows), what number between 1 and 10 would you give yourself? Note this number on Figure 2.1.

Assess Your Stress Results Physiological measures associated with increased stress include, among others, increased heart rate and increased respiration rate. Although many factors affect these rates, such as physical conditioning and recent physical exertion, you will learn in Chapter 3 why the stress response can increase your pulse and respiration rates. The pulse rate for adults ranges between 50 and 100 beats per minute with the average heart rate approximately 70–80 beats per minute. The average respiration rate is 12–16 breaths per minute. A faster heartbeat or breathing rate might be an indicator of higher-than-desired stress levels. It could also be a sign of a medical condition or recent physical activity such as running up the stairs to get to class.

Were you primarily a chest breather or an abdominal breather? Many of us are primarily chest, or thoracic, breathers. Chest breathing happens due to chronic activation of the stress response. Chest breathers tend to take shallower breaths with the unconscious intention of getting more air into the lungs more quickly in preparation for fighting or running.

FYI

Meditation Slows Breathing

Did you know that meditating can affect the way you breathe and the amount of oxygen your body needs? People who regularly practice meditation tend to have slower breathing rates and naturally breathe more efficiently, that is, their bodies use the oxygen they breathe in more effectively. Various studies have shown that oxygen consumption is reduced during meditation, in some cases by up to 55%, and that respiration rate is lessened, in some cases to one breath per minute, when twelve to sixteen breaths per minute are normal. This is a natural physiological change due to a lowered requirement for oxygen by the cells and a slower metabolism. This happens naturally during meditation.

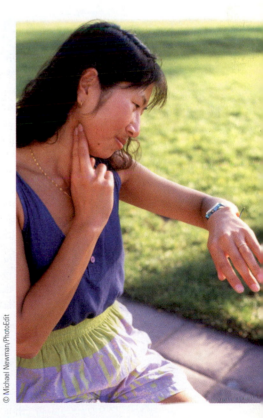

An elevated heart rate is an indication of stress. One site for counting your heart rate is the carotid artery.

Diaphragmatic, or abdominal, breathing uses the abdominal muscles to facilitate deeper breathing. This allows you to take in more oxygen with each breath. Deep breathing slows your nervous system in direct opposition to the stress response, which speeds it up. Later you will learn more about deep breathing as a relaxation technique.

Your perception of stress is instrumental in how your body responds. Results from the Stress-o-Meter increase your awareness of the level of stress you perceive in your life. When we do physical exercise, we can follow a perceived exertion scale that gives us some idea of how hard we are exercising, to determine our intensity level. Similarly, we can use the Stress-o-Meter to assess our general levels of perceived stress over the past month. You will learn later in the book how your perception of stress relates to your health and your physiological response. Whether the stress is real or imagined, your body responds the same: Your perception becomes your reality.

Look back over the results you recorded in Figure 2.1. What does this information tell you about your stress level?

Symptoms of Stress: Assessment How frequently do you find yourself experiencing problems such as headaches, difficulty going to sleep or staying asleep, unexplained muscle pain, jaw pain, uncontrolled anger, or frustration? Using Figure 2.2, assess the frequency in which you experience the symptoms of stress, by placing an X in the appropriate box.

The more often you experience these symptoms of stress, the more likely it is that stress is having a negative impact on your life. Stress is not the only factor to cause these symptoms. Athletes, for example, may experience sore muscles from training. However, when these symptoms occur for unexplained reasons, stress must be considered as a contributing factor. Like Angie in the opening vignette, you may be so used to feeling a certain way that you assume it is normal. If you don't know you are in distress, you can't change. Learning to be self-aware helps you recognize symptoms of stress early so you can take action. Look back over Figure 2.2. Do you recognize symptoms of stress in yourself that you would like to eliminate or change? In later chapters you will learn proven strategies to help you eliminate the negative symptoms of stress in your life.

FIGURE 2.2 Symptoms of Stress Form

Symptoms	Frequency of Symptoms						
	Almost all day, every day	2–3 times a day	Every night or day	2–3 times per week	Once a week	Once a month	Never
Headaches							
Tense muscles; sore neck and back							
Fatigue							
Anxiety, worry, phobias							
Difficulty falling asleep							
Irritability							
Insomnia							
Bouts of anger/ hostility							
Boredom, depression							
Eating too much or too little							
Diarrhea, cramps, gas, constipation							
Restlessness, itching, tics							
Grinding teeth, clenching jaw during sleep							
Difficulty concentrating							

Stress and Deep Sleep

In a University of Pittsburgh study reported in the journal *Psychosomatic Medicine,* researchers monitored the heart rates of 59 healthy undergraduate students while they slept. Variations in heart rate can provide clues about activity of the involuntary nervous system, which directs the function of organs such as the heart and the lungs. To trigger stress during sleep, the researchers told half of the students they would have to deliver a 15-minute speech when they woke up. The topics would be chosen for them upon their awakening.

The researchers detected significant heart rate variations between the stressed and non-stressed students as they slept. The stressed group had changes in heart rate patterns during **rapid eye movement (REM) sleep**—the sleep phase when dreaming occurs—and non-REM sleep. The heart rate variability patterns detected in the stressed students were similar to those seen in people with insomnia, suggesting similar pathways of disruption in the nervous system. This study found that stressed sleepers wake up more often and have fewer episodes of deep sleep. The link between daytime stress and restless sleep is well established, but scientists are still investigating the exact ways that stress affects sleep.

Source: University of Pittsburgh, news release, Feb. 5, 2004, *ScoutNews,* LLC, retrieved from www.healthfinder.gov/news.

Stress Busting Behavior: Stress Level Checklist

Monitor your stress levels regularly with the following list. Check the box if your answer to the question is "yes."

☐ Check your resting heart rate — is it higher than usual?

☐ Are you breathing from your chest only (rather than abdomen)?

☐ Is your rate of respiration elevated?

☐ Is your perceived stress level above a 5 on a scale of 1 to 10?

☐ Do you have any other stress symptoms, such as headaches, tense muscles, or difficulty falling asleep?

If any of the above are checked, take action to manage your stress!

Perceived Stress Scale (PSS) The Perceived Stress Scale (PSS) is represented in Figure 2.3. This classic stress assessment instrument remains a popular choice for helping us understand how different situations affect our feelings and our perceived stress. The questions in this scale ask about your feelings and thoughts over the past month. In each case, you are asked to indicate how often you felt or thought a certain way. Although some of the questions are similar, you should treat each one as a separate question. The best approach is to answer fairly quickly. Don't try to count up the number of times you felt a certain way. Rather, indicate the alternative that seems like a reasonable estimate.

The Perceived Stress Scale is interesting because it considers your *perception* of what is happening in your life as most important. Consider two students, John and Dan, who had the exact same events and experiences in their lives for the past month. John is thinking, "well, things aren't going quite how I planned, but I am learning some good lessons and things can only get better!" while Dan thinks, "things aren't going how I planned, everything is going downhill, my life is a mess and I'm a loser!" Depending on their perception, John's total score could put him in the low-stress category and Dan's total score could put him in the high-stress category.

Inventory of College Students' Recent Life Experiences Another useful scale used to measure stress levels in a different way is called the Inventory of College Students'

FYI

Lesson from the Titanic

The blockbuster movie *Titanic* has a health lesson for us all. The captain of that mighty ship was warned six separate times to slow down, change course, and take the southern route because icebergs had been sighted. But he ignored all six specific warnings, lulled into complacency by believing the ship was unsinkable. The lesson is: *Listen to your body when it sends you signals.* Symptoms and changes are warnings that you should slow down, change course, or take another route.

Source: Connections: Health Ministries Association Newsletter, "A Lesson from the Titanic," by Jean Wright-Elson, *Parish Nurse Note* (Huntington Beach, CA.).

Nothing can bring you peace but yourself.

—*Ralph Waldo Emerson*

FIGURE 2.3 Perceived Stress Scale (PSS)

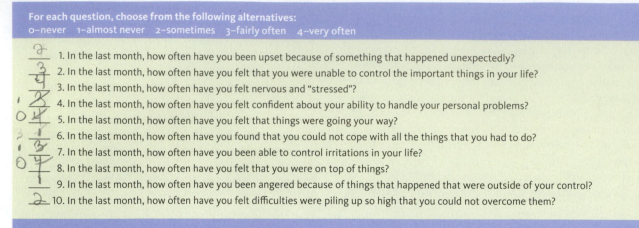

For each question, choose from the following alternatives:
0–never   1–almost never   2–sometimes   3–fairly often   4–very often

_2_ 1. In the last month, how often have you been upset because of something that happened unexpectedly?

_3_ 2. In the last month, how often have you felt that you were unable to control the important things in your life?

_4_ 3. In the last month, how often have you felt nervous and "stressed"?

_2_ 4. In the last month, how often have you felt confident about your ability to handle your personal problems?

_4_ 5. In the last month, how often have you felt that things were going your way?

_1_ 6. In the last month, how often have you found that you could not cope with all the things that you had to do?

_3_ 7. In the last month, how often have you been able to control irritations in your life?

_4_ 8. In the last month, how often have you felt that you were on top of things?

_____ 9. In the last month, how often have you been angered because of things that happened that were outside of your control?

_2_ 10. In the last month, how often have you felt difficulties were piling up so high that you could not overcome them?

Figuring your PSS score:

You can determine your PSS score by following these directions:

First, reverse your scores for questions 4, 5, 7, and 8. On these four questions, change the scores like this: 0 = 4, 1 = 3, 2 = 2, 3 = 1, 4 = 0. For all other questions, use the number you wrote down as the score.

Now add up your scores for each item to get a total.

My total score is 14.

Individual scores on the PSS can range from 0 to 40, with higher scores indicating higher perceived stress.

Scores ranging from 0–13 would be considered low perceived stress.

Scores ranging from 14–26 would be considered moderate perceived stress.

Scores ranging from 27–40 would be considered high perceived stress.

Source: A Global Measure of Perceived Stress, by S. Cohen, T. Kamarck, & R. Mermelstein, in _Journal of Health and Social Behavior_, 24(4), 1983, 385–396. Used by permission.

Recent Life Experiences (ICSRLE), represented in Figure 2.4. The ICSRLE was designed to identify individual exposure to sources of stress or hassles. This inventory also allows you to identify the extent to which you experienced those stressors over the past month. As its name suggests, the ICSRLE was developed uniquely for college students and, as you know, the sources of stress in a university environment can be different from other settings.

Ardell Wellness Stress Test   Don Ardell developed a stress assessment that is unique in its holistic approach to stress. In Chapter 1 you learned about the importance of incorporating all dimensions of health in your understanding of stress. The Ardell Wellness Stress Test, represented in Figure 2.5, incorporates physical, intellectual, emotional, spiritual, and social aspects of health for a balanced assessment. While this assessment is not as scientific as others, it provides useful information in putting together your current stress status puzzle. Your personal perception of satisfaction in factors related to body, mind, and spirit greatly impacts your quality of life.

When you have completed the Ardell Wellness Stress Test, look back and identify which items relate more to physical health, intellectual health, emotional health, spiritual health, or social health. Do you detect any patterns? For instance, are more areas of disappointment related to physical health than to social health? Again, for holistic health seek a balance in all dimensions of health.

Student Stress Scale   The Student Stress Scale (Figure 2.6) is an adaptation specifically for college-age students of the Life Events Scale developed by Holmes and Rahe.[1] This classic stress assessment was designed to predict the likelihood of disease and illness following exposure to various stressful life events and the extent to which the change impacted the individual. In the assessment, each life event is given a score indicating the amount of readjustment a person has to make as a result of the change. Events that are potentially both positive and negative are included, based on the premise that the adaptation to change is the contributing factor to disease and illness. Some studies have found that people with serious illnesses tend to have higher scores on similar assessments.[2]

This scale indicates that change in one's life requires effort to adapt and subsequent effort to regain stability. Stress is a natural by-product of adapting and then regaining

FIGURE 2.4 Inventory of College Students' Recent Life Experiences (ICSRLE)

The following is a list of experiences that many students have at some time or other. Indicate for each experience how much it has been a part of your life over the past month. Mark your answers according to the following guide:

Intensity of Experience over the Past Month			
0 = not at all part of my life	1 = only slightly part of my life	2 = distinctly part of my life	3 = very much part of my life

_____ 1. Conflicts with boyfriend's/girlfriend's/spouse's family
_____ 2. Being let down or disappointed by friends
_____ 3. Conflict with professor(s)
_____ 4. Social rejection
_____ 5. Too many things to do at once
_____ 6. Being taken for granted
_____ 7. Financial conflicts with family members
_____ 8. Having your trust betrayed by a friend
_____ 9. Separation from people you care about
_____ 10. Having your contributions overlooked
_____ 11. Struggling to meet your own academic standards
_____ 12. Being taken advantage of
_____ 13. Not enough leisure time
_____ 14. Struggling to meet the academic standards of others
_____ 15. A lot of responsibilities
_____ 16. Dissatisfaction with school
_____ 17. Decisions about intimate relationship(s)
_____ 18. Not enough time to meet your obligations
_____ 19. Dissatisfaction with your mathematical ability
_____ 20. Important decisions about your future career
_____ 21. Financial burdens
_____ 22. Dissatisfaction with your reading ability
_____ 23. Important decisions about your education
_____ 24. Loneliness
_____ 25. Lower grades than you hoped for

_____ 26. Conflict with teaching assistant(s)
_____ 27. Not enough time for sleep
_____ 28. Conflicts with your family
_____ 29. Heavy demands from extracurricular activities
_____ 30. Finding courses too demanding
_____ 31. Conflicts with friends
_____ 32. Hard effort to get ahead
_____ 33. Poor health of a friend
_____ 34. Disliking your studies
_____ 35. Getting "ripped off" or cheated in the purchase of services
_____ 36. Social conflicts over smoking
_____ 37. Difficulties with transportation
_____ 38. Disliking fellow student(s)
_____ 39. Conflicts with boyfriend/girlfriend/spouse
_____ 40. Dissatisfaction with your ability at written expression
_____ 41. Interruptions of your school work
_____ 42. Social isolation
_____ 43. Long waits to get service (at banks, stores, etc.)
_____ 44. Being ignored
_____ 45. Dissatisfaction with your physical appearance
_____ 46. Finding course(s) uninteresting
_____ 47. Gossip concerning someone you care about
_____ 48. Failing to get expected job
_____ 49. Dissatisfaction with your athletic skills

Scoring the ICSRLE

Add your total points: _____

Your score on the ICSRLE can range from 0 to 147. Higher scores indicate higher levels of exposure to hassles. From your results, focus on two key outcomes:

1. Determine your current level of stress by adding your score for each hassle and getting a total.
2. Discover which hassles play a greater part in your life. Items that you rated "3" indicate that those stressors are more of an issue for you.

Source: The Inventory of College Students Recent Life Experiences: A Decontaminated Hassles Scale for a Special Population," by P. M. Kohn, K. Lafreniere, & M. Gurevich, _Journal of Behavioral Medicine, 13_(6), 1990, 619–630. Used by permission.

internal homeostasis, or balance. Note that this assessment considers only the events that occur, not individual perceptions of these events in life. Students frequently point out, for example, that changing colleges or getting a new boyfriend or girlfriend can be stress-relieving depending on the circumstances. Change, however, does require adaptation. The value assigned to each life event can be interpreted as representing the amount of energy it takes to cope with any given change. Thus, the value in the Student Stress Scale is in increasing your awareness of potential stress-producing events and helping you understand the connection between change and health. Ultimately, your individual perception of the event has to be taken into account.

Stress Vulnerability Factors Do you think some people are just more vulnerable to the effects of stressors than others? Assessing your vulnerability to stress is another important aspect in understanding your stress experience. Vulnerability has to do with a factor, or set of factors, that increases a person's susceptibility to stress. People with low vulnerability need to experience more stress before they become distressed whereas those people with high vulnerability need much less stress to reach their tipping point to distress.

FIGURE 2.5 Adapted Ardell Wellness Stress Test for College Students

This assessment is based on your personal perception of satisfaction. Rate your satisfaction with each of the following items by using this scale:

+3 = Ecstatic	+2 = Very happy	+1 = Mildly happy	0 = Indifferent
−1 = Mildly disappointed		−2 = Very disappointed	−3 = Completely dismayed

_____ 1. Choice of college

_____ 2. Choice of major, area of study

_____ 3. Marital or relationship status

_____ 4. Friendships

_____ 5. Capacity to have fun

_____ 6. Amount of fun experienced in the last month

_____ 7. Financial prospects

_____ 8. Current ability to meet expenses

_____ 9. Spirituality

_____ 10. Level of self-esteem

_____ 11. Prospects for having impact on those who know you and possibly others

_____ 12. Sex life

_____ 13. Body—how it looks and performs

_____ 14. Relationship with family

_____ 15. Happiness with current living situation

_____ 16. Learned stress management capacities

_____ 17. Nutrition, health, and fitness choices

_____ 18. Life skills and knowledge of issues and facts related to your studies or future career

_____ 19. Ability to recover from disappointment, hurts, setbacks, and tragedies

_____ 20. Confidence that you currently are, or will be in the future, reasonably close to your highest potential

_____ 21. Achievement of a rounded or balanced quality in your life

_____ 22. Sense that life for you is on an upward curve, getting better and fuller all the time

_____ 23. Level of participation in issues and concerns beyond your immediate interest

_____ 24. Role in some kind of network of friends, relatives, and/or others about whom you care deeply and who reciprocate that commitment to you.

_____ 25. Emotional acceptance of the changes the passage of time brings

TOTAL _____

Interpretation

+51 to +75	You are a self-actualized person, nearly immune from the ravages of stress. There are few, if any, challenges likely to distract you from a sense of near total well-being.
+25 to +50	You have mastered the wellness approach to life and have the capacity to deal creatively and efficiently with events and circumstances.
+1 to +24	You are a wellness-oriented person, with an ability to prosper as a whole person, but you should give a bit more attention to optimal health concepts and skill building.
0 to −24	You are a candidate for additional training in how to deal with stress. A sudden increase in potentially negative events and circumstances could cause a severe emotional setback.
−25 to −50	You are a candidate for counseling. You are either too pessimistic or have severe problems in dealing with stress.
−51 to −75	You are a candidate for major psychological care with virtually no capacity for coping with life's problems.

Source: From _High Level Wellness: An Alternative to Doctors, Drugs, and Disease_, by Don Ardell (Berkeley, CA: Ten Speed Press, 1986). Used by permission.

So what causes the differences in people's vulnerability? What makes one person more vulnerable than another? Researchers have determined a number of factors that impact vulnerability, including:

- **Genetics**–Evidence from family studies, particularly studies involving twins, seem to show a strong genetic element. One aspect of a person's vulnerability is related to his or her genetic makeup. However this is not the whole story.
- **Coping style**–Some methods of coping with life's difficulties seem to be more effective than others. People who use effective coping skills seem to deal with stress better than those who do not. You will be learning many of these effective coping strategies.
- **Thinking style**–How people think about themselves or the world around them seems to make a major difference to their level of vulnerability to stress. This is more than simply being optimistic or pessimistic. As you will learn in Chapter 6, there are certain thinking methods that help people to cope better than others.

FIGURE 2.6 Student Stress Scale

For each event that occurred in your life within the past year, record the corresponding score. If an event occurred more than once, multiply the score for that event by the number of times the event occurred and record that score. Total all the scores.

Life Event	Mean Value
1. Death of a close family member	100
2. Death of a close friend	73
3. Divorce of parents	65
4. Jail term	63
5. Major personal injury or illness	63
6. Marriage	58
7. Getting fired from a job	50
8. Failing an important course	47
9. Change in the health of a family member	45
10. Pregnancy	45
11. Sex problems	44
12. Serious argument with a close friend	40
13. Change in financial status	39
14. Change of academic major	39
15. Trouble with parents	39
16. New girlfriend or boyfriend	37
17. Increase in workload at school	37
18. Outstanding personal achievement	36
19. First quarter/semester in college	36
20. Change in living conditions	31
21. Serious argument with an instructor	30
22. Getting lower grades than expected	29
23. Change in sleeping habits	29
24. Change in social activities	29
25. Change in eating habits	28
26. Chronic car trouble	26
27. Change in number of family get-togethers	26
28. Too many missed classes	25
29. Changing colleges	24
30. Dropping more than one class	23
31. Minor traffic violations	20
Total Stress Score	

Score Interpretation:

Researchers determined that if your total score is:

300 or more—statistically you stand an almost 80 percent chance of getting sick in the near future.

150 to 299—you have a 50/50 chance of experiencing a serious health change within two years.

149 or less—you have about a 30 percent chance of a serious health change.*

Source: *Health Awareness Through Discovery* by Kathleen Mullen and Gerald, Costello, Minneapolis: Burgess Publishing Company, 1981.

- **Environment**–The way that people deal with stress and the options they have are often related to their environment. This can include anything from a cluttered house to constant noise. In Chapter 14 you will learn how you can create a healthy environment to reduce your vulnerability to stress.
- **Social skills**–The more integrated people are in society and the more social support they experience, the less vulnerable they are to stress. The better a person's social skills the easier it is for him or her to give and receive help. People with more supportive relationships tend to do better in times of crisis.[3]

The Stress Vulnerability Questionnaire will help you evaluate some of the physical, mental, emotional, spiritual, and social factors that affect your vulnerability to stress, providing you with another piece in your stress status puzzle. Throughout this book, you will be learning many new skills to assist you in reducing your stress vulnerability.

FIGURE 2.7 Stress Vulnerability Questionnaire

This stress vulnerability questionnaire helps you determine your current vulnerability to stress and helps you identify areas where you can reduce your vulnerability to stress.

Item	Strongly Agree	Mildly Agree	Mildly Disagree	Strongly Disagree
1. I try to incorporate as much physical activity* as possible in my daily schedule.	1	2	3	4
2. I exercise aerobically 20 minutes or more at least three times per week.	1	2	3	4
3. I regularly sleep 7 to 8 hours per night.	1	2	3	4
4. I take my time eating at least one hot, balanced meal a day.	1	2	3	4
5. I drink fewer than two cups of coffee (or equivalent) per day.	1	2	3	4
6. I am at recommended body weight.	1	2	3	4
7. I enjoy good health.	1	2	3	4
8. I do not use tobacco in any form.	1	2	3	4
9. I limit my alcohol intake to no more than one drink for women or two drinks for men per day.	1	2	3	4
10. I do not use hard drugs.	1	2	3	4
11. I have someone I love, trust, and can rely on for help if I have a problem or need to make an essential decision.	1	2	3	4
12. There is love in my family.	1	2	3	4
13. I routinely give and receive affection.	1	2	3	4
14. I have close personal relationships with other people who provide me with a sense of emotional security.	1	2	3	4
15. There are people close by whom I can turn to for guidance in time of stress.	1	2	3	4
16. I can speak openly about feelings, emotions, and problems with people I trust.	1	2	3	4
17. Other people rely on me for help.	1	2	3	4
18. I am able to keep my feelings of anger and hostility under control.	1	2	3	4
19. I have a network of friends who enjoy the same social activities I do.	1	2	3	4
20. I take time to do something fun at least once a week.	1	2	3	4
21. My religious beliefs provide guidance and strength to my life.	1	2	3	4
22. I often provide service to others.	1	2	3	4
23. I enjoy my job (major or school).	1	2	3	4
24. I am a competent worker.	1	2	3	4
25. I get along well with co-workers (or students).	1	2	3	4
26. My income is sufficient for my needs.	1	2	3	4
27. I manage time adequately.	1	2	3	4
28. I have learned to say "no" to additional commitments when I am already pressed for time.	1	2	3	4
29. I take daily quiet time for myself.	1	2	3	4
30. I practice stress management as needed.	1	2	3	4

*Walk instead of driving, avoid escalators and elevators, or walk to neighboring offices, homes, and stores.

Total points: [   ]

Rating:

   0–30 points.................................. Excellent (great resistance to stress)

   31–40 points.................................. Good (little vulnerability to stress)

   41–50 points.................................. Average (somewhat vulnerable to stress)

   51–60 points.................................. Fair (vulnerable to stress)

   ≥61 points.................................. Poor (highly vulnerable to stress)

Source: *Lifetime Physical Fitness & Wellness,* by W. W. K. Hoeger and S. A. Hoeger (Belmont, CA: Wadsworth/Cengage Learning), 2009.

Tombstone Test When all is said and done, one of the most important assessments may be what we call the Tombstone Test. How do you want to be remembered? As being a workaholic? As the one who always won the argument? For making more money than your neighbor? As someone who never forgave anyone who wronged you? Or do you want to be remembered as a good parent, mate, and friend? Do you want to be remembered as someone who was whole and balanced in body, mind, and spirit? Do you want to be remembered for the service you provided to those who needed help?

Take a few minutes to write down how you want to be remembered. What do you want others to say and think about you when your life is over? List the qualities and characteristics you want to be remembered for. Are you living your life in a way that demonstrates the qualities you value?

The choices you make every single day determine your stress to a large extent. Your daily activities, which at times can feel like drudgery, actually can become stress-relieving when you view them all as part of your contribution to bigger priorities. Thinking about today, this minute, the task at hand in a positive manner can bring peace and contentment. As the story goes, two people are laying bricks. A passerby asks, "What are you doing?" The first worker answers, "Laying bricks." The other worker answers, "Building a cathedral."

Author Anecdote A Culture of Stress Our family spent two years living in Australia in the small ocean community of Torquay. Stepping out of the Midwestern culture I had grown up in was eye-opening. My Norwegian, Protestant work-ethic paradigm for viewing the world was well established. For the first time, I began to examine some of my values, beliefs, and goals.

When the annual 6-week summer "holiday" rolled around, Australians flocked to the beaches near our small community to relax and have fun. My husband saw this as an opportunity to get a summer job to supplement our meager income during this break from his teaching job. This was a foreign idea to his Australian colleagues.

"What? You want to work during your summer holidays? Why?" they asked in astonishment.

We learned a valuable lesson from our Australian friends: Take time to renew and relax. One of my favorite sayings from our time in Australia is, "She'll be right mate." That translates into something like, "Don't worry—things will work out okay."

* * *

More recently, I traveled to the Netherlands to attend a class at the University of Amsterdam. Every day as the afternoon went on, I noticed people gathering in the streetside cafes and pubs. The streets of Amsterdam in the late afternoon are alive with the sounds of people laughing, talking, relaxing, socializing, and having fun at the end of the work day.

How much of the stress we experience today is related to our cultural practices? Have we become a society of hard-working, isolated people who have lost sight of the importance of relaxing, socializing, and just having fun? Should we reexamine our culturally induced priorities? How much of our stress is a result of our self-imposed choices?

—MH

FYI

Vacation Days

Number of vacation days awarded to the average worker in France: 39

Number of vacation days awarded to the average worker in the United States: 12

Source: AARP Newsletter, September/October, 2005, p. 18.

Assess what is most important in your life. When your choices are guided by the values and goals that are most important to you, your life can be full and active, yet not stressful. Decide how you want to be remembered—and then live your life so that happens.

Daily Stress Diary

Chances are that many of you have completed a food diary at some time. Its purpose is to record everything you eat to increase your awareness of what you are eating. The information you enter can be analyzed for its caloric level and nutritional content and thereby help you evaluate your diet. The Daily Stress Diary serves the same purpose, but it relates to your stress. You will find it worth your time to complete the Stress Diary Lab Activity found at the end of the chapter.

The Stress Diary can be a real eye-opener as you become aware of stress triggers throughout your day. Watch for patterns that develop. Does your stress level go through the roof every time your roommate's boyfriend comes over and plops himself down in your favorite chair? Do you invariably feel stressed after you and your friend consume an entire family-sized pizza? Do you find that the days that seem filled with stress and the days you seem more vulnerable to stress are the days after you stay up late for the all-you-can-drink specials at the bar?

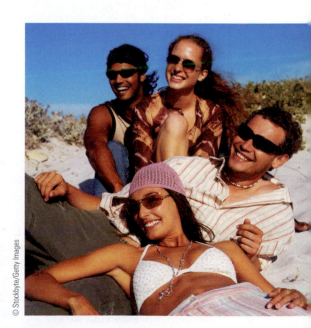

© Stockbyte/Getty Images

Culture is a major influence on our choices for relaxation.

Conclusion

In this chapter you have had the opportunity to assess your stress using several different measures. Look back over each of the assessment activities, surveys, and tools. You will see that these tools measured stress from a variety of perspectives, including:

- Physiological indicators of stress
- Your perception of what is happening in your life
- Sources of stress and the frequency of hassles
- Your level of satisfaction with the events in your life
- Life events you have experienced
- Your vulnerability to stress

The real impact of this chapter will come from what you do with the information you learned about yourself. Each of the assessments is like a piece of a puzzle: When you put all the pieces together, you have a complete picture. You can translate this picture into a plan to help reduce stress and enhance the quality of your life.

2.1 Daily Stress Diary

ACTIVITY Each stress assessment in this chapter provides you with information you can use to better understand the impact of stress on your life. The Stress Diary provides an additional opportunity to assess your personal routine and the situations you encounter on a daily basis. For one day, keep a diary.

I. Throughout the day, list the situations or events initiating the stress response (sources of stress). For each event include:

   1. Source of stress.
   2. Time and Place.
   3. Level of perceived stress (1 = Slight, 2 = Moderate, 3 = Strong, 4 = Intense).
   4. Thoughts and feelings about the stressor.
   5. Coping strategies you used to deal with the stressor.

II. At the end of the day, reflect on:

   1. What was your major source of stress for the day?
   2. What is your personal assessment of how you managed stress today?

2.2 Stress Profile

You have completed a variety of stress assessments aimed at providing you with a comprehensive evaluation of your current stress status. Compile your results for each assessment by completing a paper including the following information. You can also find this Stress Profile at the Premium Website.

I. ASSESSMENT RESULTS

1. Assess Your Stress

Resting Heart Rate _____ Beats per minute

Breathing Pattern _____ Abdomen _____ Chest _____ Both

Respiration Rate _____ Breaths per minute

Stress-o-Meter 1 2 3 4 5 6 7 8 9 10

2. **Symptoms of Stress**

   What are the three symptoms of stress you experience most frequently?

3. **Perceived Stress Scale**

   My total score is _____. This puts me in the _____ (low, moderate, high) perceived stress range.

4. **Inventory of College Students' Recent Life Experiences**

   My total score is _____.

   List the hassles that you rated "3".

5. **Ardell Wellness Stress Test**

   My score is _____.

   What does the interpretation of my score indicate?

6. **Student Stress Scale**

   My total score is _____.

   Based on my score, my chances of experiencing a stress-related health change in the near future is _____ %.

7. **Vulnerability Questionnaire**

   My total score is _____.

   What are the top three behaviors you would like to change to decrease your vulnerability to stress?

8. **Tombstone Test**

   What are the top three qualities or characteristics for which you want to be remembered?

II. ANALYSIS OF RESULTS

1. For each of the 8 assessments listed above, briefly explain the following:
   a. What aspect(s) of stress did the assessment measure, in other words, what is the specific purpose of this assessment as compared to others? What unique information does it provide?
   b. What did you learn from the assessment? Did the results surprise you? Do you agree or disagree with the results?

2. Which assessments were most relevant and valuable to you?

3. Reflect on the overall picture of your current stress status. Give this some careful thought as you reflect on what you learned about yourself from this comprehensive assessment of many dimensions of stress. This learning is critical for you to understand if you are to move toward a more balanced, less stressed life. What three important insights or ideas did you gain from completing this assignment?

Key Points

- The first step in developing a plan to reduce and manage stress is assessment.
- Stress can trigger physiological changes such as increased pulse and increased respiration rate.
- Physical symptoms of stress can be headache, muscle tension, insomnia, and a host of other warning signs.
- When assessing stress, perception is key. The same situation can elicit very different stress responses in different individuals because of the individual's *perception* of the experience.
- Another way to measure stress is to evaluate the frequency of exposure to different stressors and hassles.

- Several factors affect your vulnerability to stressors. Successfully managing these factors can help you become less susceptible to the harmful effects of stress.
- A Daily Stress Diary can be a valuable tool for increasing your awareness of stressors in your life.
- Because no single survey or tool can provide the whole picture when it comes to assessing stress, the results from several assessments are needed to give you a better understanding of your personal stress level.

radial pulse
carotid pulse

respiration rate
rapid eye movement (REM) sleep

Discussion Time For Critical Thinking/Discussion Questions please visit this book's Premium Website.

Notes

1. "The Social Readjustment Rating Scale," by T. H. Holmes and R. H. Rahe, *Journal of Psychosomatic Research,* *11* (1967): 213–218.

2. "The Relationship between Life Events and Indices of Classroom Performance," by K. DeMeuse, *Teaching of Psychology 12* (1985): 146–149.

3. "Understanding Stress and Vulnerability," by S. Sorenson, Mental Health Sanctuary 2002, http://www.mhsanctuary.com/articles/ustress.htm, retrieved September 12, 2008.

3 The Science of Stress

- Why do I need to understand the *science* of stress? I just want to learn to relax. ■ What is the purpose of the fight-or-flight response? ■ What really happens in my body when I am feeling stress? ■ Is the physiological response to stress different in males and females?

Study of this chapter will enable you to:

1. Describe the human fight-or-flight response to stress.
2. List the physiological changes associated with the stress response.
3. Identify the stages of the general adaptation syndrome.
4. Explain how the science of stress relates to stress management and prevention.

STUDENT OBJECTIVES

To understand the stress response, we must possess a fundamental knowledge not only of psychology but of physiology as well.

—*George Everly*

Superwoman Have you ever heard stories of people displaying almost superhuman powers when confronted with an emergency situation? How can we explain this superhuman response that releases power and strength beyond anything we have imagined or experienced previously? What physical and psychological factors are responsible for these amazing abilities? Here is a true story that Sarah shared in class one day.

* * *

Sarah raised her hand and told of a time when her mother and sister were out working on their farm. Her mother was driving a big farm machine designed to cut the hay that was growing in their field. Her mother didn't see the youngster, who was playing in the tall wheat stocks, and she accidentally ran over her young daughter. Noticing the unusual sensation as she struck her daughter, she quickly shut off the engine and hurried to see what she had run over. Realizing it was her daughter, she panicked, not knowing what to do. No one was around to help.

In this moment of extreme alarm, she lifted the heavy machine off her daughter and pulled her out with one mighty motion. Carrying her daughter, she ran all the way back to the farmhouse to call for help. Afterward, the mother collapsed from exhaustion, unable to generate any energy. In those few moments of her daughter's peril, she had become superwoman.

The Science of Stress

The story of stress is a long one, beginning with our ancestors many generations ago. Throughout history, people have experienced stress related to everything from war to poverty to disease to money. The quest for understanding stress has resulted in a surge of research during the past half-century. More is known about the physiology and psychology of stress than ever before.

This chapter and the next one provide a scientific foundation on principles, theories, and models of stress to help you understand the physiology and psychology of stress. In keeping with the experiential focus of this book, the intent of this chapter is not to teach you everything there is to know about the physiology of stress. Entire books have been written on this subject. The purpose of this chapter is to provide you with sufficient knowledge to understand how stress affects your body.

Discovering what actually happens in your body and your mind will help you understand the mechanics behind the stress-prevention and stress-management skills you will be learning. Knowledge of the science and theory of stress provides strong, credible support for why and how stress-management techniques work.

Stress and the Big Bear

Why do you feel stress in the first place? What is the purpose of this complex interaction among nerves, muscles, hormones, organs, and body systems that leads to unpleasant symptoms such as headaches, fatigue, feeling emotionally upset, and a host of other side effects? To answer these questions, we have to go back a few thousand years to see what life was like then. This will help us understand how our bodies are programmed to respond to threats and danger today.

In order to understand the origins of this programming, consider the following scenario: Imagine that you and I live in a remote place many thousands of years ago, where we find no trace of modern conveniences. We do not have comfortable homes, telephones or television, indoor plumbing, electricity, or any of our modern-day comforts. For the sake of this story, let's say we live in caves that are out in the "wilds" of some remote area.

I have invited you to my dwelling because we just killed a large animal and are roasting it in a pit. Several of our friends are outside of my cave enjoying a relaxing round of Kick the Rock. We are having a great time.

Suddenly we notice a rustling of bushes in the distance. Then, charging mightily—or hungrily—toward us emerges a huge, ferocious-looking bear. This enormous creature has smelled our food and wants some of it for itself. It is a menacing creature that could easily put us out of commission with a single swipe of its mighty forearms.

* * *

As you imagine yourself in this scenario, one of the first thoughts that likely will pop into your mind is something like: "Uh-Oh! I'm in trouble here!" or "I'm in danger and I'm likely to feel some pain!" These immediate thoughts are followed closely by the next thought: "Run!" You sense the immediate need to get away from this ominous animal. You don't want to be its dinner. Or your next thought could be, instead, "I need to kill this creature to protect my family, myself, and my friends! *Fight!*"

The Fight-or-Flight Response

After the initial awareness of danger, a surge of physiological processes immediately floods the body automatically and precisely. This is a state of physiological and psychological hyperarousal. The cascade of nervous system activity and release of stress hormones lead to immediate responses that help a person deal with danger by either fighting or running.

Harvard physiologist Walter Cannon coined the term **fight-or-flight response** to describe the body's automatic response anytime we perceive a threat or danger. This primitive response gives us strength, power, and speed to avoid physical harm. As you read in Sarah's story in the opening vignette, the fight-or-flight response can be activated to protect both ourselves and others when we perceive danger.

The fight-or-flight response is designed to help us do one thing, and only one thing, very well: *survive!* Physiologically, the stress response is characterized by activation of the sympathetic nervous system, which results in the secretion of chemicals into the bloodstream, mobilizing the behavioral response. Whether the response culminates in "fight" or "flight" depends on whether we perceive the threat or stressor as surmountable or insurmountable. Thus, an appropriate stress response is essential to survival. Figure 3.1 illustrates the fight-or-flight response.

Because we are designed for survival, our body systems react to protect us from pain and death in life-threatening or dangerous situations. In the short run, this response is a powerful and useful process. If kept "on" for a longer period, however, it can produce serious problems.

Scientists use the term **homeostasis** (homeo = the same; stasis = standing) to define the physiological and emotional limits in which the body functions efficiently and comfortably. Stress disturbs homeostasis by creating a state of imbalance. When we are in homeostasis, we are in a state of balance. Then something happens in our surroundings—something equivalent to a big bear charging out of the forest. This perception of danger automatically initiates the fight-or-flight response.

Once we sense no more danger, we experience exhaustion and fatigue because we have expended a tremendous amount of energy while running or fighting. We are exhausted, and the stress response is no longer activated. Because we feel safe again, the functions in the body that activate the stress response are turned off and we gradually return to normal (homeostasis).

The fight-or-flight response is generally regarded as the prototypical human response to stress. The tend-and-befriend theory, as explained in the Research Highlight, provides some intriguing food for thought, but this research is still in the early stages. Although

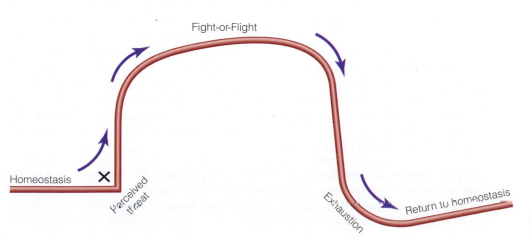

FIGURE 3.1 Fight-or-Flight Response

Tend-and-Befriend, Not Fight-or-Flight

For the last five decades the fight-or-flight theory has dominated stress research. Our understanding of how the body responds to stressors has increased dramatically during this time. Note that the biobehavioral fight-or-flight theory has been disproportionately based on studies of males. This is attributable in part to the fact that females experience natural, cyclical variations in hormonal and neuroendocrine responses, which can lead to confusing and often uninterpretable results. Therefore, the processes involved in stress responses in females are less well understood.

A team of scientists supported by the National Institute of Mental Health formulated a theory that characterizes female responses to stress by a pattern it terms **tend-and-befriend** rather than fight-or-flight.* This research supports the premise that female stress responses have evolved selectively to simultaneously maximize the survival of self and offspring. Thus, the tend-and-befriend pattern involves females' nurturing offspring under stressful circumstances, exhibiting behaviors that protect their offspring from harm (tending), and befriending (creating and joining social groups to exchange resources and provide protection). The scientists propose that these responses build on the biobehavioral attachment–caregiving processes that depend in part on oxytocin, estrogen, and other sex-linked hormones.

In addition, the literature on human and nonhuman primates alike provides evidence of substantial female preference to affiliate, or make close connections with others, under stress, as compared to males. The tend-and-befriend pattern likely is maintained by social and cultural roles, in addition to sex-linked, neuroendocrine responses to stress. This new theoretical model opens a fresh field of inquiry into research on stress.

A Neuroendocrine Model Explains Gender Differences in Behavioral Response to Stress (Bethesda, MD: National Institute of Mental Health, June 7, 2001).

Source: "Biobehavioral Responses to Stress in Females: Tend-and-Befriend, Not Fight-or-Flight," by S. Taylor, L. Cousino-Klein, B. Lewis, T. Gruenewald, R. Gurung, and J. Updegraff, in *Psychological Review, 107*(3) (2000), 411–429.

we know that there may be some differences in how males and females respond to stress physiologically, we also know that the male and female responses have many similarities. The fight-or-flight response explains most clearly the chain of events that occur in most people in response to stress.

Physiological Response to Stress

When the stress response is initiated, immediate and powerful changes come about because a branch of the nervous system called the **autonomic nervous system** (ANS) is activated. The ANS is responsible for many functions in the body that typically occur involuntarily, such as digestion, heart rate, blood pressure, and body temperature. The activity of the autonomic nervous system takes place primarily beyond our conscious control. It is automatic.

The two branches of the ANS are designed to regulate the fight-or-flight response on a constant basis:

1. The **sympathetic nervous system** (SNS) is the part of the ANS responsible for initiating the fight-or-flight response each time we have a thought of potential or actual danger or pain. We need only to think that we are in danger and the flood of physiological and emotional activity is turned on to increase power, speed, and strength.

2. The **parasympathetic nervous system** (PNS), the other branch of the ANS, is designed to return the physiology to a state of homeostasis, or balance, after the threat, danger, or potential pain is no longer perceived to be imminent. The example of our state of mind as we enjoyed a primitive barbecue is a good example of how homeostasis works. The parasympathetic branch is responsible for counterbalancing the body's sympathetic activity, which restores calm, promotes relaxation, and facilitates digestive functions, energy storage, and tissue repair and growth.[1] Breathing is slow, as is the heart rate. Blood pressure and body temperature drop. In general, muscle tension decreases. During parasympathetic activity (general relaxation), the body regenerates and restores for future activity.

The autonomic nervous system is controlled by the **hypothalamus,** located in the **diencephalon** area of the brain. The diencephalon is the central portion of the brain and is responsible for regulating emotions, among other things. The hypothalamus plays a key role in the stress response because it is the chief region for integrating sympathetic and parasympathetic activities. When the hypothalamus receives the message of danger from the higher-order thinking part of the brain, it is like an alarm system going off deep in your brain, which delivers a message through the nervous system that connects to every other system of the body.

The hypothalamus also delivers a message to the endocrine system to initiate the secretion of hormones. The stress hormones, including epinephrine and cortisol, flood the bloodstream and travel throughout the body, delivering information to cells and systems that will aid in generating the body's ability to be more speedy and powerful, as demonstrated in Sarah's story in the opening vignette.

These stress hormones are produced by the **adrenal glands,** two triangle-shaped glands positioned on top of the kidneys. **Epinephrine** (adrenaline) and **norepinephrine** (noradrenaline) are released into the bloodstream from the **adrenal medulla. Cortisol,** the other key stress hormone, is released from a portion of the adrenal glands called the **adrenal cortex.** Together, these hormones flood every cell in the body with the specific message to prepare for fight-or-flight—for more power and speed—when we are faced with an imminent threat. The dual response of the nervous and endocrine systems constitute the stress response. In an instant, with the interpretation of a stimulus as potentially threatening, your body leaps into alert mode. This reaction gave early humans the energy to fight aggressors or run from predators. It helped the species survive.

Consider this scenario:

A dry twig in the jungle snaps and our common ancestor—your father, my father, 1,500 generations ago—leaps into alert mode. Adrenaline floods his system, causing lipid cells to squirt fatty acids into his bloodstream for quick energy. His breathing becomes shallow and rapid, and his heart beats faster, increasing the flow of oxygen to his muscles, enhancing his strength and speed. His blood vessels constrict, minimizing bleeding if he's injured, and his body releases natural coagulants and painkillers. His sweat glands open, leaving his skin slippery and hard for a predator to grasp. His hair stands on end, making him appear larger and more threatening. His pupils dilate, increasing his ability to scan dark jungle terrain. All this happens in less than a second, and—zip—Dad's off and running, far enough ahead of the tiger, to ensure that your bloodline, and mine, makes it to the next generation.[2]

All these responses served to prepare the person for emergency action. This response is believed to be an adaptive, evolutionary response that remains with us still today.

Autonomic Nervous System Responses

Figure 3.2 shows the effects of stress on the human body. The immediate physiological changes that result from activating the sympathetic nervous system are:

- Increased central nervous system (CNS) activity
- Increased mental activity
- Increased secretion of adrenaline (epinephrine), noradrenaline (norepinephrine), and cortisol into the bloodstream and to every cell in the body
- Increased heart rate
- Increased cardiac output
- Increased blood pressure
- Increased breathing rate
- Dilation of breathing airways
- Increased metabolism
- Increased oxygen consumption
- Increased oxygen to the brain
- Shunting of blood away from the digestive tract and directing it into the muscles and limbs
- Increased muscle contraction, which leads to increased strength
- Increased blood coagulation (blood-clotting ability)
- Increased circulation of free fatty acids
- Increased output of blood cholesterol
- Increased blood sugar released by the liver to nourish the muscles
- Release of endorphins from the pituitary gland
- Dilation of the pupils of the eyes
- Hair standing on end

Brain becomes more alert.
- Stress hormones can affect memory and cause neurons to atrophy and die.
- Headaches, anxiety, and depression
- Disrupted sleep

Digestive system slows down.
- Mouth ulcers or cold sores

Heart rate increases and blood pressure rises.
- Persistently elevated blood pressure and heart rate can increase potential for blood clotting and risk of stroke or heart attack.
- Weakening of the heart muscle and symptoms that mimic a heart attack

Adrenal glands produce stress hormones.
- Cortisol and other stress hormones can increase central or abdominal fat.
- Cortisol increases glucose production in the liver, causing renal hypertension.

Skin problems such as eczema and psoriasis

■ = Immediate response to stress
■ = Effects of chronic or prolonged stress
■ = Other possible effects of chronic stress

Breathing quickens.
- Increased susceptibility to colds and respiratory infections

Immune system is depressed.
- Increased susceptibility to infection
- Slower healing

Digestive system slows down.
- Upset stomach

Reproductive system.
- Menstrual disorders in women
- Impotence and premature ejaculation in men

Muscles tense.
- Muscular twitches or nervous tics

FIGURE 3.2 Effects of Stress on the Body

Source: "The Effects of Stress on Body," Figure 3.2 in *An Invitation to Health*, 2009–2010 Edition, by Dianne Hales, (Belmont, CA: Wadsworth/Cengage Learning, 2009), p 60. Used by permission.

- Blood thinning
- Increased brainwave activity
- Increased secretion by sweat glands
- Increased secretion from apocrine glands, resulting in foul body odor
- Constriction of capillaries under the surface of the skin (which consequently increases blood pressure)

When the fight-or-flight response is activated, the nervous system processes in the body decrease in the following ways:

- Immune system is suppressed
- Blood vessels are constricted, except the vessels that go to the muscles used for running and fighting
- Reproductive and sexual systems stop working normally
- Digestive system stops metabolizing food normally
- Excretory system turns off
- Saliva dries up
- Pain perception decreases
- Kidney output decreases
- Bowel and bladder sphincter close

To enable us to escape from threatening situations, we do not need this last set of functions and systems to operate at high capacity. Their work, therefore, is suppressed to divert energy to the vital systems involved in increasing speed and power. In contrast to the fight-or-flight response is a principle called the rest-and-digest response. In short, if you are required to run from a mugger, both nap time and lunch—the rest-and-digest response—can wait. The SNS and PNS often operate simultaneously in response to stress. For example, the heart rate increases (SNS) while the digestive system shuts down (PNS).

Understanding the nervous system's response to stress is important in explaining the stress-related diseases and conditions covered in the next chapter.

The Stress Response in Today's World

In a vast majority of cases, today's stressor does not require us to fight or flee. Harvard cardiologist Herbert Benson remarked that "the fight-or-flight emergency response is inappropriate to today's social stresses."[3] Many situations other than imminent physical danger can trigger the stress response. This is because *our bodies are unable to distinguish between life-threatening dangers and more mundane sources of stress, such as a disagreement with a friend, credit card debt, or a major exam.*

Our ancestors survived by running away from or fighting their predators. Few situations in modern life require this response. Today we face traffic jams and deadlines, loneliness and lack of money, arguments and exams—different types of stressors, which do not demand that we run or fight. Most situations today benefit from a calm, rational, controlled, socially sensitive approach. In effect, then, our fight-or-flight response is an outdated mechanism to which our primitive systems have not yet adapted. In the short term, we need to control our stress response to be effective in our daily life. In the long term, we need to keep it under control to avoid the consequences of burnout and poor health. Understanding this dynamic validates the importance of being proactive, rather than just reactive, in coping with the effects of stress.

Acute Stress The way the stress response works in the short run helps us generate great strength, focus more clearly, increase our speed, and perform at a higher level when a threat is present. Occasionally we can use this source of immediate energy to help us when we do find ourselves in actual danger, facing potential pain or even death.

Imagine this scenario that Ashley shared in class.

* * *

My apartment mate, Julie, had left earlier in the day to spend the weekend with her family. After a quiet evening at home, I locked the doors and settled into my cozy bed feeling safe and secure. Sometime during the night I woke suddenly with a strange feeling that something wasn't right. There, standing next to my bed, was a tall, dark figure. My body instantly responded as I jolted from the bed and let out a scream that would wake the dead. I grabbed my telephone from my bedside table and flung it in the direction of the intruder. The shadowy figure turned quickly and dashed out through the open window.

* * *

Ashley's stress response may have saved her life. The threat imposed by this stranger activated her stress response in an automatic and powerful manner. You probably can think of times when your body has responded to a danger in a manner similar to Ashley's response.

Author Anecdote Self-Induced Fight-or-Flight When I was a teenager, I lived in an area of town with nothing but homes and parks for many blocks. One part of this neighborhood had a large hedge about 4 feet high next to a somewhat busy street. During the winter months my friends and I assembled behind this hedge and prepared for oncoming cars. When they came close to our location, we unloaded a barrage of snowballs on the unsuspecting cars. (This was how we kept our arms in shape for baseball season during the off-season!) The person who was awarded the highest honors was the one who could make the best "dent" sounds in the car or truck that was passing by. Even more exciting than the dent sound was the rare occasion when the car or truck would stop and the driver of the car would jump out and start chasing after us.

Of course, nobody knew our neighborhood like we did, so the possibility of our getting caught by even the swiftest of pursuers was remote. But what we did notice, as we were being chased through our neighborhood, down the streets, and across the parks, was that in those times of pursuit, we suddenly were gifted with incredible speed and power. We were able to jump over high fences with ease, and run down streets and through parks with the velocity of Olympians. We even noticed that during those times, our ability to see where we needed to go to make it to safety (this activity always took place after the sun had set and darkness prevailed) improved dramatically. I am not proud of those days and find myself irritated at teens who do the same thing to my car nowadays, but I learned some powerful lessons about the fight-or-flight response in those early years.

—MO

The irony is this: Our bodies react to stress in exactly the same way whether or not we have a good reason for being stressed. The body doesn't care if we're right or wrong. Even in those times when we feel perfectly justified in getting angry—when we tell ourselves it's the healthy response—we pay for it just the same.

—Doc Childre

Pressure and stress
is the common cold
of the psyche.
—*Andrew Denton*

Here is a sampling of circumstances of acute stress in which the demand, danger, or threat is immediate and very real:

- Being chased by an angry dog
- A blown tire on the highway
- A trip and fall down a steep hiking trail
- An earthquake
- A lightning strike

You get the point. Occasionally we experience acute stress. Activation of the stress response at these times is beneficial and may even save your life. In reality, however, these types of experiences are rare in the typical daily life. Unless you work in a high-risk occupation such as police officer, soldier in combat, firefighter, or whitewater rafting guide, your days will not likely entail threats to your life.

Contrary to how our world may appear from watching the evening news, our society today is not largely one in which *real* acute threats or dangers are a daily occurrence. An upcoming exam or being late to work may make us feel like we are in danger, but in reality we don't need our primitive survival forces of fight-or-flight to manage these situations. The concept of perceptions will be explained more fully in Chapter 5.

Chronic Stress If the stress response is allowed to stay in the "on" position longer than necessary to escape danger, the result can be damaging to health. If stressful situations pile up one after another, the body has no chance to recover. "Chronic stress" is the term we use to describe this state of continued sympathetic nervous system activation. Instead of returning to homeostasis, the fight-or-flight response is activated for an extended time. This long-term activation of the stress-response system can disrupt nearly all body processes. Figure 3.3 illustrates chronic stress.

Our body is a wise instrument. It is designed to give us feedback about the choices we make. Consider the person who deliberately gets drunk during an evening of partying. When he wakes up in the morning hung over from the excessive alcohol, his body sends messages of discomfort, including headache, nausea, unclear thinking, and muscle pain. This feedback provides a clue that drinking was not a healthy decision. Or when someone eats too much sugar at one time, she may experience feelings of nausea, tiredness, and irritability. By contrast, a jog or walk can result in your feeling balanced, alert, refreshed, and energized. The body is sending messages that running was a healthy decision. The body lets us know what is good and what is bad for us—what is healthy and what isn't.

Our body gives us feedback about unhealthy chronic stress with a host of signals indicating imbalance. Some of those signals, if not heeded, can damage parts of our system. Although stress is not listed among the top 10 causes of death in the United States, it is linked to many illnesses. This does not necessarily mean that stress *causes* the problem, but it does mean that stress contributes to the problem. Additional problems associated with chronic activation of the stress response will be explored in Chapter 4.

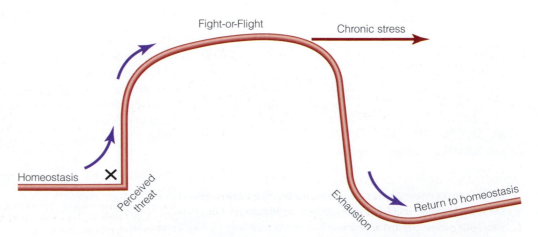

Fight-or-Flight

Chronic stress

Homeostasis

Perceived threat

Exhaustion

Return to homeostasis

FIGURE 3.3 Chronic Stress

The General Adaptation Syndrome

One of the best known biological theories of stress is the **general adaptation syndrome** (GAS), a process by which the body tries to adapt to stress. The general adaptation syndrome provides a summary of the physiological changes that follow stress as the body attempts to return to homeostasis.

History of the General Adaptation Syndrome
Stress pioneer Dr. Hans Selye developed the GAS theory as a result of his research on the physiological effects of chronic stress on rats. Whenever he injected an animal with a toxin, he observed some specific responses:[4]

- The animal's adrenal glands enlarged.
- The animal's lymph nodes shrank.
- Eosinophils (white blood cells) dropped significantly.
- Severe bleeding ulcers developed in the animal's stomach and intestine.

Ten years earlier, as a medical student, he had noticed similar responses in people. Selye theorized that the same pattern of changes occurs in the body in reaction to any kind of stress and that the pattern is what eventually leads to disease conditions, such as ulcers, arthritis, hypertension, arteriosclerosis, or diabetes. Selye called the pattern the general adaptation syndrome. For decades, researchers have studied the syndrome, and Selye's theories have held up to scientific scrutiny.[5] Figure 3.4 depicts the stages of the general adaptation syndrome.

Stages of the General Adaptation Syndrome
Dr. Selye identified three stages of the general adaptation syndrome:

1. *Alarm stage.* When a stressor occurs, the body responds in what has been described previously as the fight-or-flight response. Homeostasis has been disrupted. Several body systems are activated, especially the nervous and endocrine systems, to prepare the body for action. If the stressor subsides, the body returns to homeostasis.
2. *Stage of resistance.* If the stressor continues, the body mobilizes its internal resources in an effort to return to a state of homeostasis, but because the perception of a threat still exists, the body does not achieve complete homeostasis. The stress response stays activated, usually at less intensity than during the alarm stage, but still at a level to cause hyperarousal. For example, if you learn that your mother has been diagnosed with cancer, you may respond intensely and feel great stress at first. During the subsequent weeks, you struggle to carry on, but this requires considerable effort.
3. *Stage of exhaustion.* If the stress continues long enough, the body can no longer function normally. When chronic stress persists, organ systems may fail and the body breaks down in a variety of ways. Continuous stress that causes the body to adapt constantly can become a threat to health. A state of wellness is difficult to maintain over time when our body energy is channeled into coping with stress.

Application of the General Adaptation Syndrome
In their book, *Lifetime Physical Fitness and Wellness,* Werner and Sharon Hoeger provide this excellent application of the GAS to college test performance.

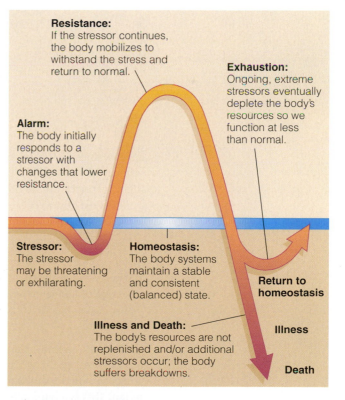

Resistance:
If the stressor continues, the body mobilizes to withstand the stress and return to normal.

Exhaustion:
Ongoing, extreme stressors eventually deplete the body's resources so we function at less than normal.

Alarm:
The body initially responds to a stressor with changes that lower resistance.

Stressor:
The stressor may be threatening or exhilarating.

Homeostasis:
The body systems maintain a stable and consistent (balanced) state.

Return to homeostasis

Illness and Death:
The body's resources are not replenished and/or additional stressors occur; the body suffers breakdowns.

Illness

Death

FIGURE 3.4 The Three Stages of Selye's General Adaptation Syndrome

Source: "General Adaptation Syndrome," Figure 3.1 in *An Invitation to Health*, 2009–2010 Edition, by Dianne Hales (Belmont, CA: Wadsworth/Cengage Learning, 2009), p. 59. Used by permission.

As you prepare to take an exam, you experience an initial alarm reaction. If you understand the material, study for the exam, and do well (eustress), the body recovers and stress is dissipated. If, however, you are not adequately prepared and fail the exam, you trigger the resistance stage. You are now concerned about your grade, and you remain in the resistance stage until the next exam. If you prepare and do well, the body recovers. But if you fail once again and can no longer bring up the grade, exhaustion sets in and physical and emotional breakdowns may occur. Exhaustion may be further aggravated if you are struggling in other courses as well.[6] Stressors, whether they are threatening or exhilarating, require adaptation. If you watch closely for manifestations of the exhaustion stage, you can take action to return to a state of homeostasis.

Stress Busting Behavior: Fighting Stress Exhaustion

Check those that apply to you.

☐ You recognize the symptoms of the fight-or-flight response.

☐ You are aware of how often this response is triggered in you.

☐ You are aware that if the stress continues long enough, or the stress is habitual, you will reach the stage of exhaustion.

☐ If you experience the stage of exhaustion, you take action and reprioritize:

   • Are you doing too much?

   Yes ☐   No ☐

   • Are all the things you "need to do" REALLY necessary?

   Yes ☐   No ☐

   • Can you cut back on your commitments?

   Yes ☐   No ☐

   • Can you put your health first, and plan a schedule that is lower in stress?

   Yes ☐   No ☐

The Stress Response and You

So how does all this relate to you? You may have never been chased by a big bear, or any other wild animal for that matter. Still, tuning in to your body's response to the fight-or-flight response and to the three stages of the general adaptation syndrome can help you understand how to prevent the ill-effects of chronic stress.

Physician Dan Beskind wrote:

> There is no doubt that the human body is exquisitely adapted to deal with stress in brief doses. Our fight-or-flight response is one example of the way that short bursts of heightened energy and vigilance can actually save our lives. But we aren't well adapted to deal with surges of adrenaline and cortisol day after day. In evolutionary terms, traffic jams, two-career marriages, and kids involved in six after-school activities were not part of the plan.[7]

The bottom line is that we need to take responsibility to slow down and carefully assess our choices for living wisely. Many of us feel completely stressed out much of the time. The common denominator is that we often feel overloaded. Many of us are trying to do too much. This is a hard habit to break because our culture views multitasking as the normal way of getting things done. If we are not juggling a dozen different commitments at once, we tend to think something is wrong with us or we are lazy.

Ask yourself these important questions: Have you created a culture of busyness that keeps your stress response unnecessarily activated? If so, what can you do about it? This book will guide you in answering these questions.

The Culture of Busyness

One of the major goals of this book is to help you reduce stress in your life. You would assume that everyone would have the same desire to have less stress, but it's not necessarily so! In certain modern subcultures, it's not unusual to hear a conversation like the following:

"I am sooo busy. I haven't had time to get my hair cut, water the plants, or walk the dog for the past three weeks."

"Oh, I can top that! I spend all day driving the kids to school and activities, running errands, and getting the house remodel going, so I have to do my work at night. Usually I get only four hours of sleep a night. I sure never have time to be bored!"

Are these two people actually competing to be the most stressed-out person in their circle of acquaintances? It sounds that way. Why would anyone want to be "the winner" in an event that the rest of us are trying to avoid altogether?

This phenomenon seems to appear in fairly well-to-do areas where people spend a lot of time in competitive environments. In the San Francisco Bay Area culture of the mid-2000s, people routinely compete with each other to purchase homes in one of the costliest housing markets in the country. They compete for employment in a job market that has been shrinking since the dot-com bust of the late 1990s. Their kids have to interview to enroll in kindergarten at private schools, competing for a limited number of openings. Competition is almost as routine as breathing.

This also seems to be a result of wanting to have it all. While salaries in the Bay Area are high in comparison to the rest of the country, the cost of living is even higher.

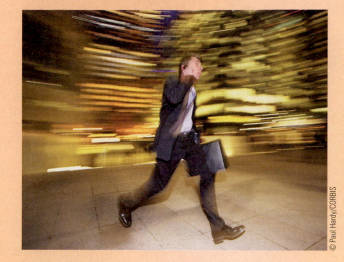

Have we created a culture of busyness?

© Paul Hardy/CORBIS

Even in families with considerable incomes, both parents in most families work so they can afford the SUVs, private schools, and luxury vacations that most of their friends have.

In some cases, players in the "stress competition" are bluffing and simply going along with the one-upmanship game so they don't feel left out. But other players appear genuinely harassed. They clearly haven't had a haircut in weeks and look as if they are suffering from lack of sleep. Money doesn't seem to be buying happiness. Maybe they could put aside some time and some of that money for a trip to a spa, at least!

Source: Personal communication, Anne Scanlan-Rohrer, March 3, 2005.

Conclusion

Your body is designed to respond to acute stress in a predictable manner for one outcome—your survival. This response, the fight-or-flight or stress response, is critical for your ability to survive life-threatening situations throughout your life. Through the actions of the autonomic nervous system, your body is programmed for a response that will protect you from harm.

In today's world, many of our challenges are not acute, physical challenges. Today our stressors are primarily psychological and social, such as having too much to do, financial debt, concern for a loved one, loneliness, or unhealthy relationships. The physiological response is not well suited to deal with these types of stressors. When our bodies stay in a state of physiological hyperarousal without release, negative health consequences accumulate.

Take a few minutes to think about the relationship between the concepts presented in this chapter. Consider the relationship between the fight-or-flight response, acute and chronic stress, and the general adaptation syndrome. Connecting these concepts to events in your life will help you see the relevance of the science of stress to your understanding of how stress affects you. This knowledge also will give you a foundation for understanding how relaxation techniques have the potential to intercept the stress response. In Chapter 4 you will learn more about the powerful mind/body connection and its impact on health and disease.

3.1 Fight-or-Flight

ACTIVITY

1. Review the immediate physiological effects of the fight-or-flight response. Think about how each of the responses is designed to help a person survive physical danger. List one reason why each of the following immediate physiological responses would happen when we need to deal with a real threat:
   - Increase in heart rate
   - Increase in breathing rate
   - Large (fighting and running) muscles become tense
   - Increased tolerance for pain
   - Increase in blood sugar levels
   - Suppressed immune system
   - Digestive system stops metabolizing food normally

2. Clearly, the stress response becomes your best friend when you find yourself in a dangerous situation. The immediate speed, power, and quickness that come from fight-or-flight activation can save your life. Write down a situation you, or someone you know, found yourself in where you had no other desire than to stay alive by escaping.

3. Describe how your body reacted in ways that are similar to those described in this chapter with your immediate activation of the stress response.

4. Consider the following situations that people commonly perceive to be stressful. Take a moment to evaluate whether or not the event is one that warrants activation of the stress response in order to escape from it to stay alive. First, list the situations in which there is no real physical threat involved. Next, list the potentially life-threatening situations.

   - Taking a test
   - Having an argument
   - Escaping from a house fire
   - Arriving late for a class
   - Being chased by a mugger
   - Giving a prepared speech to a crowded room of people
   - Sliding down a steep mountainside while hiking
   - Being rejected when asking someone out on a date
   - Getting a bad score on a test
   - Getting ready for a very important ball game

5. How do you explain the fact that you feel stressed in situations where there is no real danger involved? What can you tell yourself in these situations in order to put the stressful event in perspective and keep your stress response in proportion to the actual risk?

Key Points

- The fight-or-flight response is the body's way of helping us survive.
- The fight-or-flight response involves a complex interaction of many body systems and organs. This response activates needed functions and minimizes unnecessary functions during times of stress.
- The autonomic nervous system (ANS) is responsible for a large number of commonly occurring functions in the body that occur involuntarily, such as digestion, heart rate, blood pressure, and body temperature.
- The two branches of the ANS are the sympathetic nervous system and the parasympathetic nervous system. The sympathetic branch is responsible for expending energy. The parasympathetic branch is responsible for conserving energy.

- The autonomic nervous system is controlled by the hypothalamus.
- Although the fight-or-flight response is essential to our survival during times of acute physical stress, this response can have unhealthy consequences during times of ongoing social or psychological stress.

- The general adaptation syndrome describes a process in which the body tries to accommodate stress by adapting. This process consists of three stages: alarm, resistance, and exhaustion.

Key Terms

fight-or-flight response
homeostasis
tend-and-befriend response
autonomic nervous system
sympathetic nervous system

parasympathetic nervous system
hypothalamus
diencephalon
adrenal glands
epinephrine

norepinephrine
adrenal medulla
cortisol
adrenal cortex
general adaptation syndrome

Discussion Time For Critical Thinking/Discussion Questions, please visit this book's Premium Website.

Notes

1. *The Stress Effect*, by R. Weinstein (New York: Avery, 2004).
2. "What Doesn't Make Us Stronger Kills Us," by S. Perrine, *Men's Health,* July/August 2004.
3. *Mind/Body Health: The Effects of Attitudes, Emotions, and Relationships* (3rd ed.), by K. Karren, B. Hafen, N. Smith, & K. Frandsen (San Francisco: Benjamin Cummings, 2006).
4. *Breaking the Stress Habit*, by A. Goliszek (Winston-Salem, NC: Carolina Press, 1987).
5. *Mind/Body Health: The Effects of Attitudes, Emotions, and Relationships* (3rd ed.), by K. Karren, B. Hafen, N. Smith, & K. Frandsen (San Francisco: Benjamin Cummings, 2006).
6. *Lifetime Physical Fitness and Wellness* (10th ed.), by W. Hoeger and S. Hoeger (Belmont, CA: Wadsworth/Cengage Learning, 2009).
7. "Juggler's Syndrome," by D. Beskind, *Utne Reader, 122*, March/April 2004, p. 16.

4 The Mind/Body Connection

■ How do my thoughts and feelings change my physical condition? For instance, can stress really change my cells? ■ Why do I get sick after I go through a stressful time? ■ What is the placebo effect and does it really work?

STUDENT OBJECTIVES

Study of this chapter will enable you to:

1. Describe the role of stress in disease.
2. Discuss how stress can affect body systems including the cardiovascular, nervous, digestive, and immune systems.
3. Explain the concept of psychoneuroimmunology.
4. Explain the placebo effect as an example of the power of the mind over the body.

It is more important to know what sort of a person has a disease than to know what sort of disease a person has.

—*Hippocrates*

© Mick Powell/CORBIS

Physician and Scientist For so many thousands of years, the popular culture believed that stress could make you sick, and that believing could make you well. People believe what they feel, but scientists need evidence. Until recently, however, there really wasn't any good, solid scientific evidence to prove these connections, nor was there a good way to measure them, and scientists believe only what they can actually measure. Once scientists and physicians believed that there was a connection between the brain and the immune system, they could then take it to the next step: that maybe there is a connection between emotions and disease; between negative emotions and disease, and between positive emotions and health.

We can then say, okay, maybe these alternative approaches that have been used for thousands of years—approaches like meditation, prayer, music, sleep, dreams—all of these approaches that we know in our heart of hearts really work to maintain health.... Maybe there is a scientific basis for them.

Excerpted from the Website www.nlm.nih.gov, National Institutes of Health video, *Celebrating American Women Physicians*.

The Mind/Body Connection

More than 300 years after he made his observation about happiness. John Locke's insight into health and happiness still has relevance. Even though we may have widely differing experiences with stress, one thing is certain: What is going on with your mind and emotions is at least as important, if not more so, than what is happening in your body. Actually, what is going on in your mind *determines* what is happening in your body.

When you look in the mirror, what do you see? You see your body, your hair, your skin, your muscles, your face. We can see and understand how the body works. We can measure blood pressure and hormones and heart rate and body fat, but what about your mind? Can we measure an emotion? Can we see a thought? Can we prove that outlook changes the level of stress? For decades scientists have studied how stress affects the body. As you learned in previous chapters, the body of knowledge explaining the physiology of stress is substantial. More recently, researchers have been studying the mind/body connection to understand how thoughts and emotions relate to our experience with stress.

A sound mind in a
sound body is a short
but full description
of a happy state
in this world.

—*John Locke,
philosopher, 1693*

Psychological Health

Psychological health, which encompasses both our emotional and mental health, is instrumental in determining physical health. In Chapter 1 you learned, from the definitions of the dimensions of health, that emotional health relates to feelings and the ability to achieve emotional balance while mental health relates to a state in which the mind is engaged in lively, healthy interactions both internally and with the world around you. Psychologically healthy people develop awareness and control of their thoughts and feelings. The outcome is a healthy and satisfying quality of life.

Today we know beyond question that the mind and emotions have a powerful and very real impact on the body. James Gordon, M.D., Director of the Center for Mind–Body Studies in Washington, DC, says:

> The mind clearly can have a profound effect on every aspect of physiologic functioning....
> Individuals who are chronically pessimistic, angry, anxious, or depressed are clearly more susceptible to stress and illness, including heart disease and cancer.[1]

Similarly, almost every medical illness affects people psychologically as well as physically.

Clearly, stress affects your body, your physiology. In Chapter 3 you learned about how the stress response activates a specific physiological process in your body. But what part does your mind play in your experience with stress? *A complex physiological process, the stress response, always starts with a single thought.* Your thoughts, your feelings, and your emotions have a profound impact on the quality of your life.

There is nothing
either good or
bad, but thinking
makes it so.

—*Shakespeare*

Psychological Health

43

In this chapter we will explore the fascinating relationship between the mind and the body to better understand the role of stress in both disease and health. You will read about scientific studies that provide a solid foundation of scientific evidence explaining the connection between the body and the mind. You will see how you can use this information to go beyond preventing disease to also promote optimal health.

The Role of Chronic Stress in Disease

Stress is an everyday fact of life for most people. It is becoming common knowledge, however, that stress at too-high "doses," and/or for too-long periods of time, can cause health problems. Hundreds of studies over the last 30 years have shown that stress contributes to a significant percentage of all major illness, including the number-one cause of death in America, cardiovascular disease. Cancer, endocrine disease, emotional disorders, and a vast array of other stress-related disorders account for many visits each year to healthcare providers.

Healthy People 2010, the document containing the health promotion goals for our nation, reports the continuing trend that health problems related to stress are among the most pressing concerns in public health. Five of the ten Leading Health Indicators (high-priority public issues) identified by the Office of Disease Prevention and Health Promotion are significantly interrelated with stress. These include mental health, obesity, smoking, physical activity, and substance abuse.

Direct and Indirect Effects of Chronic Stress   Evidence supports the premise that stress can affect health either directly by way of physiological changes in the body, or indirectly through a change in a person's behavior. The clearest connection between stress and disease is demonstrated by the release of hormones by the endocrine system during the alarm reaction stage of the general adaptation syndrome. The cardiovascular, immune, and other systems of the body are affected.[2] In Chapter 3 you learned that chronic stress could result in exhaustion, the final stage of the general adaptation syndrome. If the fight-or-flight response remains activated for an extended time, we start to experience physical and emotional effects.

The indirect effects of stress on health occur when those who experience high levels of stress respond with unhealthy behaviors. For example, it has been shown that individuals under stress in general consume more alcohol, smoke more cigarettes, and drink more coffee than those who are under less stress. Use of these substances has been associated with higher risks for heart disease and cancer, as well as trauma and death from unintentional injuries.[3] In Chapter 15 you will learn more about how lifestyle habits and daily choices affect stress.

Chronic stress can be the result of many repeated rounds of acute stress, such as several semesters with an especially heavy load (episodic acute stress), or a life condition, such as a difficult job situation or chronic disease. In either case, the stress response remains activated as if we are responding to physical danger. The thought of threat, on a continual basis, sends the message to body systems that the survival mechanisms of fight-or-flight have to be activated continually. As a result, the normally functioning systems of the body cease to function well.

What feedback might your mind and body give you that indicates continued activation of the stress response? Awareness of both the medium-term and long-term effects of chronic stress can help you understand why preventing and managing stress is essential to good health.

We are what we think. All that we are arises with our thoughts. With our thoughts we make the world.

—*Buddha*

Medium-Term Chronic Stress

When we recognize what is happening during the stress response, we can understand why medium-term health effects of stress happen. Many functions in the body turn off because they are not needed to deal with danger. Other functions in the body are activated to higher than normal levels. When we are not in danger, however, continued activation of the stress response is not necessary. You only need to *think* you are in danger for the stress response to activate.

Effects of Medium-Term Chronic Stress
Effects of medium-term chronic stress include, among others, muscle tension, headaches, fatigue, upset stomach, difficulty sleeping, bruxism, sore throat, and colds. Each of these conditions is briefly explained in relation to stress.

Muscle Tension and Pain
Do you ever feel like your muscles are so tight that your shoulders are pulled up around your ears? Do tight neck muscles cause you stiffness and pain? Normally, a muscle is not in the contracted state for a prolonged time. A muscle is supposed to contract only when it receives a message to contract. When a muscle is told to continue contracting for a prolonged time, two obvious results are pain and fatigue. When a muscle stays contracted, it activates nervous system pain receptors that deliver the message of pain.

Headaches
A headache may result from muscles that tighten longer than intended in response to a threat. If the contracting muscles are "head muscles," or posterior neck muscles, the result is a headache. This explains why people take muscle relaxants to ease the pain of the headache. A headache can provide feedback that our thoughts are causing tension.

Fatigue
Another effect of continued muscle contraction is fatigue. Have you ever come home from a rough day at work or school totally exhausted, even though you have exerted little physical effort? When a muscle is continually receiving the message to be ready for action, fatigue will result. Considerable energy is required for muscles to remain contracted.

Upset Stomach
In fight-or-flight situations, we do not need the digestive system, so it ceases to efficiently coordinate all of the processes necessary to break down food. When the stress response is activated continually, the digestive system won't transport food from the digestive system to the bloodstream as effectively. An upset stomach is the result.

Difficulty Sleeping
We should not require more than a few minutes to start sleep. We also should sleep comfortably through the entire night without waking up several times. Sleeping should come naturally. If we are having a hard time falling asleep, it may be because our minds are thinking too much about things not associated with sleeping. Troublesome thoughts of today's activities or worrisome thoughts of tomorrow's send messages to the mind that resemble threats. Consequently, the body remains aroused and alert. One physiological response of fight-or-flight is altered brainwave activity. Sleep-inducing brainwave activity can happen only when we are able to turn off the stress response. Stress can hurt you doubly because it affects the ability to sleep, which in turn affects the ability to cope with stress and anxiety.

Bruxism
Bruxism is the term for grinding, gnashing, or clenching the teeth during sleep or during situations that make the person feel anxious or tense. This condition is the third most common form of sleep disorder. Getting an estimate of how many people suffer from bruxism is difficult because it relies primarily on self-reporting. Most estimates indicate that bruxism affects about 10% to 20% of the population. Although physiological conditions can cause bruxism, more often the causes are psychological, including anxiety, stress or tension, suppressed anger or frustration, or aggressive, competitive, or hyperactive personality characteristics.[4]

If you grind your teeth because of stress, you may be able to prevent it through strategies that promote relaxation, such as exercise and meditation. Cutting down on consumption of alcohol, tobacco, and caffeine also may help, as the condition seems to worsen with the use of these substances.

Cold or Sore Throat
We do not need the immune system for fight-or-flight situations, so it turns down its high-functioning protection. The immune system is our internal defense mechanism that keeps us from contracting a cold or the latest flu that is going around. Without a strong immune system, the virus can get the upper hand. We will discuss the role of stress on the immune system in more depth when we look at long-term effects of stress.

The Cold, Hard Facts

The common cold is not an equal-opportunity attacker, according to research from psychologist Sheldon Cohen. Why do some people seem to rarely catch a cold in spite of being exposed to hoards of sneezing, sniffling cold-sufferers, while others seem to catch every bug that comes along? A growing body of evidence suggests that factors such as personality, stress, and social life can all affect our vulnerability to the common cold.

Cohen's research involved exposing volunteers to colds by dropping rhinoviruses into the nose. The subjects then were quarantined and monitored for the development of infection and cold symptoms. After 5 days of quarantine, medical exams and questionnaires revealed the following:

- Happy, relaxed people are more resistant to illness than those who tend to be unhappy or tense. Adults with the worst scores for calmness and positive mood are about three times more likely to get colds than the more relaxed and contented adults. When happy people do get sick, their symptoms are milder.
- Serious work-related or personal stress that lasts at least a month increases the chances of catching a cold. In the lab, the longer that people lived with bad stress, the more likely they were to catch a cold.
- The rates of respiratory infection and clinical colds increased in a dose-response manner (as stress levels increased, so did the number of colds) with the extent of psychological stress the person had experienced in the previous year.

From this research, we apparently can add "fewer colds" to the list of the benefits of stress management.

Source: "Psychological Stress and Susceptibility to the Common Cold," by S. Cohen, D. Tyrrell, and A. Smith, in *New England Journal of Medicine, 325* (1991), 606–612.

Additional symptoms associated with medium-term effects of chronic stress include unpleasant conditions such as the following:

Upset stomach, problems retaining food	Rashes, hives, skin irritation
Change in appetite	Increased blood pressure
Tightness in chest, back, shoulders	Excessive sweating
Aching jaw, tight forehead	Menstrual problems, missed menstrual periods
Shortness of breath, dizziness	
Sweaty palms	Feelings of anxiety
Tingling sensation in fingers or toes	Anger
Nervous tension all over	Concentration problems
Heart palpitations	Depression
Diarrhea or constipation	Lack of interest in food
Constant low grade fever	Any number of other symptoms

Role of the Immune System

Have you ever noticed that you tend to get sick more frequently after you go through a stressful experience? Because the immune system is unable to work as effectively when you are stressed, you are more susceptible to the diseases and illnesses that cross your path. In a 3-month study of daily moods and illness, adults had more antibodies to counteract infection on days with positive events. The worse the day, the fewer the antibodies, according to psychologist Arthur Stone. In Stone's studies, adults got sick three to five days after their roughest days.[5]

Animal research may explain why people often get through acute stress but fall ill afterward, says Esther Sternberg from the National Institute of Mental Health. Stress unleashes adrenaline-like hormones first, and these stimulate the immune system. Then the body releases cortisol, a hormone that battles inflammation but weakens immunity. Sternberg explains:

> For a while, both hormones are going full steam ahead. When the stress ends, the adrenaline hormones shut down first, leaving hormones that suppress immunity to hang around alone, and in these few days illness may take hold.[6]

Cortisol in particular lingers in the body and weakens the body's immune response. This helps explain why people frequently get sick following a stressful event.

In short, the medium-term symptoms of chronic stress result when the stress response causes imbalances throughout normally functioning body systems. These symptoms signal to us that we should make some changes. We should keep in mind that whatever system turns on or off is a direct response to what we would need for flight-or-fight. When this goes on for an extended period, health suffers.

Long-Term Chronic Stress

While the medium-term effects of chronic stress are unpleasant and annoying, the long-term effects are dangerous and contribute to disease, suffering, and even death.

Stress and the Heart Cardiovascular disease is the number-one cause of death in the United States. One of the most devastating results of long-term chronic stress may turn out to be its link to cardiovascular disease. What is the relationship between cardiovascular disease and stress?

Increasingly, evidence suggests a relationship between the risk of cardiovascular disease and environmental and psychosocial factors. These factors include job strain, social isolation, and personality traits. More research is needed to fully understand how stress

FYI

The Price of Chronic Stress
A dramatic change in the health of the American population in the last decade has been the sharp decline in the health of African Americans. Possibly the most disadvantaged person in the nation in terms of health is the African American male, whose life expectancy is steadily decreasing.* The exact causes of the worsening health of African Americans have not been identified conclusively, but strong evidence suggests that they are at greater risk because of higher rates of smoking, high blood pressure, high cholesterol levels, alcohol and other drug intake, excess weight, and diabetes—health problems often associated with lower income and stressful life circumstances.**

Medical Sociology (5th ed.), by W. Cockerham (Englewood Cliffs, NJ: Prentice Hall, 1992).
**Health Assessment and Promotion Strategies Through the Life Span* (6th ed.), by R. Murray, and J. Zentner (Stamford, CT: Appleton & Lange, 1997).

contributes to the risk for heart disease and whether stress acts as an independent risk factor for cardiovascular disease. Acute and chronic stress may affect other risk factors and behaviors, such as high blood pressure and cholesterol levels, smoking, physical inactivity, and overeating.[7]

While the research continues, researchers have made some significant advances in understanding the association between stress and cardiovascular disease. Here are some of the findings:

- Mental stress increases oxygen demand because blood pressure and heart rate are elevated.
- Vascular resistance and coronary artery constriction during mental stress decrease the blood supply, resulting in decreased blood flow to the heart muscle.
- As a result of stress, blood tends to clot more easily. Your body is designed so you won't bleed to death, but increased blood clotting in the blood vessels that surround the heart or blood vessels in the brain can increase the chances that one of those clots may lodge itself on the wall of a blood vessel. If a clot is too big and the diameter of the blood vessel is too small, and if we add to that an increase in blood pressure, which weakens the blood vessels, the result may be a heart attack or a stroke.
- Chronically high levels of cortisol may affect cardiac health by promoting inflammation that causes heart attacks.

Stress and the Immune System
Stress has a profound impact on the immune system—the network of organs, tissues, and white blood cells responsible for defending the body against disease. The immune system includes lymphocytes, monocytes, and chemical messengers called **interleukins,** which allow the lymphocytes to communicate with each other. Stress causes cortisol to slow production of lymphocytes, as well as to suppress the release of interleukin. Stress hormones inhibit the immune system, making the body less capable of fighting disease and infection.

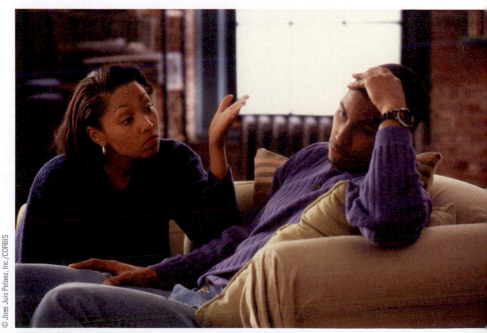

© Jose Luis Pelaez, Inc./CORBIS

African American men are among the populations at higher risk for the negative effects of stress.

Surprise Attack

Myocardial stunning refers to a unique medical condition in which severe emotional stress causes heart abnormalities, including heart failure. A small, descriptive study was conducted to identify possible causes for myocardial stunning. The subjects were previously healthy patients presenting to a medical center with chest pain or heart failure following an episode of acute emotional stress. The most common emotional stressor that initiated cardiac stunning was the news of an unexpected death, although some subjects had experienced the condition following an event such as a surprise party or a surprise reunion.

Authors of the study propose as possible causes for the myocardial stunning:

- Coronary artery spasm from increased sympathetic tone due to mental stress
- Microvascular spasm within the heart in response to a sudden release of stress hormones.

This study provides objective measures that emotional stress can injure the heart. Studies such as these can help us understand the powerful effect of stress on the body. You might want to think twice before you plan the surprise 90th birthday party for Grandpa Joe!

Source: "Emotional Stress May Precipitate Severe, Reversible Left Ventricular Dysfunction," by L. Barclay and C. Vega, in *Medscape Medical News*, February 9, 2005; retrieved from http://www.medscape.com.

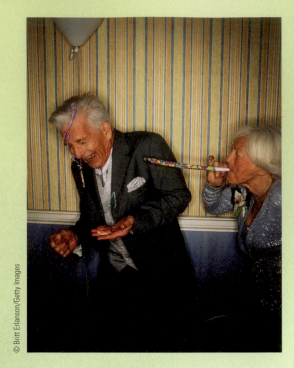

© Britt Erlanson/Getty Images

Surprise! You might think twice about surprising Grandpa Joe. Sudden emotional stress can damage the heart.

Stress Busting Behavior: Stress and Your Health

When you are under stress, your immune system is weaker than usual. Do you do the following to avoid getting sick in times of stress? Circle the item that is your "weakest link" in times of stress.

- ☐ Avoid increased use of alcohol or cigarettes
- ☐ Avoid increased use of caffeine
- ☐ Avoid increased use of sugar
- ☐ Eat balanced meals
- ☐ Get regular physical activity
- ☐ Get a good night's sleep
- ☐ Use meditation, prayer, and other stress-reducing activities
- ☐ Try to maintain a calm and positive attitude

Simply stated, stress hinders the immune system's ability to produce and maintain **lymphocytes** (the white blood cells necessary for killing infection) and **natural killer cells** (the specialized cells that seek out and destroy foreign invaders), both of which are crucial in the fight against disease and infection.[8] Impaired immunity makes the body more susceptible to many diseases, including infections and disorders of the immune system itself, such as the autoimmune disease rheumatoid arthritis.

Stress and Aging

If you have looked at "before" and "after" photos of U.S. presidents, you won't be surprised that research supports the premise that prolonged stress can age people prematurely. Some emerging research suggests that over-the-top stress actually can injure cells of the body.

In a study published in the *Proceedings of the National Academy of Sciences*, the research team found that chronic stress seems to accelerate the aging process by shortening the life

RESEARCH HIGHLIGHT

Chronic Stress and Immunity

Researchers at Ohio State University in Columbus have discovered a link between chronic stress and a body chemical associated with the development of serious and even deadly conditions. Dr. Janice Kiecolt-Glaser, a professor of psychology and psychiatry, and colleagues studied a group of 119 men and women who were dealing with the stress of caring for a spouse with dementia. These caregivers were compared with a control group of 106 individuals of similar age and health status who did not serve as caregivers. Over the 6-year study, blood tests showed that a chemical known as interleukin-6 (IL-6) dramatically increased in the caregivers as compared to the noncaregivers.

IL-6 is a chemical known as a cytokine that is involved in the body's immune system. Overproduction of IL-6 has been associated with the development or progression of a number of medical conditions, including heart disease, type 2 diabetes, certain types of cancer, osteoporosis, arthritis, and functional decline. Even if the spouse of the caregivers died, the increased levels of IL-6 persisted for several years in the group of caregiving spouses.

This research offers one possible explanation for the link between stress and illness by suggesting that stress may increase the risk of many typical age-associated diseases by altering the immune response. These data underscore the need for stress management and control of chronic stressors.

Source: *Chronic Stress and Age-related Increases in the Proinflammatory Cytokine IL-6*, by J. Kiecolt-Glaser, K. Preacher, R. MacCallum, C. Atkinson, W. Malarkey, and R. Glaser, Proceedings of National Academy of Sciences (USA), July 2, 2003.

span of cells, opening the door to disease. The cells of people under high stress aged the equivalent of 9 to 17 years more than the cells of people under little stress. The study involved mothers caring for chronically ill children and, as a control, mothers with healthy children. The longer a mother had been caring for an ill child, the higher was her stress level and the more severe her cellular decline.

Even in the control group, women who simply *thought* they were stressed also showed significant cellular deterioration. "It's not just that you're a caregiver," says Elissa Epel, one of the psychologists who co-authored the study. "It may be more or equally important how you view your life and cope with demands, and what kind of support you have."[9] Caregivers who viewed their situation positively didn't seem to suffer the ill effects of stress. Epel concluded that a positive outlook on life and the support of friends might help buffer a damaging stress response.

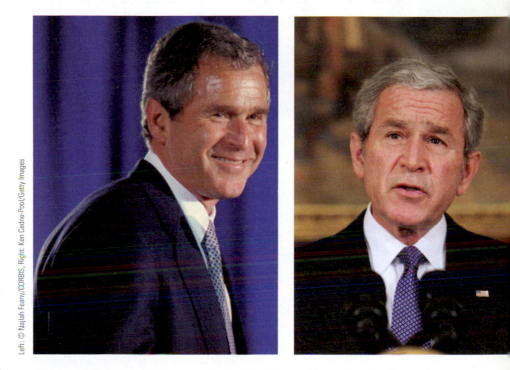

Left: © Najlah Feanny/CORBIS, Right: Ken Cedno-Pool/Getty Images

Stress contributes to premature aging. Look at the pictures of former President Bush at the beginning and the end of his presidency and see if you agree.

The link between stress and premature aging has major implications for health. The specific cellular changes identified in this study could become a warning sign to help doctors prescribe life-extending therapies. That means that people at risk for high stress could slow cell aging through exercise, meditation, prayer, or other forms of stress reduction.[10] We have long known that a common factor among people who live to be at least 100 years old is that they handle stress well.

Other Disease Conditions of Stress Long-term chronic stress adversely affects health beyond increasing the risk for cardiovascular disease and compromising the immune system. Studies suggest that high levels of stress can trigger a large number of diseases and conditions—from obesity to ulcers. These and other stress-related diseases sicken millions of people each year, says brain researcher Bruce McEwen at Rockefeller University in New York.[11] Chronically high cortisol levels lead to a number of health effects, including insulin resistance and poor sleep patterns. This can reinforce bad eating habits that can then trigger fatigue, which saps our desire to exercise. It is a vicious cycle. The list of stress-related conditions is long, as you can see.

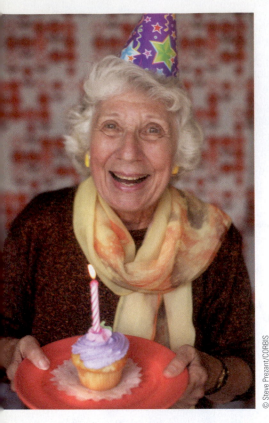

A common factor among people who live to be at least 100 years old is that they handle stress well.

© Steve Prezant/CORBIS

50

Abnormal heartbeat (arrhythmia)
Alcoholism
Allergies
Angina pectoris
Arteriosclerosis
Asthma
Atherosclerosis
Autoimmune problems
Birth defects
Breast cancer
Bruxism
Burnout
Cancer
Carpal tunnel syndrome
Cholesterol levels elevated
Chronic backache
Chronic fatigue syndrome
Chronic obstructive pulmonary
    disease (COPD)
Chronic tension headaches
Chronic tuberculosis
Cold sores
Common cold
Coronary heart disease
Coronary thrombosis
Depression
Diabetes
Eczema
Endocrine problems
Epileptic attacks
Erection problems
Fertility problems
Fibromyalgia
Gastritis
Gastroesophageal reflux (GERD)
Headaches

Heart disease
High blood pressure
HIV
Hives
Hypertension
Hyperthyroidism
Immune system disturbances
Impotence
Infertility
Insomnia
Irritable bowel syndrome
Kidney disease
Loss of interest in activities
Memory loss
Menstrual problems
Migraine headache
Multiple sclerosis
Myasthenia gravis
Night eating syndrome
OCD (obsessive-compulsive disorder)
PMDD (premenstrual dysphoric disorder)
Pancreatitis
Premature aging
Psoriasis
Raynaud disease
Respiratory ailments
Rheumatoid arthritis
Shingles
Social anxiety disorder
Stroke
Systemic lupus
    erythematosus
TMJ (temporomandibular joint)
    syndrome
Ulcerative colitis
Ulcers

The American Institute of Stress issued this statement about the long-term effects of stress:

> Many of these effects are due to increased sympathetic nervous system activity and an outpouring of adrenaline, cortisol, and other stress-related hormones. Certain types of chronic and more insidious stress due to loneliness, poverty, bereavement, depression, and frustration due to discrimination are associated with impaired immune system resistance to viral-linked disorders ranging from the common cold and herpes to AIDS and cancer. Stress can have effects on other hormones, brain neurotransmitters, additional small chemical messengers elsewhere, prostaglandins, as well as crucial enzyme systems, and metabolic activities that are still unknown. Research in these areas may help to explain how stress can contribute to depression, anxiety, and its diverse effects on the gastrointestinal tract, skin, and other organs.[12]

You can clearly see that the effects of stress have a profound impact on body physiology. The scientific evidence confirming stress-related disease is strong. Understanding how stress contributes to disease is facilitated by exploring how the mind and body communicate.

How the Mind and Body Communicate

An ever-increasing body of research documents the way in which attitudes, thoughts, and emotions impact health. Growing awareness of the role that thoughts and emotions play in health opens some exciting possibilities into our ability to prevent disease and

In a Climate of Overwork, Japan Tries to Chill Out

Stress in Japan has made headlines around the world and purportedly claims the lives of 10,000 Japanese men a year.* *Karoshi* in Japanese means "death by overwork." *Karoshi* is a rising social concern that has resulted directly from the well-known Japanese hard-working society that produced the highest productivity for its economy in the late 20th century. The Japanese government reported a significant increase in fatal heart attacks and strokes attributable to overwork, with the hardest-hit professions being information technology experts, doctors, teachers, and taxi drivers. Also reported was a record high number of suicides, many related to the economic downturn. In its evaluation of working practices in the 6 months before death, the Japanese Health, Welfare and Labor Ministry found that the *karoshi* victims were working an average of more than 80 hours each week.

The good news is that many Japanese workers and businesses are starting to look for options to help relieve *sutoresu,* the Japanese word for stress. English gardening, aromatherapy, reflexology, pets, and herbs have joined the traditional leisure pursuit of hot-spring bathing in a boom in *iyashi,* a word that conveys a mixture of healing, calming, and getting close to nature. Until 10 years ago, *iyashi* was largely unknown outside of the psychiatric profession, in which the term was used to denote a form of healing and relaxation for those who were overworked and over-stressed. Now, many Japanese, especially young women, want to relax and enjoy the fruits of their labor.

The bad news is that the ingrained belief that a worker should sacrifice personal well-being for the company means that even the most *iyashi*-conscious consumers have to compromise. Compounding the situation is that an obsession with work is often seen as a virtue in Japanese culture, and weariness a sign of weakness. "Americans and Japanese work the most in the world, but the work ethic is much more extreme in Japan because of the patriarchal legacy of loyalty between the samurai and feudal lord," says Dr. Relko Homma True, a psychologist and consultant to many Japanese mental health organizations.*

Despite the *iyashi* boom, Japan seems to be working harder than ever. Labor statistics show that the average worker takes only 49.5% of his or her 18-day vacation allowance. Ironically, this hard work is creating economic as well as psychological problems because many in the workforce do not have enough free time to spend their money, which slows economic activity.**

Source:
*"Health & Productivity Management on the March in Europe," by W. Kirsten, in *Health & Productivity Management,* (March 2005), *4*(1).
**In a Climate of Overwork, Japan Tries to Chill Out," by J. Watts, *Lancet* (2003), *360* (9337), 932.

heal ourselves. Awareness of the thoughts and emotions that contribute to stress and the conscious effort to control and change those factors can clearly result in improved health.

Author and physician Deepak Chopra sums it up in saying:

> Sad or depressing thoughts produce changes in brain chemistry that have a detrimental effect on the body's physiology, and likewise, happy thoughts, loving thoughts of peace and tranquility, of compassion, friendliness, kindness, generosity, affection, warmth, and intimacy... each produce a corresponding state of physiology via the flux of neurotransmitters and hormones in the central nervous system.[13]

To help you understand how the mind and body communicate, we will explore three areas of study: psychosomatic illness, the placebo and nocebo effect, and psychoneuroimmunology. This knowledge will help you discover the power of the mind techniques for relaxation, which you will be introduced to in later chapters.

Psychosomatic Illness

You might have heard someone say, "She's not really sick. It's all in her head." For years the common perception of psychosomatic illness was that it was not real, that somehow the person imagined that he or she was sick or didn't feel well. The belief was that all illness was caused by things like germs, radiation, tobacco, or diet. How could diseases such as cancer and heart disease, or even a stomachache or the flu, be the result of how our mind interprets events in life? Our mind could not actually be the cause of our ill health, could it?

Experience tells us otherwise. Have you ever wanted to avoid participating in some activity and as a result had the incredible power of creating a short-lived sickness that got you out of the event? We do have the power to make ourselves sick.

Fortunately, we have come a long way in our understanding of psychosomatic conditions. The term **psychosomatic** originates from the core words *psyche,* meaning the mind, and *soma,* meaning the body. Conditions that have a mind and body component are often called psychosomatic. Today, psychosomatic conditions also are called **psychophysiological** to avoid the negative connotation that the condition is somehow imagined.

For as a man thinketh in his heart, so is he.
—*Proverbs 23:7*

It has become evident that our bodies are thinking and feeling bodies. Research by Candace Pert, Research Professor in the Department of Physiology and Biophysics at Georgetown University Medical Center, has demonstrated that our thoughts and feelings affect our health. She wrote:

> As I've watched as well as participated in this process, I've come to believe that virtually all illness, if not psychosomatic in foundation, has a definite psychosomatic component. Recent technological innovations have allowed us to examine the molecular basis of the emotions, and to begin to understand how the molecules of our emotions share intimate connections with, and are indeed inseparable from, our physiology. It is the emotions, I have come to see, that link mind and body.[14]

Deepak Chopra recognized the mind/body connection in relation to health and disease when he said:

> Conventional medicine already recognizes that ordinary experience can play a complex role in disease. For example, statistics show that single people and widows living alone are more likely to get cancer than people who are married. Their loneliness is called a risk factor—one could just as truly call it a carcinogen. Then why isn't curing loneliness a cure for cancer? It may well be, but in a different kind of medicine than we now practice.[15]

The Placebo and Nocebo Effects One of the best-researched examples of the power of the mind to create physical changes in the body is the **placebo effect,** a phenomenon whereby an inactive substance or treatment is used to determine how the power of suggestion affects the psychology, physiology, or biochemistry of experimental participants.[16] The placebo effect is created by a person's belief that he or she will benefit from an intervention.

Placebos frequently are used in studies to test new medications. Some subjects are given the medication and, as a control, some are given a placebo—an inert substance—and the results are compared. In study after study, across a broad range of medical conditions, 25% to 35% of patients consistently experience satisfactory relief when they receive placebos instead of regular medicines or procedures. The research supports the premise that belief that a treatment works *does* result in increased effectiveness.

A study reported in the highly respected *Journal of the American Medical Association* involved a review of pain treatments over the previous 20 years, encompassing both medication and surgery. The researchers found that placebo response rates varied greatly and frequently were much higher than the expected 25% to 35%. The study concluded that the quality of the interaction between the patient and the physician can be extremely influential in patient outcomes and in some cases, perhaps many cases, patient and provider expectations and interactions may be more important than the specific treatments.[17] These researchers are saying that when the patient and the healthcare provider expect a treatment to be successful, the likelihood of success increases.

Here are other examples demonstrating the placebo effect:

- *Hair growth in balding men.* Men who believed they were receiving a drug that would increase hair growth actually experienced such growth even when given an inert substance, a placebo.[18]
- *Cure for nausea and vomiting.* Pregnant women were cured of their nausea and vomiting when given a substance they were told would prevent these conditions. Even more amazing is that the substance used as the placebo was not simply an inert substance, but in fact Ipecac—which is actually used to induce vomiting.[19]

If our thoughts and emotions have a positive impact on health, it makes sense that they also might affect us in negative ways. The **nocebo effect** explains the causation of sickness and death by expectations of these negative outcomes and by associated emotional states.[20] For example, when people who are susceptible to poison ivy are exposed to a harmless look-alike plant and told it is the real thing, they can develop a rash.

In another study, cancer patients experienced hair loss when they were given a totally inert substance and were told it was a powerful anticancer medicine that causes hair loss.[21] The scientific evidence that our thoughts can affect our health negatively is demonstrated in studies such as these.

FYI

What's Lipragus?

Larry Dossey, MD, writes about an early experience with the placebo effect while he was working in a hospital pharmacy during his college days. Curious to learn about the most popular medications prescribed in the hospital, he encountered the medication Lipragus.

He learned that Lipragus was sugar pil(l) spelled backward. Healthcare providers have long understood the impact of the placebo effect.

Source: From his book *Meaning and Medicine* (New York: Bantam, 1991).

Studies on both the placebo and nocebo effects provide strong support for the connection between thoughts and feeling and physical health. The literature is filled with examples demonstrating the placebo and nocebo effects. As you will learn in Chapter 5, The Power of Perceptions, an understanding of the power of our mind has important implications for stress prevention and management. This information can empower us to understand the role our thinking plays in our health. And, as has been demonstrated, expectation affects reality.

Psychoneuroimmunology

Today, entire areas of science are studying the relationship between the body and mind. One interesting field of scientific inquiry studies the chemical basis of communication between the body and mind as it relates to the nervous system and the immune system. This area of study, called **psychoneuroimmunology** (PNI), seeks to understand the complex communications between and among the nervous system, the psyche, and the immune system, and their implications for health.

As you have learned, the effects of a compromised immune system are far-reaching, and extend to everything from susceptibility to the common cold, to the rate of wound healing, and even a link to developing breast cancer. Following is a brief summary of several studies linking stress to its effect on the immune system.

- PNI research has shown that traumatic stress, such as the death of a loved one, can impair the person's immunity for as long as a year.
- Studies of university students and staff in the United States and Spain have implicated stress and a generally negative outlook as increasing susceptibility to the common cold.[22]
- By inflicting small cuts in volunteers who then were subjected to controlled stressful situations, researchers have shown a significant delay in healing among those who were under stress.[23]
- People who were shown films of Mother Teresa consoling the poor and the sick experienced increased levels of Salivary Immunoglobulin A, one of the body's first lines of defense against invading pathogens. The levels of this substance in children have been shown to increase through relaxation and self-hypnosis. In adults, the levels increased when humor was introduced.[24]
- In research on women with metastatic breast cancer, psychiatrist David Spiegel found that stress hormones played a role in the progression of breast cancer. The average survival time of women with normal cortisol patterns was significantly longer than that of women whose cortisol levels remained high throughout the day (an indicator of stress).[25]
- Dr. Janice Kiecolt-Glaser, a National Institute of Health-funded researcher, reported that her team administered a small puncture wound to a group of dental school students, doing so once during an exam period and then again during a vacation period. They examined how the wounds healed. All the students took longer (on average, 3 days longer) to heal their wounds during exams than during vacation; the researchers attribute this to stress. "If you're wounded and you're stressed," Dr. Kiecolt-Glaser commented, "you take longer to heal. You also have a greater chance of infection."[26]

Dr. Candace Pert says:

> The immune system, like the central nervous system, has memory and the capacity to learn.
> Thus it can be said that intelligence is located not only in the brain but in cells that are
> distributed throughout the body, and that the traditional separation of mental processes,
> including emotions, from the body is no longer valid.[27]

Author Anecdote Power of the Mind In the early days of my nursing career, I worked on a busy orthopedic unit in a Midwestern hospital. One of our repeat patients, George, suffered from long-term back pain of unknown origin. Despite physical therapy, medications, and even surgery, George didn't feel relief from his chronic pain. Injection of a high-potency analgesic drug was the only thing that seemed to provide relief, yet these drugs come with negative side effects.

George's healthcare team decided to see if a placebo would work. Without his knowledge, the plan was to alternate the narcotic injections with an inert water injection. I remember feeling conflicted with the idea of "tricking" George this way and was sure the placebo would not result in pain relief. No one doubted that his pain was very real. But sure enough, the placebo injections did result in pain relief. Through some complex mechanism that we are only now beginning to understand, George received pain relief because he expected it. This was an amazing lesson to me in the power of our mind on our body.

—MH

Psychoneuroimmunology Finds Acceptance as Science Adds Evidence

According to Margaret Kemeny, an associate professor of psychiatry and biobehavioral science at the University of California, Los Angeles, psychoneuroimmunology (PNI) research has exploded in the last decade, demonstrating that hormones and neurotransmitters released under stress can change immune cell behavior. These various cells actually have receptors to "hear" the signals, allowing the nervous, endocrine, and immune systems to "talk."

For example, studies with a group of medical students focused on the effects of academic stress and response to a hepatitis B vaccine that would mimic the response to an infectious agent. These studies demonstrated that antibody and immune cell responses were diminished in subjects with more anxiety, higher stress, and less social support.

Source: *The Scientist* (1996, Aug. 19), 10(16), 14.

The evolving research opens up new ways of thinking about how the mind and emotions, the nervous system, and the immune system are inextricably interconnected. The science is complex and has tremendous ramifications for how we view health and illness.

Author Anecdote

If Only … Laura was a graduate student, a wife, a mother of two young children, and a happy, giving person. She was training to run her first marathon when she was struck with a rare and aggressive form of cancer. Laura and her family pursued every avenue of treatment, both conventional and unconventional, yet the cancer spread.

In her final days of life, Laura shared with me her feelings: "I feel so guilty and responsible. Could I have prevented this by thinking more positively or by having a better attitude? I really believe how I think affects my health, so I keep wondering what I did to cause this."

Although many studies show that in some cases a positive approach does make a difference, disease cannot always be prevented. There comes a time when accepting that fact can help make the journey easier.

—MH

Blaming the Victim

We cannot conclude this chapter without making an important point about the relationships between body, mind, and disease. In spite of our best efforts to manage stress and have a positive outlook on life, disease happens. The mentality that disease is the victim's "fault" is not a productive approach to health. This line of thinking, also called "blaming the victim," reinforces the attitude that if the person would have just tried harder, he or she could have prevented the illness. Although this may be true at times, a more constructive approach to health is to acknowledge that even though how we think and feel do have an impact on our health, some disease and death are inevitable. There is a 100% chance that we will die. But our thoughts and emotions can make a difference in the quality of our journey through life.

Conclusion

In this chapter we explored the relationship between the mind and the body to better understand the role of stress in disease and health. The bottom line is that the body is affected by what the mind experiences and the mind is affected by what the body experiences. Scientific studies provide a solid foundation of scientific evidence explaining the associations between the body and the mind. In his book, *Mind as Healer, Mind as Slayer*, Kenneth Pelletier summed it up in writing, "Generalized, and unabated, stress places a person in a state of disequilibrium, which increases his susceptibility to a wide range of diseases and disorders."[28]

We cannot predict which maladies will develop from too much stress in our lives, because so many factors are involved. One thing we can know with certainty, though, is that keeping the stress response activated increases our risk for many diseases and decreases the quality of life. A positive outlook can reduce the impact of stress on health.

The mind is a powerful weapon in the battle for health. The mind can be both *healer* and *slayer* because thoughts, feelings, and perceptions have profound implications for health and disease. Understanding the power of the mind will empower you to prevent some diseases and also to promote optimal health.

4.1 Body Signals

REVIEW Think about a health concern that you, or someone you know, might be experiencing right now in which stress has likely played a part in its development. This health problem may be a headache, insomnia, or it may be something more serious like depression or ulcers.

1. What is the condition?
2. Based on what you have read in this chapter, explain why chronic stress may have been the primary cause of the problem.

RESPOND Our body always gives us signals indicating that we are in balance or out of balance (and as we know from these two chapters, chronic stress is an imbalanced state). These signals tell us when we've done something that is good for us, like the way we feel after we've worked out, eaten a healthy salad, or helped someone with a problem. We also receive signals from our body letting us know when we have chosen unhealthy behaviors, like the hung over feeling from drinking too much, the stuffed feeling from over-eating, or the negative feelings following a stressful argument.

1. Consider what your body is telling you about the way you've been treating it. Do you feel perfectly balanced and terrific or are there conditions you have been struggling with that are telling you that something's not quite right, and that stress is the likely culprit?
2. Next, intentionally participate in a healthy behavior. Examples might include going for a pleasant walk with someone you love; eating a balanced healthy meal, but eating a little less than you normally would; doing something that you thoroughly enjoy with no other motive than to involve yourself in that activity; helping someone who needs some assistance without letting anyone else know about it. Explain the activity that you selected.
3. Focus deliberately on the way your body feels during and after doing the healthy activity that you selected. What signals does your body give you indicating that it was a beneficial activity? Write down your observations.

REFLECT Finally, write a paragraph reflecting on how frequently you listen to the feedback your body is giving you. When was the last time you felt terrific? When was the last time your body-mind felt completely centered, balanced, harmonious, and whole? Explain how you can do more listening to the wisdom of your body to make choices that help you feel tremendous rather than terrible.

Key Points

- Psychophysiological conditions have a mind and body component that is supported by science.
- Chronic stress is a contributing factor to many illnesses and diseases.
- Medium-term stress results in an array of unhealthy signs and symptoms including muscle pain, headaches, fatigue, and sleep disturbances.
- Long-term stress results in serious health problems, including cardiovascular disease, compromised immune function, and digestive disorders.

- Conditions that have a mind and body component are called psychosomatic.
- The placebo and nocebo effects demonstrate the power of the mind on the body.
- Psychoneuroimmunology is the field of study that seeks to understand the complex communications between the nervous system, the psyche, and the immune system, and their implications for health.

Key Terms

psychological health	natural killer cells	psychophysiological
bruxism	*karoshi*	placebo effect
interleukins	*sutoresu*	nocebo effect
myocardial stunning	*iyashi*	psychoneuroimmunology
lymphocytes	psychosomatic	

Discussion Time For Critical Thinking/Discussion Questions, please visit this book's Premium Website.

Notes

1. *An Invitation to Health* (2009–2010 edition), by Dianne Hales (Belmont, CA: Wadsworth/Cengage Learning, 2009).
2. *An Introduction to Community Health* (3rd ed.), by J. McKenzie, R. Pinger, and J. Kotecki (Boston: Jones and Bartlett Publishers, 1999).
3. McKenzie et al., note 2.
4. http://www.mayoclinic.com
5. "In the War on Colds, Personality Counts," by M. Elias. Rretrieved from: http://www.usatoday.com/news.
6. Elias, note 5.
7. "Can Managing Stress Reduce or Prevent Heart disease?" American Heart Association fact sheet. Retrieved from http://www.americanheart.org.
8. *Wellness Guidelines for a Healthy Lifestyle* (3rd ed.), by W. Hoeger, L. Turner, and B. Hafen (Belmont, CA: Wadsworth/Thomson Learning, 2002).
9. "Bulletin Board—Stress," by C. Le Beau, *AARP Bulletin,* (Jan. 2005), pp. 3–4.
10. Note 9, "Bulletin Board."
11. "Stress Can Ravage the Body, Unless the Mind Says No," by K. Fackelmann, *USA Today,* March 22, 2005, p. 7D.
12. "America's Number One Health Problem; How Can Stress Cause So Many Diseases?" Retrieved from http://www.stress.org.
13. *As Above, So Below: Paths to a Spiritual Renewal in Daily Life,* by R. Miller (New York: Putnam, 1992).
14. *Molecules of Emotion: The Science Behind Mind–Body Medicine,* by C. B. Pert (New York: Touchstone, 1997), pp. 18–19.
15. *Quantum Healing: Exploring the Frontiers of Mind/Body Medicine,* by D. Chopra (New York: Bantam Books, 1989), p. 142.
16. *Mosby's Complementary & Alternative Medicine: A Research-Based Approach* (3rd ed.), by L. Freeman (St. Louis: Mosby, 2009).

17. "The Importance of Placebo Effects in Pain Treatment and Research," by J. Turner et al., *Journal of the American Medical Association 271*(20) (1994): 1609–1614.
18. "Placebos Prove So Powerful Even Experts Are Surprised: New Studies Explore the Brain's Triumph Over Reality," by S. Blakeslee, *New York Times,* Oct. 13, 1998.
19. "Effects of Suggestion and Conditioning on the Action of Chemical Agents in Human Studies: The Pharmacology of Placebos," by S. Wolf, *Journal of Clinical Investigation 29* (1950): 100–109.
20. "The Nocebo Phenomenon: Concept, Evidence, and Implications for Public Health," by R. Hahn, *Preventive Medicine* (1997), *26*, 607–611.
21. *The Spirit and Science of Holistic Health,* by J. Robison and K. Carrier (Bloomington, IN: AuthorHouse, 2004).
22. "Stress and Susceptibility to the Common Cold," by B. Takkouche et al., *Epidemiology 11* (1991): 345.
23. "Stress, Cytokine Changes and Wound Healing," by A. Rubin and S. Karageanes, *Physician and Sportsmedicine, 28*(5) 21.
24. *The Spirit and Science of Holistic Health*, by J. Robison and K. Carrier (Bloomington, IN: AuthorHouse, 2004).
25. "Social Support and Salivary Cortisol in Women with Metastatic Breast Cancer," by J. Turner-Cobb et al., *Psychosomatic Medicine 62*(3) (May–June, 2000): 337.
26. "Researcher Explains Stress-Inflammation Link," by J. Kiecolt-Glaser, *CAM at the NIH*, Volume XV, Number 3, October 2008.
27. *Molecules of Emotion: Why You Feel the Way You Feel*, by C. Pert (New York: Scribner, 1997).
28. *Mind as Healer, Mind as Slayer*, by K. R. Pelletier (New York: Dell Publishing, 2002).

5 The Power of Perceptions

■ Is my life really stressful, or is it all in my mind? And if it is in my mind, can I think about things differently and not experience so much stress? ■ Why does one of my classmates thrive while balancing a full class load, a job, and an active social life, while another classmate in the same situation burns out? ■ I feel like I'm being pulled in too many directions, but I don't see that I have any choices. How much of my stress is the result of my thinking, and what can I do about it?

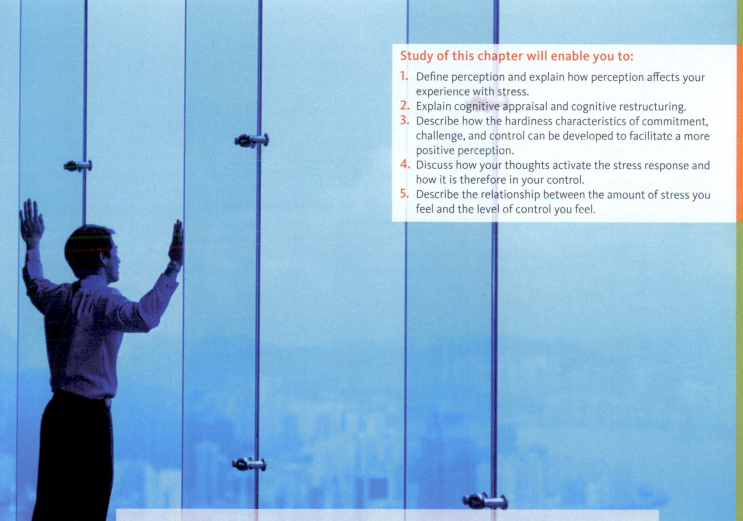

© Walter Hodges/CORBIS

Great men are they who see that spiritual force is stronger than any material force, that thoughts rule the world.

—*Ralph Waldo Emerson*

It's All How You See It *Jerry's story:* "I worked hard during high school, both at school and at my job after school at a grocery store. I have always wanted to go to college and knew it was up to me to make it happen. My parents were always supportive, but with four kids to support and not great jobs, I knew early on that I couldn't expect any financial help from them. I really like college and appreciate the opportunity I have to learn and grow. I think college will help me accomplish my goals, and even though it's hard, I'm determined to learn as much as I can and make the most of this opportunity."

* * *

John's story: "College seems like a waste of time to me. The teachers expect too much and don't seem to understand that students want to have a life besides studying. Most of my classes seem to have nothing to do with the real world, and the assignments are a bunch of busy work. This really is a waste of my time."

* * *

Jerry and John attend the same university, have the same major, and take many of the same classes. Jerry views school as an opportunity. John views school as a burden.

The Power of Perceptions

Have you ever wondered why people react to the same situations differently? Some people get nervous before a test, or a big game, or speaking in front of a group of people, while others enjoy the challenge. Could it be genetics, perception, personality, or attitude that makes the difference? Yes, yes, yes, and yes—and probably other reasons, too. Your experience with life's events depends on your strategies for coping with stress, your previous experience with stress, your genetic makeup, and your level of social support. Most important, however, is how you perceive the events in life. A shift in perspective is the first critical step toward improving how you experience stress. Understanding how the mind interprets and perceives incoming information is the key to stopping stress where it starts—in your own mind.

But can you actually change the way you perceive things? Can you learn to *think* differently? Absolutely! Changing the way you think is no small matter, yet this goes to the heart of where stress begins. In this chapter and the next we will explore the power of the mind and the power of perceptions. You will learn specific and proven methods, including cognitive restructuring, levels of responding, and rational emotive therapy, to help you *prevent* stress. These tools will help you perceive events in life more accurately and effectively. You will learn how your mind affects your experience with stress.

When you finish reading these chapters, you will know the answers to these two questions:

1. How do my thoughts relate to the way I experience stress?
2. What tools and techniques can help manage my thoughts and perceptions to prevent stress and enhance the quality of my life?

The story about Nonoko illustrates that individuals can have the same experience but with very different results, depending on their thinking. Like Nonoko, you can learn to think about the events of life in a positive, life-enhancing manner to prevent stress and greatly improve your quality of life. Think back to the dimensions of health introduced in Chapter 1. Recall that the intellectual, or mental, dimension

Nonoko's Story

Once upon a time there was an old Zen master named Nonoko who lived alone in a hut in the woods. One night while Nonoko was sitting in meditation, a powerful stranger came to the door and, brandishing a sword, asked Nonoko for all his money. Nonoko continued to count his breaths while saying to the stranger, "All my money is on the shelf behind the books. Take all you need, but leave me ten yen. I need to pay my taxes this week."

The stranger went to the shelf and removed all the money except ten yen. He also took a lovely urn on the shelf.

"Be careful how you carry that urn," said Nonoko. "It can easily crack."

The stranger looked around the small, barren room once more, then began to leave.

"You have forgotten to say 'thank you,'" said Nonoko.

The stranger said "thank you" and left.

The next day, the whole village was in an uproar. Half a dozen people claimed they'd been robbed. When a friend noted that Nonoko's urn was missing, he asked Nonoko if he, too, had been a victim of the thief.

"Oh, no," said Nonoko. "I loaned the urn to a stranger, along with some money. He said 'thank you' and left. He was pleasant enough but careless with his sword."

Source: From *The Book of Est*, by L. Rhinehart (New York: Holt, Rinehart & Winston, 1976).

of health relates to thinking and the emotional dimension relates to feeling. The intellectual dimension of health is the focus of this chapter.

Perception

Perception, a person's cognitive (mental) interpretation of events, is perhaps the most critical aspect in preventing unnecessary and unhealthy stress. Experts who study stress agree that in nearly all cases, the events themselves are not what cause us to feel stress but, rather, *the way we perceive or interpret those events is what causes us to feel stress.*

Are You in Danger?

Ask yourself this important question: In the past month of your life, how much of your time was spent in life-threatening situations? Taking into account every minute, how much of the time was your life really in danger? Perhaps you were in a car accident or some other incident that briefly involved a dangerous situation. Maybe you were hiking and lost your footing in a dangerous place along the path. Maybe you were at risk of being mugged or attacked. We all can recount occasional instances when we have been in danger. Sometimes the danger is rational and can be interpreted as threatening. This distress can lead to positive action that is necessary for you to avoid pain or danger.

If we take into account every waking moment of our lives, we can immediately realize that we are rarely in any kind of danger in which our life is at risk or in which we will feel physical pain from an outside source. Certainly there are exceptions. Some of us live in places where real danger regularly looms large. But for most of us, if we analyze our situations accurately, we have to acknowledge that our lives do not involve many life-threatening experiences.

In the previous chapters you learned about the effects of stress on the physical body. You also learned that the stress response begins with a thought. The thought sends an initial message to your various body systems that you are in danger. This message activates a state of physiological arousal, the fight-or-flight response. This fight-or-flight response is an automatic reaction to the sensation that you are in danger.

Refer to the Stress-o-Meter self-assessment that you completed in Chapter 2. This was a general assessment of the level of stress you felt during the last month. You gave yourself a ranking between 1 and 10. What was your score? Was it higher than a 2 or 3? At this point, we must ask the key question: If you are in real danger so infrequently, if you have so few genuinely threatening experiences when you need extra energy, speed, or power to survive, why would you report any score higher than 2 or 3 on the Stress-o-Meter?

Author Anecdote How Stressed Are You *Really?* In my classes, I begin this discussion by asking each of the students the following question: "In the past month, how much of your time was spent in situations where your life was really in danger?" Usually, three or four students went through something serious like being in a car accident or running out of air while scuba diving. One student told me she was camping and a big brown bear really did show up in her campground.

I go around the room asking each student this question, and as I do this, I do some math. A class usually has about 30 students, and I multiply that number by 30 days in a typical month multiplied by 24 hours in a day multiplied by 60 minutes in an hour. This adds up to 1,296,000 total minutes of life accumulated by the members of our class during the last month. Then I total the number of minutes they spent in a situation when their life was in honest-to-goodness danger. The top number so far has been 15 minutes.

Continuing with the math, I take the number of minutes during which the class experienced stress from true danger and divide that number by the total number of minutes lived during the last month. The results invariably come out to be far less than 1%. Then I go a step farther and ask the students what percent of their time they feel stressed. They report anywhere from 30% to 90% of each day feeling unpleasant stress.

—MO (to be continued)

Author Anecdote How Stressed Are You *Really?*

(continued) . . . At this point, I usually ask someone from the class to come to the front of the room and stand beside me. Let's say I have chosen Susan. I ask her if she knows "The Star Spangled Banner." I tell her to think of that song in her mind so she is clear how it goes. Next, I ask her to sing that song to the rest of the class at the very top of her lungs, much like the singer does at the beginning of a major league baseball game—just barrel it out!

Occasionally someone will be courageous enough to go for it, but most of the time, the students become red in the face (either in anger at me or in embarrassment, or both), fidget a lot, and try to talk their way out of my request for them to sing.

After a few long moments I ask Susan to sit down, and I thank her for volunteering. Then I ask her this important question: "Susan, if you were at home and nobody else were around—in other words, you knew nobody would hear you—perhaps you were in the shower or vacuuming your house, would you have any problem singing 'The Star Spangled Banner' at the top of your lungs?"

Invariably the response is, "No, I would have no problem if I were at home all by myself."

My next question to the class is this, "What is the difference between being at home and being in front of a classroom full of people? Aren't you singing the same song in both places? You're essentially doing the exact same thing both times."

I ask Susan what initial thought went through her head when I asked her to sing. Usually it is a sense of panic. Susan will report that she felt her heart rate increase, her face become flushed, her breathing change, and many other internal sensations, all of which are natural responses when we feel like we are in danger. But her life was not in danger in any way up there in front of the class.

—MO (to be continued)

Author Anecdote   How Stressed Are You Really?

(continued) . . . In my class, I next ask the students to name a few stressors—events they think cause them to feel stress. They usually respond with things such as finances, homework, tests, not enough time to do everything, or family and relationship problems. Then I choose one of those stressors, such as taking tests. I ask the class if it is possible for them to study for and take the test without feeling any distress.

"No way!" is the common roar in return.

I rephrase the question and ask, "Even though it may not be likely, is it humanly possible for someone to study for and take the test without feeling any anxiety?"

A few students usually have caught on by now, but the most vocal ones still emit a resounding "Impossible!"

Then I ask the students if I, as a teacher at the university, would feel any stress if I were to take the test. What if I were to study hard and then take the test? Or what if my 6-year-old son were asked to complete the test? Why in the world would he or I feel any stress about taking the test? A few more students have caught on by now.

—MO

FYI

What Makes You Nervous?

Can you guess the top four situations that people perceive as stressful? Here is what Bernice Kanner, author of *Are You Normal?*, says:

1. Making a speech
2. Getting married
3. Getting divorced
4. Going to the dentist

What makes your top 10 list of situations that you interpret to be stressful?

Source: From *Are You Normal?: Do You Behave Like Everyone Else?* by Bernice Kanner. (New York: St. Martin's Press, 1995).

Remember—the only purpose of the stress response is to keep you alive. But if you are in danger so infrequently, why would you need to activate the stress response? To be honest, why would you ever feel stressed?

Stress Comes from Within

As typified by the student who was asked to sing in front of the class, the chronic stress that we feel is rarely, if ever, the result of a truly threatening situation. The point of that example was to demonstrate that our stress almost always stems from situations that are not, by their nature, sufficient to put us in real danger. The outcome that we think is going to do us harm usually doesn't. As a result, we create in our bodies a false sense of emergency.

This leads to an important conclusion about the stress we feel: *The perception or the interpretation of an event is what initiates the fight-or-flight response. The event itself is not what causes us to experience stress.* As stress theory has evolved, the notion that human stress is a direct response to external stimulus is no longer credible. Whether we feel stressed or not seems to depend on how we view what is happening. Interpretation of stressors, not the stressors themselves, causes distress. This is not a new idea, as the quotations below reveal.

In his book *Creating Health*, Deepak Chopra explains that we commonly assume that stress is something outside of us, that stress is speed, noise, and chaos. This view is in error, he says. Stress comes from within. Chopra quotes Dr. Daniel Friedman, an authority on stress, who says:

Stress is a coupled action of the *body and mind* involving *appraisal* of a threat, an instant modulation of response. The triggering mechanism is the individual's *perception* of threat, not an event. Perception is modified by temperament and experience.[1]

Dr. Friedman goes on to say that we all respond to outer threats in our own way, depending on our previous level of arousal and ability to adapt. Appropriate stress helps the individual to adapt. Inappropriate stress, by contrast, serves no useful purpose and may result in disease. So stress is subjective and the individual's perception of threat, not the event itself, is what triggers stress.

Whenever we sense a potential for pain or danger of any kind—emotional, social, spiritual, or physical—our body reacts in its perfect way to help us survive. *The only way the body knows to do this is to turn on the fight-or-flight response.* We do not have any other natural way to handle a perceived threat. Certainly we can learn other ways, but our body inherently knows only one way that is immediate, fast-acting, and guaranteed to produce powerful results.

The reality of an exam is that it has no power to turn on the fight-or-flight response. It is merely a piece of paper with words printed on it. The stressor is based entirely on what that test means to us and how we interpret it. If a stranger—someone who was not in the class—were

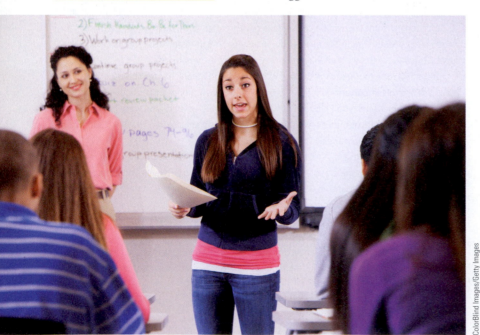

Public speaking can be a stressful experience.

to be given the same test, she probably would interpret it as some interesting questions with no other meaning to her personal well-being. If you were to give it to a young child, he might see it as a piece of paper that he could easily transform into a paper airplane. Students who feel stressed about a test are the ones who interpret it as critical to their future because a low score may pose a threat to their well-being.

The World is NOT a Stressful Place

The summarizing point and the essential concept in preventing stress is that *no event in life is inherently stressful*. Rather, we make stressful *interpretations* of the events of our days. No event in life causes stress universally for everyone. We have decided that some facet of the situation will inflict pain or discomfort, which may be physical, emotional, or spiritual. The situation also may be seen as a threat to our sense of well-being and comfort.

This understanding shifts the influence of what causes stress from external factors to internal control. Although some situations, such as the Asian tsunami, a gulf coast hurricane, an incurable illness, or being attacked, will be interpreted as stressful almost universally, we usually have the power to take control of how we interpret any event in life.

This concept might be fairly easy to capture intellectually, but to make it a working principle in daily life is quite another thing. We are not trained to think this way. From our earliest days we are taught commonly accepted statements such as these:

- This test is stressing me out.
- You make me mad.
- This class makes me bored.
- He hurt my feelings.
- She is so irritating.
- Life is stressful.

We simply accept the mistaken notion that what happens outside of us affects how we feel inside. Life events happen, and our reactions seem to be automatic.

The following real-life scenarios demonstrate how interpretation and perception are the deciding factors in the outcome.

* * *

Lindsay steps up to the foul line, puts the basketball in her shooting hand, lofts the ball into the air, and watches it sail through the hoop. She scores. When would this situation—standing at a foul line shooting foul shots—be stressful? One answer would be "when she is shooting to win the game." If she misses, her team will lose.

In our culture, we have decided that losing is painful. When will this not be stressful? Lindsay probably will feel no stress when she is in her backyard shooting foul shots by herself. She is doing precisely the same thing in both circumstances (at the end of the game or in the backyard). The only reason one situation is stressful and the other is not is because she has interpreted one differently than she has interpreted the other.

During the game Lindsay is thinking of all the negative consequences if she misses. Because she is thinking about avoiding future pain, her body automatically turns on the stress response. When she is shooting in her backyard, she doesn't sense any negative consequences if she misses the shot. In the absence of a perception of potentially negative consequences, she will not feel any effects of the stress response. The way she has interpreted the event is the key point.

* * *

See if you can relate to the following example:

Imagine that you are driving down a narrow, winding road behind someone who is driving slowly. You are in a hurry, but she, apparently, is not. Imagine that you are late for an important exam. This exam is so important that you may fail the course if you are late. You are definitely in a rush. The driver in front of you, though, is on a leisurely drive with her husband and kids.

Now imagine that an elderly man, who is driving a large car, pulls out just in front of this family. He is in even less of a hurry than the family in the car in front of you. The driver in front of you slows down so that her car doesn't run into the old man. You are forced to slow down as well.

The speed at which this older man is moving is driving you bananas. Soon you are in a rage, pounding the steering wheel, honking your horn, shaking your fist; your face has turned red

Stress is an ignorant state. It believes that everything is an emergency.
—Natalie Goldberg

If you are distressed by anything external, the pain is not due to the thing itself but to your own estimate of it; and this you have the power to revoke at any moment.
—Marcus Aurelius
(121–180 AD)

Everything good and bad comes from your own mind. To find something beyond the mind is impossible.
—Bodhidharma
(470–543 AD)

> Everything in life is but a challenge. Challenges can never be good or bad; we make of our challenges what we will.
>
> —*Toltec teachings book*

Point Of Positive Perception = Prevention

—*Margie Hesson*

and you are noticeably irate. If we ask why you are so upset, you might say something about how that man is making you stressed out. He is upsetting you because he is driving too slowly. In reality, you are upset, stressed, and out of balance because of how you are interpreting the situation. The older gentleman isn't making you feel stress. The other driver, the one with her family in the car, is on the same road, driving at the same speed behind the same slow-driving man, and she is not feeling upset, out of balance, or the least bit stressed. Why not?

These two drivers are not stressed because they have interpreted the situation differently. The second driver may see the situation as an opportunity to move even more slowly so she can catch more of the wonder of this beautiful drive. You interpret the slow-driving man as a major hindrance to you. In his thoughtless leisure, he is possibly causing you to flunk your test. That thought, for you, is painful. The event is not what causes you stress. What causes you stress is the meaning you give to the event.

Events themselves are not inherently stressful. This idea is illustrated concisely by this Taoist story of a farmer whose horse ran away:

> Upon hearing the news, all the neighbors came over to lament the loss. "What bad fortune!" they exclaimed, to which the farmer's reply was, "Maybe."
>
> The next morning the farmer awoke, and to his surprise he saw his horse had returned, and with it had come six wild horses. The neighbors came over, and with astonishment, congratulated the farmer on his good fortune.
>
> The farmer's reply was simply, "Maybe."
>
> The following day, the farmer's only son was trying to saddle and ride one of the new horses when he fell off and broke his leg. Again, the neighbors came to offer their sympathy for the misfortune. Again, the farmer simply said, "Maybe."
>
> The next day, the officers from the army came to recruit every young man to help fight in the war, but because of the broken leg, the farmer's son was rejected. When the neighbors came in to say how fortunate the father was that everything had turned out, his reply to them was, "Maybe."[2]

As you can probably guess, this story goes on and on. The events themselves did not make the farmer feel any particular way. How he interpreted these events was what led to his serene attitude toward the events that others viewed as tragedies.

In short, the examples provides in this chapter are intended to emphasize the idea that the events in the surrounding environment are not what precipitate stress in most people; interpretations are what actually trigger the stress response.[3] The connection between perception and physiology is incredibly strong. We can set off the stress response just by imagining confrontation with a teacher, for example. When we feel stress, we do it to ourselves. It is our own doing. Knowing this one single thing gives us complete power to *undo* it. If we are feeling stress, we can immediately take responsibility and take positive measures to stop the stress. This puts us back in control! Cognitive restructuring will help you learn how to do this.

Author Anecdote

POPP Formula for Prevention

Over the years, I have taught stress-management workshops in large corporations and in small churches, to nurses, teachers, farmers, students, and executives, from coast to coast and overseas. One of the most important ideas in each and every workshop is this: Your perception becomes your reality. I developed the POPP formula for prevention to help participants in my workshops remember this critical concept.

POPP is an acronym for Point Of Positive Perception. Let this idea POPP into your mind every time you find yourself in a potentially stressful situation:

- There is an actual **point** in time when your thoughts initiate the stress response.
- You can choose a **positive** thought to respond to the events in your environment.
- This positive **perception** will stop the stress response from activating.
- You have **prevented** unhealthy and unproductive stress.

There is power in the simplicity of this formula. We are not talking about managing stress, or coping with stress. We are talking about preventing stress.

—*MH*

Cognitive Restructuring

Cognition is a mental process that consists of thinking and reasoning skills. The ability to think and learn makes us uniquely human. It enables us to be rational, make good judgments, interpret the world around us, and learn new skills. Without cognitive functions, we could not interpret our daily lives, adapt and make changes, and develop the insights to make those changes.[4] Cognitive functioning allows us to react individually to the same situation. **Cognitive appraisal**—our interpretation of a stressor—is the deciding factor in our reaction.

Cognitive restructuring refers to the mental act of changing the meaning or our interpretation of the environmental stressors in life. This is sometimes called **reframing.** This approach substitutes our perceptions of stressors from thoughts that are threatening to thoughts that are nonthreatening. The source of excess stress is **cognitive distortion,** in which perceptions become distorted and magnified out of proportion to their seriousness. Cognitive restructuring entails first awareness, and then correction, of these stressful, maladaptive thoughts.

Hardiness

Hardiness research[5] suggests that the combination of three personality traits works together to dramatically reduce the perception of stress in individuals possessing these traits. The premise is that some individuals have traits that actually facilitate a more positive perception of daily events. **Hardiness** is the term used to describe this combination of personality characteristics and includes the traits of commitment, challenge, and control. A "hardy" individual is described as one who:

1. views potentially stressful events as interesting and meaningful (commitment),
2. sees change as normal and as an opportunity for growth (challenge), and
3. sees oneself as capable of having an influence on events (control).

Individuals strong in *commitment* believe in the truth and value of who they are and what they are doing. They have a sense of meaning and purpose in work and relationships. Therefore they remain committed and deeply involved rather than allowing themselves to become alienated by fear, uncertainty, or boredom. The term *challenge* reflects an outlook on life that enables an individual to perceive change as an opportunity for growth rather than a threat to one's sense of security or survival. Change, rather than stability, is seen as the common mode of life. The term *control* reflects a belief that one can influence the course of life events within reasonable limits. Hardy individuals have an internal sense of personal mastery, confronting problems with confidence in their ability to implement effective solutions.[6]

Studies suggest that the hardy personal traits of commitment, challenge, and control can be learned. Understanding these hardiness characteristics is important because if you don't always perceive situations in the most positive manner, these are areas you can focus on to improve your perceptions. In the pages to come, you will learn more about how to develop these traits to help you gain a more positive perspective on the events that contribute to your stress.

Commitment—Turning Problems into Opportunities

It is not what happens to you in life but what you do with what happens to you in life that determines the outcome. Listen to the experience of world-class cyclist and Tour de France winner Lance Armstrong, who in his mid-20s was diagnosed with cancer:

> The most interesting thing about cancer is that it can be one of the most positive, life-affirming, incredible experiences ever. When somebody is in that position, he starts to really focus on his life, on his friends and family, and what's really important. You experience a different emotion and feeling than the guy who has woken up for thirty years in perfect health and gone to work or school and never had to worry about anything. That guy forgets that every day when you wake up, it's really a gift. . . . I love what I am doing by a factor of at least a hundred.[7]

How many of us would think of cancer as a positive, incredible experience? Remember, commitment, your ability to view potentially stressful events as interesting and meaningful, influences your perception and your perception becomes your

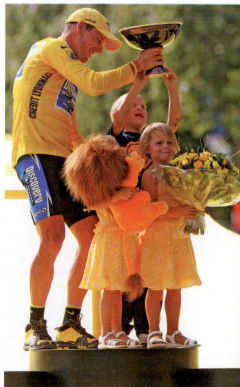

Lance Armstrong learns that life is about more than a bicycle race. He says, "The most interesting thing about cancer is that it can be one of the most positive, life-affirming, incredible experiences ever. When somebody is in that position, he starts to really focus on his life, on his friends and family, and what's really important."

Fear of Failure Most anxiety is based on personal perception, says Paul J. Rosch, M.D., president of the American Institute of Stress. "The Chinese word for 'crisis' consists of two characters—danger and opportunity," he says. "If you fear failure, you are under the kind of constant, slow-burning stress that can deplete your energy and corrode your health. If you can learn to see your failures as opportunities to learn and grow, the danger is gone and stress evaporates."

Source: Quoted in "Contents Under Pressure," by M. Zimmerman and S. Tuck, in *Men's Health*, August 2004, p. 176.

reality. Lance Armstrong's story clearly illustrates that an event such as being diagnosed with cancer, which normally would be considered very bad luck, can be interpreted as a positive, life-enhancing gift. His commitment to finding meaning and purpose through this life-changing experience affected his perception, and ultimately the quality of his life. The cancer is not what causes stress. The meaning we give to the cancer is what determines the outcome. So, even when we cannot change the things that cause us stress, we can change our perception.

Challenge—Change as Challenge Rather Than Threat

You probably have heard the aphorism, "The only constant in life is change." Yet most people like constancy. Change can disrupt the normal flow of life and create a stressful environment. One must be prepared for change, because change will happen whether we want it to or not. You can adopt one of two reactions to change: Either resent and fear change or embrace it and see new opportunities for growth in it. The first way leads to frustration, anger, and bewilderment, the other to excitement, awe, and challenge.

When you approach life with a more accurate interpretation of events around you, this positive perception halts the initiation of the stress response and the resulting disease and ill health, and you also learn that you can turn problems into opportunities to reawaken your enthusiasm for life.

Thomas Edison perceived things in a positive manner when he said, "I have not failed 10,000 times. I have successfully found 10,000 ways that will not work." It's all how we look at things.

Author Anecdote I Can See Clearly Now A few years ago, for the first time, I got glasses. I was amazed and surprised at how clear and sharp the world around me became when I put on my glasses. Had the world around me changed? No. The difference was that I could now see the world clearly. My perspective had changed. I had become so accustomed to the dull and blurry view that I was not even aware of what I was missing. The world didn't change. I did.

Have you become accustomed to a dull, blurry view of the world? Do you expect your day to be filled with stress? Can you learn to see things in your life differently to make your life better? We tend to think we are objective and how we see the world is how it really is. But more accurately we see the world not as it is but as we are. We are conditioned to see things in a certain, sometimes stressful, way. We must look at the lens through which we see the world and understand that the lens shapes how we interpret the world. It has been said that the real voyage of discovery consists not in seeking new landscape, but in having new eyes.

One of my students shared with me that after reading this anecdote, he made the decision to use the act of putting on his glasses each morning as a reminder that he could choose how he saw the events of each and every day.

—MH

Control

An important aspect of how we perceive our environment has to do with the level of control we feel over our environment. Not only is control one of the characteristics of a hardy personality, but it is also key to understanding how you view the events in your life. Think of **control** as a deeply held belief that you can directly impact a situation. There is a relationship between the amount of control we think we have and the corresponding amount of stress that we feel. The more control we feel we have over our circumstances, the less stress we tend to feel. As our sense of control diminishes, stress levels tend to rise.

To understand this concept of control, let's explore what can and can't be controlled. There are some things in life over which we have no control. These are things such as the stock market, natural phenomena such as weather, earthquakes, and storms, and some forms of disease. We do not have control over other people. Although we can influence others, we do not have control over other people's thoughts, feelings, or actions.

We do our best to try to control how someone is thinking, feeling, or acting. As examples, we may act like a martyr or try to make someone feel guilty or angry in attempts to control someone else's thoughts and feelings. Ultimately, we do not have the power to control anyone else, even though we may spend a lot of time trying. The healthy response to things over which we have no control is acceptance, allowance, and a go-with-the-flow attitude.

By contrast, we do have total control over some things. These things are related primarily to ourselves—our thoughts, feelings, behaviors, and actions. At times, we may not feel that we are in control of these things, but ultimately, nobody but you can control your inner life. Your perception of what is happening in your life has a lot to do with whether you believe you are in control and have power over what is happening, or whether you believe external factors are controlling your life.

Self-Limiting Beliefs In between those things over which we have no control and those things over which we have total control are various situations over which we have some degree of control. In many instances, we have much greater control than we realize. In many areas of life, we frequently create beliefs, or feelings of certainty, about our limitations. For example, we might have a belief that we are not smart enough or capable enough to go to graduate school. We tend to act on that belief and not achieve what we would like to. The belief that we couldn't possibly be a concert pianist—even though this would be an appealing goal—may stop us from even trying to learn how to play the piano.

Thinking in this way comes from faulty notions that a person does not have the ability to carry out a specific task. These are called **self-limiting beliefs.** Our culture promotes beliefs that prevent people from pursuing worthy goals. Some examples of self-limiting statements are:

- I'm too old.
- I'm too young.
- I'm too fat.
- I'm not smart enough.
- I'm too shy.
- I'm not strong enough.
- I don't have enough willpower.
- I won't be successful, so why try?
- I can't control how I feel when this or that happens.

Statements such as these may not be accurate self-assessments, but because we believe them, we tend to act on these beliefs and bring about results that coincide with the limiting beliefs. Psychologists call these types of beliefs **premature cognitive commitments.** We commit prematurely to an inaccurate belief about ourselves. Richard Bach made an astute statement about what happens when we have these self-limiting beliefs when he said, "Argue for your limitations, and sure enough, they're yours."[8] Our beliefs become our reality, regardless of how true or false they may be.

If the need or desire is great enough, we can control a lot more than we think. If someone were to give you a hundred dollars to sit next to a crying baby during a 2-hour airplane flight, or to wait patiently in the supermarket line while the woman in front of you spends 20 minutes digging through her coupons, or to listen to the guy next to you in the library smack and pop his gum while you are trying to study, could you do it? Of course you could. Could you do it without feeling stressed? Suddenly it is not so awful, is it? Events that seem irritating and stress-producing take on new meaning.

RESEARCH HIGHLIGHT

Out of Control

Job stress can raise blood pressure over the long term, according to a study in the *American Journal of Epidemiology*. Men working 25 or more years in a demanding job where they felt they had little control had higher blood pressure at work and home than those who felt they had more control. The deterioration of health was not a result of the job itself but, rather, to the lack of control the worker felt. Feeling in control of our life reduces the unhealthy physiological changes induced by the stress response.

Source: "Life-course Exposure to Job Strain and Ambulatory Blood Pressure in Men," by P. Landsbergis, P. Schnall, T. Pickering, K. Warren, and J. Schwartz, in *American Journal of Epidemiology*, 157(11), 998–1006.

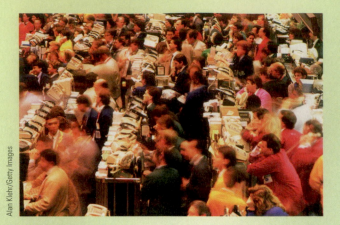

Alan Klehr/Getty Images

Perceived lack of control contributes to job stress and health problems, like high blood pressure.

When we are highly motivated, we can take control and prevent the event from initiating the stress response. If you could control your stress response for a hundred dollars, would you do it for a lifetime of less stress and better health? Again, we see the principle of perception and interpretation at play in virtually all events.

Locus of Control   An additional concept related to control, known as **locus of control (LOC),** refers to the way we ascribe our chances of success or failure in a future venture to either internal or external causes. People with an **internal locus of control** see themselves as responsible for the outcomes of their own actions. People with an **external locus of control** believe that whatever happens to them is unrelated to their own behavior—making it beyond their control.

Your perception of control has a profound impact on your motivation and your health. Researchers theorize that as far as a sense of control is concerned, a person is somewhere along a continuum of internal and external control. For example, if your thinking is more toward the internal LOC end of the continuum you might say, "The grade I receive in this class is entirely dependent on the work, study, and effort I exert toward each of the assignments and tests." People with an internal LOC tend to participate in behaviors that positively affect their health, such as exercising, eating healthy food, and doing relaxation exercises.

Stress is a response and therefore can be controlled. All it requires is changing your perception of what truly requires a stress response. You have the power to control the stress in your life. Decide to control the stressor; don't let the stressor control you. Since we cannot change reality, let us change the eyes which see reality.

—*Nikos Kazantzakis*

If you tend to think from a more external LOC perspective, you might think or say, "I'll get a good grade in this class because the teacher likes me or is in a good mood when she's giving out grades." People with an external locus of control would consider the condition of their health as being independent of their behaviors. If they remain healthy or get sick, it is because of luck, chance, or circumstances.

People with a tendency to think from an internal LOC perspective are more likely to take responsibility and believe they can influence what happens to them. Moving toward this style of thinking will positively affect your ability to reduce the stress in your life. If you think you can control the stress you are experiencing, you are well on your way to doing so. This idea relates to the next concept we will discuss: self-efficacy.

Self-Efficacy   Changing our perceptions depends on the belief that we can change and will succeed. **Self-efficacy** describes the belief in our ability to accomplish a goal or change a behavior. When we truly believe we can do something, we often find we can. Have you read the children's story, "The Little Engine That Could"? The little engine is famous for saying, "I think I can, I think I can, I think I can," as it pulls the train up the mountain. This is self-efficacy. The little engine did not say, "I wish I could" or "I might be able to" or "I hope I can" or "No way—I'm too small." If you have the courage and the faith to believe in yourself and your abilities, you can control the stress in your life if you think you can.

You might be saying to yourself that this surely sounds nice, but it isn't that easy to change how a person thinks about things. True, it isn't easy, but people can and do take control of their thinking and their perceptions every day. As a result, they change their behavior, even in the most difficult-to-change thinking patterns.

Think of someone who has addictive behaviors. An addiction is a perception that we cannot do without something and still function normally. This is a strongly held belief. But people control addictions all the time. All around us we see people who quit smoking, people who stop taking drugs, people who stop being angry, and people who change many other behaviors that some believe are nearly impossible to change. Many people come to realize the control they have over their thoughts and feelings. They recognize that they are not at the mercy of forces outside of themselves. Regardless of the environmental situations, they can control their thoughts and, therefore, their feelings and behaviors.

As we were discussing this concept of control in class, one student offered an enlightened insight: "If you have control over something, there is no need to worry about it. If you can't control something, there is also no need to worry about it. There is nothing else . . . so there really is *nothing to worry about.*" These are wise words. Understanding this balance is the key to preventing stress.

Stress Busting Behavior: A New Way of Thinking

Practice incorporating these new modes of thinking into your everyday life:

1. "I don't need to be stressed about this. I'm not in any danger."

2. "It's not a problem, it's a challenge and a chance to grow."

3. "It's not a failure, it's a learning experience."

4. "Change is good. It brings new opportunities."

5. "I can't control how others behave, but I can control the way I think about it. And I can give others the benefit of the doubt."

6. "I think I can!"

7. "I am in control of my own destiny."

8. "I never think, 'I'm too old,' or 'I'm not smart enough,' or 'I could never do that.' I can do anything if I put my mind to it."

9. "Success depends on me; I am the one in control."

Which of these are already part of your usual mode of thinking (list the numbers)?

_____

Which of these modes of thinking will be most difficult for you to switch to (list number)?

_____

Pick one of these modes of thinking and describe a recent experience where it would have helped if you had used it.

_____

_____

_____

_____

Author Anecdote An Immediate Change in How We Viewed the Situation We had been waiting 45 minutes beyond the scheduled start time for my daughter's soccer game to begin. As each minute passed the fans along the sidelines were getting angrier and angrier because the referee was late. The shared attitude of the crowd was "How could this guy waste our day like this?" They were furious that he would take so long to arrive. I heard many comments about all the mean things these parents were going to say and do to this guy when he finally decided to show up.

Then came a phone call from the referee to one of the other referees in the game. It turns out that his son had been in a really bad car accident and he needed to attend to that situation before he could come to the game. Upon hearing this news instantly a collective change in attitude toward this man occurred. In one moment he was an evil person who deserved the maximum amount of wrath they could throw at him. And the next, he was the subject of their greatest sympathies. A change in how they looked at the situation completely changed the way they felt about it.

—MO

Putting It All Together

What can we do with this chapter? How can we apply the information? When we find ourselves becoming tense, we can ask ourselves the following questions to help diffuse the stress response.

1. *Is this stressor real?* Am I really in danger, or am I just imagining or creating the danger or pain? If we look at the situation with a rational eye, we find that rarely is the danger or pain real. This does not mean that the things we involve ourselves in are not important and worth pursuing. What it does mean is that we can do the important things that we choose to do without the added anxiety levels and accompanying stress. If we do not sense any danger, we will not feel any threat and, as a result, the stress response will not have to activate to prepare us for any potential of peril. We then can function in a more balanced way.

2. *Can I handle this situation?* One sure source to determine if we can handle something, and therefore diffuse the need to turn on the stress response, is our past experience. We have taken hundreds of tests, met thousands of people, done many unknown things that seemed scary at first, and we have survived them all. Why should this situation be any different? If we can handle something, there is no need to feel threatened by it. Our past experience tells us that we can handle most potentially stressful situations successfully.

3. *Can I think about this differently?* As events happen, we have a choice about how we view it or what it means to us. Depending on how we interpret the situation will lead to feelings of calmness or stress. In Chapter 6 we expand on this idea.

Conclusion

Here is how perception influences the stress level:

1. Perception, or interpretation of events, determines the stress outcome.
2. Events are perceived as stressful if the expected outcome is threatening or painful.
3. We are actually in real danger less than 1% of the time; therefore, we rarely need the stress response for protection.
4. By changing how we interpret events, we can prevent the stress response from activating.
5. Preventing unnecessary stress will promote health, improve quality of life, and prevent disease.

If you allow it, stress can bring out the best in you. You should view the changes in life as energizing opportunities to grow. Recognize that your perception becomes your reality. Embrace the powerful idea that you, and you alone, are in control of your thoughts, and that you can learn to think in a positive, stress-preventing manner. Learn to let go of the stressors that are not in your control. The bottom line is that you have a choice about whether life events will cause you stress or not. You can decide whether the stressors in life will control you or you will control the stressors.

5.1 POPP

REVIEW AND APPLY Review and apply the POPP formula for prevention. For one day, deliberately focus on applying the POPP formula every time you feel your stress response begin to activate. When you feel yourself becoming stressed, stop and deliberately think of how you can perceive the situation in a positive manner so the stress response never activates. Use a cue, like wearing a Hawaiian shirt or switching your watch to the other wrist, to remind you that you are applying the POPP formula for the day. You will need to really pay attention to be alert to the events that are initiating your stress response and you will need to think carefully about how your perception of that event can change the outcome for you. Here is an example:

> Adam experienced stress on nearly a daily basis due to the lack of parking spaces at his university. This was not a good way to start his day. Adam applied the POPP formula when he was driving around the parking lot looking for an open space. At the point when he began to feel his hands gripping the steering wheel and his thoughts turning to frustration, he took a deep breath and deliberately changed his perception of the situation. He reminded himself that he could park a few blocks away. This would allow him to get some exercise, enjoy a nice morning walk to class, and appreciate the beautiful morning. He prevented his stress response from activating.

1. Describe the events you encountered throughout the day that would typically initiate your stress response and your usual way of perceiving the situation.

2. Explain how you changed your thinking (perception) in each situation to change your outcome.

3. Explain your experience with applying the POPP formula. Include how you felt when you perceived potential stressors in a positive way as opposed to how you typically feel when you respond by becoming stressed.

4. At the end of the day, reflect back on how applying the POPP formula affected your day.

5.2 Locus of Control

IDENTIFY Identify each of the following statements as representing either internal or external LOC thinking. Put an "I" in front of the internal examples and an "E" in front of the external examples.

_____ 1. "I flunked my psych exam because the teacher didn't tell us what to study."

_____ 2. "I wouldn't drink so much if my parents didn't put so much pressure on me."

_____ 3. "I didn't get enough sleep last night because I didn't organize my time and set my priorities."

_____ 4. "I didn't get enough sleep last night because my teachers give too much homework."

_____ 5. "I gained 3 pounds last week because when my sister visits we just have to go to the all-you-can-eat pizza buffet."

_____ 6. "I gained 3 pounds last week because I went to the pizza buffet twice and didn't exercise."

(Continued)

_____ 7. "I was late for class because this university does not provide enough parking for students."

_____ 8. "I was late for class because I did not get up in time to allow for unexpected emergencies."

Consciously monitor your thinking and talking for a day to determine how your thinking affects your level of stress. Do you tend to think with more an internal or external LOC focus? Select one specific situation you can shift from external to internal LOC.

(Results: External—1, 2, 4, 5, 7. Internal—3, 6, 8.)

Key Points

- The first critical step to improving the stress experience is to shift your perspective.
- Understanding how our mind interprets and perceives incoming information is the key to stopping stress where it starts—in the mind.
- The perception or the interpretation of an event, rather than the event itself, is what sparks the fight-or-flight response.
- We are in actual danger infrequently, yet because of our perception, we frequently feel stressed.
- When our motivation or desire to change is high enough, we can control more than we typically think we can.

- Self-limiting beliefs can have a negative effect on perception.
- The hardiness characteristics of commitment, challenge, and control can be developed to facilitate a more positive perception.
- Locus of control explains the extent to which a person believes he or she can influence the external environment.
- Self-efficacy describes the belief in one's ability to accomplish a goal or change a behavior.

Key Terms

perception
cognition
cognitive appraisal
cognitive restructuring
reframing

cognitive distortion
hardiness
control
self-limiting beliefs
premature cognitive commitments

locus of control
internal locus of control
external locus of control
self-efficacy

Discussion Time For Critical Thinking/Discussion Questions, please visit this book's Premium Website.

Notes

1. Friedman as cited in *Creating Health: Beyond Prevention, Toward Perfection*, by D. Chopra (Boston: Houghton Mifflin, 1987).

2. *Tao: The Watercourse Way*, by A. Watts (New York: Pantheon Books, 1975).

3. *How To Make Yourself Happy and Remarkably Less Disturbable*, by A. Ellis (New York: Citadel, 1999); *Cognitive Therapy of Personality Disorders*, by A. Beck (New York: Guilford Press, 1999); *Cognitive therapy: Basics and Beyond*, by J. Beck and A. Beck (New York: Guilford Press, 1995).

4. *Essentials of Mental Health Nursing* (3rd ed.), by K. Fountaine and J. Fletcher (Redwood City, CA: Addison-Wesley Nursing, 1995).

5. *Stressful Life Events, Personality, and Health: An Inquiry into Hardiness*, by S. Kobasa, Journal of Personality and Social Psychology 37:1–11, 1979.

6. *The Relationship of Hardiness, Coping Strategies, and Perceived Stress to Symptoms of Illness*, by M. Soderstrom, C. Dolbier, J. Leiferman, & M. Steinhardt, Journal of Behavioral Medicine, Vol. 23, No. 3, 2000.

7. *The Right Words at the Right Time*, by M. Thomas (New York: Atria Books, 2002), p. 16.

8. *Illusions: The Adventures of a Reluctant Messiah*, by R. Bach (New York: Dell Publishing, 1977).

6 Thinking and Choosing

■ Can I really control how I think? Stressful thoughts automatically pop into my mind. I'm looking for some simple strategies that can help me reduce stress by changing how I think. ■ My first thoughts always seem to be to see the negative side of things. Can I learn to be more optimistic in how I think about things? ■ Can I do anything to change how I respond to stressful events?

Study of this chapter will enable you to:

1. Experience and apply a variety of cognitive techniques to prevent unhealthy stress.
2. Distinguish between effective and ineffective ways of responding.
3. Respond to situations in the most effective way that will result in inner peace.
4. Explain how rational thinking differs from irrational thinking.
5. Identify specific types of thought patterns you engage in that have positive or negative effects on your handling of stress.
6. Evaluate how your thinking influences your emotions and stress.

STUDENT OBJECTIVES

Mind is the Master power that molds and makes
And Man is Mind, and evermore he takes
The tool of Thought, and, shaping what he wills,
Brings forth a thousand joys, a thousand ills:
He thinks in secret, and it comes to pass,
Environment is but his looking glass.

—*James Allen*

A Wake-Up Call Motivational speaker and author Earl Nightingale relates this story:

* * *

Some years ago, a friend of mine played a trick on his wife that changed her life. Over the years, his wife, Karen, had formed the habit of shouting at the children, particularly in the morning. She screamed at them to get up and get dressed, to come to breakfast, to get ready for school, to catch the school bus. This was a scene that no doubt is duplicated in thousands, perhaps millions, of homes every morning.

But it left my friend, John, and the children with jangled nerves every morning, with a great desire to get as far from the house as possible in the shortest possible time. Each morning, John found himself heaving a sigh of relief as he left the wild confusion and noise of his home for the quiet drive to his office.

On one such drive, John began to think of ways in which this situation could be changed. It was absurd to think that every member of his family had to start each day with an unhappy scene of shouting and confusion. Suddenly he got an idea he thought might work.

The next morning, unbeknownst to Karen, John hid in the kitchen a tape recorder with the volume turned up. Throughout the frenetic tableau of shouting and imprecations, the silent machine recorded every word. Then, after the children had left and Karen was sitting limply in her chair with a cup of coffee, catching her breath after her morning drillmaster duties, John played the tape for her.

For a few moments, Karen looked at him in curious amazement. Then she suddenly realized that the strident, shouting, barking, unhappy voice was her own. For the first time, she heard herself as she sounded each morning to her husband and children. Her face flamed in wounded embarrassment as the awful sound of her own voice again filled the kitchen. Long before the tape was over, she had put her head in her arms and begun to cry.

John turned off the tape recorder and put his arms around her. When she raised her tear-streaked face to look at him, it was filled with resolve. She said quietly, "John, I'll never make another sound like that as long as I live."

The next morning the children were dumbfounded but delighted. Their mother was smiling happily. She spoke to them in normal tones. After the children, still dazed by the smiling stranger who looked like their mother, had left for school, John and his wife sat and talked over a cup of coffee. She explained that she had been operating on autopilot and needed a wake-up call.

Source: "To See Ourselves," by Earl Nightingale, in *Nightingale-Conant's Insight, 100* (Chicago: Nightingale-Conant Corp., pp. 37–38).

Thinking and Choosing

Do you think your love life is a failure? How about your job? And what about your less-than-perfect body? You probably don't need a psychologist to tell you that what you think creates how you feel. In nearly all situations, the stress you are feeling begins with a thought. This is the bottom line of cognitive therapy. The way you think—your ideas, values, perceptions—all affect your stress level. Your thoughts shape the events and circumstances of your life. Thoughts relieve stress and, moreover, can result in extraordinary life changes.

Cognitive (thinking) techniques can transform stress-producing thought patterns into thought patterns that actually prevent stress. In the last chapter you were introduced to the concepts of cognitive restructuring, including perception and control. In this chapter you will learn a variety of cognitive techniques, from simple to challenging, that you can use to change how you view the events and situations in your life. These techniques help you reduce stress mentally by showing how your mind contributes to every stressful event you experience. You will learn simple techniques such as thought-stopping and power language. Four additional, detailed remedies to faulty thinking that will be explained are conditioned-response, levels of responding, rational emotive behavior therapy, and the ABCDE technique.

Cognitive Distortions

What are some of the thinking errors that give rise to stress in the first place? The term *cognitive distortion* was introduced in Chapter 5. Cognitive distortion occurs when thoughts are magnified out of proportion to their seriousness, resulting in excess stress. You might have the habit of magnifying negative thoughts. If you do, you are not alone. Many people who react strongly to mental stress find they have developed self-destructive thought patterns. Inspirational speaker Zig Zigler calls this "stinkin' thinkin'"—which is quite descriptive. This negative thinking can turn everyday events into plagues of anxiety. See if any of these relate to you.

- *All-or-nothing thinking.* You either did the work perfectly or you totally messed up. Everything is seen as an extreme (good or bad), so there is no middle ground. *Example:* "I can't believe I blew that test. I'm a terrible student."
- *Personalizing.* This is the tendency to assume responsibility for things that are out of your control. Personalizing can lead to feelings of needless guilt. You constantly ask yourself, "What did I do wrong?" The answer might be *nothing. Example*: "Brad walked right by my desk this morning without saying hello. I must have made him mad."
- *Discounting the positive.* Are you the type of person who cannot accept a compliment? Many people feel they are undeserving of praise. *Example*: You played a great ballgame or performed well in an artistic endeavor. Afterward, someone compliments you on your performance. Rather than saying "thank you," you respond, "It was pure luck" or "It was nothing."
- *Assuming the worst.* Some people think they know what others are thinking or how things will turn out—and it's never good. This is also called **pessimism** or **awfulizing.** The awfulizer predicts disaster and lives as if it is inevitable. Awfulizers spend much of their life feeling upset. *Example:* "I think that guy is staring at me. He must think I'm weird-looking." This thought is quickly followed by, "I'm the ugliest person I know."

Distortions in thinking often lead to feelings that are associated with stress. Learning to think in new ways is an outcome of cognitive therapy. **Cognitive therapy** is intended to focus on cognitive distortions and relearning thought processes as a way to alter negative emotions, to raise self-esteem, and to gain hope for the future. Cognitive therapy has been used with groups as well as with individuals. Here is what one student reported after participating in cognitive therapy to help her deal with stress, "I've been doing outstanding. Not every day is good. But now I know that if one thing goes wrong, I don't have to have a bad day; I can have a bad moment." Cognitive therapy can be a remedy for both distorted thinking and more serious disorders such as depression.

Thinking Errors

Similar to the concept of distorted thinking, psychologist Albert Ellis identified 12 irrational ideas he calls "thinking errors." These ideas, common to our culture, are inaccurate and irrational and may lead to problems. The beliefs and conditioned-responses often take the form of absolute statements. Instead of responding with a preference or a desire, we make unqualified demands on others or convince ourselves that we have overwhelming needs. Ellis also presents disputing ideas that successfully counter the irrational ones. These new ideas allow us to move forward with confidence and without unreasonable stress and anxiety.

Negative thinking can be a learned response resulting from negative comments children hear every day.

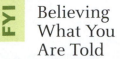

FYI

Believing What You Are Told

In a study that observed parent–child interactions over several days, researchers found that, on average, there were 400 negative comments for every positive one spoken to the child. The researchers concluded that negative thinking may be a learned response that can be carried into adulthood.

Source: "Self-Esteem and Peak Performance," by J. Canfield (Nyack, NY: Vantage Communications, 1988).

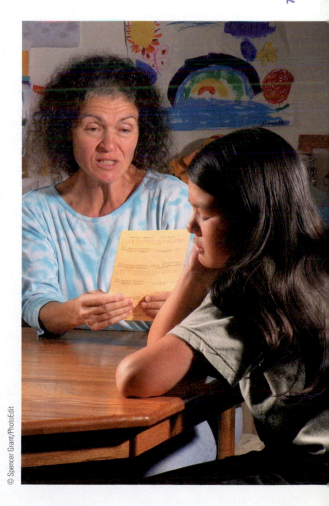

© Spencer Grant/PhotoEdit

Out of the Darkness

A study was conducted to determine the effectiveness of cognitive therapy on depressed nursing-home residents. Depression affects approximately 50% of people older than 65 years of age. With the current expansion of the elderly population in the United States, the problem is likely to increase. The depressed person perceives situations negatively when more positive interpretations are equally valid.

In this study, one control group received music therapy for 60 minutes twice weekly. The second control group received the nursing care normally provided. The experimental group received a 10-week program of cognitive therapy in which the subjects attended each 90-minute session twice weekly.

The results indicated that residents' attendance at the cognitive therapy group was significantly higher than at the music group. The improvement in depression scores in the cognitive therapy groups was significantly higher than in the control groups. All outcomes of the study were positive, including those measuring physical function as well as thought processes.

Implications of this study are that cognitive group therapy is effective with depressed elderly people, and is one way to help them feel more satisfied about their life. As this study shows, it is never too late to change our thinking.

Source: "Out of Darkness: Group Cognitive Therapy for Depressed Elderly," by J. Zerhusen, K. Boyle, and W. Wilson, *Journal of Psychosocial Nursing* (1991), *29*(9), 16–21.

> When one door closes, another door opens: but we often look so long and so regretfully upon the closed door.
>
> —Alexander Graham Bell

12 Irrational Ideas That Create and Add to Stress

1. *Irrational idea:* I must be loved by everyone and everyone must approve of everything I do.
    Rational disputing idea: I can't possibly please everyone. I will be true to my own values, as I strive to be loving, creative, and productive. Others may like me, or they may not, but I choose not to be anxious about their opinions of me.

2. *Irrational idea:* Certain acts are awful or wicked, and people who perform such acts should be severely punished.
    Rational disputing idea: People's poor behaviors do not make them rotten individuals. There are things that others do that I wouldn't. But they are not bad people. Blaming and punishing does little, if any, good and often can be harmful. People usually do what they feel is the best thing to do in most situations. This applies both to me and to everyone else. I can allow for that.

3. *Irrational idea:* It is horrible when things are not the way we like them to be.
    Rational disputing idea: Many different things happen in the world. It is not possible for all of them to be to everyone's liking. I can accept that the things that take place might never be exactly the way I would like them to be. That's just how life is.

4. *Irrational idea:* Human misery and unhappiness are always externally caused and are forced on us by outside people and events.
    Rational disputing idea: Most, if not all, unhappiness I experience is not caused by the unpleasant aspects of the events of life but is created internally by the things I say to myself about those events. I may be able to control parts of external events, but I can control all of my internal responses to those events. That part is mine to choose.

5. *Irrational idea:* If something is or may be dangerous or fearsome, we should be terribly upset and endlessly obsess about it.
    Rational disputing idea: I cannot control or prevent events from happening in the world. Worrying about them will not positively affect them in any way. Strangely, most of the things I worry about don't happen anyway. If an unpleasant event does happen, I'll approach it realistically, deal with it appropriately, and move on.

6. *Irrational idea:* It is easier to avoid difficulties and responsibilities in life than to face them.
    Rational disputing idea: I can face my problems squarely and solve them to the best of my ability. An enjoyable life is not one without problems; it is one where I meet challenges and successfully overcome them.

7. *Irrational idea:* I absolutely need something or someone stronger or greater than me, on whom I must rely, to succeed.
    Rational disputing idea: I easily take appropriate risks and trust that my skills and abilities will rise to the surface to succeed. I enjoy other people in my life, but I have no complete need for anyone.

8. *Irrational idea:* We should be thoroughly competent, intelligent, and achieving in all possible respects.
    Rational disputing idea: I don't need to be perfect in everything. In fact, it is impossible to be truly perfect at anything because there's always room for improvement. I will strive for achievement and accomplishment. I will make mistakes, and that's okay. I will learn from those and move on.

9. *Irrational idea:* Because something once strongly affected our life in the past, it must determine our present and future behavior; the influence of the past cannot be overcome.
    Rational disputing idea: I can certainly learn from my past experiences, but I don't need to be overly attached to or prejudiced by them. The past does not equal the future. I am not the same person I was before. I am constantly changing. I can choose to see things in a different light.

10. *Irrational idea:* We must have certain and perfect control over things.
    Rational disputing idea: The world is full of probability and chance and we can still enjoy life despite this. Because I can't control most of what happens around me, I might as well flow with it instead. I choose to let go and flow.
11. *Irrational idea:* Human happiness can be achieved by inertia and inaction.
    Rational disputing idea: I am happiest when I am venturing out of my comfort zones to practice creative pursuits and devote myself to people or projects outside of myself.
12. *Irrational idea:* We have virtually no control over our emotions; we are their victim and cannot do anything about how we feel when things happen.

    Rational disputing idea: I do have control over my emotions. I am responsible for how I feel and I always choose the emotion that I experience based on my own thoughts about what is happening.

Source: "The Essence of Rational Emotive Behavior Therapy (REBT): A Comprehensive Approach to Treatment," by Albert Ellis; retrieved from *http://www.rebt.org.*

Reflect carefully on Ellis' 12 irrational ideas and decide which three relate the most to your way of thinking. We all practice irrational thinking to some degree. Think of personal examples that demonstrate this thinking. Think about the related rational disputing idea and how you could integrate this new way of thinking.

Making a conscious effort to change or reframe the way you think or to focus on the positive thought is an important element in stress management. Eliminating "stinkin' thinkin'" involves first awareness, and then correction, of these erroneous thoughts. The goal is to create positive feelings of challenge rather than negative feelings of stress. Implementing cognitive techniques can help get you started.

Stress Busting Behavior: Think Right!

Follow these tips to change your mindset and reduce your level of stress. Check all that you already follow or that you are committed to trying.

☐ **Accept shades of gray.** Just because something is not perfect doesn't mean that it's terrible.

☐ **Don't take it personally.** Sometimes things go wrong. Sometimes people won't like you. That's normal, and it doesn't mean that there's anything wrong with you.

☐ **Accentuate the positive.** Play up the good aspects of your life and your achievements; downplay the negative aspects and the mistakes.

☐ **Accept compliments.** Don't deny that you deserve the praise; just say thank you!

☐ **Assume the best.** Think positively about your current situation and the future.

☐ **See the best in other people.** Assume that they have good reasons for what they do, even if you think they are misguided. Give people the benefit of the doubt.

☐ **Refuse to worry.** Do your best to achieve a positive outcome, but then be ready to accept whatever life has in store for you. Whatever will be, will be, and worrying doesn't help!

☐ **Believe in your ability to control your emotions.** You get to choose how you feel in response to what happens in your life.

Cognitive Techniques That Help Overcome Distorted Thinking

Some helpful cognitive techniques include positive self-talk, thought-stopping, power language, and going with the flow.

Positive Self-Talk   **Self-talk** describes the messages you send to yourself, your internal dialogue. This flow of thoughts, sometimes called **stream of consciousness,** often determines how you interpret events in your life. Becoming aware of this stream of consciousness and listening to what you are thinking is the first step in mastering your self-talk. Many of us don't even realize how often our self-talk is negative. Our brain thinks faster than we

Silver or Bronze?

Three research psychologists published an interesting article demonstrating that what you think affects how you feel. They observed Olympic silver and bronze medal winners as they stood on the podium receiving their medals and they rated them according to how happy they appeared to be. Who do you think looked happier: the silver or the bronze winners?

The findings may surprise you. The bronze winners, even though they had performed worse than the silvers, appeared happier. The researchers found that the silver medal winners tended to compare themselves up to the gold medal winners, thinking "If only I'd been a second faster, I'd be the best in the world. Now, I'm a loser." The bronze medalists, on the other hand, tended to compare themselves to all the rest of the competitors. They were thrilled to be on the podium when they could easily have been just one of the many competitors.

How you feel depends upon what you say to yourself, especially when comparing yourself to others. So next time you're stressed about how little money you have, or how your car is about to fall apart, think bronze and be thankful for what you have. According to the research, it's good psychology.*

*"**Winning** a Bronze Medal May be Better in the Race for Happiness," by S. Brody, *Los Angeles Times*, 2004.

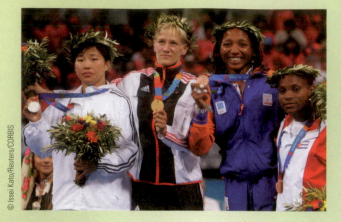

Bronze Olympic medal winners appear happier than silver medal winners. Researchers found that silver medalists felt like losers because they tended to compare themselves to the gold medal winners. Bronze medalists were thrilled to be on the podium, realizing they could have been one of the many competitors not to medal. How you think about an experience greatly impacts the resulting feelings.

Source: "Are Smiles a Sign of Happiness? Gold Medal Winners at the Olympic Games," by F. Dols, J. Ruiz-Belda, and M. Angeles. *Journal of Personality & Social Psychology* (1995), 69(6).

can talk, so if we are in the habit of thinking negatively, these thoughts will enter the mind so quickly that we may not even be aware of them. Becoming aware of your self-talk is the first step to mastering it.

Much of the internal dialogue in the mind is a result of habit. Because we are used to thinking in certain ways, changing this pattern may be challenging. You can learn to manage your self-talk by becoming more aware of the things you say to yourself. Do you tend to put yourself down?

- "I'm too fat. No one thinks I'm cute."
- "I'm late again. I can't get anywhere on time."
- "If I weren't such an awful parent, Jeff wouldn't have turned to alcohol."
- "I'm too stupid. I'll never pass this math course."

Negative self-talk is largely habitual. With frequent repetition of any negative judgment about ourselves, we begin to believe it. Try talking to yourself like you would to a friend you care about.

- "I have a lot to offer in a relationship."
- "I'm a smart and capable person. Tomorrow I'll leave early enough to get to work on time."
- "Even though Jeff has made some poor choices, I've always been a loving parent."
- "I'll have to work hard, but I've successfully passed other tough classes and I can pass this class, too."

Here is an example to demonstrate the impact self-talk can have on stress. See if you can relate to Joe's experience.

Joe has just received his final grade in chemistry, and he is furious. He was only one point away from receiving a B, and a C has now blown his GPA. He can hardly believe that his rigid teacher will not cut him some slack and give him one point to raise his grade. He is also mad at himself. "I'm so stupid. I slept in one day and missed a quiz that ended up ruining my grade." Joe is stressed and angry.

Joe could choose to think about this situation in a more positive way to reduce his stress. His grade will remain the same either way, but the way he feels will be different. "I'm disappointed that I earned a C in chemistry, but that's what I got. I learned a lot about the importance of attending every class and turning in all my assignments. I won't make the mistake again of missing class, especially when my grades are this important. I'll raise my GPA next semester, and I know I can do it."

Think about a recent experience when you felt angry or frustrated. Then describe your self-talk during that experience. Now try rethinking the whole situation using positive self-talk.

Positive self-talk can improve self-esteem and eliminate the chronic, nagging stress that destroys people from the inside out. Your thoughts generate your feelings. When you think negative thoughts about yourself, this affects your self-esteem. The results are negative, stress-producing emotions such as guilt, anger, anxiety, and fear. Conversely, when you think positively about these learning experiences, it affects your self-esteem similarly, but in a positive way. As a result, your stress-reducing emotions are positive, including happiness, peace of mind, confidence, and self-control. Mental health professionals promote the conscious use of positive self-talk as a powerful force for changing the way individuals think, feel, and act.

Thought-Stopping
Thought-stopping is just what it sounds like—stopping negative thoughts when they enter your stream of consciousness. When an unconstructive thought creeps into your mind, you can recognize your choice to think, and say "Stop!" In doing so, you replace the stress-producing, negative statement with a positive statement. The key to success is to believe the positive statement. Although this may take some practice, you actually can change the way you think.

Suppose you start to think, "I'll never be able to learn how to use this computer. I'm too old." Say, "Stop!" and replace the negative, stress-producing thought with, "I've learned difficult things before. I can do this." This simple technique works in part because it increases awareness. Consciously analyzing the thoughts that pass through your mind brings greater awareness to the messages those thoughts contain. Thought-stopping also brings an immediate end to negative messages and the resulting emotions that follow faulty thinking.

Because what we say is a result of what we think, you also can apply this technique to what you speak. Ask friends and family to help by saying, "Stop your negative self-talk" when they hear you putting yourself down. Before long you will be acutely aware of negative-talking.

The outcome of positive self-talk and thought-stopping is **learned optimism.** Psychologist Martin Seligman explains, "We have a choice about how we think. Optimism is a learned set of skills. Once learned, these skills persist because they feel so good to use." Seligman contends that by learning to challenge automatic negative thoughts that enter our brains and asserting our own statements of self-worth, we can transform ourselves into **optimists** who see what is right rather than **pessimists** who forever focus on what is wrong.[1]

Power Language
Power language is a way of speaking that helps you boost your feeling of control simply by changing the words you use. Words can create a feeling of powerlessness or a feeling of control. Compare these two statements:

"I can't handle this deadline."
"I won't handle this deadline."

"I won't" is a choice you make—an act of will—resulting in a sense of control rather than helplessness. You are no longer the helpless victim of the events around you.

Author and lecturer Anthony Robbins said, "Simply by changing your habitual vocabulary—the words you consistently use to describe the emotions of your life—you can instantaneously change how you think, how you feel, and how you live."[2] He suggests making slight adjustments to our internal conversations with examples like those shown in Table 6.1.

As you can see, the words you use to describe your emotions will have a noticeable affect on how you feel. You do have the power to change how you feel by changing the words you use.

TABLE 6.1 Transforming Negative Internal Conversations into Positive Conversations

Confused	transforms into	curious
Failure	transforms into	learning
Angry	transforms into	disenchanted
Furious	transforms into	passionate
Hurt	transforms into	bothered
I hate	transforms into	I prefer
Lonely	transforms into	available
Overwhelmed	transforms into	many opportunities
Rejected	transforms into	misunderstood
Stressed	transforms into	energized

Source: *Awaken the Giant Within: How to Take Immediate Control of Your Mental, Emotional, Physical, and Financial Destiny,* by A. Robbins (New York: Summit Books, 1991).

Going with the Flow **Going with the flow** or accepting situations we cannot control is a cognitive technique that we sometimes overlook. Maybe we tend to overlook acceptance because it can be difficult. Psychologist Robert Eliot says, "If you can't fight it or flee it… flow with it," expressed eloquently in the *Serenity Prayer*, widely credited to St. Francis of Assisi:

> God grant me the serenity to accept the things I cannot change,
> the courage to change the things I can,
> and the wisdom to know the difference.

Consider the metaphor of the bamboo plant and the grass reed. When it is full-grown, the bamboo plant stands tall and stiff. The grass reed similarly grows tall but has more flexibility in its shaft. When the fierce winds come, the bamboo tries its best to continue standing tall and strong, resisting the force of the wind. But the power of the wind snaps the long shaft from the lower parts of the plant. The reeds encounter the same stiff wind. They simply bend and flow as the wind pushes them around violently. In the end, after the winds have calmed, the reeds have survived. They flowed with the circumstances they could not control and have emerged better off than the bamboo. The resistance of the bamboo plant is the cause of its demise.

Underlying Theories and Techniques

Becoming increasingly aware of how you think and then implementing techniques to replace stress-producing thought patterns can have a great impact on how you feel. Positive self-talk, thought-stopping, power language, and going with the flow are tools to develop a stress-relieving thinking pattern. Now that you have some tools for improving your thinking, we will look in more detail at some underlying theories and therapies that help explain stressful thinking. Conditioned-response, levels of responding, rational emotive behavior therapy, and the ABCDE technique provide better understanding of how to prevent stressful thinking.

Conditioned-Response One theory that describes why people make the choices they do has at its core the well-known concepts of stimulus-response and conditioning. This **conditioned-response theory** proposes that when things happen in our environment, we are conditioned to respond in certain ways.

In the 1890s, Russian physiologist Ivan Pavlov conducted a series of experiments dealing with salivation responses in dogs. He would introduce a stimulus of food to a dog, and immediately the dog would begin to salivate. This is a natural response: Salivation helps the dog digest food.

Pavlov then introduced a sound (he used various sounds such as whistles and tuning forks) simultaneously when he introduced the food. With the introduction of that paired stimulus—the food and the sound—the dog still responded with salivation. Finally, Pavlov introduced the sound but without the presence of the food. He found that the dog was

WHAT ELSE CAN I DO?

Turn Needs into Preferences Our basic physical needs are air, food, water, and maintaining an appropriate body temperature. All the other things in life are things we simply want but don't necessarily have to have. Downgrade your needs to preferences, and release your attachment to the things you think you need but really just want. Instead of saying, "I need," say, "I want." Say "I choose to" instead of "I have to." Notice how differently you feel when you speak to yourself this way.

conditioned to salivate to the sound because it associated the sound with the food. When the food was not present, the dog still salivated. This, and other similar studies, became the basis for our understanding of why people sometimes react the way they do.

Most experts agree that people are conditioned to a large extent. We respond to stimuli in our environment in learned ways that are almost automatic. For example, we tend to eat at certain times of the day. In the United States, we drive our cars on the right side of the road rather than the left. Most of us sleep during the night and are awake during the day. When the telephone rings, we pick up the receiver expecting to talk with someone. These are all learned behaviors, and many of them serve us well—for example, driving on the same side of the road. Having to relearn the mechanics of driving a car every time we want to go somewhere would be tiresome and inconvenient. Not having to think about many of the things we do is helpful.

Some other patterns of behavior (conditioned-responses) that we perform automatically do not serve us quite so well. For example, if someone yells obscenities at us, we likely will get angry, offended, and defensive. When we are driving behind someone who quickly cuts in front of us, we probably will get frustrated or upset at that person. When we are sitting in a class or a meeting and the speaker goes on and on in a monotonous tone, we will tend to get impatient or bored. These are conditioned or learned responses. They are not inherited tendencies. We do not have angry, bored, or easily offended genes. We are not programmed from birth to automatically respond in that way.

In the chapter opening story about Karen and John, Karen's surprise when she heard herself on the tape recorder indicates that she had become conditioned to react to the morning demands in a predictable way without much thought or awareness on her part. She reacted by yelling at her family. The result was stress and pressure on Karen and her family.

This conditioned-response is like an elephant that gets trained for the circus. When the elephant is born, the trainer puts a huge clamp around one of the elephant's legs as soon as it is able to walk. Attached to this clamp is a chain. At the other end of this chain is a pole to which the chain is attached. The trainer teaches the elephant to walk in circles around this pole. After several weeks of this training (conditioning), the elephant comes to believe that whenever it has a clamp around its leg, it can go only so far away from the pole. You could tie a flimsy string from the clamp to the pole and this big, strong elephant would still remain in the circle. It has been conditioned to accept its limitations.

In much the same way, we tend to grow attached to our beliefs. As a result, we limit ourselves to our own self-made borders. These ways of responding are learned behaviors. This is both good news and bad news. The bad news is that we did it to ourselves. For example, when we are offended by someone else's words or behavior, the truth is that the other person does not have the power to offend us. Instead, we make the choice to be offended. Our own thoughts about what the person says or does are what make us feel offended. We choose to feel offended. We decide how we interpret what is happening and the feelings we get from that experience.

The good news is that if we learned to respond in a certain way to something that happens, we can unlearn it. We can remove that way of responding from our thoughts and behaviors. We are not stuck to any pattern of conditioned behavior. We can retrain ourselves to respond in ways that will be more productive and less stressful.

Choice   As conscious and aware human beings, we have the capacity to place something between the stimulus and the response that immediately puts us in control of how that situation will affect us. That important element is *choice*. In any situation, we have the power to choose our response to what is happening. We do not automatically have to react with anger toward the person who is yelling at us. We have a choice in the matter, and we can choose a different reaction. We can choose to return this person's anger with our own, or to remain calm, or to turn and walk away. Just because the driver in front of us quickly swerves doesn't mean we have to respond with irritation. We can choose to ignore the driver. Or we can choose to respond with kindness. Or we can choose to smile and wave. It really is our choice. As Master Yoda, the Star Wars character, appropriately said, "We can unlearn what we have learned."

Choosing to respond in a way that is different from how we are conditioned can be challenging and requires deliberate intent, but it can be done. One of the most profound

No one can make you feel inferior without your consent.
—*Eleanor Roosevelt*

WHAT ELSE CAN I DO?

Make more mistakes! In reality, there are no such things as failures, only outcomes. You decide whether or not you failed at something. When you have done something you feel was a mistake, learn from it. There is no point in getting upset over it. Time has passed and you can't undo what happened. The only valuable thing that you can do with that which has passed is learn the lesson the experience is giving to you, make amends where appropriate, and choose differently next time.

examples of being responsible (response-able) is that of Victor Frankl, a prisoner of war in the Nazi concentration camps of World War II. In his book *Man's Search for Meaning*, he tells how he came to realize that, regardless of what his Nazi captors did to him, he had the total and complete choice of how to respond. He reached the following conclusion:

> The experiences of camp life show that man does have a choice of action. There were enough examples—often of a heroic nature—which proved that apathy could be overcome, irritability suppressed. Man can preserve a vestige of spiritual freedom—of independence of mind—even in such terrible conditions of psychic and physical stress. We, who lived in concentration camps, can remember the men who walked through the huts comforting others, giving away their last piece of bread. They may have been few in number, but they offer sufficient proof that everything can be taken from a man but one thing. The one thing that can never be taken away is the last of the human freedoms—to choose one's attitude in any given set of circumstances, to choose one's own way.[3]

Frankl's message is that whenever we are upset, angry, bored, nervous, anxious, embarrassed, shy, or experience any other emotion, it stems from our thoughts, not the event that is happening. Rather than blame the teacher for the boring feelings you have during class, or pin your rage on that driver who cuts in front of you, you have a choice in how to react.

James Allen made the following statement more than 100 years ago, and it still rings true:

> Man is made or unmade by himself; in the armory of thought, he forges the weapons by which he destroys himself. He also fashions the tools with which he builds for himself heavenly mansions of joy and strength and peace. By the right choice and true application of thought, man ascends to the Divine Perfection; by the abuse and wrong application of thought, he descends below the level of the beast. Between these two extremes are all the grades of character and man is their maker and master.[4]

Levels of Responding   Things happen over which we have absolutely no control. We can do nothing to affect their progression or outcome. Typical examples or circumstances are natural occurrences, other people's actions, and world events that we view on television. When we notice these uncontrollable events, we have a tendency to react before we think about how we are reacting. We are on autopilot.

For example, a person is eating lunch at a restaurant. The waitress brings him some food and a drink. As the waitress hands the man his drink, it spills on his lap. This is an event that has happened, and he can do nothing to undo the spill. His tendency may be to become angry. But he could react differently, and how he reacts will affect his emotional state and his stress level.

Even though individuals respond to events in a variety of ways, we can categorize how people respond to uncontrollable events in two broad categories:

1. *effective responding,* and
2. *ineffective responding.*

These responses are designated as effective or ineffective based on whether they result in feelings associated with relaxation, such as joy, peace of mind, balance, growth, and happiness, or if they result in emotions such as anger, fear, frustration, imbalance, boredom, and chaos.

Within those two categories, seven subcategories of **levels of responding**

Author Anecdote   Funerals and Feelings   One place where we see how our choices and perceptions affect how we feel is clearly demonstrated during the grieving period after the death of a loved one. Many in our society believe that death is the absolute end of life. They think that when someone dies, their consciousness ceases to exist beyond that point. Others believe that this person continues to live in some other dimension, and without the body that he or she had while on Earth.

Those who believe that life ends at death have a hard time at funerals. The belief that they will never see this person again, that he or she is gone for good, creates intense emotion that can be almost unbearable. Conversely, those who believe that at some time in the future they will meet the loved one again, that the person continues to exist, view death in an entirely different way. They see it more as passing through a door to another existence and reuniting at some future time. These people have a more hopeful attitude at funerals. Certainly they mourn for the temporary loss of this loved one, but they don't view this as such a catastrophe. I've seen both examples and the differences are glaringly obvious.

The important point here is not to debate which view is accurate—whether life ends or continues elsewhere—but how the bereaving person interprets the situation. If the person views death as a catastrophe, that thought will generate some painful emotions that may include severe depression, heartache, and possibly the need for counseling. If a person views death as another step in the progress of the person who died, this thought will result in more positive healthy and less stressful emotions as part of the grieving process.

—MO

TABLE 6.2 Levels of Responding

Usefulness	Degree of Inner Peace	Ways We Respond to Events	Sounds Like (what we say to ourselves)	How We Feel—What We Get: Our Resulting Emotional State
Effective Leads to feelings associated with relaxation	More Peace	Gratitude	I appreciate . . .	Joy, serenity, contentment
		Allowance/Acceptance	It's okay . . . I embrace . . . I can live with this . . . I can go with the flow	Peace, release, relaxation, freedom
		Discovery	I wonder . . . What would happen if . . . ? What can I learn from this?	Inquisitiveness, curiosity, growth
		Observation	I am noticing . . .	Calm
Ineffective Leads to feelings associated with stress	Less Peace	Resistance/ Complaining	I wish things were different (complaining)	Boredom, fatigue, anger
		Judgment/Criticism/ Blaming	This is really a /He is really a (insert a negative noun) . . .	Guilt, shame, low self-worth, false pride
		Attachment/Rightness	This *must* be a certain way . . . Use words like must, have to, need to, should have	Mistrust, anxiety, anger, disappointment

help clarify the best ways to respond: gratitude, allowance/acceptance, discovery, observation, resistance, judgment, and attachment. Table 6.2 shows the ways we typically respond to situations we can't control and the results we get when we respond in those ways.

Let's explore each way of responding beginning with the least effective and moving to the most effective response. To help clarify the differences in the levels of responding, we will relate each category to a situation in which a person, Jenny, finds herself but doesn't have much control in changing. She is waiting in a long line to buy tickets to an upcoming concert. The line is outdoors and rain is starting to fall. She has been in the line quite a while and the line is moving slowly. Further, she has a class in 30 minutes, for which she will be late if the line doesn't move any faster. To get the tickets, she must be the one who pays for the tickets when it comes to her turn, but that will not be happening soon. Jenny simply has to wait in line. Let's consider how her possible responses to the situation will affect how she feels about what is happening.

Attachment/Rightness Attachment/rightness occurs when we clutch emotionally to ideas, concepts, or situations. When we become emotionally attached to ideas and situations, we think that we know what is best and cling emotionally to that view. We carry the attitude that we are *right* and that *we* know what is best for us or someone else. When we attach ourselves to opinions, to ideas, and to how we think things "ought to be," we find ourselves in arguments; we mistrust people who do not think as we do; and we are disappointed when our expectations aren't met. People who respond with attachment to events tend to become quickly anxious, angry, and fearful. Their need to be *right* supersedes their desire to be happy. When things aren't as they *ought to be*, they get angry and tense. They translate being wrong to a loss of self-esteem.

In our scenario, Jenny feels that the line to buy tickets should be moving faster. She processes in her mind thoughts that might sound like this: "If these people knew what they were doing, they would have made several lines—and done it inside where it isn't raining!" Jenny feels things should be different than they are. As a result of this way of thinking, Jenny will generate feelings associated with stress.

Judgment/Criticism/Blaming Judgment, criticism, and blaming describe the mental act of putting a label on something and then trying to make that label the reality. People who react in this way tend to judge, criticize, and blame things, people, circumstances, and situations. For example, blaming the hostess who spilled the drink at the restaurant as "sloppy" or "clumsy" would be an ineffective way of responding for a number of reasons.

First, we have no possible way of accurately judging a situation or a person based on limited experiences. Consider how many life experiences every one of us has had from the first moment of consciousness to the present moment. Every one of those life experiences has had some impact on our current behaviors and decisions. We cannot capture the essence of every one of those life experiences and confine them into an accurate moment of judgment or criticism.

Second, when we judge, we essentially have closed off other possible ways of seeing that person or situation. When we label someone we know who is careful with money as a "tightwad," we limit our ability to see him as economical or frugal.

Third, the act of judging is a mental process in which we are elevating our worth to a higher level than the person we are judging. When we call a thrifty person "penny-pincher," we are saying to ourselves that we are better than she is because of her obvious flaw that has to be pointed out.

Our judgments of others may reflect our own feelings of inadequacy. In reality, no one has more worth than anyone else. People who have the highest self-esteem tend to be complimentary of others. They do everything possible to try to build up other people because they realize, perhaps unconsciously, that they do not have a need to inflate their own self-esteem artificially by putting someone else down. Responding judgmentally or critically to situations results in feelings of guilt, shame, low self-worth, and false pride.

If Jenny responds with judgment, criticism, or blaming, she might say things about the situation that sound something like, "Those idiots! They don't have the slightest idea what they're doing." As you can imagine, calling the ticket sellers names is ineffective in improving the situation and likely will serve only to escalate Jenny's stress.

Resistance/Complaining Resistance is the mental process of wishing things were different than they are. The problem is that frequently things cannot be different than they are. Many things are completely out of our control and happen as they do. But resistance says that we wish things were otherwise. Resistance is demonstrated in saying to yourself, "I'm in this situation, but I wish I were somewhere else right now." But here *is* where you are, and this *is* what is happening. Wishing otherwise just adds to levels of stress. We can notice if we are resisting what is happening in several ways.

One obvious resistance factor is *anger*. When we are angry, we are saying that something is not happening according to our expectations. The subject of anger is treated more thoroughly in Chapter 8.

Another way to determine resistance is if we are bored or tired. *Boredom* is the emotion that results from thoughts of, "I wish this were happening differently." As an example, when we are bored while listening to someone, we are resisting what the person is saying or how he is saying it. We are wishing that he would speak in a different way or do something else.

Another way that we can tell when we are resisting something is by noticing how rapidly or slowly *time* seems to be moving. If we notice that time is moving slowly through an event, we probably are resisting it. When we are in a traffic jam and we are resisting it, the traffic seems to take forever to get where we are going.

Have you ever spent a few short minutes talking with another person and it seemed like the conversation would never end? Conversely, have you ever spent time talking with someone and before you knew it, several hours had passed? In the first instance, you were resisting the experience. You didn't want what was happening to be happening. In the second instance, you were completely allowing what was happening to happen.

If Jenny responds to the slow ticket line with resistance—if she says to herself that this line should be moving faster than it is (which isn't reality)—time will seem to drag by. Jenny's feelings of anger and stress will fester as a result.

Observation Instead of these negative ways of responding, more positive responses—responding above the line—are effective because they automatically lead to positive feelings of relaxation, well-being, calm, and inner peace. We are not always trained to respond in these ways, and we may lack role models who demonstrate this type of responding. If you watch television shows such as *Jerry Springer*, the way people respond to situations and circumstances is almost entirely below the line. Many people are taught, from an early age, to exchange blow for blow, to give others "what they deserve," to react negatively. Responding above the line involves a shift in awareness toward a conscious focus on choice rather than reacting by habit and conditioning.

A Taoist Perspective on Resisting

Chuang Tzu, one of the greatest of the Taoist writers, tells this witty story of what sometimes happens to a person who wishes things were different than they are.

***

There was a man who was so disturbed by the sight of his own shadow and so displeased with his own footsteps that he determined to get rid of both. The method he hit upon was to run away from them. So he got up and ran. But every time he put his foot down, there was another step, while his shadow kept up with him without the slightest difficulty. He attributed his failure to the fact that he was not running fast enough. So he ran faster and faster, without stopping, until he finally dropped dead. He failed to realize that if he merely stepped into the shade, his shadow would vanish, and if he sat down and stayed still, there would be no more footsteps.

Source: *The Way of Chuang Tzu*, by T. Merton (New York: New Directions Publishing Corp., 1965), p. 155.

The first positive response, observation, is the simple act of noticing something without adding anything. Our senses bring us data from the outside world, and we simply become aware. We might respond by saying something like, "Hmm . . ." or "I'm noticing or observing . . . (whatever my senses bring into my awareness)." We are taking in the information that presents itself. We are not adding anything more. This is how we function when we are being mindful, as you will learn in Chapter 7. Initially this may sound strange or ineffective. What is the value in spending our moments remarking on what we are noticing?

In our example, if Jenny is responding by observing, her thinking goes something like this, "Hmm, I'm noticing that this line isn't moving very fast and I might not arrive at my class on time." She does not add any emotion. She simply observes *what is*. With this attitude, Jenny is able to remain calm. The value of responding by simply observing has tremendous power in keeping us free of stress.

Discovery Discovery is based on observation and adds the additional component of learning, of seeking to understand—of discovery. When we respond in this way, we become like the artist, the poet, or the scientist. We observe what is happening, and we seek to find out what we can learn from it. We focus on how this can add to the enjoyment of our experience of the present moment rather than hinder or act as an obstacle. At this level of responding, we live in the questioning mode.

Taking this approach, Jenny would maintain an attitude of playful discovery that might sound like this: "I wonder what cool things I can notice about the other people who are in this line." "How many boys are in this line compared to girls?" "How many are blond, brunette, redheaded, or bald?" "What can I learn about this experience so next time I'm not waiting in a line making myself late for class?" "If I look up at the clouds, perhaps I can tell how long this rain will last." Imagine how much better standing in this line will be for Jenny if she has thoughts that are in the discovery mode of responding. This way of thinking will not generate stressful thoughts and emotions.

Allowance/Acceptance Allowance and acceptance occur when we emotionally embrace what is happening as the way things are and we are okay with them. We are essentially saying "yes" to *what is*. Acceptance says we allow and even embrace what is happening. Acceptance is realizing that what is happening is how it is and it isn't any other way—and that is okay.

In this mode, as Jenny stands in line, she notices the speed at which it is moving and accepts that this is how concert ticket lines sometimes move. In doing this, Jenny retains her equanimity and her ability to think rationally. When we respond to events and circumstances with acceptance, we experience the positive emotion of peacefulness naturally.

Consider the metaphor of a cork drifting down a stream. It is moving along easily as the current takes it gently down to some endpoint. On its way, it approaches a huge rock stationed in the middle of the river. What the cork *does not* do when it encounters this rock is to begin yelling at the rock for getting in the cork's way, thinking it should not be there (resistance). It also does not whine and moan because of its beliefs that rocks should not impede this cork's path (attachment/rightness). The cork also does not call the rock angry

> To acquire knowledge, one must study; but to acquire wisdom, one must observe.
> —*Marilyn vos Savant*

> When it rains, I let it.
> —*113-year-old man in response to a question about the secret of his longevity*

Happy Gratitude   Sonja Lyubomirsky, psychology professor at the University of California, Riverside and author of *The How of Happiness* says, "In my studies, I have found that gratitude leads to increased happiness, even in stressful times." Through research in which participants pen letters to people who have shown them kindness, Lyubomirsky discovered that people who express gratitude get happier because they feel more connected and more in control.

Source: "Living Thanksgiving—Science Shows Gratitude Can Have Wide-Ranging Health Benefits," by E. Schneider. *Energy Times*, November/December, 2008.

WHAT ELSE
CAN I DO?

Count Your Blessings   Start a gratitude journal. Make a list of things you are grateful for at least three times weekly. Robert Emmons PhD, psychology professor and author of *Thanks! How the New Science of Gratitude Can Make You Happier* encourages people to focus on "simple everyday pleasures, people in your life, personal strengths or talents, moments of natural beauty or gestures of kindness from others." Based on his research, Emmons has made some striking discoveries, most notable that people who keep gratitude journals are 25% happier than those who do not. If you look at the bright side of things and see all that is wonderful in your life, you won't be so tempted to concentrate on failure, disappointments and unmet expectations.

Source: "Living Thanksgiving—Science Shows Gratitude Can Have Wide-Ranging Health Benefits," by E. Schneider. *Energy Times*, November/December, 2008.

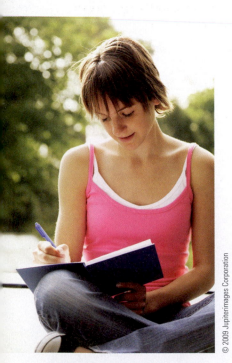

Keeping a gratitude journal can help you feel happier.

names for getting in its path (judgment). The cork simply follows the current that flows around the big rock and continues on its way (acceptance/allowance).

Gratitude   Gratitude means, after witnessing an event, showing appreciation or thankfulness for the opportunity to experience this moment. In this frame of mind, we see each moment as a gift with something in it that will help us grow, develop and enjoy life even more. The results of having an attitude of gratitude? Contentment, peace, and joy. These feelings are diametrically opposed to those below the line of stress—tension and anxiety. When we are thankful for what is happening, we need not bother about what is *not* happening. We appreciate, and that is sufficient for us in that moment.

Jenny might respond with appreciation by saying, "I'm sure glad I'm healthy enough to remain standing here as long as I am" or "I'm usually in such a hurry. This is an ideal time to slow down and enjoy not doing anything for a little while. What a great feeling!" If Jenny were to respond to the slow-moving ticket line in this way, how calm and serene she would feel! Gratitude, thankfulness, and appreciation are enormously powerful responses in creating and maintaining inner feelings of well-being and serenity.

When we respond above the line, we remain in greater control of our inner environment and, as a result, we prevent stress from happening. We are in charge of our inner life regardless of what is happening outside of us.

If we find ourselves in a situation that does require change or action, and we *can* do something to improve it, we should do what is necessary to make the appropriate change. For example, if a person walks past an alley and sees someone getting robbed, the response of taking action to change what is happening (calling 911 for example) is far more appropriate than going with the flow and accepting what is happening. This focus on how to respond does not imply an attitude that allows people or situations to get the best of us. Sometimes getting serious and taking positive action or being attached to a right way to do something can be the most valuable way of responding to a situation or event.

In the discussion here, we are dealing with situations over which we have no control. If you are sitting in a traffic jam, for example, you will want to choose effective ways of responding to remain calm and enjoy the experience more fully.

The way we respond to the events in life results in either an empowering proactive attitude or a disempowering, reactive attitude. Effectively incorporating these ideas into your daily activities takes practice. We typically are not conditioned to respond at the more effective levels. If we respond ineffectively, we create a chaotic inner environment that will activate the stress response. If we respond effectively, we will maintain inner peace. Realizing this, we understand that our inner experience is completely within our control.

Rational Emotive Behavior Therapy

Albert Ellis developed **rational emotive behavior therapy** (REBT) based on the premise that stress-related behaviors are initiated by self-defeating perceptions that can be changed. Viewing situations and events consciously gives a clearer look at events to see them in more effective and productive ways. REBT emphasizes replacing defeating, victimizing thoughts and feelings with more accurate and powerful thoughts. The result of this approach to how we think is a more peaceful and happy life. Individuals take responsibility for their emotions, resulting in the power to change and overcome unhealthy behaviors that interfere with the ability to function and enjoy life.

REBT is based on the following few simple, but profound, principles:

1. You are responsible for your own emotions and actions.
2. Your harmful emotions and dysfunctional behaviors are the product of your own irrational thinking.
3. You can learn more realistic views and, with practice, make them a part of you.
4. You will experience a deeper acceptance of yourself and greater satisfactions in life by developing a reality-based perspective.

According to REBT, difficulties are of two different types: **practical problems** and **emotional problems.** Practical problems relate to things that result in feelings of being treated unfairly by others or being in undesirable situations. These usually are experiences over which you have little, if any, control. Unfortunately, our human tendency is to get emotionally disturbed about these practical problems.

For example, you might be on an underground subway train that has stopped and the lights have dimmed considerably. You find yourself getting angry, frightened, annoyed, or overwhelmed at the situation in which you find yourself. This emotional disturbance unnecessarily creates a second order of problems—emotional suffering. According to REBT, these are disturbances over which you have total control.

Responding to Garbage

One day I was riding my road bike on a highway. After a pleasant ride of about 25 miles, I looked back to see a truck approaching very close to where I was riding on the road. As it got even closer, I sensed that it was slowing slightly. As the truck came beside me, I felt something hit my shoulder. The young boys in the truck had hurled their bag of fast-food garbage at me. I was surprised by the action, but the bag didn't hurt me at all. As I continued riding, I watched the boys in the car laughing and speeding ahead as fast as their old truck could go.

Now was my chance to respond. At this point, I could do absolutely nothing to affect these kids. Even on my best days, I couldn't possibly catch their speedy truck. I was left to myself to respond in whatever way I chose. Let's consider each of the following ways of responding to see how my thinking would affect my emotional state.

- *Attachment*: Young kids like those shouldn't be allowed to drive on this stretch of road. There should be a law against kids driving so close to bikers. (*anger, mistrust, stress*)
- *Judgment*. Those idiot, good-for-nothing kids are so rotten and worthless! (*false pride, stress*)
- *Resistance/Complaining*. I wish those kids weren't riding on this road. It's too narrow anyway. Why did they choose to ride here today and throw their garbage at me? (*frustration, anger, resentment, stress*)
- *Observance*. Hmm—I noticed those boys threw something out of the truck, and it happened to hit me. I noticed they kept right on going without bothering to pick it up. (*calmness*)
- *Discovery*. I wonder where those boys ate lunch today. Based on the bag, it looks like a burger and fries. If I would have hit my brakes really hard just as I saw the bag coming, I wonder by how far the bag would have missed me. (*curiosity, growth*)
- *Acceptance*. Those kids were just trying to having some fun. And I'm not hurt. I can fully accept them for being how they are. They're just doing what kids do. I probably did something like that when I was younger. Soon enough, they will learn from their actions what brings joy and what brings pain. I'm fine with that. (*peace, freedom, relaxation*)
- *Gratitude*. I'm so grateful that I didn't get hurt and that I have the good health to be out on my bike riding on this beautiful day. I'm riding a great bike, and I get to enjoy riding on such nice roads. Sure, odd things happen, but I appreciate being able to have odd things happen to me in the first place so I can learn to be more in control of my thinking. (*joy, happiness, freedom*)

In place of this situation, we could substitute any other event and we will get the same opportunity to choose—and the same resulting emotional states.

—MO

REBT Guidelines You begin taking control, and thereby minimizing emotional suffering, by following these guidelines:

1. *Take responsibility for your emotional upsets and distress.* Only you can upset yourself about events. The events themselves, no matter how undesirable, can never upset you. They do not have this power. Recognize that neither another person nor an adverse circumstance can ever disturb you. Only you can. Others can cause you physical pain—by hitting you over the head with a tennis racquet, for example—but you create your own emotional suffering, or self-defeating behavioral patterns, about what others do or say.
2. *Identify your "musts."* Once you admit that you alone alter your own emotions and actions, determine precisely how to alter them. The reason usually lies in one of the three core "musts":
   - Must #1 is a *demand on you*: "I *must* do well and get approval or else I'm worthless." This demand causes anxiety, depression, and lack of assertiveness.
   - Must #2 is a *demand on others*: "You *must* treat me reasonably, considerately, and lovingly or else you're no good." This demand leads to resentment, anger, hostility, and violence.

- Must #3 is *a demand on situations*: "Life *must* be fair, easy, and hassle-free or else it is awful." This thinking is associated with hopelessness, procrastination, and addictions.

  Determine what you are demanding of yourself, of other people in your life, or of your life's circumstances. Once you have figured out the "must" behind your emotion, you are able to move forward and effectively reduce your distress.

3. *Determine the reality of your "musts."* The only way you will remain disturbed about difficulties is by persistently agreeing with one of these three "musts." Once you have come to a conclusion about what "must" you are demanding, you can confront and question your demands. Begin by asking yourself: "What is the evidence for my *must?*" "How is it true?" "Where is it etched in stone?" And then by seeing: "There is no evidence." "My *must* is entirely false." "It is not carved indelibly anywhere." Make your view *must-free*, and your emotions will heal.

4. *Upgrade your "musts" to preferences.* Now you proceed with your thoughts based on preferences:
   - Preference #1: "I strongly *prefer* to do well and get approval, but if I fail, I will accept myself fully."
   - Preference #2: "I strongly *prefer* that you treat me reasonably, kindly, and lovingly, but because I do not run the universe and it is a part of your human nature to err, I cannot control you."
   - Preference #3: "I strongly *prefer* that life be fair, easy, and hassle-free, and it's frustrating that it isn't, but I can bear frustration and still enjoy life considerably."

Rational emotive behavior therapy provides for conscious, controlled thinking. This cognitive restructuring can give you the tools you need to dispute negative thoughts at the moment they occur.

ABCDE Technique   The **ABCDE technique** is a simple way of remembering the REBT mental process. Dr. Ellis devised this method of coping with anxiety, which consists of examining irrational beliefs.[5] The technique involves first examining irrational beliefs that make us anxious, then changing those beliefs and envisioning more positive consequences of our actions. The ABCDE technique consists of the following steps:

A	=	Activating event (identify the stressor)
B	=	Belief system (identify rational and irrational beliefs)
C	=	Consequences (mental, physical, behavioral)
D	=	Dispute irrational beliefs
E	=	Effect (change consequences)

When an activating event (A) occurs, it can cause a reaction or consequence (C) in a person. After careful examination, however, we may find that A did not actually cause C. What really caused C to happen was the person's belief system (B). Following are a couple of examples to demonstrate how this works.

A person performs poorly on a test. That event is A, what actually happened. This fact might activate the belief system that sounds something like, "I really did poorly on that test. That is just horrible! *I always* do that. I'm really incompetent at everything I do. I'll never succeed. I'm worthless." The emotional result of thinking this way might include anxiety, loss of self-esteem, and even depression. We sometimes call this type of negative, irrational thinking *awfulizing* (which you learned about earlier in the chapter). This person is overreacting to the facts of the situation.

Consider another example in which a normal college student asks a girl out for a date and she turns him down (A). Irrational thinking based on a faulty belief system might sound like this: "I must not be good enough for her. Girls always turn me down. I'm such a loser." The emotional feelings (C) this person will experience may include anxiety, depression, and low self-esteem. This way of thinking might even lead to a vicious circle of additional events that reinforce this student's negative belief system about his inability to have a comfortable situation with the opposite sex. As a result, he may avoid asking another person out on a date or avoid social situations altogether.

This irrational way of thinking, however, can be fixed by learning to successfully dispute (D) the irrational thought. In rational thinking, the student who did poorly on the test could change her way of thinking to a more accurate series of thoughts, which sound something like this: "Boy, that test was rough! Everybody struggles occasionally on tests. The important thing is that I learn from today's experience. How can I improve my performance on the next test?" With these thoughts running through her head, she will feel powerful, assertive, and ready to continue pursuing her academic activities.

The young man who is turned down for the date might more accurately say these things to himself: "She must have a lot going on in her life. There are a lot of other girls who would be happy to spend some time with me. Everyone gets turned down occasionally. It's no big deal." He will be confident enough to find another person to go on a date and will feel much better about himself. He will feel more courageous, confident, and self-assured with these thoughts foremost in his mind.

Once we dispute (D) the irrational belief, we are free to enjoy the positive psychological effects (E) of the more rational belief. By reinforcing realistic, self-benefiting beliefs, you can eliminate your emotional and behavioral problems in the present and avoid future problems of that sort. In the process, you'll experience far less stress.

Conclusion

How we think matters! When we find ourselves under stress, our first reaction is often to look outside ourselves for something or someone to blame. However, as you have learned in this chapter, stress is not created by external events; it is created within us by our own thoughts. Thoughts give you the power to control experiences. Once you understand this idea, you can move on to transcend your sense of victimization and reach a place of control and empowerment.

Managing our self-talk, stopping negative thoughts, and going with the flow are powerful mental tools to help us prevent the stress response from activating. These tools help you tap into the power you already have to be a more centered, confident person. Awareness of our levels of responding, rational emotive behavior therapy, and other cognitive techniques introduced in this chapter can help you take control of your thoughts and help you experience inner peace.

> The basic difference between an ordinary man and a warrior is that a warrior takes everything as a challenge, while an ordinary man takes everything as a blessing or a curse.
> —Carlos Castaneda

LAB

6.1 A Day Above the Line

ACTIVITY Spend an entire day focusing on the principle of present moment acceptance and responding to every situation in ways that are above the bold line. Refer to the Levels of Responding Chart in this chapter. Do this activity on a busy day when you will have many opportunities to select your response.

Amidst all your other activities of the day, keep in mind a constant awareness of the more effective ways of responding to people, situations, and experiences (noticing, discovering, accepting/allowing, and appreciating). Work to avoid responding to situations ineffectively (judging, criticizing, being right, complaining, and resisting). Use some type of cue to remind yourself throughout the day to respond effectively. This may be a rubber band on your wrist, a particular shirt, or some other unique reminder. As you start your day, this cue also helps you prepare to purposefully start the activity.

At the end of the day, write about your experience. Include:

1. Each opportunity you had to choose between effective and ineffective responding.
2. Several examples of "Above the Line" choices that you deliberately made.
3. What you noticed about your sense of inner peace, harmony and happiness.
4. Any additional challenges and insights that you had about yourself while you focused on responding more effectively.

6.2 Choosing to Respond More Effectively

ACTIVITY As an alternative to Lab 6.1, reflect on a past situation. The purpose of this activity is to give you a clearer view of how you can choose to respond to situations in more effective, less stressful ways. Refer to the Levels of Responding Chart in this chapter.

Recall a situation in which you recently found yourself experiencing some version of one of the following emotions: Anger, frustration, boredom, guilt or some other unpleasant emotion. Notice which of the ways listed in the Levels of Responding Chart describe how you were responding to what was happening, for example, getting angry because things weren't happening the way you thought they should be happening.

Take a moment and relive the situation or event and describe how you could have responded differently based on the effective ways of responding on the chart. Describe what might have happened had you responded in the above-the-line ways and how you would have felt emotionally as a result of responding more effectively.

Go through each way that you could respond to that situation and how you could see the situation differently by reconstructing your thoughts according to the table below:

Ways We Respond to Events	Sounds Like (what we say to ourselves)	What you might say to yourself
Gratitude	I appreciate… I'm thankful for…	
Allowance/Acceptance	It's okay… I embrace… I can live with this… I can go with the flow	
Discovery	I wonder… What would happen if…? What can I learn from this?	
Observation	I am noticing…	
Resistance/Complaining	I wish things were different (complaining)	
Judgment/Criticism/Blaming	This is really a /He is really a (insert a negative noun)…	
Attachment/Rightness	This *must* be a certain way… Use words like must, have to, need to, should have	

Key Points

- Psychologist Albert Ellis identified 12 irrational ideas, called "thinking errors," which can create and add to stress.
- Several cognitive techniques, among them positive self-talk, thought-stopping, power language, and going with the flow, can be used to help prevent and reduce stress.
- Conditioned-response theory proposes that when things happen in our environment, we are conditioned to respond in certain ways.
- Conscious choice gives us the capacity to choose a healthy response to stressful events.

- The levels of responding concept explains the range of responses, both effective and ineffective.
- Rational emotive behavior therapy (REBT) is based on the premise that stress-related behaviors are initiated by self-defeating perceptions that can be changed.
- A method of coping with anxiety that consists of examining irrational beliefs is called the ABCDE Technique.

Key Terms

pessimism	learned optimism	levels of responding
awfulizing	optimists	rational emotive behavior
cognitive therapy	pessimists	therapy
self-talk	power language	practical problems
stream of consciousness	going with the flow	emotional problems
thought-stopping	conditioned–response theory	ABCDE technique

Discussion Time For Critical Thinking/Discussion Questions, please visit this book's Premium Website.

Notes

1. *Learned Optimism,* by M. Seligman (New York: Knopf, 1991).
2. *Awaken the Giant Within: How To Take Immediate Control of Your Mental, Emotional, Physical and Financial Destiny,* by A. Robbins (New York: Summit Books, 1991), p. 211.
3. *Man's Search for Meaning,* by V. E. Frankl (New York: Simon & Schuster, 1963), pp. 103–104.
4. *As a Man Thinketh,* by J. Allen, originally self-published 1900; available online at http://www.asamanthinketh.net/
5. *A Guide to Rational Living,* by A. Ellis and R. Harper (North Hollywood, CA: Melvin Powers, Wilshire Book Co., 1975).

7 Mindfulness

■ I think of mindfulness as living in the moment. If I do this, how can I plan for the future and accomplish my goals? ■ How does mindfulness relate to meditation? ■ Does mindfulness mean living recklessly for the moment?

Study of this chapter will enable you to:

1. Explain the relationship between mindfulness and reality.
2. Distinguish between mindfulness and mindlessness.
3. List the qualities of mindfulness.
4. Explain the benefits of mindfulness.
5. Experience mindfulness as a tool to unclutter the mind and bring about mental tranquility.

© Caterina Bernardi/zefa/CORBIS

Ten thousand flowers in spring,

The moon in autumn,

A cool breeze in summer,

Snow in the winter,

If your mind is not clouded by unnecessary things,

This is the best season of your life.

—Wu-men, 12th-century Chinese scholar

Mindfulness in Action

Trina

When students were discussing what they had learned from their assignment on mindfulness, Trina made a profound statement: "I looked everywhere for what was missing in my life, and I found out it was me." She went on to explain that she came to realize that she was almost never "in the moment." She was missing out on the moments of life because her mind was somewhere else—worrying about something that might happen or what she had to do or feeling guilty about something she had done in the past. Mostly, her mind was so full of thoughts of what she had to get done that she rarely focused on the moment at hand. Through deliberately applying the qualities of mindfulness to her daily life, Trina was able to find what was missing—herself.

* * *

Ryan

Ryan shared his story about how he was able to incorporate mindfulness into his daily life:

I was first introduced to the idea of mindfulness in my stress-management class. One of our assignments was to actually try being mindful during some activity of our choice. I was feeling a lot of frustration and stress about the amount of time I spent studying for my algebra class. I was especially stressed because even though I spent lots of time studying for this class, I wasn't getting good grades on the tests. So I decided to give it a try and be mindful while I studied.

It helped that I went to the library and found a quiet study area. I started by closing my eyes and taking a couple of deep breaths. I focused on being present in the moment—right here, right now. I opened my book and concentrated on what I was reading. I even tried to picture the important formulas like they were on a movie screen and I was watching them. When thoughts about things other than algebra entered my mind—and they did—I noted the thought and then returned my focus to algebra.

After lots of practice, this has gotten easier. One of the things I learned as I think back is that even though I was spending much more time studying before I used mindful studying, I wasn't really paying attention. I would study at home, often with my music playing, and with constant interruptions. I would get so frustrated. I now accomplish more in a couple of hours of mindful studying than what used to take me most of a day. I feel much less stressed because I feel like the time I spend studying really matters. Plus I'm doing better in school and have more time to do other things I want to do.

* * *

Both Trina and Ryan learned that stress can be prevented and life can be improved by conscious, present-moment awareness and a mindful approach to living.

Mindfulness

Two monks were walking through the woods when they came upon a woman standing by a stream. "Please, sir, would you kindly help me across the stream?" she asked. One monk silently nodded his head, hoisted the woman on his back, and walked across the stream with her. She bowed, thanked him, and walked on. The two monks watched her walk out of sight and then continued on their journey. Many miles and hours later the monk who had not carried the woman said, "I've been thinking, how could you have touched that woman? You know our order frowns on touching women." The other monk smiled and said, "I put her down a long time ago. Why are you still carrying her?"

The Nature of Reality

We begin our discussion about mindfulness with this question: What is reality? Or to ask it a slightly different way, what is real? You might say that reality includes our thoughts, our dreams, our desires, our imaginations, God, and the physical stuff that surrounds us,

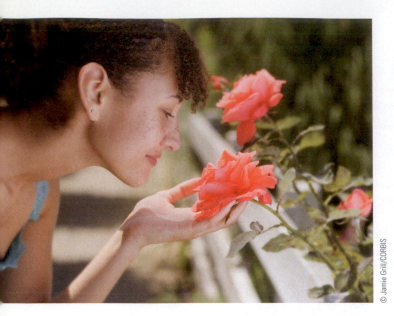

Take time to stop and smell the roses. It is good for your health.

A simple definition of **reality,** which we will use for the purposes of this text, is this: Reality is *what is.* Reality is *what is happening.* **Unreality,** then, is what is not (happening). Some people call unreality illusion.

How do we determine what reality is? Put another way, how do we know what is happening? The answer is found in two places.

The first place to locate reality is through our senses. The sounds we hear are reality. We see a bird flying and clouds floating behind the bird. This view of what we are seeing is reality. When we touch the top of the table with our hand, the sensation of touch tells us of the hardness of the table. We hear a dog barking, or we smell chocolate chip cookies baking in the kitchen. The word that clues us in to reality is *experience.* What we are experiencing is reality. The book you are reading right now is reality.

A second place we can look to find out *what is happening* is internally. Many sensations are happening right now within us. Sensations such as balance, equilibrium, and physiological processes such as digestion, our heart beating, and breathing, all are examples of our internal experience.

The things that are *not* reality are the things we make up, our judgments, our opinions, or ideas *about* our experience. For example, we see a car driving at a certain speed in front of us. That is reality. Our senses of sight and hearing and the inner sensation of movement through space capture the information about what is happening in our environment.

Ideas that we create in our minds about this situation are not reality. These thoughts are our own creations about the situation. We might think that the slow-driving person ahead of us is old and incapable of driving properly, that this person is keeping us from getting to where we want to go at a faster pace, and that old people should not be on the road in the first place. These are thoughts we make up about the situation, not the reality of what *is happening.*

The Here and Now

The next question is not difficult but it is one whose answer we often forget, which can lead to much stress: Where are you right now? The only correct answer to this question is *here.* Where are you *not* right now? The only correct answer is *everywhere else.* How do you know you are *here*? Because your senses, your experience, verify that this is the case. Right here is reality.

At what point in time are you? The only correct answer to this question is—*now.* At what point in time are you *not*? The correct answer to this question is your *future* and your *past.* This moment right now is reality.

Every moment of our life, we are in our here and now. That is all life is for each of us—successive present moments of *here-and-now* experiences. It will never be different for anyone. This is reality. You cannot transport yourself into your past or your future. You also cannot possibly be somewhere else than right *here.* Certainly, you may do so in your mind, but based on our discussion of reality, that is your creation, something you are making up.

Alan Watts spoke of this here and now concept this way:

> Take it that you are not going anywhere but here, and that there never was, is, or will be any other time than now. Simply be aware of what actually is without giving it names and without judging it, for you are now feeling out reality itself instead of ideas and opinions about it.[1]

So what does all of this have to do with managing stress?

Wherever you go,
there you are.
—*Jon Kabat-Zinn*

© Jamie Grill/CORBIS

Understanding Mindfulness

Understanding the concept of mindfulness will help us understand how to become more focused on the present moment and, as a result, more relaxed and peaceful. **Mindfulness** is commonly defined as the state of being attentive to and aware of what is taking place in the present.[2] Mindfulness is the process of cultivating appreciation for the fullness of each moment we are alive. It is present-moment awareness. When we are mindful, we are paying attention, on purpose, non-judgmentally. It is an acceptance of present-moment reality. It is waking up to the fact that our lives unfold only in moments.

But why is it so important to devote an entire chapter to our ability to focus on the present moment? Why do we need to consider the fact that our experience of here and now is our only reality? Because *there is no stress in the present moment.* When our attention is focusing directly on this here-and-now moment, there is no threat, and the result is no stress. But we aren't trained to think in this way. This chapter will finally teach you how.

Jon Kabat-Zinn, founder and director of the Stress Reduction Clinic at the University of Massachusetts Medical Center, described mindfulness as a conscious discipline that can be explained as the intentional cultivation of non-judgmental moment-to-moment awareness.[3] Mindfulness may be thought of not so much as a technique but as a way of life. Mindfulness approaches are not considered relaxation techniques but, rather, a form of mental training to reduce vulnerability to reactive modes of thinking that heighten stress and emotional distress.[4] The result is that stress can be prevented through conscious living.

Mindfulness is based on the ancient contemplative tradition called **vipassana,** which means "seeing clearly." Mindfulness is the process of learning how to be fully present in all experiences while being less judgmental and reactive. Mindfulness practices include self-reflection, acceptance, self-care, and opening to difficulties without avoidance. Mindfulness suggests being present in the here and now, attending to and listening for whatever arises, and remaining focused and relaxed.[5]

We can begin to understand mindfulness with an example of how we function mentally when we are driving our car and notice that a police officer is driving immediately behind us. His lights are not flashing to pull us over. He is just following us. When we drive with this level of alertness, we are completely aware of everything that is going on. We are aware of the distance between our car and the one in front of us. We are aware of how fast we are driving. We are totally aware of aspects of driving such as how soon before the intersection we will have to turn on the signal to indicate that we are making a turn, how quickly we shift lanes, if our lights are on, and slowing down to the proper pace. In essence, we are completely tuned in to our immediate environment.

> Man looks without seeing, listens without hearing, touches without feeling, eats without tasting, moves without physical awareness, inhales without awareness of odour or fragrance and talks without thinking.
>
> *—Leonardo da Vinci*

Mindlessness, by contrast, is demonstrated when we are driving along a stretch of road, and before we realize it, we have traveled 15 miles and have no idea about the stretch of road we have just driven. We suddenly catch ourselves and marvel that we didn't have an accident for failing to pay attention. **Mindlessness** occurs when our thoughts are not in the present moment and when we tune out what is happening. Our mental focus is on times and places other than the here and now. We ignore the present moment because our attention is focused elsewhere. This is what Trina was talking about in our opening vignette when she said, "I looked everywhere for what was missing in my life and I found out it was me."

Qualities of Mindfulness

The focus of mindfulness is on the experience. Professor Stefan Schmidt, of the University of Freiburg in Germany, identified attitudinal qualities that facilitate mindfulness, including *beginner's mind, non-judging, acceptance, non-attachment*, and *non-striving*.[6] These five qualities can be cultivated as you develop a more mindful approach to life.

Beginner's Mind: Thinking Like a Child Mindfulness entails openness in how we observe experiences. Rather than observing experiences through the filter

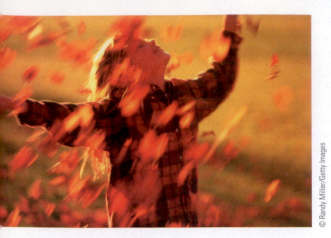

© Randy Miller/Getty Images

Celebrating life!

of our beliefs, assumptions, expectations, and desires, mindfulness involves seeing things "as if for the first time," a quality often referred to as "beginner's mind."[7] It is an observation full of curiosity, interest, and joy.

We can regain the quality of beginner's mind. We say "regain" because this is how young children operate. They don't concern themselves with "what if" and "if only." Consider how silly it would be if a 1-year-old who is learning how to walk starts questioning the notion that walking has advantages over crawling. She starts thinking things such as, "I don't know if I should try this, because if I learn to walk, I'll be much more likely to fall down the stairs, and that will really hurt." Or equally as silly would be this thought, "I fell when I tried walking last time. I'm a rotten walker because last time I tried it, I fell flat on my behind. I might as well give up because I'll never be able to walk." This, fortunately, is not how children think. They look at the present moment, see what's in it, and experience it fully.

Mary Maisey-Ireland shares this story:

She runs barefoot around the yard, arms outspread, hair streaming behind her, face upturned to the rain. I am witnessing radiant, unadulterated joy, completely expressed by my 9-year-old daughter.

I stand transfixed at the kitchen window, soapy plate in my hands, moved by her happiness. She celebrates wind, too. And sunsets and moonrises and flowers and kittens and, well, life.[8]

Gerald Jampolsky explains how our best model for living mindfully is a child:

I have often thought that we have much to learn from infants. They have not yet adapted to the concept of linear time with a past, present, and future. They relate only to the immediate present, to right now. . . . As we become older, we tend to accept the adult values which emphasize projecting past learning into the present and anticipated future. It is difficult for most of us to have even the slightest question about the validity of our past–present–future concepts. We believe that the past will continue to repeat itself in the present and future without the possibility of change. Consequently, we believe we are living in a fearful world where, sooner or later, there will be suffering, frustrations, conflict, depression, and illness.[9]

Jampolsky contends that we can choose to experience this instant as the only time there is, and live in a reality of *now*.

Non-Judging The quality of non-judging represents straightforward observation. It means that one should not infer from what one is observing, and should not evaluate the observation in any way. One should just observe with calmness the immediate experiences as they are.

WHAT ELSE

CAN I DO?

Become Like a Child Our best model for living a low-stress life would probably be that of a young child. Think of how a child operates in a typical day. His thoughts are always on what is happening right now or what is coming up next. He does not worry about whether he will be able to pass a bicycle-riding test later in the day. He isn't concerned about what other people are thinking about the clothes he is wearing. He isn't thinking of all the things that he might have done to his friends yesterday that might have made them think about him in a certain way. He accepts everyone as they are. He may have emotional upsets, but he gets over them. He doesn't let the minor disturbance of yesterday get in the way of the fun he will have the next time he plays with his friend, the same one who upset him yesterday. He doesn't have any need to be more powerful or more important than anyone else.

Here are some more characteristics that are typical of being like a child:

Risk taker
Adventurer
Fun lover
Humorous
Playful
Creative
Curious
Enjoys being loved
Teachable
Trusting
Vulnerable
Likes most things about life
Free from guilt
Free from worry
Lives now, rather than in the past
    or the future
Realizes that the moments between
    the events are just as important as
    the events themselves

Not threatened by the unknown
Independent
Enjoys privacy
Absence of approval seeking
Knows how to laugh
Accepts himself and others
Enjoys and appreciates the natural world
Doesn't engage in useless fighting
Honest; doesn't blame others
Little concern with order, organization,
    or systems
High energy levels
Not afraid to fail
Lack of defensiveness
Views all people as human, and places
    no one above or below himself
    in importance.

It is not likely that you will immediately incorporate all of these traits into your own nature. But by considering each one individually, and by thinking of each trait frequently, little by little, you can develop the qualities that will help you live more freely, more happily, and more contentedly, like a child. For example, when you find yourself in situations where you could choose being a risk taker over being too conservative, if it is appropriate, choose to take the risk.

Source for the above list: *Your Erroneous Zones*, by W. Dyer (New York: Avon Books, 1976).

We can become more mindful by eliminating our need to judge. When we simply observe, without adding the mental analysis of the situation, we free ourselves to see things more accurately. As we discussed in Chapter 6, we never can judge another person truly accurately. Because we cannot do this, we might as well release our need to judge. We do this by simply staying in an observational state of mind without judgment or expectations.

This is called **detached observation.** Thoughts enter consciousness objectively and without judgment or emotion. A detached and non-evaluative observation is not cold-hearted. Mindful awareness is warm and accepting. Think of it like the mind being a wide movie screen with your thoughts projected on the screen. You observe them without judgment or analysis. The result is often increased awareness.

Awareness is not limited to any one focal point, as is common in many forms of meditation, but, rather, encompasses mind, body, environment, and whatever arises in the field of awareness. The object of focus is not the point. Instead, it is the quality of awareness of what passes through the individual's consciousness. The outcome is a way to experience life directly, without it being filtered through beliefs, expectations, and preconceptions.

Imagine calling someone on the phone. This person is having a particularly rough day. You ask her if she would like to join you for lunch. She snaps back angrily, letting you know she doesn't have time for you, or for lunch. In an instant you notice yourself becoming angry and judgmental about her and the rude way she treated you. The reality of this situation (what is happening) is that she said some words to you about not going to eat lunch with you. All the misguided things you conclude about her, all the judgments you create about her, are what you make up but *are not what is happening.* Her anger had nothing to do with you, but your mind races with all of the thoughts about her and your apparently faltering relationship. Letting go and not judging means simply dropping the need to have all of those unnecessary thoughts racing through your mind.

Acceptance of What Is Happening
Non-judging is the basis for accepting what is happening. Acceptance is holistic and unconditional. Acceptance means we acknowledge experiences as they are. To bring our focus more into the present, we can simply turn off the mind chatter that is racing through our minds of what is not happening—about the future and the past, about thinking we always have to be somewhere else, about our opinions, judgments, and things we make up about an event. It is attending to and allowing what is happening now.

Ron Smotherman commented on the usefulness of mindfulness in saying:

> All the confusion clears up when we realize that there is only one "time" and that time is *now.* If you are willing to experience the truth that it is right now, your "problems" about the past and future will clear up. Why? Because there is no past or future; there is only right now. If you are stuck in what you call the "past," you are stuck right now. If you spend your time daydreaming about the "future," you do that process right now. You can't even go to these places called the "past" and the "future." They are not real.[10]

We also can simply attend to *what is* with all of our senses. It is almost a passive observing of what is happening around you. We observe, we notice, we watch, we become sensory-aware of what is happening in our environment. When we notice ourselves getting wrapped up in our thoughts, we simply step back and let the moments unfold, observing and not trying to change anything. We allow ourselves to be content, to be sufficient with this moment.

Non-Attachment
The quality of non-attachment refers to the non-identification with the object of our attention. It means not getting carried away with thoughts or feelings and not holding onto experiences. The observation is detached from the object.

This important aspect of mindfulness involves resisting the need to cling emotionally to anything—ideas, events, or periods of time to which we release our attachment. We give up the need for things to be a certain way. We let things be as they are.

A Culture of Doing

Physician William Thomas says that simple observation has led him to regard life as the dynamic and unfolding interplay between the state of "being" and the state of "doing." He explains how, as a function of culture and shared expectations, we move through transitions starting with infants, who are the purest form of being. Adolescence is a transition to adulthood, from the joyfulness of play to a preference for *doing* over *being*. In adulthood the emphasis on *doing* over *being* increases. One of the first questions adults ask when they meet is "What do you do?"

Thomas says, "Elderhood brings us full circle to a life that favors being over doing. This is a gift of great value.

Watching older and younger people together, you get the sense of a secret collusion that excludes adults. I remember visiting a nursing home that also had a child daycare center. A group of older people and children were painting flowerpots when the adult overseer announced that time was up. All but one of the children trooped out of the room. Andrew, who was curled up in an elder's lap, wouldn't move. As he was being prodded to leave, I heard him say, 'I want to be with Frank.' The time they were spending together soothed them both. The adults could not be expected to understand."

Source: *The Search for Being*, by W. Thomas, *AARP Bulletin*, Nov. 2004, pp. 30–31.

Author Anecdote Here and Now I enjoy spending time with my son on the deck of our house. He looks up into the sky and sees the clouds come to life with shapes of all the animals in the zoo. As he does this, I catch myself thinking of so many other things that aren't happening. I stop and just look with him. It is a freeing feeling to simply observe and accept what is happening.

—MO

Author Anecdote Peace in the Moment This concept of being mindful hit me with such power on one occasion that it changed my entire outlook on life. I was in the middle of work on my bachelor's degree and was preparing to take a major test for one of my classes. Much of my grade for the class, and ultimately for my succeeding in that major, depended on this test. I studied like a madman for this test. I thought I knew all I needed to know.

The day came to take the test. I parked my car and walked to the testing center. Talk about stress—300 people in a large room all doing nothing but taking tests! I gave the person my ID card. I got my test and Scantron answer sheet and found a little desk, where I would spend the next few hours. It was a tough test, but I thought I knew the material. Finally I finished and turned in my completed test. I waited a few minutes, then got my results.

Sheer anger, horror, regret, and anguish all hit me at once as I saw that I had gotten a "D" on this test. "How could this professor have been so evil?" "I can't stay in the major with a 'D' hanging over me!" "What am I going to do now?" These and a multitude of similar-sounding questions and derogatory remarks flew through my head like a river gushing down a steep mountain.

As I was walking back to my car in this sour state, I happened to look up. It was late October and the trees were changing colors. Off in the distance, to the west, the sun was getting ready to set and its reflection was bouncing off the large lake that rested on the other side of the city. Looking the other way, to the east, the enormous mountains reflected the hues of the setting sun in a way that made them look flaming reddish-gold. Nature offered me an extremely spectacular sight that afternoon.

In that moment I caught myself in my tirade of unpleasant thoughts. It occurred to me that I had a choice. I could continue to work myself into a frenzy over this test, which was over, and my now-uncertain future, or I could stop and watch this beautiful scene of dazzling colors, of trees, mountains, lake, sunset, and unparalleled beauty in front of me. Fortunately, I chose to sit on a bench and watch that wondrous event of day turning to evening. After it was complete, I walked to my car in a most peaceful state of mind. I was different. I somehow knew that everything would turn out fine.

—MO

Non-Striving The quality of non-striving is not goal-oriented. Non-striving implies giving up our need to try to change anything. We simply give ourselves permission to allow this moment to be exactly as it is, and allow all things to be exactly as they are. For just a moment, we are no longer doing, we are just being. We let go of wanting something else to happen. We let go of our need to *do* anything. We are content with *being*. It has been said that we might more aptly be called "human doings" rather than human beings, as most of us are more inclined to be *doing* than *being*.

We live in a culture that encourages doing. By nurturing mindfulness, we can learn to be better at being. Jon Kabat-Zinn said it best: "Mindfulness involves intentionally doing only one thing at a time and making sure I am here for it."[11]

Let's look at an example of how Kabat-Zinn's quote plays out in daily life. Every morning when you wake up, you take a 10-minute shower. During those 10 minutes you can be thinking about all you need to do that day. You can worry about the psych test you have to take, and you can feel guilty that you watched a movie last night instead of studying. Or you can spend that same 10 minutes being fully aware and present in the moment. You can enjoy the feel of warm water and the smell of the soap. You can listen to the water running and notice that you relax when the water hits your shoulder muscles. You can be grateful for hot and cold running water. Either way, you have spent 10 minutes of your life in the shower. The result can be that you are barely aware of the experience and come out feeling rushed and stressed, or you can come out having had a pleasant experience and feeling relaxed and refreshed.

Mindfulness as a Way of Being

Mindfulness can be practiced in all facets of daily life by bringing awareness to all activities and to all experiences. Mindfulness in daily life simply means to be present in all of one's activities and interactions.

Thich Nhat Hanh, a Vietnamese Buddhist monk, spoke about mindfulness when he said:

> If while washing dishes, we think only of the cup of tea that awaits us, thus hurrying to get the dishes out of the way as if they were a nuisance, then we are not "washing the dishes to wash the dishes." What's more, we are not alive during the time we are washing the dishes. In fact we are completely incapable of realizing the miracle of life while standing at the sink. If we can't wash the dishes, the chances are we won't be able to drink our tea either. While drinking the cup of tea, we will only be thinking of other things, barely aware of the cup in our hands. Thus we are sucked away into the future—and we are incapable of actually living one minute of life.[12]

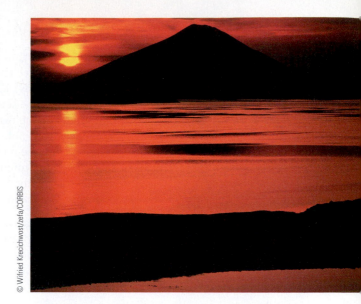

© Wilfried Krecichwost/zefa/CORBIS

Mindfulness brings peace to the moment. Don't miss the beautiful moments in life because your mind is elsewhere.

Thich Nhat Hanh was speaking of something so completely mundane, so seemingly mindless, to describe his experience of being mindful.

Washing dishes and riding a thrilling roller coaster and every other event in life all offer the opportunity to choose between living fully in the present and experiencing all that is available or focusing on the unrealities of our past and future, which increases our likelihood for avoidable stress. The choice is, once again, ours.

Ken Keyes spoke about this idea when he said:

> Serenity is the end—and serenity is also the means—by which you live effectively. By fully tuning in to the now moment in your life, you will discover that you always have enough to enjoy every moment of your life. The only reason you have not been happy every instant is that you have been dominating your consciousness with thoughts about something you don't have—or trying to hold on to something that you do have but which is no longer appropriate in the present flow of your life. Here and now is the key to the optimal interaction pattern between you and the people and things in the world around you.[13]

Author Anecdote California Screamin' Recently I was at Disneyland with my family. We went on a ride called "California Screamin'," which was a total blast of a ride. After our turn had ended and we were discussing how much fun we had, it occurred to me why the ride was so much fun. While we were zooming through the twists and turns, the high speeds and the upside-down loops, we had no focus on the future or the past. Our only awareness was of the exhilaration of that moment and what was happening here and now.

Imagine how silly it would have been to be zooming around on this ride, having the time of our lives, and at the same time worrying about whether we would find a parking spot when we went to our hotel, or which restaurant we would go to that evening, and if all of our kids would find something on the menu they would like to eat or if we would have to go somewhere else to please their appetites. Equally absurd would be a thought process that focused on the angry conversation I had with one of my daughters and how I should have been more considerate of her feelings, which led to my own character flaws as a father. If my mind were to go in either direction, I would miss the ride completely. With my thoughts wrapped up with images of future and past I certainly wouldn't be able to enjoy the thrill of the ride as I flew through its joyous speedy voyage.

—MO

When we live mindfully, focusing our attention on what is happening here and now, and allowing ourselves to be totally absorbed in the activity at hand, we become more effective and productive, whatever the task, be it skiing down a tricky ski slope or doing our best on a tough test. The extra mind chatter of future and past and the associated emotions of fear, worry, guilt, and anger seem to diminish. As we do this, in as many moments as possible, we begin to understand that there is no other moment in time or point in space but that which is happening here and now.

When we are operating mindfully, we become the witness to the events that are unfolding around us. We simply notice things as they are. The words we use when we are focusing on what is happening in this moment are, "I am noticing . . ." We then allow our senses to bring to our awareness whatever things, people, or situations they come into contact with.

Why Be Mindful?

Focusing on the moment helps to clear the mind of clutter. The mind juggles many thoughts, produced both internally (memories, worry) and externally (conversations, traffic, TV broadcasts), all of which compete for attention. This can lead to a frazzled attempt to concentrate on several thoughts at once. As these thoughts accumulate, our minds get cluttered, and the result is **sensory overload.** Sensory overload is like a blackboard filled to capacity with notes, scribbles, and information that is difficult to organize and understand. A cluttered mind becomes a stressed mind. Practicing mindfulness is like an eraser that cleans the mind's blackboard. Mindfulness unclutters the mind and brings about mental tranquility.[14]

Joseph Goldstein, founding teacher of Insight Meditation Society, says:

> Cultivating an active mindfulness of one's experience, moment to moment, is the path to awakening: taking a step, standing up, reaching for a door. When we're not mindful, different things happen. We can be going through the daily activities of life completely lost in thinking about the past or the future, about our hopes, our worries, our anxieties—without being present at all.[15]

Robert Pirsig said it this way in his book, *Zen and the Art of Motorcycle Maintenance:*

> Mountains should be climbed with as little effort as possible and without desire. The reality of your own nature should determine the speed. If you become restless, speed up. If you become winded, slow down. You climb the mountain in equilibrium between restlessness and exhaustion. Then, when you're no longer thinking ahead, each footstep isn't just a means to an end but a unique event in itself. This leaf has jagged edges. This rock looks loose. From this place the snow is less visible, even though closer. These are the things you should notice anyway. To live only for some future goal is shallow. It's the sides of the mountain that sustain life, not the top. Here's where things grow. But of course, without the top, you can't have any sides.[16]

We can apply anything we do the same way Pirsig describes climbing the mountain. He mentions that we need the top of the mountain—the goal toward which we are shooting. But the important part is where we are on the way to the goal. Every step along the way is where we are. If we leave the focus on each step, we miss what joy, beauty, and wonder it has for us to discover.

> No one imagines that a symphony is supposed to improve in quality as it goes along, or that the whole object of playing it is to reach the finale. The point of music is discovered in every moment of playing and listening to it. It is the same, I feel, with the greater part of our lives, and if we are unduly absorbed in improving them we may forget altogether to live them.
>
> —*Alan Watts*

Timothy Gallway wrote of the consequences of allowing ourselves to lose focus on the present moment. He was speaking of what happens during a tennis match, but his thoughts apply to most of the situations in which we find ourselves. These are the natural consequences of letting our minds dwell on future and past and elsewhere instead of here and now:

> The greatest lapses in concentration come when we allow our minds to project what is about to happen or to dwell on what has already happened. How easily the mind absorbs itself in the world of what-if's. "What if I lose this point?" it thinks; "then I'll be behind 5–3 on his serve. If I don't break his serve, then I'll have lost the first set and probably the match. I wonder what Martha will say when she hears I lost to George." At this point it is not uncommon for the mind to lapse into a little fantasy about Martha's reaction to hearing the news that you have lost to George. Meanwhile, back in the now, the score is still 3–4, 30–40, and you are barely aware that you are on the court; conscious energy you need to perform at your peak in the now has been leaking into an imagined future.[17]

One of the Jedi Masters in the *Star Wars* films clues us in to this notion of mindfulness. The trainee Obi-Wan is talking with his master Qui-Gon during a tense moment. Qui-Gon advises him about the mind and where to focus.

Obi-Wan: I have a bad feeling about this.

Qui-Gon: I don't sense anything.

Obi-Wan: It's not about the mission, Master, it's something . . . elsewhere . . . elusive.

Qui-Gon: Don't center on your anxiety, Obi-Wan. Keep your concentration here and now where it belongs.

Obi-Wan: Master Yoda says I should be mindful of the future.

Qui-Gon: But not at the expense of the moment. Be mindful. . . .

Benefits of Mindfulness

You learned in earlier chapters that, apart from those rare events of real danger, we live our present moments without any real threat or danger. The present moment usually involves no concern for stress. Stress occurs only when we allow our minds to think of things other than what is happening in our current experience. We focus our thoughts on potential future events, about the past, and about things that might be happening elsewhere. When we associate any kind of pain or discomfort with those thoughts of other times and places, we initiate the stress response as a natural reaction to the perception of a false emergency. Mindfulness turns off the stress response and, as a result, facilitates relaxation, reduces stress hormones, and boosts the immune system.

In a review of the studies investigating the physiological and psychological benefits of mindfulness focusing on Kabat-Zinn's mindfulness-based stress reduction program, author, educator, and researcher Dr. Lyn Freeman concluded:

> **FYI** Mindful Meditation **Mindfulness-based stress reduction**
> (MBSR), developed by Jon Kabat-Zinn and his colleagues at the University of Massachusetts, is a participatory wellness program based on mindfulness meditation. Participants in MBSR are taught how to work with aspects of awareness. MBSR has been used successfully to decrease a wide range of physical and psychological symptoms and increase clients' well-being. Studies with well populations link MBSR to improved physical, emotional, social, and mental health.
>
> **Sources:** "Evaluation of a Wellness-based Mindfulness Stress Reduction Intervention: A Controlled Trial," by K. Williams, M. Kolar, B. Reger, and J. Pearson, in *American Journal of Health Promotion* (2002), *15*, 422–432; "Student Nurse Health Promotion: Evaluation of a Mindfulness-based Stress Reduction (MBSR) Intervention," by L. Young, A. Bruce, L. Turner, & W. Linden, *Canadian Nurse* (2001) *97*(6), 23–26.

> MBSR may be effective for general stress reduction with nonclinical populations and for managing stress and mood disorders in patients with cancer. The evidence for benefits with clinical populations is suggestive, but more research is needed. On its face, MBSR appears to have great potential as an intervention in clinical and medical settings. Well-designed studies to support the uncontrolled findings must be performed before final conclusions can be drawn.[18]

Although the mechanism through which mindfulness enhances psychological and behavioral functioning remains unclear, research indicates that the enhancement of mindfulness is associated with a variety of well-being outcomes such as reductions in pain, anxiety, depression, binge eating, and stress.[19]

Research that examined the impact of MBSR on perceived stress, positive state of mind, pain, and mindfulness self-efficacy found that, at the conclusion of the MBSR intervention, the participants reported significantly reduced perceived stress and enhanced positive states of mind, compared to baseline results. The researchers concluded that the practice of mindfulness meditation may have helped study participants reduce their perception of stress, maintain non-judgmental awareness during different situations, and experience higher levels of positive states of mind.[20] A study that explored the relationship between MBSR and stress in college students found that college students who participated in the MBSR intervention reported an increased overall sense of control and utilization of an accepting or yielding mode of control in their lives, two variables that conceptually can be associated with reduced stress.[21]

Attending to the present moment simultaneously combines an internal focus and attention to the outer world. Incorporated in mindfulness practice are attitudes such as proceeding without judgment and expectation. Calming the mind and body allows us to gain insight and become aware of repetitive cognitions and feelings and habitual behaviors.[22]

RESEARCH HIGHLIGHT

Does Mindfulness Decrease Stress?

A pilot study of baccalaureate nursing students explored the effects of an 8-week mindfulness-based stress-reduction course on stress and empathy. The course was intended to provide students with tools to cope with personal and professional stress and to foster empathy through intrapersonal knowing.

Participation in the intervention significantly reduced students' anxiety. Favorable trends were observed in a number of stress dimensions including attitude, time pressure, and total stress. The authors concluded that being mindful may reduce anxiety and decrease tendencies to take on others' negative emotions. By attending to oneself in the present moment, and then expanding one's awareness to include the environment and other people, one paradoxically becomes less focused on oneself.

When students use mindfulness to quiet their minds, bodies, and emotions, and to observe what is present, they may be better able to reach out to distressed clients and respond with empathy without suffering emotional contagion.

Source: "Does Mindfulness Decrease Stress and Foster Empathy Among Nursing Students?" by A. Beddoe and S. Murphy, *Journal of Nursing Education*, (2004) 43(7).

Because mindfulness involves self-monitoring that helps increase awareness of what is going on from moment to moment, it has been used effectively in a number of stress reduction programs, including those at the University of Massachusetts, Harvard, and the University of Utah.[23]

Experiencing Mindfulness: Testing the Principle

Whenever our thoughts are not focused on what is happening in the present moment, we increase the chances of activating the stress response. When we turn our mental focus exclusively to what is happening in the present moment, the stress response turns off. Here is an exercise to demonstrate this:

Sit at a desk or table with a pen and piece of paper. Place your nondominant hand in a position where you can easily see it, and write down everything you notice about your hand. Using your senses of sight, touch, hearing, smell, and even taste, write down everything your senses tell you about your hand. Continue doing this for several minutes. When you think you have gotten everything, stop and observe again with all of your senses, and continue writing.

When students do this in the classroom, a couple of questions facilitate their learning this principle.

1. "How long do you think you could continue doing this and still come up with things to write?" Some reply that they could have gone on for much longer. Others claim that they got it all.
2. (mainly to those who say they wrote down everything about their hand) "How many of you wrote down that you have four fingers and a thumb?" Usually only about 5% to 10% say they noticed that specific detail. This seems so obvious, yet so few notice.

The point of this exercise is not to discover our hands again but, rather, to make an observation. This activity requires students to be totally focused on something here and now. When asked how much stress they felt as they were doing this activity, students report that they did not feel stressed.

This simple activity demonstrates a powerful principle: When we focus our attention on what is happening, when we keep our awareness on the here and now, what we get is an experience without stress. Because stress occurs when we are associating a future pain or discomfort with some event (worrying) and the need to prepare for it with the fight-or-flight response, when we think mindfully, we eliminate the possibility of stress turning on in the first place.

> You must live in the present, launch yourself on every wave, find your eternity in each moment. Fools stand on their island opportunities and look toward another land. There is no other land, there is no other life but this.
>
> —Henry David Thoreau

Focusing fully on the present moment is depicted in the Zen story of a monk who was being chased by two tigers. He came to the edge of a cliff. He looked back, and the tigers were almost upon him. Noticing a vine leading over the cliff, he quickly crawled over the edge and began to let himself down by the vine. Then, as he checked below, he saw two tigers waiting for him at the bottom of the cliff. He looked up and observed that two mice were gnawing away at the vine. Just then he saw a beautiful strawberry within arm's reach. He picked it and enjoyed the best-tasting strawberry in his whole life![24]

A Simple Mindful Exercise

This exercise invites you to experience how it feels to be mindful as it has been described to you in this chapter. Follow Stress Management Lab 7.1 at the end of the chapter to guide you in completing this activity. Take about 45 minutes to an hour to do this. *You are not to speak to anyone during this exercise!* You can do it either sitting or walking around, but make sure that you are entirely by yourself, with paper and pen in hand. Anywhere that you find yourself is an appropriate place to practice this exercise. The process is the same regardless of location.

During this time, you will focus entirely on mentally noticing, observing, and sensing what is (reality). You do this by stating to yourself again and again, "I am noticing . . ." or "I am aware of . . ." or "I am sensing. . . ." You finish each statement by describing whatever shows up in your present-moment experience.

Tune in both to your senses and to your internal activity (your thoughts as well as physiological and other internal activity) and discover whatever is presented to you. Notice the unfolding of everything before you. Use all your senses to experience mindfully what always has been around you but you may have never really noticed. Don't look for anything—just look. Move your attention back and forth from what your senses present to you to what is happening in your internal environment.

Externally notice everything you see, hear, touch, smell, and even taste. It might help to repeatedly ask, "What do I see *now*?" "What do I hear *now*?" "What do I smell *now*?" "What do I notice about the taste of what's *now* in my mouth?" "What information does my sense of touch bring to me *now*?" (This sense of touch includes every part of your body.)

Internally, observe things such as your breaths and your heart beating. Notice how gravity is keeping you where you are, and combine that with your ability to remain balanced as you move. Tune in to any feelings of physical pain or discomfort, and simply notice these feelings as a detached observer. Internally, you also can focus on the flowing of your thoughts as they come and go (thought-watching). Observe if these thoughts consist of memories, thoughts of the future (plans), and judgments or criticisms about anything. If you notice yourself criticizing or becoming judgmental of the exercise, simply treat those thoughts as you would everything else that you are observing.

Your single function during this time is to explore, watch, and observe. If you have ever just sat and watched a sunset or a sunrise and done nothing more than observe it happen, that gives you a hint of how this process feels.

Author Anecdote This Moment Is All You Have! Many people come to me wondering why they are so stressed. When I give them this exercise to do for 45 minutes to an hour, they write it off as something silly and stupid. They think they should be doing something seemingly worthwhile, something much more important.

My response is usually something like this:

"If you are to ever be at peace, you must come to accept, even embrace, what is happening here and now. And the only way to really experience the present moment is to stop analyzing, stop judging, stop trying to figure everything out, and just look. Just stop and observe. *To be fully present in this moment is to be at peace. To be out of this moment, thinking we are somewhere else, doing something else is precisely why we feel so much stress.* To say this is a silly exercise is to say life is silly. Look at your experience. There is never a time when it is not this moment, right here, right now."

"All of life consists of successive moments of the present. We always can choose what we want to see in this moment. To choose to be mindful instead of mindless is wisdom of the highest order. In my mind, it is one of the grand keys to becoming peaceful, contented, and stress-free. But it must be practiced. So practice, for the rest of your life, because that is all you have—this moment."

—*MO*

On your paper, write down everything you notice. Use as many pages as you need. If you begin to get bored or feel yourself resisting the process, stop and just be present with what is, notice what shows up, and then continue writing what you experience. At the conclusion of this activity, complete the questions found in Stress Management Lab 7.1.

Inner Mindfulness Meditation

Inner mindfulness meditation, also called thought-watching, focuses the mind internally rather than externally through the five senses. It differs from other forms of meditation, which suggest that thoughts and images be developed and created to either relax or create positive images (discussed in Chapter 20, Guided Imagery, and Chapter 21, Meditation). Thought-watching encourages non-judgmental observation of thoughts and images for heightened awareness. One's awareness is not limited to any one focal point but, instead, is allowed to view one's thoughts as one would view a movie that is happening inside one's own mind, from the perspective of a detached observer.

A mindful meditation proceeds this way: With the eyes closed, take a moment to tune in to your thoughts. Allow yourself to non-judgmentally watch your thoughts as they seem to come and go. As you keep your eyes closed, separate your awareness from the many thoughts that pop in and then leave your mind. Watch how some thoughts come into your awareness from nowhere, and then watch them expand and develop and lead to other thoughts. Watch these thoughts fade away as others replace them. See if you can differentiate thoughts that come and go. Notice that some thoughts focus on the past while others focus on the future. Watch for those thoughts that are making judgments about or are critical of anything.

Continue to watch your thoughts passively as if you were pulling up a chair and sitting next to your thoughts. If you notice judgmental thoughts about this process, passively observe those thoughts you are having as well. If your mind wanders and you lose your focus, gently bring it back. Practice this inner awareness of watching your thoughts for as long as you feel comfortable doing it. Start with 5 minutes, then increase it for as long as 20 minutes. When you are finished, take a little time returning to normal awareness.

Mindfulness Self-Efficacy

Mindfulness self-efficacy relates to the question, "How confident are you that your ability to maintain moment-to-moment non-judgmental awareness will keep you peaceful?" Think about situations that represent common sources of stress that can interfere with experiencing non-judgmental awareness. This might include frustration during goal-oriented activities (such as shopping, driving, and school); interpersonal problems and receiving criticism; and physical or health stressors (such as fatigue, pain, sleep, and hunger).

Stress Busting Behavior: Mindfulness in Daily Life

Mindfulness self-efficacy is your confidence in your ability to remain mindful and "in the moment" when you encounter potentially stress-producing events throughout the day. The moment-to-moment non-judgmental awareness can help keep you peaceful, but it takes practice. Check those situations where you feel confident in your ability to remain calm, non-judgmental, and in the moment.

☐ When you wait in the express line at the grocery store as the person in front of you has too many items

☐ When you are hungry and see yourself reaching for junk food

☐ When your teacher gives you an extra assignment due by the next class

☐ When you have a fight with a friend

☐ When you are caught in slow traffic

☐ When you are having trouble sleeping and have a big test the next day

☐ When your boss is telling you that you have done a task incorrectly

☐ When someone you love hurts you deeply

☐ When the person next to you in the restaurant is speaking loudly on his cell phone

Researchers Frederic Luskin and Mark Abramson[25] have developed a mindfulness self-efficacy scale to help you assess how confident you are that your ability to maintain non-judgmental awareness will keep you peaceful in situations. Rate your confidence in handling situations such as those presented in the Stress Busting Behavior feature.

Imagine yourself in these or other situations where you might experience stress. Think deliberately about how you can apply mindfulness to that situation by simply observing and being aware, rather than reacting in a stress-producing way. Imagine how different your experience with stress will be. As you practice mindfulness and apply it in your daily life, your self-efficacy will increase.

Ways to Practice Being More Mindful

The following are some suggestions that you may use in your quest to become more mindful.

- Choose an activity that you do in a less than mindful way, and focus on involving yourself completely in the experience. For example, practice eating mindfully. Absorb yourself in the sensations that are part of eating. Take in the smells, the tastes, the colors, the textures of the food. Spend time with each bite enjoying chewing—combining saliva with the food, feeling the food as it is transformed from large pieces to tiny sizes as you chew, feeling your food traveling from your mouth to your stomach.

  There are other opportunities to practice being fully present in the here and now; you may try commonplace activities such as taking a shower, driving, walking from one place to another, talking to a friend or a family member, or spending time in nature. Compare your experience of being mindful with how you normally operate in these common experiences and see if there is any difference in how you feel and how you relate with the things in your experience.

- Pay attention to things that are happening around you. Rather than thinking about so many things, try simply observing all that is showing up for you in your experience. Just watch, without concern for how you think things ought to be. Observe how things *are*. Do this with all your senses. Notice all the sounds, the different things to see, the textures to touch and feel, the varieties of smells. Be careful to avoid making judgments of what is unfolding before you.

- Consciously speak to yourself, saying something like: "In this moment I allow myself to be here now. I cannot be anywhere else right now, nor can I be in my past or future, so I might as well relax and enjoy what is happening, here and now."

- If you find yourself in a setting that is mundane or always the same, take time to rearrange things. For example, change the layout of your bedroom or other rooms in your house. Changing your scene from time to time allows you to see things in different ways and therefore become more interested and observant of them.

- Take "mindfulness breaks" in which you do nothing but engage yourself in a certain place and time. Nature is an excellent place to practice mindfulness breaks because it offers so much to tune into and experience. The variety, along with the slower pace of nature, adds to our sense of enjoying the moment more fully. Try an "emotional walk-about" in which you walk without caring where you are going and with no purpose in mind other than to be present in the moment.

- Try a new sport or hobby. Totally engage yourself in learning a new skill.

WHAT ELSE CAN I DO?

Regularly Have Fun When you are doing something you absolutely enjoy, your mind usually leaves the negative stressors behind. When we do our most preferred activities, we are more mindful and focused on the present moment. This focus promotes relaxation.

In our hectic days, we frequently forget to include time for those things that bring us the most joy. We tend to relegate those activities to far lesser importance, as they aren't urgent-action items. Much of the tension we build up at school or at the office can be released by participating in a pleasurable activity away from the source of tension. Including our favorite activities in our planning and goal-setting time assures that we spend moments effectively meeting our deepest needs.

Each of us has activities we would classify as hobbies. Our minds turn to the activity, and we are absorbed in it. Some hobbies require a certain amount of tension, such as sky-diving, river rafting, and rock climbing. This is the kind of stress, however, that causes us to participate at high levels. It is the eustress rather than distress. Other hobbies, such as crafts, art, and most sports, allow for mindful experiences.

- Change your normal routines slightly. Go to school a different way than you normally do. Bike rather than walk to a close destination. Shop at a different supermarket or drugstore. Eat at a restaurant where you have never eaten before. Each time you experience these out-of-the-ordinary occasions, you open yourself up to new and exciting ways of experiencing life.
- When you are involved in, or notice others engaging in, situations with heightened emotion, step back and simply become an observer rather than becoming emotionally involved in the incident. Become a passive observer, watching what is happening, rather than diving in and getting overly worked up. As you do this, notice that you are much more able to solve problems calmly rather than to create bigger problems by adding to the drama.

Planning for the Future

Mindfulness does *not* mean living with reckless abandon *for the moment*. It means living fully *in the moment*. A discussion on living in the moment and mindfulness frequently raises questions such as: What are we to do about planning, setting goals, and creating our own future? Where does that fall into this discussion on mindfulness?

Living mindfully does not mean that you ignore planning for the future or setting goals for what you want to accomplish. Planning for the future and creating goals entail bringing future moments into the present so you can apply appropriate control toward achieving them. This is a visionary process that constructively focuses on the future in this present moment. It is worthwhile and appropriate.

Conversely, worrying about a future event and directing our attention to the potentially painful outcomes of a future event is not productive. Planning involves arranging future events in the way that we prefer. When we plan something, we use our imagination constructively to create a future reality. When we worry about something, we use our imagination destructively. Worry happens when we think of a future event and then, while that image is on our mind, we also add to the image some pain or discomfort that we believe will happen to us as part of that future event. We make up these thoughts and tend to spend our present moments dwelling on them. It is not a very useful way to spend our present moments. Worrying will be covered more thoroughly in the next chapter.

One of the leading social fears in our culture is speaking in front of a group of people. When we *plan* for that event, we carefully pin down all the things we will say and how we will say them. When we worry about the public speech we will be giving, we imagine all the mental spears that those in the audience will throw our way while we are speaking. The difference between worrying and planning is treated more fully in later chapters.

Putting It All Together

Think of mindfulness in two stages. The first stage involves self-regulating one's attention to maintain it on immediate experience. The second stage requires adopting a certain orientation toward one's experiences in the present moment, an orientation characterized by curiosity, openness, and acceptance.[26]

Although we are not likely to be fully mindful every minute of every day, we can have more moments of mindfulness. Start with one activity in your day—going for a walk, taking a shower, eating lunch, or even studying. Deliberately concentrate on being mindful for that time. When we step back and observe our thoughts and feelings, as well as the external environment around us, we gain a new perspective. Mindfulness teaches us to see things as they really are, not the way we think they should be. With practice, mindfulness soon becomes a peaceful way of living.

> Let him who would enjoy a good future waste none of his present.
> —*Roger Babson*

Author Anecdote In the Moment Our daughter's friend Christy told us about a simple technique to remind her to be more mindful. She carries a special, small, smooth rock with her every day. She keeps it with her keys, so every day when she gets ready to leave for work, she puts it in her pocket. During the day when something stressful happens or she starts to feel tense and feels her mind filling with stressful thoughts, she takes a deep breath and gently rubs the smooth rock. This is a simple reminder to be in the moment. Mindfulness won't happen by accident. Think about a simple trigger that you can use throughout the day to remind you to be in the moment.

—*MH*

Conclusion

Mindfulness—the ability to enjoy the present moment—is one of the essentials for stress management, yet this ability to fully experience and appreciate the moment is elusive for many. Learning to practice mindfulness has the potential to reduce one's perception of stress, to enhance one's ability to maintain non-judgmental awareness in stressful situations, and to experience increased levels of positive states of mind.

To be at peace with oneself, learn to replace thoughts that produce unhealthy emotions such as guilt, worry, fear, and anger with a mental focus on the present. Mindfulness combines an internal focus with attention to the outer world. Each day offers thousands of moments to let go and focus directly on the here and now. Benefits result when we learn to separate thoughts and emotions of everyday life from the essence of who we are. As our awareness increases, emotional states lose their power and ability to cause stress. In the words of Thich Nhat Hanh, "Be part of the miraculous moment."

> Finish each day and be done with it. You have done what you could do; some blunders and absurdities have crept in; forget them as soon as you can. Tomorrow is a new day; you shall begin it serenely and with too high a spirit to be encumbered with your old nonsense.
>
> —Ralph Waldo Emerson

7.1 Full Mindfulness Activity

PURPOSE The purpose of this activity is to allow you to experience mindfulness using your ability to observe with all your senses.

DESCRIPTION OF ACTIVITY Psychologists tell us that we normally take in about 1% of all of the stimuli that is available to us in any given moment. The primary reason for this is because we simply aren't paying attention. Our thoughts are constantly on other things, other places, other times than here and now. This activity helps us tune in to the other 99% of the stimuli that our senses usually miss. Focusing on the present moment has a profound impact on stress.

DIRECTIONS During this activity, you are going to go somewhere **completely by yourself.** You will NOT talk to anyone. NO SPEAKING ALLOWED! For about an hour, do nothing but observe. This activity can be done virtually anywhere but somewhere outdoors may be more appealing.

At the top of your page write "I AM NOTICING . . ." just once, then for an hour finish the sentence over and over based on what your senses bring to you. You will begin each moment with the simple statement, "I am noticing . . ." as you discover all the things that present themselves to you. Use all your senses to experience mindfully what has always been *here and now* but you may have missed because your thoughts were focused on some other time and somewhere else. Don't look *for* anything—just look. On your paper, write down the things that you observe with each of your senses. If you find yourself getting bored or resisting the process, stop, look, notice what shows up, and then continue.

When you are finished, summarize your experience by responding to the following:

1. What setting did you select for your mindfulness activity? Why?
2. What were some of the main things that you observed, especially those things you wouldn't normally notice?
3. What did you notice about your thoughts?
4. What did you notice about your feelings?

(Continued)

LAB

5. What insights did you gain about yourself and about mindfulness as you were practicing being mindful?

6. What did you notice about your stress levels as you immersed yourself fully in your experience?

Key Points

- Mindfulness is the process of cultivating appreciation for the fullness of each moment we are alive. It is present-moment awareness.
- Mindlessness occurs when our thoughts are not in the present moment. We ignore the present moment because our attention is directed elsewhere.
- Mindfulness is a tool to unclutter the mind and bring about mental tranquility.

- Detached observation means simply staying in an observational state of mind without judgment or expectations.
- Mindful awareness is not limited to any one focal point, as is common in many types of meditation but, rather, encompasses mind, body, environment, and whatever arises in the field of awareness.
- Mindfulness does not mean living with reckless abandon *for the moment*. It means living fully *in the moment*.

Key Terms

reality
unreality
mindfulness

vipassana
mindlessness
detached observation

sensory overload
mindfulness-based stress reduction
mindfulness self-efficacy

Discussion Time For Critical Thinking/Discussion Questions, please visit this book's Premium Website.

Notes

1. *Tao: The Watercourse Way*, by A. Watts (New York: Pantheon Books, 1975).
2. "The Benefits of Being Present: Mindfulness and Its Role in Psychological Well-Being," by K. Brown, and R. Ryan, *Journal of Personality and Social Psychology 84*(4) (2003): 822–848.
3. *Full Catastrophe Living: Using the Wisdom of Your Body and Mind to Face Stress*, by J. Kabat-Zinn (New York: Delacorte, 1990).
4. "Mindfulness: A Proposed Operational Definition," by S. Bishop, et al., *Clinical Psychology: Science and Practice 11*(3) (2004).
5. "Does Mindfulness Decrease Stress and Foster Empathy Among Nursing Students?," by A. Beddoe, and S. Murphy, *Journal of Nursing Education 43*(7) (2004).
6. "Mindfulness and Healing Intention: Concepts, Practice, and Research Evaluation," by S. Schmidt, *Journal of Alternative and Complementary Medicine 10*, Suppl. 1 (2004).
7. Bishop.
8. "Choose Joy," by M. Maisey-Ireland, *The Black Hills Art Anchor*, September 2003, p. 12.
9. *Love is Letting Go of Fear*, by G. Jampolsky (Berkeley, CA: Celestial Arts, 1979).
10. *Winning Through Enlightenment*, by R. Smotherman (San Francisco: Context Publications, 1980).
11. Kabat-Zinn.
12. *The Miracle of Mindfulness: A Manual on Meditation*, by T. N. Hanh (Boston: Beacon Press Books, 1976).
13. *Handbook to Higher Consciousness*, by K. Keyes (Coos Bay, OR: Living Love Center, 1985).
14. *Stress Management*. National Safety Council (Boston: Jones and Bartlett Publishers, 1995).
15. "Awakening to the Dharma," by J. Goldstein. In B. Shield and R. Carlson, *For the Love of God* (San Rafael, CA: New World Library, 1990).
16. *Zen and the Art of Motorcycle Maintenance*, by R. Pirsig (New York: Bantam Books, 1974).

17. *The Inner Game of Tennis*, by W. T. Gallway (New York: Random House, 1974).

18. *Mosby's Complementary & Alternative Medicine: A Research-Based Approach* (2nd ed.), by L. Freeman (St. Louis, MO: Mosby, 2004).

19. "The Effects of Mindfulness-Based Stress Reduction Program on Stress, Mindfulness Self-Efficacy, and Positive States of Mind," by V. Chang, O. Caldwell, N. Glasgow, M. Abramson, F. Luskin, M. Gill, A. Burke, and C. Koopman, *Stress and Health 20* (2004): 141–147.

20. Chang.

21. "Stress Reduction Through Mindfulness Meditation: Effects on Psychological Symptomatology, Sense of Control, and Spiritual Experiences," by J. Astin, *Psychotherapy and Psychosomatics 66*(2) (1997): 97–106.

22. Beddoe.

23. *Mind/Body Health* (2nd ed.), by K. Karren, B. Hafen, N. Lee, and K. Frandsen (San Francisco: Benjamin Cummings, 2002).

24. Keyes.

25. Chang.

26. Bishop.

8 Managing Emotions

■ Am I realistic to think I can eliminate negative emotions such as fear and anger? ■ I have always wanted to go on a study abroad program for a semester, but I'm afraid I might not be able to handle being so far from home. I feel like I'm missing out. What can I do to overcome my fear? ■ My grandma is a worrier, my mother is a worrier, and I'm a worrier. Is worrying a result of heredity or environment? ■ Sometimes I get so angry I think I'll explode. What can I do to control my anger?

Study of this chapter will enable you to:

1. Explain how negative emotions such as guilt, worry, fear, anger, and hostility relate to stress.
2. Describe the physiological manifestations of certain emotions.
3. Distinguish between guilt and worry.
4. Explain the differences between anger and hostility.
5. Take action to prevent and control stress-causing emotions.

If you think the problem is outside of you, that thought is the problem.

—Stephen Covey

© Mike Powell/CORBIS

Fear Factor Lyn Freeman relates this story about fear:

* * *

Theresa was rock climbing in an area indigenous to rattlesnakes. She was careful to wear protective leg gear so she would be safe while climbing to the top of the bluff. Upon reaching an especially precarious part of the climb with only one good handhold left, she was tired. With as much force as possible, Theresa jammed her fingers into the rock crevice and prepared to swing herself up to the top. At that moment she heard a rattling sound. In an instant, she was gripped with fear.

In a split second, the thought of being snake-bitten several times, the fear of pain, a picture of her hand swelling, and the fear of an agonizing death—all raced through Theresa's mind and body. Her heart began to pound, and she began to pant and sweat profusely. Her body stiffened as her gaze froze on a shadow in the crevice. Her thoughts focused like a laser on her predicament.

"Don't let go!" a voice screamed in her head. She thought she might survive a snakebite, but never a 2000-foot fall. With all her will, Theresa strengthened her finger grip on the crevice and with tremendous effort swung herself to the top of the bluff. She ripped off her climbing gloves and checked for signs of a bite. Her hand was unblemished. Safe, her bodily responses slowly began to return to a more normal state.

A few minutes later, the climber just behind Theresa pulled himself onto the bluff. "Did you encounter the rattler?" Theresa asked.

"Oh, do you mean this?" the climber responded. He reached into his shirt and pulled out a chain with snake rattles attached to the end. Shaking the rattles, he said, "This is my good-luck charm."

Source: *Mosby's Complementary and Alternative Medicine: A Research-Based Approach* (3rd ed.), by Lyn Freeman (St. Louis: Mosby, 2009).

Managing Emotions

Do you control your emotions, or do your emotions control you? The ability to experience a wide range of emotions is part of what makes us uniquely human and keeps life interesting. We get angry. We get scared. We feel guilt and worry. How boring life would be if we never were to experience the ups and downs of emotions! Like most things in life, we need a healthy balance for optimal well-being. Chronic guilt and worry, fear that prevents us from living life fully, an attitude of hostility and anger—all are negative and stress-producing. You will learn in this chapter that you can control your emotions so they don't control you. The focus is on the emotional dimension of health.

As Theresa's story demonstrates, strong emotions may or may not be based on reality, but the powerful physiologic response to fear is the same whether the rattlesnake is real or imagined. Negative emotions such as anger and fear have a very real and profound impact on quality of life. To think that we can eliminate all negative emotions is unrealistic. In this chapter we will learn how to control and eliminate many of the negative consequences of these emotions. The key to better health and a more contented life lies not in which emotions seize us but, instead, in our ability to express and control our emotions.

The Physiology of Emotions

Researchers have discovered that certain emotions can make us more susceptible to stress and disease. These negative emotions, including worry, guilt, fear, anger, and other strong emotions, can activate the sympathetic nervous system division of the autonomic nervous system, evoking the stress response—as is so clearly demonstrated in Theresa's story at the beginning of this chapter. Fear put Theresa's body on alert. Powerful hormones, including cortisol and epinephrine, flooded her body. Her blood pressure soared and her heart raced.

Theresa's experience had a profound physiologic and biochemical effect on her. Will this intense one-time scare have long-term effects on Theresa's health? Probably not.

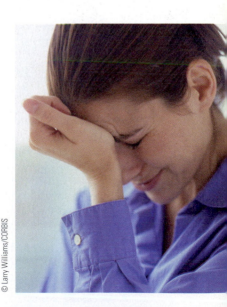

Experiencing a range of emotions is part of the human experience.

It isn't the experience of today that drives men mad. It is the remorse for something that happened yesterday, and the dread of what tomorrow may disclose.

—*Robert Jones Burdette*

You wouldn't worry so much about what other people think if you realized how seldom they do.

—*Eleanor Roosevelt*

These emotions can be used for protection. The emotions of fear and anger have been linked to the fight-or-flight response, where they can serve a protective function. Fear relates to "flight," in which we realize that sometimes running from or escaping from a potentially dangerous situation can protect us. Anger relates to "fight," in which the stress response is useful to confront and resist that which we perceive as dangerous.

The problem comes when long-term emotions such as fear and anger affect health in much the same way that long-term stress affects health and longevity. Emotional stress is clearly a significant factor in creating vulnerability to disease by disrupting normal homeostasis. A growing body of research indicates that as many as half of all patients who visit physicians have physical symptoms directly caused by emotions. Some research findings even put that figure as high as 90% to 95%. These are not imaginary, but real, physical symptoms. What this tells us is that the root of many of today's illnesses and diseases is mental and emotional rather than organically physical.[1]

When worry or fear or anger become a typical emotional response to life, health deteriorates and life loses some of its joy. Learning how you can manage the primary stress emotions can prevent that from happening.

Guilt and Worry

Wayne Dyer states that one of two emotions, guilt or worry, is associated with virtually every stressor we perceive. Dyer believes that guilt and worry are the most ineffective coping techniques for stress management because they perpetuate the avoidance of stress-related issues that require resolution.[2]

Guilt is the conscious preoccupation with undesirable past thoughts and behaviors. Guilt is an expression of self-anger detected by internal dialogue that includes self-talk such as, "I should have. . . . " While guilt keeps the mind occupied with thoughts and behaviors from the past, **worry,** a manifestation of fear, keeps the mind focused on events yet to come.

Clinical psychologist Thomas Pruzinsky says, "Worry is a state in which we dwell on something so much it causes us to become apprehensive. It differs from the far stronger emotion we call fear, which causes physical changes such as a racing pulse and fast breathing. Worry is the thinking part of anxiety."[3] So, as opposed to worry, **anxiety** is the psychological and physiological response to worry. When worry and anxiety escalate, the outcome is fear.

Letting Go of Worry   When you watch young children play, you become aware that they rarely demonstrate guilt or worry. These are habits we develop. Imagine how silly it would sound if one youngster were to say to another, "I'm so worried about coming to your house later today. We might get hurt, or your mom will yell at us, or we may disagree about how a front flip is done on your trampoline."

Kids don't let thoughts of what may or may not happen dominate their thinking. They are too busy attending to what is happening right now and enjoying their present-moment activities to use up their consciousness on some unlikely future event. Children can teach a lesson about worry that many adults need to learn.

Guidelines to Help You Manage Worry   The following seven ideas can help you when you feel the urge to worry.

1. *Most things we worry about are out of our control.* Many of the things we worry about have to do with events or situations over which we have no control. Even if we can change some aspect of the things we worry about, worrying is not the way to do it. We worry about war, the economy, the possibility of coming down with some illness, about losing our job; we worry about whether someone likes us; we worry about the people we love; we worry about our weight, or whether we will get a good grade in a class. We worry about getting old and even dying. The list of the things we worry about is endless.

2. *Worry is not the same as caring.* We have no control over most of the things we worry about, but we have been taught, and accept as true, the notion that worrying is the same as caring. This is a learned response. We are not born worriers, but we may be taught at an early age that if we care about someone that means we worry about them. We believe that if we don't worry, we must not care very much.

Worry and the Mind

Stress emotions can affect our cognitive abilities. When we are overcome with emotions, we have trouble thinking clearly, and long-term worry can produce lasting decline. In a study reported in *Neurology*, chronic worry was linked to an increased risk of cognitive decline. Comparing worriers with non-worriers, based on an initial assessment, 1,064 members of a community were observed 3 to 6 years later for Alzheimer disease. The results showed that obsessive worriers had more than double the risk of decline compared to their more carefree peers.

Source: "Proneness to Psychological Distress and Risk of Alzheimer Disease in a Biracial Community," by R. S. Wilson, L. L. Barnes, D. A. Bennett, et al. *Neurology, 64* (2005), 380–382.

Tip: Take time to reflect on the idea that worrying is not productive. Think of someone you worry about. Make a list of alternative ways you can demonstrate caring toward that person in productive ways. For example, if you are worried about your mother's health, take a few minutes, rather than wasting time worrying, to write her a note expressing your love and appreciation for her.

3. *Worry is not the same thing as planning.* The problem with worrying is that it does not change anything. When we plan, we bring future moments into the present so we can control those future events appropriately. When we plan, we are using our present moments in a useful way to prepare us for a future event or experience. It is essential to distinguish the difference between worrying about the future (unproductive and stress-producing) and planning for the future (productive and stress-relieving).

4. *Most worries never happen.* When we worry, we focus on the possible painful outcomes that we associate with some future event. We let our present moment be filled with what *might* happen but usually doesn't. Worry prevents thinking in the present moment because of our preoccupation with things that may, or may not, occur in our future. Mark Twain understood this when he said, "I am an old man and have known a great many troubles, but most of them never happened."

5. *Move your worries from your mind to paper.* Idle worrying is not constructive. Next time you catch yourself worrying, write down what is troubling you. Once you have moved the worry from your mind to the paper, you can identify the concern more clearly and go to work on finding a solution. You might even try making a list of everything you worry about for one day. Go back and review the list in a week, and you might be surprised to see how few of your worries ever came to pass.

6. *Practice mindfulness.* An effective way to remain free from both guilt and worry is to practice being mindful, as was explained in Chapter 7. Mindfulness keeps our attention on what is happening here and now. When our thoughts are focused on here and now, we aren't as likely to

> We worry and we worry . . . and we worry about worrying.
> —Leo Buscaglia

Author Anecdote — Worry Turned to Panic

In graduate school I had a good friend whose wife allowed worry to take pointless control of her life. For example, while she was driving home from the store, here are some of the thoughts that would run through her head:

"I wonder how things are going at home. . . . The babysitter is a good one . . . she seems to take such good care of our kids. . . . But I wonder if she's okay right now. . . . I wonder if the kids are okay right now. . . . Sometimes the babysitter isn't completely responsible. . . . I'll bet she's taken the kids to play in the park. . . . She's probably taken the kids for a walk and left them alone. That irresponsible babysitter has left the kids on their own, and they don't know how to get back home. . . . My kids are in danger! . . . Somebody is going to kidnap them! . . . The kidnapper is going to hurt my kids! . . . Things can't possibly get any worse than this!"

By this time, the woman was having a panic attack. Her hands were clutching the steering wheel, her heartbeat was soaring, her blood pressure was through the roof, and her thoughts were racing madly about all the horrible things that surely were happening to her kids. She drove home barely able to control herself for fear of what had become of her kids. She had literally driven herself to a frenzy because of her worry-filled thoughts about her kids.

Of course, when she arrived home, the kids were just fine. They were happily playing with the babysitter and enjoying a pleasant afternoon in the backyard.

This loving mother allowed her thoughts to control her consciousness to the point where she was damaging her physical and emotional well-being. Her body was flooded with stress hormones, resulting in a full-fledged stress response much like what she would need if she were truly threatened and had to protect her children.

Notice how unnecessary her worrying was. As she was driving home, she could do absolutely nothing about what was happening with her kids and the babysitter. Her worrisome thoughts were immobilizing her and preventing her from enjoying her ride home.

—MO

dwell on thoughts of the past and the associated guilt, or thoughts of the future and the associated worry and fear.

7. *Remember—worry is a habit.* Negative habits such as worrying are learned, and they can be unlearned or replaced with healthy, positive habits. When you become aware that you are worrying, say to yourself, "Worry is a habit, and I choose to break this habit." Focus your mind on a relaxing image or a stress-relieving affirmation.

Tip: If worry is a habit you can't seem to break, give yourself designated "worry time." It sounds crazy, but by limiting your worry time, you can prevent worry from consuming your thoughts.

Stress Busting Behavior: No More Worry Wart

Review the 7 helpful ideas for when you feel the urge to worry. Prioritize these ideas from the most helpful for you (1) to the least helpful (7). Circle your number 1 idea. This week each time you feel the urge to worry, focus on the idea you rated as most helpful to reduce and/or eliminate the negative emotion of worry.

☐ Most things we worry about are out of our control.

☐ Worry is not the same as caring.

☐ Worry is not the same as planning.

☐ Most worries never happen.

☐ Move your worries from your mind to paper.

☐ Practice mindfulness.

☐ Remember, worry is a habit.

Letting Go of Guilt Guilt can be a destroyer or a teacher. When we reflect on our actions, we can learn important lessons from them. Hindsight is a great teacher if we are willing to listen.

Several of the seven ideas for how to manage worry also relate to how to manage guilt. For example, you can remember that guilt is a habit. When you are feeling guilty, you can change the focus of your thinking and focus on mindfulness. To manage stress and enjoy life, remember that we can learn from our past experiences, and we can plan for our future. Worry and guilt will not help unless we use those emotions to motivate us for positive change.

Fear

What is fear and what is happening in our minds when we fear something? **Fear** is a state of escalated worry and apprehension that causes distinct physical and emotional reactions. When worry becomes intense, we feel fear. Fear usually involves a focus on the future. We create in our mind thoughts that something in our future, some event or experience, is going to involve pain, danger, or discomfort and therefore is to be avoided. Psychologists report that fear is one of the chief reasons people seek their help. Fear may be the single most potent stressful emotion.

TABLE 8.1 Types of Fear with Examples

Fear	Examples
Change	Afraid to move to a new city, change majors, or break up with a boyfriend or girlfriend
Pain or physical suffering	Fearful of going to the dentist or getting a shot
Failure	Afraid of not being selected for the track team or not being accepted into graduate school
Some *thing*	Afraid of snakes or spiders or being mugged
The unknown	Fearful of going away to school or of people who are different from you
Death	The biggest unknown of all

Types of Fear

Common types of fear and examples of each are given in Table 8.1.

Fear can paralyze and incapacitate us and can stop us from going after our desires. In succumbing to fear, we settle for less and get less than what we really want. As an example, you probably know of someone who wants to interview for a job, try out for the golf team, ask someone out on a date, or audition for a play, but because of that person's feelings of fear, he or she does not realize those desires. The belief that these activities will be painful in some way stops the person from moving forward toward a desired outcome.

It's about Growing

To understand fear, we must ask an ominous-sounding question: *Why are you here*? This question is not the same as asking: Why are you where you are right now? The deeper questions are: Why do you think you are alive on this planet at this time? What is your purpose for being? For what are you living? These might seem like strange questions to include in a chapter about fear and emotions, but stay with us—this is important. Some typical replies to these questions are:

- To learn everything I can
- To enjoy life to the fullest
- To make a difference in other people's lives
- To serve others
- To have and support a family and provide a quality life for my kids
- To develop my skills, talents, and natural abilities
- To have a good time
- To be happy
- To work toward and reach the goals that I set for myself

All these purposes are worthwhile and have great value. When we look at them, we notice a common theme: the general desire among humans to grow, to develop, to serve, and to enjoy. We have a natural tendency to want to expand, to become more of who we are. Even people like the great physicist Albert Einstein, at the point of death, decried the fact that so little of him had been realized. We have great untapped potential.

Comfort and Discomfort Zones

In contrast to our innate need to grow and expand is another natural law of behavior: We tend to gravitate toward our comfort zones. A **comfort zone** is any place, situation, relationship, or experience where we do not feel threatened. It usually is a known place or situation where we feel safe and in control. Examples of comfort zones are our homes, especially certain rooms or places in our homes, our jobs, the family and friends we spend time with, the types of food we eat, the places we go to exercise, the make of car we drive, and the routes we commonly travel. We prefer being in places, being around people, and doing things that are more comfortable to us. Figure 8.1 shows a circle representing ourselves within a comfort zone. This is where we prefer to be most of the time.

When we are in our comfort zone, we experience little growth or progress. To grow, we must leave our comfort zone and move out into our **discomfort zone.** The word *discomfort* implies that we do not feel especially comfortable "out there." Discomfort zones are those places where we *do not* naturally gravitate. We usually try our best to avoid our discomfort zones. Figure 8.2 represents movement into our discomfort zones.

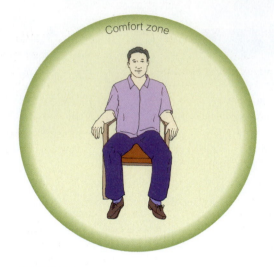

FIGURE 8.1 Comfort Zone

FIGURE 8.2 Discomfort Zones

Although moving out of a comfort zone can help us progress in the direction of our potential, it has a catch: This growth takes effort. Included in this effort usually involves overcoming or dealing with some type of fear.

When we venture out of our comfort zones, we sense the emotion of fear because we believe that some kind of pain or discomfort might be lurking out there. But the reality is that *there is no pain in our discomfort zone.* When we move out into our discomfort zones, we rarely are hurt in the true sense where physical pain is involved. On rare occasions this can happen. Some people live in environments where physical danger can be a real threat. In these situations, fear can protect us. In the vast majority of situations that we feel fear, however, we are not really in danger of having pain inflicted on us. We mentally manufacture the pain we experience. So while the fear we experience is sometimes justified and prompts us to take action, most of the time, we create the false need to prepare for some pain that simply isn't going to happen. Consider the following example that looks at one of our top social fears—public speaking.

Imagine that you have been asked to speak in front of a large group of people. Because this is something you are not comfortable doing, you prepare for several days. As the time approaches for you to speak, you notice that you are feeling more and more nervous. Finally you find yourself at the meeting where you are to be the next speaker. You feel prepared, yet prior to being introduced, you notice that your knees are shaking, your mouth is dry, and you are having trouble thinking clearly. Your mind races with thoughts of what the people in the audience might think of you once you start speaking. You notice yourself sweating, feeling extremely uncomfortable. You almost feel like crying or running away as your name is announced.

With some difficulty, you make your way to the podium. At first, it seems like you barely can get any words out, but soon you settle into a nice flow and you end up giving your speech without any problems. The attendees are attentive, nodding, smiling, and even laughing at your jokes. At the end of the speech, you notice that the crowd is applauding. You return to your seat with a smile on your face, relieved that you are finished.

Fear is a feeling based on the thought that you want to avoid potential pain in the future. So let's analyze where the pain can be found in the process of giving your speech and why doing so seemed so unpleasant. If you felt fear at any point as you approached this speech, we must ask the crucial question: *Where* was the *real* pain during the speech? Going through each phase of giving the speech, where would we find pain? No real pain was happening while you were sitting in your seat waiting to get up or while you walked over to the podium. No real pain occurred as you were speaking. Nor did any pain accompany you as you went back to your seat after you finished speaking. At no point during the entire event was there *real* pain. If giving this speech in reality is a pain-free experience, why would you feel any fear?

Your fear was based on your thoughts about the people who were there. You interpreted the potential reactions of the audience in a certain way. They could have disagreed with you or thought mean things about you. That thought, to you, was psychologically painful.

Lean into your fears, dare them to do their worst and cut them down when they try. If you don't, they'll mushroom 'til they surround you, choke the road to the life you want. Every turn you fear is empty air dressed to look like jagged hell.

—*Richard Bach*

Remember that thoughts always happen before emotions. Your thought was that those people's opinions mattered to you, and rejection hurts. The fear you felt is the emotion that follows the thought of wanting to avoid *that* pain. But remember that there was nothing painful about the speech itself.

You can do a test to show that this is a working principle, that your fear is based entirely on your thoughts and not on the process of giving the speech: Do the same speech again in the same room, but this time do it without anyone present in the audience. Similar to the first situation, you are doing exactly the same thing— sitting, walking to the podium, speaking, and then sitting down again when you are finished. Your experience this time will be far different than the first.

What can we do with this understanding? Anytime we find ourselves afraid of something, we can mentally examine each step prior to the event and the event itself, and remove any unreal pain. By realizing that no real pain is involved except that which we create in our own minds, we can choose to think differently about it, as we have discussed. Once we have recognized that no real pain is involved, we are much more likely to move forward in the direction of our desire without fear or apprehension. We become free to move confidently toward any outcome that we choose.

Putting It Together

1. Most of us believe we are here not to be stuck in a rut of comfort but, rather, to grow and move in the direction of our potential.
2. Our natural inclination is to be comfortable—to remain in our comfort zone.
3. We need to balance our need to grow with our desire to feel comfortable.
4. Overcoming fear is necessary for growth, and growth takes effort.
5. Moving toward your potential results in feelings of accomplishment and gives meaning to life.

Author Anecdote Moving Out of My Comfort Zone

I was out of shape and overweight. With each pregnancy, I added fat to the previous excess fat. The fatter I got, the worse I felt about myself and the less motivation I felt to change. I knew exactly what I needed to do to rid my body of the excess fat, yet I was stuck in the rut of apathy and inactivity. It was easier to keep doing what I was doing. I couldn't seem to gather the energy to change my routine, to move out of my comfort zone.

One day I decided to change the way I was living and feeling. The choice was mine. I was sick and tired of feeling sick and tired. I needed to stop thinking about changing and actually *do* something. I loaded the kids in the car and headed for the track. My goal was to run 1 mile. Well, I couldn't. But I did run half a mile—and walked the other half. That marked the first baby step out of my comfort zone.

Two years from that day at the track, I ran a marathon. I crossed the finish line with tears of joy (and maybe a little pain) as my family cheered me on. When I started, I wasn't sure I could finish the marathon. Running 26 miles had seemed like an impossibility only 2 years earlier. Although I was afraid I might fail to finish the marathon (fear!), I decided to find success and growth in the process. This was important to me: Even if I didn't finish the marathon, I had grown in many ways from taking on the challenge.

People have asked what got me moving in the right direction. The turning point related to the question: Why am I here? My motivation related to my spiritual belief that we are here for a reason and to my belief that I was doing this not only for myself but also so I could be a healthy role model to my children. I believed that one of the reasons I was here was to set an example that might help others move from comfort to growth. If I could do it, so could they. Here is what worked for me:

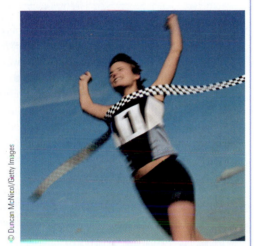

© Duncan McNicol/Getty Images

Don't let fear stop you from experiencing the abundance that makes life worth living. What have you done to step out of your comfort zone?

1. I decided to focus on what I could do rather than what I could not do.
2. I decided to enjoy exercise and think of exercise as something I was privileged to do, not something I had to do. I thought about the time I spent exercising as a gift I gave myself.
3. I was motivated by something more than the desire to shed the fat. I wanted to be a healthy role model for my children. This was a deeply ingrained value.
4. I set goals to move gradually out of my comfort zone and toward my potential.
5. Even though I was afraid I might fail, I told friends and family what I was doing. This was motivating to me and I received support and encouragement.

Finishing the marathon gave me courage to step out of my comfort zone in other areas of my life and was literally a life-changing event. It took courage to get courage. Don't let fear stop you from experiencing the abundance that makes life worth living. Dare to try.

—MH

We need courage to shift from comfort to discomfort. Moving out of our comfort zone implies facing our fears. But if we are to expand and grow, we must face our fears.

Fear Factors Four principles for managing fear can shape our understanding of fear and guide us in taking control of our choices.

Go for It! I was eating dinner at a restaurant with one of my daughters and my son. My daughter told me she was thirsty and wanted another drink of water. I told her to go ahead and ask the waitress, the next time she walked by, to bring a drink of water to her. My daughter's face went sour and her eyes lowered. I could tell she had some reservation about asking for another glass of water. She was afraid of asking but had no idea why she was afraid. I tried to help her understand that she was fully capable of following through on a task that she feared. I suggested to her that she not let her fears stop her from getting what she wanted.

Similarly, we see something that we want, but our thoughts of painful or uncomfortable outcomes keep us from going after it. As in the case with my daughter, most of the things we fear are based on empty ideas about what might happen to us, but usually don't. In her case, there was no threat. There would be no future pain. With most of the things that we fear, the same is true. For most of the fears that we deal with daily, the only real pain we will experience is the pain and discomfort that we create in our own heads.

—MO

Facing Fear In class, I ask the students to think of something that they fear—not something that will barely edge them just outside their comfort zones but something that will move them way "out there." The item they decide on must be something that they ought to do, something that would add real value to their lives, but they have not done it for fear of the perceived painful outcomes. Next I ask them to take the next 2 weeks outside of class and actually follow the steps that will move them through that experience or event they feared. They are to do that thing they fear.

At the conclusion of this assignment, I continue to be amazed at the breakthroughs as well as the insights of the students who choose to really "go for it." I frequently hear comments like these: "I can't believe I was afraid of something so silly." "I feel so alive and free ever since I did that." "What a relief to know that I can do that which I never thought I could or never tried because of my fear." The final part of the above assignment involves the student, immediately upon completion of breaking through one fear, moving to the next one and going for that one as well.

—MO

> The meaning I picked,
> the one that changed
> my life: Overcome
> fear, behold wonder.
> —Aeschylus (525–456 BC),
> Greek tragic dramatist

1. *Fear can motivate positive action.* If you are afraid of flunking a test, you can use that fear to initiate a plan of action. One student, Dave, related in class that he remembered the day he received his credit card bill in the mail and realized that he was scared. He felt absolute terror about the debt he had accumulated and feared that he would not be able to get out of debt because of the choices he had made. Dave was able to use his fear to initiate change. He sought financial advice and received help in setting up a budget. Dave used his fear for positive change.

   Fear also can serve a protective function in times of real physical danger, such as the fear of burning our hands when we touch a hot oven or the fear of being attacked if we walk alone at night. As a result, we don't touch the hot oven, and we don't walk alone at night.

2. *Nothing in the world is inherently fearful.* Like stress, there is nothing "out there" that universally causes fear. Fear is an internal experience. Many people are scared of snakes, while others are content to have the critters as pets and feel no fear as the snake slithers around their neck. The snake is not causing the fear. The fear is the result of what the person believes about the snake. When we associate a snake with pain and danger, fear is the result. The emotion of fear is the result of the thoughts we create inside our minds.

3. *Fear is learned.* Psychologists tell us that newborn babies have a natural fear of falling and loud noises. Others disagree, saying that babies are simply reacting to these stimuli without a capacity to associate pain with an experience. Regardless, most of what we learn to fear is a result of either personal experience or our belief in someone else's experience. For example, if your neighbor tells you about the time she went to the dentist and experienced excruciating pain, you may decide to do everything in your power to avoid going to the dentist. When we experience something painful, such as getting stung by a bee, in the future we will associate the past experience of pain with the presence of the buzzing bee.

   If fear is learned, it follows that fear also can be unlearned. Within our capacity is the potential to release our attachment to our fears, to let them go. If one person can overcome a fear, such as a fear of high places, or speaking in front of a group, or meeting a new person, so can others.

4. With practice and experience we can learn to overcome our fears. We get better at handling fear through practice and experience. Little by little, we develop the confidence and self-trust to risk more frequently and to do more things that seem frightening. We could talk about all the reasons we feel fear, but until we actually step out of our comfort zone, look that which we fear straight in the face, and move toward it, we will not rid ourselves of our fears.

Remember when you were learning to drive a car? Most of us were intimidated the first time we got behind the wheel of a car. And why wouldn't we be? Driving a car is a big responsibility and one of the most potentially dangerous things we can do. Yet, we overcame our fear. Through practice and experience, we gained confidence for one of the most dangerous things we ever do. Our familiarity with this activity determined our level of fear.

You can familiarize yourself with a frightening activity without actually participating in it. For example, if you are deathly afraid of the upcoming speech you know you will have to present in speech class, start by reading about how to give a good speech. Talk with friends who have been successful. You might even try videotaping yourself giving the speech. As you practice your speech under controlled circumstances, you will gain confidence.

We can reinforce the feeling of assurance that we can handle whatever we need to reach our goal by looking at our past experiences. The fact that you are alive is proof that you are a capable person. This is not a frivolous statement. It is an accurate one. You know you can handle life's challenges because you keep handling things every day. Why should some future event be any different from the millions of previous ones? Unquestionably, things are uncertain at times, but you still come out alive, unhurt, and capable of handling more. Curiously, most of us find that we can handle the things that we go after and, moreover, that we enjoy them, that they bring us pleasure. The pain that we perceived rarely happens, but the joy of going for what we want frequently does.

Strategy for Overcoming Fear
The following is a proven strategy for overcoming fear:[4]

1. *First, admit you are afraid.* List the things that cause you to feel fear. As you mentally re-create those things, try to imagine them without the emotion of fear. Learn to disassociate the pain from the event. This takes some practice, but you can do it.
2. *Next, confront your fear.* Do whatever it is that you are so afraid of. Realize that your fear will intensify as you face it, but do it anyway. Go back to your mental pictures and try to imagine that the situation is not fearful.
3. *Do whatever you are so afraid of at least three times.* Chances are that you will be less afraid each time. Chances are even better that you were afraid because you were unsure.
4. *As you confront your fear, call it something else*—excitement or a challenge, for example.

Momentum carries tremendous power. If we settle for one little victory, the growth stops there. To continue the progress, plan another visit into your discomfort zone and venture out again. Little by little, you will realize that fear is an illusion. With practice, you can adopt the feeling of assurance that you can handle it. One common thought that precedes the emotion of fear is a lack of trust in ourselves. We can allay a fear of failure with a sense of self-assurance and self-efficacy.

The Fear–Faith Connection
The more we believe that our lives are about something, that things happen for a reason, and that we are meant to benefit from the experience of our journey, the more courageous and less fearful we are when we are confronted with difficult situations. The more we are guided by fear, the weaker our faith. The stronger our faith, the less we fear. We are not talking about only a faith related to the belief in a higher power but also about the faith you have in yourself and your abilities. Pushing through fear is less frightening than living with the underlying fear that comes with a feeling of helplessness. Underlying all of our fears is a lack of trust in our ability to handle something. We need to remember we can handle it.

WHAT ELSE CAN I DO?

Ask Questions Don't let the fear of asking a question keep you from acquiring needed and helpful information. Be sure you completely understand what is communicated to you. Asking questions can help you get additional directions or clarify what is being asked of you. If you feel afraid to ask for help, summon your nerve and go for it anyway!

Fear knocked at the door. Faith answered. Nobody was there.

—*English Proverb*

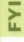

Scared to Death

Throughout medical history, examples abound about people who have been literally frightened to death. If fear is intense enough, all systems can be overloaded fatally, as the following examples demonstrate:

- Barbara Reyes was spending her Memorial Day weekend floating on a raft on Georgia's peaceful Lake Lanier. The calm of the peaceful, warm afternoon was shattered when a man riding a motorized jet ski roared within a foot of the 40-year-old Reyes. In a panic, she paddled to shore, collapsed, and died. Randolph Simpson, the Gwinnett County coroner who examined Reyes, said, "There's no question she was literally scared to death." The man who roared by on the jet ski was arrested and charged with involuntary manslaughter.
- A 45-year-old man died of fright as he stepped to a podium to give a speech.
- An elderly man sitting on his lawn collapsed and died when a car jumped the curb and appeared to be heading straight for him.
- Panamanian dictator Omar Torrijos reportedly amused himself by killing a prisoner with an unloaded gun; the sound of the blanks firing was enough to scare the man to death.

Source: *Mind/Body Health: The Effects of Attitudes, Emotions, and Relationships* (2nd ed.), by K. Karren, B. Hafen, and K. Frandsen (San Francisco: Benjamin Cummings, 2002).

You will never overcome all your fears, but you can conquer the fears that prevent you from living your life to the fullest. Set out to tackle the fears that are holding you back. Viewing life as an adventure and an opportunity to grow can help reduce the fear of venturing into new, unknown territory. Helen Keller said, "Life is either a daring adventure or it is nothing." Have you ever given up on a hope, a dream, a goal, or an adventure because you were afraid of failing? Pushing ourselves out of our comfort zone can energize us and help make life an exhilarating adventure. Some of life's greatest stress is a result of regret, of being afraid to stretch for fear of failure.

Shakespeare once said, "A coward dies a thousand deaths, a hero only one." Cowards live the potential outcomes repeatedly in their mind, continually bringing up the associated pain. The hero simply moves in the direction of the feared thing. As you move through your fears, celebrate your victories. The more you associate pleasure and positive feelings with risking, the more you will be inclined to risk again. We are not talking about unnecessary, dangerous risk but, rather, the risk to move out of your comfort zone and grow. Experiencing success in overcoming fear in one area of life can encourage you to challenge your fear regarding other personal limitations, and thereby to risk again and grow in unpredictable and exciting ways.

Risking

To laugh is to risk appearing a fool.
To weep is to risk appearing sentimental.
To reach out for another is to risk involvement.
To expose feelings is to risk exposing your trueself.
To place your ideas, your dreams, before the crowd is to risk their loss.
To love is to risk not being loved in return.
To live is to risk dying.
To hope is to risk despair.
To try is to risk failure.
But risks must be taken because the greatest hazard in life is to risk nothing.
The person who risks nothing . . . does nothing . . . has nothing . . . is nothing.
You may avoid suffering and sorrow, but you simply cannot learn, feel, change, grow, love . . . live.
Chained by your certitudes, you are a slave; you have forfeited freedom.
Only a person who risks is free.

—Ralph Waldo Emerson

Anger

Work rage, road rage, sideline rage—you can hardly watch the news or read the paper without learning about yet another example of out-of-control anger. Whether it is the basketball player who leaps into the bleachers and starts punching an unruly fan, or the soccer mom who ends up in jail for assaulting the referee, or the disgruntled college student who opens fire on his teachers and classmates, or the guy who rams full-speed into the car that passed him—all seem to be reacting with anger to these stressful times. None of us is immune to the ravages of anger. Have you ever felt like throwing your cell phone out the window because you were disconnected after being on hold for half an hour? And more than one of us has shouted profanities at our computer when it locked up and we lost 3 hours of work.

Road Rage

Americans aren't the only ones feeling stress on the road. According to a study published in the *Journal of Sociology*, road rage is a problem on the roads of Sydney, Australia, as well. **Road rage** is a term used to describe a range of aggressive and dangerous driving behaviors directed at other motorists. Uncontrolled temper and the open display of anger and frustration are typical of road rage.

The research conducted on drivers in Sydney showed that motorists viewed driving as a source of autonomy, pleasure, and self-expression—meanings that often were frustrated by the travails of negotiating the road system. Road rage was represented as a response to the stresses of urban living, not only driving in a crowded road system but also the pressures exerted by factors such as a competitive work environment and lack of time. The findings revealed that the expression of anger in road rage is conceptualized negatively because of the challenges it poses to the idea of the "civilized self," but also that such expression is seen as understandable in the context of an urban environment replete with stress.

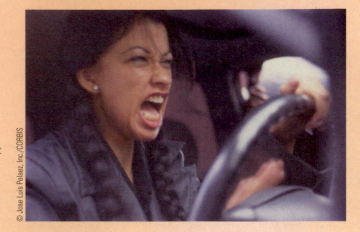

© Jose Luis Pelaez, Inc./CORBIS

Road rage—an unhealthy outcome of anger and hostility.

Source: "Road Rage: Drivers' Understandings and Experience," by D. Lupton, *Journal of Sociology* (2002), *38*(3), 275.

Anger is a transient emotional response based on the way one chooses to think about events, usually triggered by perceived provocation or mistreatment. Anger is tricky to define, but here are some common elements of anger:

- Everyone experiences anger, although to widely differing degrees.
- Anger is considered a temporary emotion.
- Anger combines physiological and emotional arousal.
- People express anger along a continuum from simple resentment or jealousy to full-blown, out-of-control rage.
- Anger is not the same as hostility (discussed later).

Anger comes in many forms including abuse, ridicule, physical violence, temper tantrums, sarcasm, and even the silent treatment. We might say things such as, "He infuriates me!" or "You really tick me off!" Jealousy is a form of anger, as are rage, annoyance, irritation, blaming, and frustration. Even guilt, as you learned earlier in this chapter, is a form of anger—in this case, self-anger.

Sources of Anger

Sybil Evans, a conflict-resolution expert in New York City, has identified three primary factors contributing to our ever-increasing anger: time, technology, and tension. She says:

> Americans are working longer hours than anyone else in the world. The cell phones and pagers that were supposed to make our lives easier have put us on call 24/7/365. Since we're always running, we're tense and low on patience. And the less patience we have, the less we monitor what we say to people and how we treat them."[5]

Stress doesn't necessarily cause us to be angry, but it certainly makes us more vulnerable to overreacting.

Dr. Wayne Dyer describes some common circumstances in which people select anger as the main emotion of the moment.[6]

- *Anger in the automobile.* While driving, we get upset at how we believe other people ought to be driving.
- *Anger in competitive games.* In every sport, we find people getting upset at opponents, teammates, referees, and even themselves.

Can't you see
My temperature's
rising, I radiate more
heat than light.
—*Neil Peart*

Mad Driver Disease The American Automobile Association's Foundation for Traffic Safety says that incidents of violently aggressive driving—sometimes called "mad driver disease"—rose 7% a year in the 1990s.

Source: "Why Are We So Angry?" by D. Hales, *Parade Magazine*, Sept. 2001, pp. 10–11.

Author Anecdote Letting Go of Anger I almost never get angry. It is an emotion I rarely experience—except when I am driving. For years I would cuss and fuss at what I considered inconsiderate drivers. You know the ones—the drivers who desperately pass, cut in quickly, then put on the brakes to slow down and turn.

Then, one day I came across a quote from Buddha: "Holding on to anger is like grasping a hot coal with the intent of throwing it at someone else—you are the one who gets burned."

What an insight! When I get angry, I'm the one who suffers. Why should I let someone I'm never going to see again control my mood and ruin my day? Inconsiderate drivers may not have any idea that they have done anything wrong, or maybe they simply don't care.

Although my initial reaction is hard to shake, when I encounter a "bad" driver now, I think of this quote. Sometimes I wave and smile. Sometimes I think about reasons why that driver did what he did. Maybe she just had a call that her child was injured at school, or maybe he is an EMT rushing to an accident. The point is that when you hold on to anger, you are the one who gets burned.

—MH

- *Anger at those things that seem to be out of place.* We have thoughts that things ought to be in certain places, and when they aren't, we lose control. An example is the driver who believes the bicyclist should not be on the road and crowds him off the road.
- *Anger about taxes.* The anger we create about something over which we have no control is senseless, but we allow ourselves to get angry over it nonetheless.
- *Anger over the tardiness of others.* The anger over people being late occurs when we believe that others ought to function according to our timetables. We immobilize ourselves with this thought: "I have a right to be angry. She kept me waiting for an hour."
- *Anger at the disorganization or sloppiness of others.* Again, this is an attempt to modify someone else's behavior according to our rules for how they ought to behave.
- *Anger at inanimate objects.* You feel your anger rise as a car alarm honks endlessly or your computer freezes up.
- *Anger over the loss of objects.* No amount of anger will turn up a lost key or a wallet.
- *Anger over world events and conditions beyond your control.* Regardless of how much you approve or disapprove of what is happening in the world, your anger will not change the situation. Similarly, your anger at the conditions of Mother Nature is unproductive. Becoming irate because the day is too hot or too cold, too windy, too rainy, or too sunny is a waste of present-moment energy.

Effects of Anger
Anger causes physiological and psychological arousal effects including:

- Increase in cortisol and adrenalin
- Increase in blood pressure
- Increase in blood sugar
- Faster pulse
- Constriction of blood vessels
- Increased serum cholesterol levels
- Decreased immune function
- Insomnia and fatigue

If this sounds a lot like the stress response, it is. Dr. Redford Williams and other researchers at Duke University found that anger is closely related to heart disease, sudden heart attacks, and chronic high blood pressure. They found that the harmful effects of anger may be more dangerous to health than the stress response.[7]

The Only Reason We Get Angry
As with all emotions, the feeling of anger comes from how we are thinking. Depending upon how we interpret what is happening, we create the emotion of anger. The feeling of anger is based on the perception that what is happening, or what might happen, or what already happened, occurred differently than how we think it should have. Anger is a reaction we have when expectancy is not met. Anger occurs when we wish some aspect of the world, or somebody in it, were different than it is.

In life we have many rules or agreements of how things ought to be. The laws by which we abide are a vast collection of rules. These tend to serve the population toward our common good. Without these rules, we would experience chaos daily. Rules of this kind bring order to our lives.

A basketball player who dribbles the ball, stops dribbling, then starts dribbling again is guilty of double-dribbling and will lose possession of the ball. Basketball has many rules. Rules for sports and games help make the games fun and competitive.

We also have individual rules that we decide are the way things ought to be. A rule is our belief or sense of surety that something should be a certain way. Anger happens when someone breaks one of our rules. Whether we get angry at other people, at things, or at situations, we are responding to a perceived need to have things our way. Give it some thought and you'll discover that *every time you have been angry, it was because you were not getting your way.* Our thought about the event usually includes the words *should, ought to,* or *must*.

Here are some examples of rules we make about everyday events:

- Dogs shouldn't bark too loudly.
- Cats shouldn't throw up on my living room couch.
- The room should be quiet when we are practicing meditation.
- The music you are playing shouldn't be too loud.
- I was here first, so the waitress ought to take my order first.
- It should not rain on my wedding day.
- I should be able to talk to a real, live person when I call the airlines.
- This professor should be on time and should be interesting.
- My computer should work as it was designed to.
- People should have the good sense not to ram their grocery cart into my heels.
- People should not drive slowly in the fast lane.
- I made an appointment, so I shouldn't have to wait.

These are everyday rules that *we make up for ourselves.* No natural or cosmic law says the house must be quiet so you can meditate. No universal rule says that the person we have asked out on a date must say "yes." We have simply decided that this is how things ought to be. Anger is the emotion we create when something happens that conflicts with how we believe things ought to be, when something happens contrary to our rules. The event, of itself, does not make us angry any more than events can cause us to be stressed, fearful, or have any other emotion. The way we construct the event mentally in our minds, what it means to us, determines if we will become angry.

Therefore, anger is often the result of our decision about how people should act. Think back to our discussion of levels of responding from Chapter 6. Remember the scenario of Jenny standing in line waiting for a concert ticket. Had she held firm to her rule that the line should be moving more quickly than it was, the result may have been feelings of anger. Reacting in anger would cause unnecessary stress and may even result in Jenny doing something inappropriate.

This doesn't mean we should never get angry. If we notice ourselves feeling that something ought to be different than it is and we are in a position to make positive changes, we can channel our anger into productive action. Sometimes anger can be channeled into productive action on an even larger scale. When enough people have the same rules and agree that the rules are necessary for the safety and well-being of the entire population, those rules may become laws. This is the case with traffic laws and the laws restricting smoking in public places, for example.

Given this understanding, we can immediately defuse any bout of anger simply by reexamining our rule and being aware that our rule, not the event itself, is what is causing us to choose anger. For example, if you notice the cat has thrown up on the couch, rather than letting anger cause you to do something you will regret later, you can immediately look at the situation and recall the rule you have set up in your mind as the real cause of anger—the rule that cats should not throw up on the couch. With this awareness, you can operate from a more positive emotional state in regard to the cat, the mess it made, and everything else around you. As long as we stay focused on who or what we think made us angry, we will remain upset. Once we understand that we create our anger with our thoughts, we can take steps to reduce our anger.

Expressing Anger Is it best to hold your anger in or let it out? The answer depends on who you ask and how your anger is expressed.

The Research Highlight suggests that expressing anger is healthy, but how you express that anger may be even more important to your well-being. Research by Brad Bushman, a psychology professor at Iowa State University, suggests that letting anger out may make people

Anger Expression

Expressing anger may help protect men from heart disease and stroke, a new study shows. The risk of a nonfatal heart attack was cut by more than 50% in men with moderate levels of anger expression, and they also were less likely to have a stroke, compared to men who rarely expressed anger, according to the study published in *Psychosomatic Medicine.* It's possible that the men who rarely expressed anger were suppressing the emotion, and that may have led to a higher risk for heart disease and stroke. The study also indicates that the relationship between anger and cardiovascular disease may be more complex than previously thought.

Source: "Anger Expression and Risk of Stroke and Coronary Heart Disease Among Male Health Professionals," by P. Mona Eng, G. Fitzmaurice, L. Kubzansky, E. Rimm, and I. Kawachi, *Psychosomatic Medicine* (2003), 65, pp. 100–110.

more aggressive, not less. He says, "Many people think of anger as the psychological equivalent of the stream in a pressure cooker: It has to be released or it will explode. That's not true. The people who react by hitting, kicking, screaming, and swearing just feel more angry."[8]

You need only to watch a chair-throwing *Jerry Springer* show to see how inappropriate expressions of anger can lead to escalation. So "venting" may make you feel better, but only for the moment. You might want to think twice before you kick the dog or scream at your roommate. Venting your anger could:

1. Make you feel worse
2. Cause your situation to escalate
3. Lead to new problems you might have to fix later

Anger Blocker In Chapter 10 you will learn forgiveness techniques that can help you express and release anger in a healthy manner. When you find yourself in a tense situation, give yourself some time to breathe. Walk away from the situation and remind yourself that it might be best to consciously decide not to get angry in the first place. "Anger blockers" can help you do that.

Here are some tips for keeping anger in check:[9]

- First and foremost, get in touch with your thoughts at the time of your anger, and remind yourself that you don't have to think that way simply because you've always done so in the past.
- Try postponing your anger. If you typically react with anger in a specific circumstance, postpone the anger for 15 seconds, then explode in your typical fashion. Next, try 30 seconds, and keep lengthening the intervals. Once you see that you can postpone anger, you will have learned control.
- Don't try to delude yourself into believing that you enjoy something you find distasteful. You can dislike something and still not have to be angry about it.
- Remind yourself at the moment of anger that everyone has a right to be what he or she chooses and that demanding that anyone be different will simply prolong your anger. Work at allowing others to choose, just as you insist on your own right to do the same.
- Ask someone whom you trust to help. Have this person let you know when he or she sees your anger, either verbally or with an agreed signal. When you get the signal, think about what you are doing and then try the postponing strategy.
- Keep an anger journal, and record the exact time, place, and incident in which you chose to be angry. Be diligent with the entries; force yourself to record all angry behavior. You will soon find that the very act of having to write down the incident will persuade you to choose anger less often.
- After you have had an angry outburst, announce that you have just slipped and that one of your goals is to think differently so you don't experience this anger. The verbal announcement will put you in touch with what you have done and will demonstrate that you are truly working on yourself.
- Try being physically close to someone that you love at the moment of your anger. One way to neutralize your hostility is to hold hands—despite your inclination not to—and keep holding hands until you've expressed how you feel and dissipated your anger.

- Defuse your anger for the first few seconds by labeling how you feel, and how you believe your partner feels as well. The first 10 seconds are the most critical. Once you've passed this window of time, your anger will often have subsided.
- Get rid of unrealistic expectations. For example, remind yourself that the basic nature of children is to be active and loud occasionally.
- Love yourself. If you do, you won't want to burden yourself with self-destructive anger.
- In a traffic jam, time yourself. See how long you can go without exploding. Work at the control aspect. Use the time creatively to write a letter or a song, or devise ways to get out of the traffic jam, or relive the most exciting experience of your life, or, better yet, plan to improve on it.
- Instead of being an emotional slave to every frustrating circumstance, use the situation as a challenge to change it, and you will have no present moment time for the anger.
- Keep in mind that although the expression of anger may be a healthy alternative to storing it up, the healthiest choice is not to have it at all. Once you stop viewing anger as natural or "only human," you'll have an internal rationale for working to eliminate it.

Hostility

Hostility and *anger* are not interchangeable terms even though they frequently are used that way. Anger is considered a temporary emotion, usually in response to a specific event, and hostility is an attitude motivated by hatefulness and animosity. Hostility often is considered as anger that is projected outward at something or someone in an aggressive or antagonistic way. Although hostility usually is not considered an emotion, it is worthy of mention here because of the important relationship between hostility and health.

Researcher Dr. Meyer Friedman thinks hostility can best be defined by its manifestations, including:[10]

- Irritation or anger at the minor mistakes of others
- Looking for whatever might go wrong
- Inability to laugh at what other people laugh at
- Inability to trust others
- Suspicion that other people have selfish motives
- Frequent use of obscenities
- Difficulty in complimenting or congratulating others
- Preoccupation with the "errors" of the government, large corporations, or the younger generation.

Hostility is especially dangerous to the heart and may be a good predictor of heart attacks. Anger and hostility seem to have a dampening effect on the body's immune system. Hostility can be dangerous on the psychological level as well. People who are hostile tend to be involved in abuse and problems with marriage, higher levels of stress, less job satisfaction, and more problems in working relationships.[11]

Conclusion

The ability to experience a wide range of emotions is part of what makes us human and keeps life interesting. The challenge is in taking responsibility to control the negative emotions that can weaken our quality of life. Long-term emotions such as fear, worry, guilt, and anger can affect health in much the same way that long-term stress affects health and longevity. Don't let out-of-control emotions hold you back from experiencing the adventure of living.

Do you see life as an adventure? Do you seek opportunities to stretch and grow? Are you willing to put aside your fear of failure or change and test your limits? Are you able to face with power and confidence the unexpected challenges that come your way?

Feeling like you are stuck in a rut and living a life of drudgery can be highly stressful. You have a choice. You can choose adventurous living, or you can choose mediocrity. What will it be? What could be more stressful than letting fear prevent you from getting what you want from life? Take control of your emotions so they don't take control of you.

"Our doubts are traitors and cause us to lose the good we oft might win for fearing to attempt."
— *Shakespeare*

LAB

8.1 Feel the Fear—Go for It Anyway

PURPOSE The purpose of this activity is to allow you to overcome a fear by participating in an activity that is outside your comfort zones.

DIRECTIONS

1. Think of something that you are nervous or fearful of doing. Select something outside your comfort zone that you know should be done, but you have been avoiding because of your fears of what might or might not happen. Your assignment is to break through your fear and take a risk. To get you thinking, here are some examples of students' fear from previous classes:

- Ask somebody out on a date
- Quit a job
- Confront someone
- Forgive someone
- Interview for a job
- Speak in a public meeting
- Go rock climbing (fear of heights)
- Change majors
- Mend a broken relationship
- Tell someone who you have avoided that you love him or her
- Visit someone you don't know very well but would like to and get to know him or her better

2. Describe the thing you fear doing. Relate your thoughts and feelings about why it seems to be fearful for you.

3. After you have completed the assignment:

   1. Describe your experience from beginning to end of going for it and doing the thing you feared.
   2. Describe the insights you gained about that particular fear. Describe the insights you have gained about your own fears in general.
   3. Explain how this activity relates to stress management.

124

Key Points

- Emotional well-being requires appropriate expression of a wide range of emotions.
- Chronic guilt and worry, fear that prevents us from living life fully, and an attitude of hostility and anger are negative and stress-producing.
- Guilt is the conscious preoccupation with undesirable past thoughts and behaviors.
- Guilt keeps the mind occupied with thoughts and behaviors from the past, and worry, a manifestation of fear, keeps the mind focused on events yet to come.
- Worry is different from planning, the latter of which brings future moments into the present so we can apply appropriate control to those future events.
- The most effective way to remain free of guilt and worry is to practice being mindful.

- Fear is a state of escalated worry and apprehension that causes distinct physical and emotional reactions.
- Anger is a transient emotional response based on the way one chooses to think about events, usually triggered by perceived provocation or mistreatment.
- Anger is considered a temporary emotion, usually in response to a specific event, as different from hostility, which is an attitude motivated by hatefulness and animosity.
- Researchers have discovered that certain emotions can actually make a person more susceptible to stress and disease. These negative emotions include anger, worry, guilt, fear, and hostility.

Key Terms

guilt   fear   anger
worry   comfort zone   road rage
anxiety   discomfort zone   hostility

Discussion Time For Critical Thinking/Discussion Questions, please visit this book's Premium Website.

Notes

1. "Bringing Mind–Body Medicine into the Mainstream," by E. Taylor, C. Lee, and J. Young, *Hospital Practice 15*, (1997): 183.
2. *Your Erroneous Zones*, by W. Dyer (New York: Avon Books, 1976).
3. "Are You a Complete Worrier?" by A. Berger, *Complete Woman* (October 1987): 58.
4. *Wellness Guidelines for a Healthy Lifestyle* (3rd ed.), by W. Hoeger, L. Turner, and B. Hafen (Belmont, CA: Wadsworth/Thomson Learning, 2002).
5. "Why Are We So Angry?" by D. Hales, *Parade Magazine*, (September 2001): 10–11.
6. Dyer.
7. Williams and Williams.
8. Hales.
9. Dyer.
10. *The Healing Brain*, by R. Ornstein and D. Sobel (New York: Simon and Schuster, 1987).
11. *Anger Kills: 17 Strategies for Controlling the Hostility That Can Harm Your Health*, by R. Williams and V. Williams (New York: HarperCollins Publishers, 1993).

9 The Importance of Values

■ I'm not sure what my values are. What can I do to get in touch with my values? ■ I get frustrated when I know I make choices that are in conflict with my values. What can I do to live according to my values in my daily life? ■ What do my values have to do with stress management? ■ I nearly flunked out of college my first semester and I'm starting to think it was because I valued socializing and fitting in with the crowd more than I valued my education. What can I do to be sure this doesn't happen again?

Study of this chapter will enable you to:

1. Clarify and prioritize the values that are most important in your life.
2. Explain the connection between values clarification and stress management.
3. Explain the Niagara syndrome as it relates to feeling stuck in your life.
4. Differentiate between instrumental values and terminal values.
5. Participate in values clarification activities.

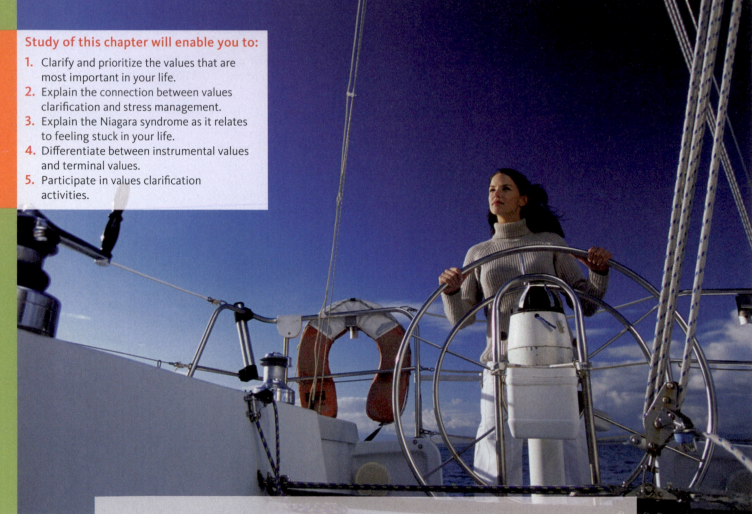

Nothing can bring you peace but yourself. Nothing can bring you peace but the triumph of principles.

—Ralph Waldo Emerson

© Southern Stock Corp Ltd/
Southern stock/Getty Images

Unchanging Principles Former President Jimmy Carter tells this story about his Plains High School superintendent, Miss Julia Coleman:

* * *

Remarkably, for a woman who never moved out of her small house in Plains, Georgia, her most important lesson was pertinent to every student who passed through her classrooms, regardless of which far-flung direction life took him. "We must adjust to changing times," she told us, "but cling to unchanging principles."

I never forgot that. She explained that we have to analyze new situations repeatedly, but whether it was choosing a spouse or selecting a career or making difficult decisions during times of stress or trial or temptation, we not only have to accommodate those new challenges but never deviate from certain ideals that we were taught, such as justice and integrity and peace and truthfulness and loyalty.

When I ran for president, I had many private conversations about what theme I should choose as my most ardent promise to the American people. I didn't want to go into complexities like supporting one specific House bill or another in my bigger speeches. My competitors did, but I said instead that I would never lie and that I would adhere to the basic principles that Miss Julia and my parents taught me. I quoted Miss Julia in my inaugural address—"Adjust to changing times but cling to unchanging principles"—committing myself and all Americans to real ideas of justice and truth, no matter what difficulties faced us.

Source: *The Right Words at the Right Time*, by M. Thomas (New York: Atria Books, 2002), pp. 44–46

The Importance of Values

Have you ever stopped to really think about who you are or how you want to live your life? This is something we do not tend to dwell on. The answers aren't always clear or easy in this sometimes confusing world. We might have a good idea of some aspects of our life, such as what we want to do academically or professionally. But many parts of our lives remain undiscovered. This may stem from our fear of finding what might be there, or maybe we simply don't know how to look. Clarifying our values and understanding what is central to defining who we are as individuals, and then living those values in our daily life, is essential to living with inner peace in an ever-changing world.

A **value** can be defined as a belief upon which one acts by preference.[1] Values guide our actions and give direction and meaning to life. When we place importance on something we cherish, we are valuing that trait, ideal, or characteristic. The decisions we make on a moment-to-moment basis create our future. Decision making comes down to how we value those things about which we are deciding. When you know what is most important to you, making the best decision is much easier. When you are unclear about what you value most, making the best decision is more difficult. The result is inner conflict and stress.

Understanding Your Values

Knowing our values, and then learning to live by them, is one of the most powerful ways to gain inner peace and decrease stress. This applies to our everyday choices as well as major decisions. Let's say you are taking a test in your math class and glance over to see your best friend, Rick, cheating. You clearly see the formulas written on his arm. When the professor isn't looking, Rick pushes up his sleeve and looks at his notes.

What would you do? Would you immediately report the cheating to your professor? Would you wait until after class to report your observations? Would you confront Rick after class? Or would you choose to do nothing, believing that in the end, cheating will hurt Rick and he will suffer the consequences eventually? Or maybe you feel no conflict and think Rick is smart for coming up with a clever strategy for cheating and decide you will try it yourself next time. Values are a strong determinant in the choices you make between competing alternatives.

Be more concerned with your character than your reputation, because your character is what you really are, while your reputation is merely what others think you are.

—*John Wooden*

Altruism—Helping Others, It Feels Good

Increasingly, students across the country are demonstrating their commitment to altruism, a value they hold high. Altruism, defined as helping or giving to others without thought of self-benefit, is put into action through student participation in community projects. Service-learning is now a student requirement in many universities. People become involved in community service for a range of reasons—for many, serving community is an altruistic act. "Today's college students have a strong altruistic bent, and are working in extraordinary ways to tackle some of our most pressing problems," said Corporation for National and Community Service CEO David Eisner. Tufts University CIRCLE (The Center for Information and Research on Civic Learning and Engagement) conducts research on the civic and political engagement of Americans between the ages of 15 and 25. Here are some findings:

- Most young people who volunteer want to help other people. For example, young people who volunteered for environmental organizations generally did so to help other people (52%), not to address a social or political problem (23%).
- Young people who grow up in a household where someone volunteers are twice as likely to volunteer regularly.
- Being asked is the top reason motivating young people to volunteer (closely followed by "because it makes me feel good").
- 87% of participants in the 2008 Civic Health Index Poll favored expanding national and community service programs so that every young American would have a chance to serve full-time for a year. Seventy six percent would like service-learning to be required of all high school students.

Volunteering and Educational Performance: The Link

It turns out that community service doesn't just feel good, it's good for you. A study correlating community service with academic success found that students who maintain a weekly community service record are significantly more likely to succeed and have a higher grade point average than those who do none at all. Investigations on the effect of school-required community service on academic performance found positive links between the two. Students who participated in school-required community service were 22% more likely to graduate from college than those who did not.

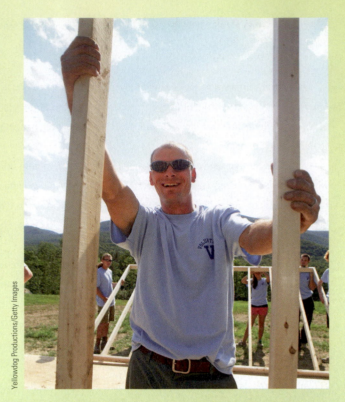

Yellowdog Productions/Getty Images

Many college students demonstrate altruism and a desire to help others by participating in service learning projects.

Examples of community service projects include (but are not limited to):

- cleaning a park;
- collecting much needed items including clothes, shoes, food, blankets, etc.;
- getting involved with Habitat for Humanity;
- cleaning up the side of the highways or roads;
- reading to the elderly in nursing homes;
- helping out a local fire or police department;
- helping out at a local library;
- tutoring developmentally disabled children for free; and
- participating in school activities that benefit the community.

If altruism is a value you hold highly, consider the benefits of volunteering to help others, and yourself.

Source: Center for Information and Research on Civic Learning and Engagement, Tufts University. Retreived from http://www.civicyouth.org, October 11, 2008.

> It is one of the most beautiful compensations of this life that no man can sincerely try to help another without helping himself.
> —*Ralph Waldo Emerson*

People who value honesty feel distress when they cheat on a test, copy a friend's paper, or shoplift from the mall. When a person places a high value on family yet finds little time to spend with the family, stress is the likely outcome. When our actions are not in line with our values, the natural emotional consequence is stress and inner chaos.

By comparison, those who value the personality traits of altruism and compassion and who devote time to volunteer for a hospice program will find deep feelings of peace and contentment because their actions are in line with their behavior. An individual who values health will gain peace and satisfaction by participating in regular exercise.

Think about the people we tend to respect the most in our culture. They usually are those who live by clearly defined values. Mahatma Gandhi, the great leader of India, is an example of someone who was entirely clear about his values, what was most important to him. Despite impossible odds, Gandhi's commitment to live according to his highest values ultimately brought about the freeing of an entire nation. Gandhi knew that his choices and behavior followed his values. He was driven by his values instead of being driven by his emotions or the circumstances in his environment. In Gandhi's words, "Happiness is when what you think, what you say, and what you do are in harmony."

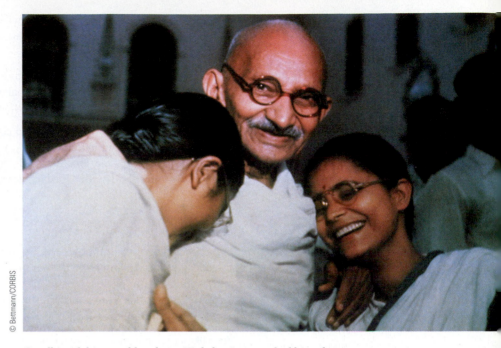

Gandhi with his granddaughters. His behaviors matched his values.

Discovering Your Values
One aspect of the complex Buddhist principle called **dharma** can be compared to a jigsaw puzzle. Consider the possibility that every person who has ever lived is a specific piece of an enormous puzzle of several billion pieces (one for each person). Consider, further, that your personal piece of this gigantic puzzle is a specific size and shape and fits correctly in only one precise place in this puzzle. Thus, you are not able to be another puzzle piece; you can be only your own.

Dharma teaches that when you find your place in the puzzle, you find satisfaction in life. You feel fulfilled, happy, and worthwhile. When a person wanders aimlessly through life not knowing where he or she fits in the puzzle, or tries to be someone else's puzzle piece, thinking that is the appropriate way to live, this person is likely to encounter confusion, unhappiness, and despair. Aimless people are not living according to their own puzzle piece, which is uniquely theirs and entirely necessary to discover. This is a source of stress.

What happens when we find our place in the puzzle? The natural consequences are inner peace, wisdom, and happiness. When we are certain about who we are, we feel fulfilled and satisfied with ourselves and the direction our life is going. We also understand that we are part of something bigger than ourselves. Every piece of the puzzle is necessary for the picture to be complete.

When we live by an agenda that is set by someone else, we easily get caught up in living someone else's life. One of the primary tasks involved in becoming an adult is to become more independent and self-directed in our thoughts and actions. Separating from the control and influence of parents and others and moving toward greater self-direction is a fundamental rite of passage into adulthood. Yet, when our values shift or when new values replace existing values, conflict and stress often result.

Cognitive Dissonance
The truth is that most people do not pay much attention to their values until they find themselves in a situation where they feel in conflict with them. The concept of **cognitive dissonance** refers to stress caused by holding two contradictory feelings simultaneously and results from situations in which our behavior is inconsistent with our beliefs, values, or self-image.

The greatest dissonance arises when the two alternatives are fairly equal. Dissonance theory is especially relevant to decision making and problem solving. A person who has dissonant cognitions is said to be in a state of psychological dissonance, experienced as unpleasant psychological tension or stress.

As an example, Mary and her best friend Sally are shopping at the mall. Sally tries on a sweater and just *has* to have it. The problem is that she has no money. Sally puts on her coat over the sweater and walks out of the store quickly. As Sally makes her getaway, the security guard races up to Mary and demands to know Sally's name. Conflict between

This above all, to thine own self be true, for it must follow as dost the night the day, thou canst not then be false to any man.
—*Shakespeare*

129

© Bettmann/CORBIS

Mary's belief that she should be faithful to her friend and her belief that it is wrong to steal results in psychological dissonance and stress.

Dissonance can be eliminated by:

1. reducing the importance of the conflicting beliefs,
2. acquiring new beliefs that change the balance, or
3. removing the conflicting attitude or behavior.

Think of an example when you experienced cognitive dissonance as a result of having to choose between competing values. When your behavior is guided by clear values, your stress is reduced. Values clarification and acquisition will help you. Before explaining those concepts, we will introduce the Niagara syndrome.

The Niagara Syndrome

What happens when we don't discover or aren't certain of our guiding principles? What are the consequences of not knowing our inner nature or of following someone else's perfect way—which is not perfect for us? Anthony Robbins, a recognized authority on peak performance, describes what commonly happens when people don't take a good look at who they are and where they are going. He calls this the **Niagara syndrome.**

> Life is like a river, and most people jump in the river of life without ever really deciding where they want to end up. So, in a short period of time, they get caught up in the current: current events, current fears, current challenges. When they come to forks in the river, they don't consciously decide where they want to go, or which direction is right for them. They merely "go with the flow." They become a part of the mass of people who are directed by the environment instead of by their own values. As a result, they feel out of control. They remain in this unconscious state until one day the sound of the raging water awakens them and they discover that they are 5 feet from Niagara Falls in a boat with no oars.
>
> At this point, all they can say is, "Oh, shoot!" But by then it's too late. They are going to take a fall. Sometimes it's an emotional fall. Sometimes it's a physical fall. Sometimes it's a financial fall. It is likely that whatever challenges you have in your life currently could have been avoided by some better decisions upstream.[2]

Stephen Covey relates a similar analogy of the person who spends his entire life climbing the ladder of success only to realize, when he arrives at the top, that his ladder is leaning against the wrong wall.[3] Throughout life, we are faced with choices that determine whether we flow in a different river or climb a different ladder. When we base decisions and actions on our values, we end up where we want to be.

Source of Values

Where do our values come from? We tend to base our values on several sources— our culture, our parental and familial influences, our teachers, friends, and other environmental influences such as television, the Internet, and a host of other media outlets. Most of our values remain at the unconscious level. We don't spend conscious time deciding if the things we see and hear are valuable to us.

Advertisers fully understand this principle. If they promote an idea for a sufficient amount of time and with enough appeal, they can convince some people to believe in nearly any value. Smoking is a good example of this. After scientific research showed the ill effects of tobacco on health, tobacco companies realized that using their product is not a healthy choice and that if people really believed this, they would not be inclined to use tobacco. But with shrewd advertising, designed to convince consumers of the value of smoking, millions

This Is My Life

On one occasion, when I was about 24, I was jogging, nearing the end of a fairly long run. The endorphins were cruising, the second wind was well in place, and I was feeling very good. I was at that place where I felt like I could jog forever. I wasn't really thinking of anything in particular when an overwhelming thought suddenly occurred to me. It sounded something like, "Damn! This is my life I'm living here! My life is nobody else's to live. I can live only this life, and all I will ever have is my life. But when I go along with the crowd, I'm not living my life. When I follow the direction that my parents, my teachers, and my coaches think is best for me, I'm not living my own life. My life is mine to choose. And if I don't start choosing, it's going to pass me by."

Then and there, I knew I didn't want to come to the end of my life and think that I had settled for mediocrity, that I had gotten so caught up in the day-to-day stuff that I had lost all awareness of what was really important to me. I didn't want my final words, when the time came to depart from this life, to be "if only."

—MO

of people have taken up a habit that most wish they had not started in the first place. If no one thought there was value in lighting up this plant and sticking it in the mouth to inhale the fumes that come from the burning plant, no one would choose to do it in the first place. The value placed on doing this determines whether a person will do it or not.

Values within Cultures

Culture is a pattern of learned behavior based on values, beliefs, and perceptions of the world. It is the lens through which we see the world. More important than the behavior is the underlying values that encourage or discourage that specific behavior. Some cultures teach, for instance, that you should stay in control of your emotions at all times. You are taught to value this control and believe that crying or expressing anger is an indication of weakness and therefore to be avoided. You are taught that men should not cry. These cultural beliefs may increase your stress because you do not feel free to express your emotions.

Another cultural value relates to what is sometimes called the "Protestant work ethic." If you value hard work to the extent that you don't feel good about yourself if you are not working and being productive, you may have difficulty participating in recreation and relaxation to manage your stress. If your identity becomes so closely linked with the work you do, you may lose sight of who you are when you are not working. Someone once said, "When who you are is what you do, then when you don't, you aren't."

Predominant Values in United States

Some of the common values in the United States are listed here.[4] Consider ways in which society promotes these values and how each may contribute to stress. Although the United States is becoming an increasingly diverse culture and not every individual will place equal emphasis on these values, studies indicate that these are accepted values in many segments of this society.

1. *Personal achievement and success.* What is good for the individual may be more important than what is good for the community or society. Emphasis is on power, competition, and wealth.
2. *Activity and work.* Hard work will be rewarded, and people who do not work hard are considered lazy, regardless of whether they have the same opportunities to achieve success.
3. *Moral orientation.* The tendency is to view things as good or bad, right or wrong, a pattern that reinforces stereotyping.
4. *Efficiency and practicality.* The short-term, quick fix is often seen as the solution to problems, rather than long-term solutions.
5. *Progress.* Change is often viewed as progress and technology is highly valued in this process. The focus is on the future rather than the present.
6. *Material comfort.* The consumer-oriented society values a high standard of living.
7. *Personal freedom and individualism.* Individual rights are highly valued, sometimes at the expense of the common good.
8. *External conformity.* Notwithstanding the value of personal freedom, pressure is applied to conform to the predominant European American, middle-class, Judeo-Christian values.
9. *Science and rationality.* The scientific, medical approach to health has led to expectations of high-tech, quick-fix solutions with less emphasis on individual responsibility.

Predominant Alaska Native Values

Compare the predominant American values with those of the Alaska Native culture.[5] Notice the similarities and the differences of the important values.

1. *Show respect to others.* Each person has a special gift.
2. *Share what you have.* Giving makes you richer.
3. *Know who you are.* You are a reflection on your family.
4. *Accept what life brings.* You cannot control many things.
5. *Have patience.* Some things cannot be rushed.
6. *Live carefully.* What you do will come back to you.
7. *Take care of others.* You cannot live without them.
8. *Honor your elders.* They show you the way in life.
9. *Pray for guidance.* Many things are not known.
10. *See connections.* All things are related.

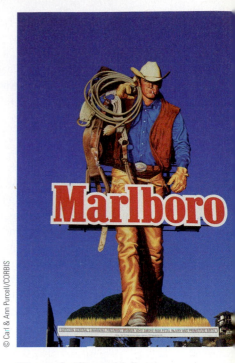

© Carl & Ann Purcell/CORBIS

We spend millions of dollars every year on products we don't need because advertisers know how to appeal to our emotions and values.

131

The Lakota Perspective of Peace and Harmony

Leonard Little Finger, great-grandson of Chief Big Foot, who was massacred at Wounded Knee, shares his perspective on Lakota values as they relate to stress management:

* * *

Throughout the Lakota history, beginning when they were known as the People of the Seven Council Fires, they understood the relationships of being interconnected with all of creation and Creator, known to them as Tunkasila, Grandfather of all. They held paramount in their belief system that the created (people and all created) were all related to one another, and all existed within a sacred circle. The flame of the council fire was likened to the flame of the sun, and the flame represented the sum of a way of life within a sacred circle, to be attained in conduct, behavior, and spiritual existence supported by law and value systems.

The sacred pipe, Cannupa, integral to all since its inception, was brought by a sacred being known as the White Buffalo Calf Woman. The rituals and ceremonies such as Hanbelciya, Vision Quest, Inipi, Sweat Lodge, Wi'wangwaci, Sundance, and the other ceremonies—are all inscribed in circles around the pipe. In addition, there are rings that denote the principal values including Kinship, Respect, Generosity, and Sharing to dictate behavior and conduct to all that is in this sacred circle.

Thus, (it dictates) the purposes to fuse an individual with his or her counterparts in the community of mankind, as well as the larger community of all. Adherence to this allows a raising or expanding of individual consciousness known to the Lakota as "Natural Law." To learn and understand this ancient and traditional spiritual knowledge sheds the isolated, individual personality and restores a conscious harmony with the universe or "Sacred Circle of Life," or "Cangleska Wakan." Peace and harmony understandings replace stress and discord. The body, mind, and spirit become one in identity.

Source: "Personal communication," Leonard Little Finger, May 9, 2005.

Reflect on the Lakota values explained in the Culture Connection. Take special note of the values of kinship, respect, generosity, and sharing that dictate behavior and conduct. Think about the impact of these different values on the perception of stress in a culture. Take time to reflect on how your cultural beliefs impact your values.

The Dynamic Quality of Values

Throughout life, we can benefit from taking time to clarify the values that guide our choices. A personal value system is not static. When we are young, our values mirror those of our parents or teachers. As we move through adolescence and young adulthood, we may challenge the values we learned as a child and develop more personal values resulting from a mix of what we learned from our parents and what we have chosen to embrace from our culture. Think of a value you have acquired that is new or different from a value your parents taught you. Has this value contributed to your well-being?

The 18-year-old college freshman away from home for the first time, the middle-aged executive who unexpectedly finds himself out of a job, the mother returning to college after 20 years of staying home to raise a family, and the elderly widower alone after 60 years as part of a couple—all may ask the same questions as they search for meaning in their lives. Who am I? What do I really want in life? What is the right path for me to take? The answer to these questions comes from understanding personal values and being true to them.

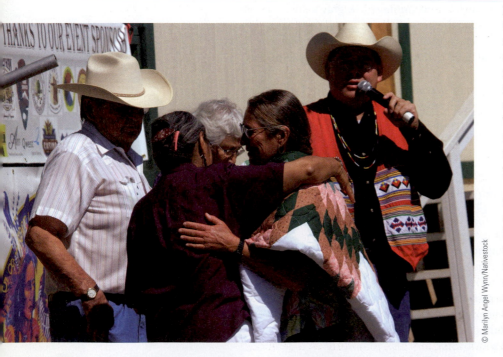

© Marilyn Angel Wynn/Nativestock

Give away ceremony honors people who made a positive difference. Some cultures hold high the value of sharing.

Acquiring Values

Many of our values are assimilated from family, friends, church, and society. **Values acquisition,** by contrast, means to consciously assume a new value. For example, a nursing student may deliberately acquire the professional value of caring or respect for human dignity as a result of education and experience. Or maybe for the first time, you have met someone you think you could spend the rest of your life with. You consciously nurture the values of love and commitment as the value of independence becomes less important to you. Values continually evolve as an individual matures in the ability to think critically and morally.

The seven steps in values acquisition are as follows:[6]

Step 1: The value is chosen freely.
Step 2: The value is chosen from among alternatives.
Step 3: The value is chosen after careful consideration of each alternative.
Step 4: The value is prized and cherished.
Step 5: The value is publicly affirmed.
Step 6: The value is acted upon.
Step 7: The value is part of a pattern of repeated action (the value is incorporated into the individual's lifestyle).

Beliefs about Values

To make positive change in the direction of our own true path, we must firmly maintain several beliefs in our mind to support us as we begin our journey.

1. We must first believe that we are capable of changing our thoughts and actions. Regardless of our current situation, we have the capacity and the ability to make any changes that we think are appropriate.

2. We also must have the belief that if we are going to create long-term change in our lives, we are responsible. Nobody else is going to do it for us. It requires our own decision, our own motivation, and our own action.

> It is better to conquer yourself than to win a thousand battles. Then the victory is yours. It cannot be taken from you, not by angels or by demons, heaven or hell.
>
> —*Buddha*

3. We must have the belief that if we set our sights in a new direction, and then move confidently in that direction, we will successfully arrive near the place we wanted to go. Henry David Thoreau wrote of his time at Walden Pond:

> I learned this, at least, by my experiment; that if one advances confidently in the direction of his dreams, and endeavors to live the life which he has imagined, he will meet with success in uncommon hours.

4. We must be clear that our values determine our actions and behaviors. We may not be clear about what we value, but our choices depend on what we believe is most important to us. All decision making is based on values clarification.

Values are the foundation for determining who we are and how we live and strongly influence the knowledge, attitudes, and beliefs that make us unique individuals.

Types of Values

Instrumental and Terminal Values Values are explained as enduring beliefs that a specific mode of conduct or end-state of existence is personally or socially preferable to an opposite or converse mode of conduct or end-state of existence. Two kinds of values are:[7]

1. **Instrumental values,** which consist primarily of personal characteristics and character traits.
2. **Terminal values,** which are the outcomes we work toward or we believe are most important and desirable.

Instrumental values involve ways of being that help us arrive at terminal values. They are ways of triggering our terminal values. Figure 9.1 provides examples of instrumental values.

Terminal values are end states of feeling. These comprise the emotional state you prefer to experience. Terminal values make our lives fulfilling and worthwhile. Figure 9.2 presents examples of terminal values.

The two listings in Figures 9.1 and 9.2 appear in a checklist format for you to use to assess your values. These lists aren't exhaustive. Rather, each provides examples of the two types of

FIGURE 9.1 Instrumental Values Checklist

- Ambitious (hard-working, aspiring)
- Broad-minded (open-minded)
- Capable (competent, effective)
- Cheerful (lighthearted, joyful)
- Clean (neat, tidy)
- Courageous (standing up for your beliefs)
- Forgiving (willing to pardon others)
- Helpful (working for the welfare of others)
- Honest (sincere, truthful)
- Imaginative (daring, creative)
- Independent (self-reliant, self-sufficient)
- Intellectual (intelligent, reflective)
- Logical (consistent, rational)
- Loving (affectionate, tender)
- Obedient (dutiful, respectful)
- Polite (courteous, well-mannered)
- Responsible (dependable, reliable)
- Self-controlled (restrained, self-disciplined)

FIGURE 9.2 Terminal Values Checklist

- A world at peace (free of war and conflict)
- Family security (taking care of loved ones)
- Freedom (independence, free choice)
- Equality (brotherhood, equal opportunity for all)
- Self-respect (self-esteem)
- Happiness (contentedness)
- Wisdom (a mature understanding of life)
- National security (protection from attack)
- Salvation (saved, eternal life)
- True friendship (close companionship)
- A sense of accomplishment (a lasting contribution)
- Inner harmony (freedom from inner conflict)
- A comfortable life (a prosperous life)
- Mature love (sexual and spiritual intimacy)
- A world of beauty (beauty of nature and the arts)
- Pleasure (an enjoyable leisurely life)
- Social recognition (respect, admiration)
- An exciting life (a stimulating active life)

values and indicates how they differ. Additional terminal values, for example, could include among many others, good health, power, passion, adventure, spontaneity, and control.

Values Clarification

Finding out what is most important to us may seem like an overwhelming task because we have so many things to consider. **Values clarification**—the process of clarifying and applying what we truly value—is helpful in reducing the stress that comes from making choices that are inconsistent with our values. Values clarification is a cognitive process that helps close the gap between what we value and what we actually do.

Clarifying and prioritizing values has great benefit. Many companies and corporations around the world have gone through the same process of finding what is most important to the company and then striving to live according to that understanding. The end result is commonly called a mission statement or a constitution.

Creating Your Personal Constitution

The following three-step process will guide you in clarifying and applying your key values. You will begin by identifying your values, next you will prioritize your values, and finally, you will write a clarifying paragraph for each of your top values. Complete the Stress Management Lab at the end of this chapter as you move through this process.

Step 1: Identify Your Values Begin by completing the following activities— Instrumental and Terminal Values Selection, and Your Funeral.

Activity #1: Instrumental and Terminal Values Selection Review the listings of Instrumental and Terminal Values found in Figures 9.1 and 9.2. Put a checkmark by each of the values listed that are important for you. Feel free to include additional values that are of importance to you.

Activity #2: Your Funeral Stephen Covey suggests another way to uncover the things that matter most to you. With your eyes closed, imagine in your mind the following scenario while someone else reads it to you:

> See yourself going to the funeral of a loved one. Picture yourself driving to the funeral parlor or chapel, parking the car, and getting out. As you walk inside the building, you notice the flowers and the soft organ music. You see the faces of friends and family you pass along the way. You feel the sense of sorrow that permeates the room for losing this special person. You also sense the shared joy of having known this person that radiates from the hearts of all the people there.
>
> As you walk down to the front of the room and look inside the casket, you suddenly come face to face with yourself. This is your own funeral and all of these people have come to honor you. They are here to express their feelings of love and appreciation for your life.
>
> As you take a seat and wait for the services to begin, you look at the program in your hand. There are to be four speakers. The first speaker is someone from your immediate family— perhaps your mom or dad, a brother, sister, aunt or uncle, a cousin or grandparent. The second speaker is one of your best friends, someone who is going to tell about the kind of person you were. The third speaker is from your work or an instructor in your school. The fourth is someone from your church or community organization where you have been involved in service.
>
> Now think deeply. What would you like each of these speakers to say about you and your life? What kind of son or daughter would you like their words to reflect? What kind of friend would you like to have others say you were? Were you there for others when they needed you? Did you care for them and trust them and have a deep respect for them? What would you best friend say about you at your own funeral? What about someone who is a neighbor who knows of you, but doesn't know you really well? What contributions would you like them to have said you made to other people's lives? What achievements would you want them to remember?[8]

Based on the Instrumental and Terminal Values and Your Funeral activities, record your results in the Stress Management Lab at the end of the chapter. In no particular order, what came to you as being your highest values. Write down all the values that came to mind. It doesn't matter how many you have. What matters is that they are yours. Look back at the Tombstone Test you completed as an assessment in Chapter 2. Compare what you wrote then to the values you have identified in this chapter.

You may find some inconsistencies—you may find that you have some values that you are not doing anything about at the present time. That is okay. List them anyway, if they are important to you. For example, you might value your health highly, but you may not be doing anything currently to improve your level of health and well-being. You still hold health as a high personal value.

Now you have a list of all your important values. Once you have identified your highest values, you can proceed to Step 2.

Step 2: Prioritize Your Values

Next, prioritize your list of values in order of importance to you. The item that is the most important goes at the top of the list. The next important value goes next, and so on through your entire list.

You may ask why this is an important step. *If you are clear about the order of your highest values, no decision is difficult.* This holds true for life's big decisions as well as the little decisions. To illustrate, imagine that you have, as one of your highest values, seeking excitement and being a thrill-seeking risk taker. You also may have security and stability as another value, but you have determined that you do not hold this latter value as highly as the first. If you happen to be in school and are studying to be an accountant who will spend most of your professional life sitting behind desks crunching numbers, you probably will find little satisfaction in that career path.

Imagine that you were offered a high-paying job requiring you to live in another country where you don't know the language and don't know anyone there. Whether you would accept the job depends on which values you ranked the highest. If you value adventure and risk taking along with an increase in your finances more highly than some of your other values, you probably would consider the proposal. If you value security, safety, and a rich family life more highly, you probably would pass up this job offer.

Knowing the order of values applies in making smaller decisions as well. Imagine that one of your values is high-level health and well-being. Another one of your values is that of being social and having a good time with friends. One of your friends calls you and says she is having a party on Friday. You know what kind of parties she throws: a lot of drinking and all the other things that go along with plentiful alcohol. Whether you will go or not is an easy decision, depending on which value you hold more highly. If you value socializing over your good health, the obvious choice is to go to the party. If you value your health more highly than socializing, you probably won't show up at the party, or you might decide to go as the designated driver.

How you prioritize your values is up to you. *This must be your decision.* The order of your values probably will change as you go through different stages of your life. For example, while you are in school and perhaps not married, you might not rank a family relationship as highly as you rank your academic development. Later on, as you perhaps create a family and develop your career, these values will become more important to you. These might be on your list now, but not ranked as highly.

Anthony Robbins suggests that you ask this important question: "If I were to design my own life, if I were going to create a set of values that shape the ultimate destiny I desire, what would they need to be?" He asks us to look at our values and see if we can rearrange them (change their order), add others and subtract some, in order to have the largest impact on our own lives.[9]

What would be the single most important value that would propel you toward living your life the most fully? What would be the next most important

---

Author Anecdote Finding the Worth of Values One day in class we were discussing this idea of prioritizing our values in a way that would propel someone toward the most fulfilling life. The reason this is so important became apparent. One student went through the entire process of finding her highest values, putting them in order, and then attaching a clarifying paragraph to each value. As I looked at her list, I saw that she had some major discrepancies between her values and her daily behavior. I also noticed that both her values and her behaviors were mediocre. The number-one value in her life was her dog. This was the most important thing to her. She really loved her dog, and I respected that fully, but she seemed to be setting herself up for long-term depression if something were to happen to the dog.

The other values she listed were uninspiring by any standards. Her life was similarly uninspiring. She was letting life happen to her like waves knocking her over, one after another. She was not the captain of her own ship. If she would have looked at her values and asked herself, "What would my values have to be to create my ultimate destiny, to be the best person I could possibly be, to have the most impact in my lifetime?" she probably would have made a far different list of values, in an order that enabled her, and motivated her, to rise above the mediocre level in which she was currently functioning. She would have charted a different destiny for herself.

—MO

value that you could integrate into your life that would have the greatest positive effect? Perhaps you have always felt that freedom is the most important thing to you. And maybe this freedom has resulted in a level of loneliness that is uncomfortable for you. If you were to include the value of intimacy as a higher value than freedom, your new focus would fill that gap you feel is currently lacking.

You now have a list ranking your important values starting with your single most important value. Again, you may or may not be living your life currently as a reflection of your prioritized values. The important learning in this step is to become aware of the values most important to you.

Step 3: Write a Clarifying Paragraph for Your Values In this step, describe what it means to be living your important values. Write a clarifying paragraph for each of your top values. Write these clarifying paragraphs as affirmations. An **affirmation** has the following three characteristics:

1. Write your affirmation as a *positive statement.* If one of your values happens to be that of maintaining high-level health, your statement might say: "I eat food that is healthy for my body, I exercise regularly, and I rest my body well to rejuvenate and recharge myself." You would not write your statement to sound like, "I don't put bad food in my body. I never go through a day without exercising, and I don't let stress get the upper hand." We are developing a mental image or picture of what it would be like in reality. It may not be happening right now, but if we have the correct picture clearly in our minds, we are much more likely to act on that picture. This happens best when we write positive statements.

2. Write your clarifying affirmations as *"I" messages,* as the examples above demonstrate. When you put yourselves into the affirmation, your mind receives the message that you are the one who is making the change.

3. Write your clarifying paragraph in the *present tense,* as if it is happening currently. For example: "I eat food that is healthy for my body, I exercise regularly, and I rest my body well to rejuvenate and recharge myself." This is instead of: "I will eat healthy food. I will exercise. I will do things to manage my stress levels." The psychology behind this principle is similar to the other two: When we tell our mind, again and again, that something is happening currently, just like the advertisers do, we tend to believe it and will be more likely to act in ways that assume this is the case. When we place the realization of that value in the future, our mind considers that it will happen in the future, not the present.

Ben Franklin's 13 Virtues
FYI

After nearly a half-century of regular practice, Benjamin finally recognized that he had realized his values. Ben Franklin showed us how powerful this process can be. When he was 27 years old, he had a midlife crisis. While working in a printing plant in Philadelphia, he felt like he hadn't accomplished anything. At that time, he asked himself some important questions that made him contemplate what his life was all about. After careful reflection, he discovered 13 values that were supremely important to him, and by living according to what he thought each one meant would cause him to, in his words, "become a perfect mortal." In his autobiography he called these his "13 virtues."

After Ben Franklin had decided on his highest values, he described each one in a short paragraph so he was absolutely clear what each of them meant to him. Then he organized his life in 13-week cycles. Each week he mentally focused on one of his values as the underlying foundation for all of his activity. He was trying to pull his performance in line with his values.

At the age of 79, Ben Franklin wrote that he had come to an important conclusion: He said he believed he had achieved oneness with his governing values. His values and his behavior were one and the same. He had earned the right to the consequential feeling of inner peace. As a result, Ben Franklin contributed a great deal to make the United States a better country, his own life more productive, and our lives happier. He created a lifetime of achievement and success based on how he lived according to the values that mattered most to him.

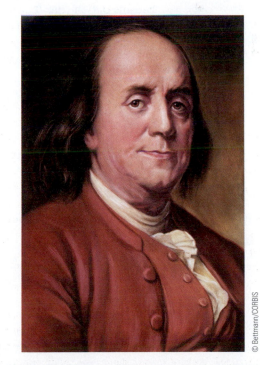

© Bettmann/CORBIS

Ben Franklin spent his life striving to live according to his highest values.

Source: *Autobiography,* by B. Franklin (London: MacMillan, 1993).

Don't be discouraged if you write a clarifying paragraph and realize that this does not represent your current reality. That is okay. You are developing a vision to guide you.

Values clarification and acquisition do not constitute a once-in-a-lifetime activity but, rather, an ongoing process of conscious reflection and deliberate action for sorting out what is most important to you. Values are more than ideals we'd like to attain; they should be reflected in the way we live each day.[10] The end result is increased awareness, focused direction, and greater inner peace.

The work of Ben Franklin and other wise individuals of his time have left a lasting legacy that affects nearly every aspect of our life today. After many months of hard work, the founding fathers of our country created the U.S. Constitution. This document of national values guides the creation of all laws that are made in every legislative body in the entire country.

Similarly, on a personal level, our own "personal constitution" can be our inner guide to all decisions we make during our lifetime. This process isn't easy—which probably is why so few people take the time to undertake it. Going with the flow and watching to see where the current takes us is easier. But those who go through this process, be it a major corporation, a family, or an individual, find tremendous value in selecting the path of their choosing. They find their own piece of the puzzle and experience the joy and satisfaction of a fulfilling life.

> The measure of a man's real character is what he would do if he knew he would never be found out.
> —Thomas B. Macaulay

Conclusion

A ship without a rudder wanders aimlessly in the sea. Similarly, if we don't know why we are alive and what is most important to us, we spend a lot of time throughout our lives wondering and wandering aimlessly. Values clarification and acquisition put the rudder in the water and help us move in the direction that is best for each of us on a personal level.

The goal of values clarification is to facilitate self-understanding. This dynamic and ongoing process results in behaviors that are consistent with values. Actions are based, either consciously or unconsciously, on values. There is tremendous power in discovering and living according to our highest values. Cognitive dissonance is reduced. Inner peace is the natural consequence.

Your values become the basis for every decision that you make. Your task now is to follow through, as Ben Franklin did, and internalize your values. By looking at your values often and thinking deeply about what they mean to you, little by little these values will become part of you. They will guide you to become the person you most want to be. You will experience the type of life you really want. You will be the captain of your ship.

LAB

9.1 Creating Your Personal Constitution

PURPOSE The purpose of this activity is to help you:

1. discover and prioritize your governing values

2. write clarifying statements for your values

3. create your personal constitution to live by

4. reduce your stress by making choices in harmony with your values

I. Identify and Prioritize Governing Values

What matters most to you and what do you value the most? What value, idea or principle has such great worth that you would dedicate your life to be able to live that value?

1. To answer these questions, begin by listing all the values that came to mind as you completed the Instrumental and Terminal Values Selection and "Your Funeral" activities in this chapter. Do not list them in any order, but simply write down all those values that seem to be worthwhile to you. List as many values as is helpful to you, but start with at least 15 values.

2. Next, prioritize your list of values according to their worth to you. As you are doing this, you may want to consider the following question, "If I were to really design my own life, if I were going to create a set of values that shape the ultimate destiny I desired, what would they need to be and in what order?"

II. Develop Clarifying Statements and Your Personal Constitution

Write a clarifying statement for at least your top five prioritized values. Answer the question, "What does this value really mean to me?" If you were living that value perfectly, what would your behavior be like and how would you describe it? Consider the following guidelines from earlier in the chapter as you write each clarifying statement:

- Write each statement as an affirmation, a *positive statement*.
- Write each clarifying statements as an *"I" message*.
- Write your clarifying paragraph in the *present tense* as if it is currently happening.

For example, a correctly written clarifying paragraph for the value of good health might sound like this:
"I am healthy and strong. My body and mind function perfectly at all times. I treat myself with respect. I eat well; I get plenty of exercise, sufficient rest, and manage my stress in excellent ways. My mind and body now function perfectly."

You may want to continue writing clarifying paragraphs for more of your values. Once you have completed this process, you will have created your own personal constitution to use as the standard for everything you do in your life.

Key Points

- A value can be defined as a belief upon which one acts by preference. Values give direction and meaning to one's life.
- Clarifying our values and understanding what is central to defining who we are as individuals will help reduce stress.
- Dharma teaches us that when we find our place in the puzzle of life, we attain satisfaction in life; we feel fulfilled, happy, content, and worthwhile.
- Cognitive dissonance results when our behavior is inconsistent with our beliefs, values, or self-image.
- Most of our values remain at the unconscious level unless we examine them consciously.

- Values acquisition, the conscious assumption of a new value, has seven criteria.
- Instrumental values consist primarily of personal characteristics and character traits.
- Terminal values are outcomes that we work toward or believe are most important and desirable.
- Values clarification, the process of applying what we truly value, helps reduce the stress that comes from making choices that are inconsistent with our values.
- The three-step action plan for values clarification provides an experiential values clarification activity.

Key Terms

value
dharma
cognitive dissonance
Niagara syndrome

culture
values acquisition
instrumental values

terminal values
values clarification
affirmation

Discussion Time For Critical Thinking/Discussion Questions, please visit this book's Premium Website.

Notes

1. *Pattern and Growth in Personality*, by G. W. Allport (New York: Holt, Rinehart & Winston, 1961).
2. *Awaken the Giant Within*, by A. Robbins (New York: Summit Books, 1991).
3. *The 7 Habits of Highly Effective People*, by S. Covey (New York: Simon & Schuster, 1989).
4. *Strangers To These Shores: Race and Ethnic Relations in the United States*, by V. Parrillo (New York: Macmillan, 1990).
5. "Health Care in Alaska Native Communities: Learning Firsthand of the Challenges" (CAM at the NIH), by National Center for Complementary and Alternative Medicine, *Focus on Complementary and Alternative Medicine* 7(2) (2005): 3–4.
6. *Interpersonal Relationships* (5th ed.), by E. Arnold and K. Boggs (Philadelphia: Elsevier Saunders Co., 2007).
7. *The Nature of Human Values*, by M. Rokeach (New York: Free Press, 1973).
8. Covey, *The 7 Habits of Highly Effective People.*
9. Robbins, *Awaken the Giant Within.*
10. *An Invitation to Health*, by D. Hales (Belmont, CA: Wadsworth/Cengage Learning, 2009-2010).

10 Spirituality

■ I have never talked about spiritual issues in any college class. What does spirituality really mean and what does it have to do with managing my stress? ■ How can I bring spirituality into my daily life in a way that will help me cope with, or even prevent, stress? ■ Can I be spiritually healthy even though I don't go to church? ■ Can prayer change anything? ■ I was deeply hurt by my best friend and can't seem to get over it. My feelings are causing me great stress. How can I learn to forgive my friend so I can get on with my life?

Study of this chapter will enable you to:

1. Describe the influence of spirituality on stress.
2. Differentiate between the terms *religiosity* and *spirituality*.
3. Discuss the research linking spirituality and health.
4. Summarize the barriers to research on spirituality.
5. Delineate five qualities of spiritual health.
6. Develop a personal plan to reduce stress through spiritual balance.

We are not human beings on a spiritual journey, but spiritual beings on a human journey.

—*Pierre Teilhard de Chardin*

Maria's Story I was in love with my high school sweetheart. We were going to get married and have six children. We were best friends. Our daily lives revolved around each other. After being together every possible moment for five years, he phoned me to say he didn't want to be together anymore. Giving no explanation, he was out of my life forever. At first I was in shock. We had been talking about marriage, and now he's out of my life. After the shock, I was in denial, then depression. How was I even supposed to live? My whole life was turned upside down. All my plans were ripped apart.

Though I may not sound like it, I'm not a stressed-out person and I've tried to avoid drama, but I didn't handle this situation well. I skipped classes and called in sick to work. I couldn't sleep and was unhealthy from lack of nutrition. I have a supportive family, yet I felt all alone. I couldn't eat, and sometimes I felt like I could hardly breathe. I felt like my life was over and I had no reason to live.

There is light at the end of this story. When I felt I had no one, I prayed. I was comforted and gradually began to understand that no one knows why bad things happen. I learned to trust that everything has a reason. God showed me to be patient because He was trying to work in my life. Shortly after our breakup, I had an opportunity to go on a life-changing mission to Jamaica. Now my life is better than ever.

In hindsight, I learned some lessons about life that I wouldn't have learned any other way. I've become a better, more understanding person because of this experience. I also have learned that because of my faith, I can handle the challenges that are part of life. I truly believe that all of the other aspects of life branch off from spirituality. I now feel fulfilled inside, and it reflects in all the other areas of my life. Spirituality is different for everyone, but for me, this is what it is and this is how I cope with stress, and with every situation in my life. This is a daily walk. I may have been happy at times before, but now I know what it feels like to be joyful.

Spirituality

Spirituality is at the heart of stress management. Your spiritual life is a potent prescription for achieving balance and health. People with a deep sense of spirituality view life differently. They have a purpose, they enjoy a sense of meaning in life, and they have a broader perspective. Spirituality buffers stress. People with a deep sense of spirituality are not defeated by crises. They are able to relax their mind, elicit the relaxation response, and heal more quickly and completely.[1]

Think back to the dimensions of health explained in Chapter 1. Here, in this chapter, we focus on the spiritual dimension. You will learn that the spiritual dimension generates a sense of peace with yourself and the world. Rather than searching outside yourself for answers, you realize that the source of your fulfillment is inside you.[2]

Discovering the contemplative, spiritual life requires not so much a radical change in lifestyle as a shift in awareness, an inner change. It is the inner intention of our spiritual essence, rather than outward circumstances of our lives, that brings peace.[3]

Relaxation is part of spiritual healing. Peace is an outcome of spiritual health.

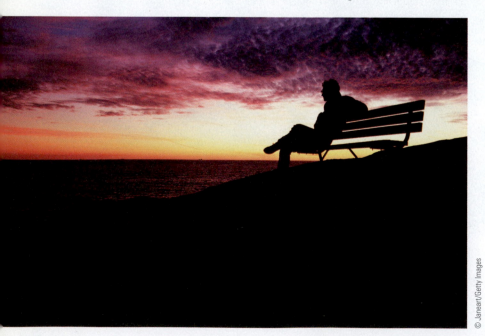

© Janeart/Getty Images

What is life all about? Pondering the vastness of the universe and what it is that brings meaning to our existence contributes to spiritual growth.

The Spiritual Quest

At a time in history when stress is said to be epidemic, our nation not surprisingly is searching for answers about the meaning of life. With the dawn of a new century, spirituality has come to the forefront in the workplace, politics, education, and healthcare.[4] Events such as the destruction of the World Trade Centers, Gulf Coast hurricanes, and the wildly fluctuating stock market, which change the lives of millions, cause us to pause and think about what is truly important in life.

Americans are looking for answers and seeking guidance on human spirituality, as evidenced by a surge in best-selling books such as *The Purpose-Driven Life, The Tao of Pooh, Handbook to Higher Consciousness, The Celestine Prophecy, The Five People You Meet in Heaven,* and *You Can Have it All.*[5] A *Wall Street Journal* article stated that the top-selling books to college students (other than textbooks) deal with spirituality.[6]

People may be tired of seeking pleasure through material gain. Some have found that they cannot buy enough to bring them peace. Turning to drugs, alcohol, and sex has not filled the void. Instead, it leaves an emptiness and continued searching. People of all ages are seeking guidance on the spiritual dimension of health in a quest for fulfillment and a meaningful life. This chapter has an emphasis on self-discovery, encouraging you to reflect on the information presented, complete the spiritual assessment, and develop an action plan to grow in the spiritual dimension of health.

Discussions of spirituality are no longer isolated in religious settings but are part of current events and daily life. Universities are offering courses such as "The Meaning of Life" and "Care of the Soul." Corporate health-promotion programs now offer courses on spiritual wellness along with courses on exercise and nutrition. Mainstream medical journals have begun to publish healing studies. Along with health care professionals' increasing acceptance of the spiritual dimension of health, we see a corresponding increase in research on prayer, meditation, and energy healing. We have come to acknowledge that wholeness of health incorporates body, mind, and spirit.

Spirituality and Religiosity

All humans have a **spiritual dimension,** a quality that goes beyond religious affiliation, which strives for inspiration, reverence, awe, meaning, and purpose even in those who do not believe in any god. The spiritual dimension tries to be in harmony with the universe, strives for answers about the infinite, and especially comes into focus as a sustaining power when the person faces emotional stress, physical illness, or death. It goes outside a person's own power.[8]

FYI

Spirituality in America

An all-time high number of Americans believe in God, 95% according to the latest in a series of national Gallup polls conducted over the last 60 years. The results also showed that most Americans consider prayer as an important part of their lives. Most people say that they believe miracles are performed by a divine power and that they sometimes are conscious of the presence of God.*

Does the trend toward spirituality apply to young adults as well? To help answer that question, a major research program underway at UCLA was initiated to track the spiritual growth of students during their college years (see the Research Highlight—Spiritual Changes in Students During the Undergraduate Years). The study revealed that today's college students have very high levels of spiritual interest and involvement. Many are actively engaged in a spiritual quest and report that to "some" or "a great" extent they are searching for meaning and purpose in life.**

Sources: *In "Spirituality and Medical Practice," by G. Amandarajah and E. Hight, *American Family Physician* (2001, Jan 1), 63(1).
**www.spirituality.ucla.edu

Author Anecdote

We've Come a Long Way

For some of you, this may be the first serious discussion on spirituality in the academic university environment. Addressing spirituality from an academic/scientific perspective may help overcome some initial reluctance by considering some of the non-theological issues of spirituality. In my classes I have found that most students are willing, even eager, to explore the spiritual dimensions of their well-being. Many of them are interested in grappling with the large questions related to who they are and what matters to them. They clearly understand the relevance of spirituality to their lives as one of my students, Marsha, so insightfully shared:

> Speaking from personal experience, I'm uplifted emotionally and physically when I attend to my spiritual needs. Our spirit is similar to our physical body, in requiring nutrition and exercise to sustain it. When I read devotions and study scripture, it is food for my spirit. When I make efforts to apply those principles in my daily life, I exercise my spirit. If I ignore my spiritual needs, my spirit becomes sick, as my physical body does when I am ill. Sometimes when I feel unhappy or sense that something is missing in my life, I reflect on scripture that has meaning for me. This scripture brings health to my spirit and comfort to my soul.[7]

Fifteen years ago it was considered inappropriate, in part because of separation of church and state, to discuss religion and spirituality in the health classes I taught at a state university. Finding a health book that mentioned spiritual health was difficult. Thankfully, we have come to understand that we can deal with questions about meaning and purpose without promoting a particular ideology. The spiritual dimension of health is just as real and valid as the physical dimension. We've come a long way!

—MH

Spiritual Changes in Students During the Undergraduate Years

Recent findings from an ongoing national study of college students' spiritual development conducted by UCLA's Higher Education Research Institute shows growth in spiritual qualities from freshman to junior years. The findings are based on comprehensive longitudinal data collected from 14,527 students attending 136 colleges and universities nationwide. The students were first surveyed as entering freshmen in the fall of 2004 and again in the late spring of 2007 at the end of their junior year.

This national study reveals that while students' attendance at religious services declines during the first three years of college, they experience significant growth along several spiritual dimensions during the same period. Compared to when they were entering freshmen, college juniors are more likely to be engaged in a spiritual quest, are more caring, and show higher levels of equanimity and a holistic worldview.

Evidence that the juniors are more engaged in a spiritual quest than they were as entering freshmen is reflected in increasing percentages who embrace the following life goals as either "very important" or "essential":

- "integrating spirituality into my life" (from 41.8% in 2004 to 50.4% in 2007)
- "developing a meaningful philosophy of life" (from 41.2% to 55.4%)
- "attaining inner harmony" (from 48.7% to 62.6%)
- "seeking beauty in my life (from 53.7% to 66.2%)
- "becoming a more loving person" (from 67.4% to 82.8%)

An increasing sense of "Equanimity" is suggested by the growing percentages of students who:

- say they have "frequently been able to find meaning in times of hardship" (from 25.9% in 2004 to 31.0% in 2007)
- describe themselves as "seeing each day, good or bad, as a gift" (from 38.9% to 45.5%) and,
- see themselves as "being thankful for all that has happened to me" (from 52.0% to 61.2%).

Growth in what the researchers call an "Ecumenical Worldview" is revealed in the students' growing endorsement of:

- "improving my understanding of other countries and cultures" (42.0% in 2004 versus 55.4% in 2007)
- "improving the human condition" (53.4% versus 63.8%)
- "feeling a strong connection to all humanity" (75.6% to 80.8%) and
- their increasing agreement with the proposition that "non-religious people can lead lives that are just as moral as those of religious believers" (from 83.3% to 90.5%).

Further evidence of increasing acceptance of persons with differing beliefs is suggested by the students' growing agreement with two other propositions:

- "most people can grow spiritually without being religious" (from 62.8% in 2004 to 74.8% in 2007) and
- "it doesn't matter what I believe as long as I lead a moral life" (from 51.1% to 57.8%).

These findings suggest that many students are emerging from the collegiate experience with a desire to find spiritual meaning and perspective in their everyday lives. The data also suggest that the collegiate experience is influencing students in positive ways that will better prepare them for leadership roles in our global society.

Source: http://spirituality.ucla.edu/news/report_backup_dec07release_12.18.07.pdf

FIGURE 10.1 Students' Views about Spiritual and Religious Matters

Source: UCLA Higher Education Research Institute, retrieved in 2005 from www.templeton.org

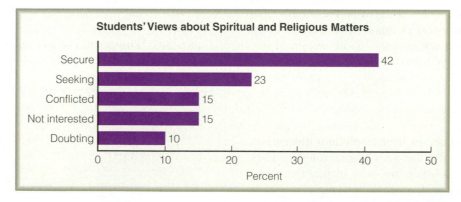

Students' Views about Spiritual and Religious Matters

	Percent
Secure	42
Seeking	23
Conflicted	15
Not interested	15
Doubting	10

Note: Figure adds up to more than 100% because students could choose more than one option.

Spirituality is a process, a journey, the essence of life principle of a person, a belief that relates a person to the world, and a way of giving meaning to existence. It is a personal quest to find meaning and purpose in life, and a relationship or sense of connection with a higher power.[9] Think of spirituality as having both a vertical dimension, which involves a transcending relationship with a higher power, and a horizontal dimension, which involves a sense of purpose and meaning in life.[10] This horizontal, human dimension involves a perspective on the self and the world within which you exist.

Spirituality is concerned with the values that we hold most dear, our sense of who we are and where we come from, our beliefs about why we are here—the meaning and purpose we see in our work and our life—and our sense of connectedness to each other and the world around us.[11] It gives rise to the actions by which we deal with the realities that surround us. Spirituality is an integral dimension of the health and well-being of every individual.[12]

Religiosity refers to the extent of participation in or adherence to the beliefs and practices of an organized religion.[13] It relates to any person who accepts the tenets of, and actively participates in, an organized religion and its practices. A religious person is one who embraces specific religious beliefs and incorporates them into his or her own worldview.[14]

Spirituality is a much broader concept that also includes non-religious beliefs and expressions. Although spirituality may involve traditional religious beliefs and practices, a person may be deeply spiritual, yet not profess a religion. For example, he or she may have a belief in and devotion to an omniscient, all-powerful God or higher power but not be affiliated or involved with an organized religious denomination or group. An individual may be highly religious but not spiritual. Perhaps this individual attends church regularly, tithes, and lives by the tenets of that church but does not pray, meditate, or have a direct experience with an omniscient God or universal power.[15]

Certainly, many people are both religious and spiritual. Religious beliefs and practices can, and often do, contribute to spiritual health. We may or may not choose to participate in a religion. Everyone has a spiritual dimension, just as everyone has an emotional, mental, and physical dimension, and many people find their religious beliefs and practices to be an integral aspect of their spiritual development.

Does our logical, scientific-thinking mind interfere with our spiritual experience? Reflecting on some important questions can help guide our understanding of how to nurture the spiritual dimension. How do we best grow spiritually? Should faith, rather than science, guide our spiritual experience? Can we ever really explain, from a scientific perspective, concepts related to something as personal as spirituality?

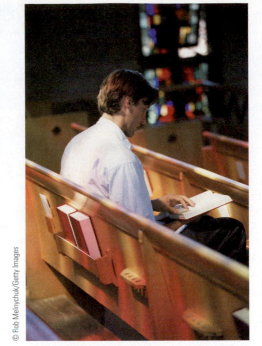

Religiosity refers to participation in or adherence to the beliefs and practices of an organized religion.

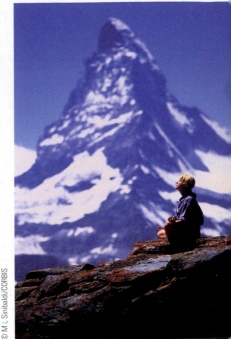

Spirituality is a personal quest to find meaning and purpose in life, and a relationship or sense of connection with a higher power.

The spiritual journey does not consist of arriving at a new destination where a person gains what he did not have, or becomes what he is not. It consists in the dissipation of one's own ignorance concerning oneself and life, and the gradual growth of that understanding which begins the spiritual awakening. The finding of God is a coming to one's self.

—Aldous Huxley

Research on Spirituality

Scientific studies have yielded findings about factors that contribute to physical health. Can these studies also determine factors that contribute to spiritual health? Do "best practices" or "evidence-based practices" apply to spiritual health? With increasing rigor, studies are being conducted to increase our understanding of how the spiritual dimension relates to health. Although we can learn from these studies, we must first consider some of the challenges related to researching individual experience with the spiritual aspects of life.

145

A Native American Perspective

Tom Brown Jr., a Native American, writes of his understanding of the spiritual nature of man. He relates the following discussion he had with another Native American whom he simply calls Grandfather, in which he is learning about the way the logical mind gets in the way of focusing on the spiritual dimension:

Grandfather said,

Man is like an island, a circle within circles. Man is separated from these outer circles by his mind, his beliefs, and the limitations put upon him by a life away from the Earth. The circle of man, the island of self, is the place of logic, the "I," the ego, and the physical self. That is the island that man has chosen to live within today, and in doing so he has created a prison for himself. The walls of the island prison are thick, made up of doubts, logic, and lack of belief. His isolation from his greater circles of self is suffocating and prevents him from seeing life clearly and purely. It is a world of ignorance where the flesh is the only reality, the only god.

Beyond man's island of ego, his prison, lays the spirit-that-moves-in-all-things, the force that is found in all things. It is a world that communicates to all entities of Creation and touches the Creator. It is a circle of life that houses all man's instinct, his deepest memory, his power to control his body and mind, and a bridge that helps man transcend flesh. It is a world that expands man's universe and helps him to fuse himself to the Earth. Most of all, it is a world that brings man to his higher self and to spiritual rapture.

As I settled back into my Quest, I began to fully understand what had been given to me. I realized that the power of the pure mind is what makes all spiritual communication

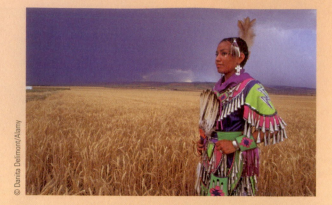

Does our logical, scientific-thinking mind interfere with our spiritual experience? Native American spirituality includes honoring nature.

pure and unrestricted. The logical mind I viewed as a barrier or filter to that communication. Any time that logical mind becomes active with its need to analyze, define, verbalize, or interpret in any way, it sets aside and imprisons the pure mind. As I sat contemplating this, I began to realize a deeper sense of duality. I now could understand that the pure mind and the logical mind were almost two separate entities. When one was active, the other was sleeping or set aside.

So, too, did I begin to understand why the logical mind was so dominant and strangling. After all, it was that mind that society wanted us to nourish. It was that mind that was like a spoiled stepchild, fed constantly by society, thus over-shadowing and smothering the spiritual mind.

Source: *Awakening Spirits: A Native American Path to Inner Peace, Healing and Spiritual Growth,* by Tom Brown (New York: Berkeley Publishing Group, 1994).

Theories abound as to why a strong spiritual faith promotes health and relieves stress. Do peace and healing result because of the intervention of a higher power or because these people believe so strongly that healing will occur that they succeed in changing their physiology and biochemistry in a beneficial way? Some key issues relate to research on spirituality, including definition of terms, the placebo effect, and lifestyle variables.

Defining Terms As we mentioned, spirituality and religion are different, yet the terminology often is used interchangeably. This leads to confusion and inaccuracies in interpreting the research on spiritual practices, religious activities or beliefs, and health outcomes.

Researchers do not always agree on the definitions of spiritual terms. Prayer, for example, has been defined in many different ways. Another issue is "dose-response": If a person prays a little, are the results different than if the person prays a lot? Spiritual health is not an exact science. Even the definition of spiritual health does not have universal agreement. As terminology becomes standardized, studies on spirituality will yield more relevant, applicable findings.

What is evident, however, is that the spiritual dimension is equal to, and perhaps even more important than, the other dimensions of health and well-being. Spiritual health is finding its way into common healing modalities such as hypnosis, biofeedback, acupuncture, massage, and reflexology. Many so-called new age and alternative therapies operate from a spiritual foundation with an emphasis on healing the spiritual aspects of the individual along with the emotional and physical. You will learn in Chapter 23, on complementary and alternative health, that these unconventional approaches to health and healing are gaining acceptance as Americans seek more holistic approaches to health.

Placebo Power A second challenge of spirituality research relates to the placebo effect. The term **placebo** describes the positive effects that are created when a person merely believes he or she will benefit from an intervention. It is generally believed that about 35% of people experience the placebo effect. For example, if a person believes a pill will make him better, he actually may feel better even when given an inert substance such as a sugar pill. When someone believes that her prayers for healing will be answered, does the prayer result in healing, or does the strong belief that healing will occur alter the mind/body response in a positive manner?

Belief that one is being healed by a divine power can produce a conditioning effect that alters stress levels, physiologic responses, and immune activity.[16] Placebo effects make the value of a treatment difficult to determine. Although the placebo effect complicates research, people receive very real benefits when they believe they will receive benefits from the intervention. The placebo effect—the power of belief—has substantial effects for many people. Theories support the premise that if modern medicine were able to bottle the placebo effects as a drug, it would be one of our most effective cures. When determining the outcomes of a spiritual intervention, the placebo effect cannot be discounted.

Variables in Religion, Health, and Lifestyle Research A third challenge for research on spirituality stems from alternative variables that may influence study results. A review of the research literature identifies a correlation between religious activities and health outcomes. Most studies suggest that religiosity is beneficial for mental and physical health and stress management and that it supports a healthy lifestyle.[17]

Based on his research, Harold Koenig, director of the Duke University's Center for the Study of Religion, Spirituality, and Health, has estimated that regular participation in religious activities and practices adds 7 to 14 years to the life span and is equivalent in benefit to not smoking cigarettes. Much of this benefit comes from the health-promoting practices of most religious groups, such as honoring the body and abstaining from drugs and alcohol.[18]

Koenig's research raises the issue of variables that must be considered when evaluating any form of healing. Do the health benefits that derive from being religious come from the intervention of a higher power, or are the benefits related to variables such as social support or healthier lifestyle choices that many religions teach?

Bottom Line on Research Scientific methods are not always adequate for exploring concepts such as faith and spirituality. Although we cannot scientifically test the mechanisms by which higher-power healing occurs, we can assess how changes in perception brought about by religious and spiritual beliefs alter physiological and psychological health outcomes. Great strides are being made in applying scientific research methodology to understanding the impact of spiritual and religious variables on health and stress management. Still, people who turn to spirituality for comfort and healing do not need scientific studies to convince them. They believe some things to be true even if they cannot be proven scientifically.

A discussion of the limitations to research on spirituality is crucial to our understanding that the paths to spiritual well-being are many. We cannot write an exact prescription for spiritual health. Spirituality points to our interiors, our subjective life. The spiritual domain has to do with what we experience privately in our subjective awareness. We must take care not to generalize about such a highly personal perspective. You can consider the information presented in the chapter and assimilate it as you choose. Research and studies can guide our understanding, but ultimately only you can choose the path that is right for you.

Stress Busting Behavior: Ways to Enhance Spiritual Health

In this chapter, you are learning about the qualities of spiritual health. To get you thinking about how this relates to you, from the following list of ways to enhance spiritual health, first, underline the two choices that you currently practice that contribute most to your spiritual wellbeing. Next, check the two choices that you most want to develop to enhance your sense of peace and wellbeing.

- ☐ Prayer
- ☐ Reflection or quiet listening to one's intuition
- ☐ Communion with nature
- ☐ Enjoyment of music, drama, art, dance
- ☐ Inner dialogue with oneself or with a higher power
- ☐ Loving relationships with others
- ☐ Service to others in need
- ☐ Forgiveness
- ☐ Empathy, compassion, hope
- ☐ Laughter, joyous expressions
- ☐ Participation in a caring community—a church, a support group, or any group that gives you a feeling of belonging
- ☐ Reading about spiritual growth from any source you find inspiring (the insights of others can help you formulate your own meaning and purpose in life)
- ☐ Quiet time each day for prayer, meditation, or thinking (silence can be healing and help restore a sense of balance)

Source: http://wellness.uwsp.edu

Five Qualities of Spiritual Health

Spiritual health refers to the ability to discover and articulate our own basic purpose in life and to learn how to experience love, joy, peace, and fulfillment. It is the experience of helping ourselves and others achieve full potential.[19]

Factors that seem to promote spiritual health include trust, honesty, integrity, altruism, compassion, and service. In addition, spiritually healthy people commune regularly with, or have some sort of personal relationship and experience with, a higher power or larger reality that transcends an observable physical reality.[20]

There are many expressions of spiritual health, just as there are many aspects of physical or emotional health. Regardless of religious affiliation, spiritual health and stress management have some qualities in common. Five qualities of spiritual health that cut across many religious and spiritual beliefs have special relevance in stress management:

1. A sense of meaning and purpose in life
2. Faith in God or a higher power—however you choose to define it
3. A feeling of connection to others and seeing oneself as part of something bigger
4. Compassion for others
5. Participation in religious behaviors or meaningful spiritual rituals.

We will examine each of these components to increase our understanding of how each of these qualities can help you manage stress.

Meaning and Purpose

"Please sir, can you tell me which way I ought to go?" asked Alice. "That depends a good deal on where you want to get to," said the cat. "I don't much care," said Alice. "Then it doesn't matter which way you go," said the cat. "…so long as I go somewhere," Alice added as an explanation. "Oh you're sure to do that," said the cat, "if you only walk long enough." (From *Alice in Wonderland* by Lewis Carroll)

Without some purpose in life, we wander aimlessly and our enthusiasm for life can be lost. Finding meaning in how we live and discovering our purpose for living brings spiritual growth and peace. Finding meaning in life can serve as a powerful inner drive for personal accomplishment and a stress-relieving sense of contentment that we are on the right path for ourselves.

One of the most influential books on finding meaning in life is *Man's Search for Meaning* by Viktor Frankl, the renowned Viennese psychoanalyst and survivor of the Holocaust. First published in 1946, this book is still life-changing for many, and millions of copies have been sold. Frankl emphasizes that, although people may be powerless to modify their environment or even their physical condition, each person does have the ultimate power to fashion his or her reactions and find *interior meaning*, even in the most difficult of circumstances. In short, how one chooses to react throughout life can be the basis of ultimate personal triumph.

Frankl encountered a stress management principle in action. He found that if he could help fellow prisoners believe that their experience—horrendous though it was— nevertheless had some meaning, he could encourage them to maintain the will to survive. He writes, "There is nothing in the world, I venture to say, that would so effectively help one to survive even the worst conditions, as the knowledge that there is a meaning in one's life. … Suffering ceases to be suffering in some way at the moment it finds a meaning."[21]

Learning that even the most difficult times in life can bring meaning can change the experience in a positive direction, as demonstrated in a study on patients with recurring cancer. Researchers in this study found that nearly half of the respondents reported engaging in a search for meaning; the greater a person's sense of meaning, the lower the symptoms of distress.[22] Often, we search for meaning during the most difficult times.

Those who find meaning, even in their suffering, are able to find peace. Maria's story in the opening vignette showed how she was able to come through a difficult time and emerge with a new sense of confidence in her ability to handle the inevitable challenges of life. The words of the philosopher Camus describe this concept: "In the depth of winter, I finally learned that within me there lay an invincible summer." Believing that your life, and all that happens in life, has meaning for you strengthens the conviction that you can handle what life brings.

Think about a difficult time in your life when you were able to grow through the experience by finding meaning in your suffering. The key message is this: Peace does not come from a lack of problems and difficulties. Peace comes from knowing that your life is in harmony with your values and beliefs and from growing and finding meaning in life's disruptions.

FYI

Survivor's Story This *USA Today* letter to the editor is a powerful testimonial of how something as devastating as cancer can actually bring peace and improve quality of living. The author writes:

* * *

I am a five-year breast cancer survivor, and my husband is a two-year prostate cancer survivor. Our lives before cancer were good. We enjoyed a loving family, a beautiful home, and successful careers. But everything was always urgent.

Our post-cancer lives are wonderful. We still have a loving family, a nice home, and rewarding careers, but we have put everything into perspective: We now look at our lives as gifts from God. Every day is special.

Has cancer made our lives better? Absolutely. Are we glad we had cancer? Of course not. The disease lurks in our minds daily. Are we going to let cancer control our lives and get us down? Never. We are working toward becoming better versions of ourselves— physically, mentally and spiritually. We are enjoying life.

Source: "Post-Cancer Experience Improved Quality of Living," by J. Dancer, *USA Today*, April 18, 2005, 14A.

Belief in a Higher Power The term **spiritual** describes a belief in, and devotion to, a higher power beyond the physical realm. This belief in a higher power is the cornerstone of every major religion and social science. Christians call this higher power God; Hindus call it Prana; Chinese call it Chi; Native Americans call it the Great Spirit; Taoists call it the Tao; a philosopher may call it "infinite intelligence"; a psychologist may call it the "collective unconscious" or "superconscious"; a mental health counselor might call it our "higher self"; a quantum physicist might call it the "unified field." Jedi Masters of the *Star Wars* movies call this all-pervading energy the Force. All of these relate to a single unifying connecting spirit as the basis for all things in the universe.

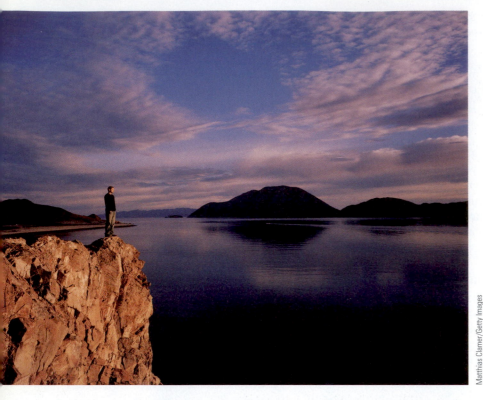

Matthias Clamer/Getty Images

Faith is the belief in or commitment to something or someone seen or unseen that helps a person realize a purpose. By definition, faith is belief without proof. Each person chooses what to believe. Faith is universal, a part of living, a part of acting, and a part of self-understanding.[23] A strong spiritual faith can promote health and relieve stress by alleviating the stressors of uncertainty and insecurity. Cardiologist and author George Sheehan credits faith with an almost unequaled power to relieve stress by providing an inner sense of calm and tranquility and a sense that no defeat is final. The result is a sense of lasting security from making connection with a higher power.[24]

Research with workers in the health and medical fields showed that faith is an important aspect of the spiritual dimension of health. It allows us to acknowledge that some power is at work, a power other than the natural and rational. We acknowledge that such a power is the cause behind the natural workings of the universe. Our perceptions and faith can bring pleasure and convince us of our ability to survive.[25] A strong faith can alleviate the stressors of uncertainty and insecurity.

Important to stress management is the question of control. On one hand, we have learned that we do have some control over things that happen in our lives. Feeling empowered and in control can be stress-relieving. On the other hand, believing that some things are not in our control is stress-relieving, too. Believing that we can release to a higher power some things that are beyond our control relieves stress by providing a sense of tranquility and security.

Author Leo Booth says about spirituality: "It is related to the word spirit—not a child's concept of a white-sheeted Holy Ghost flying in and out of our lives, but an inner attitude that emphasizes energy, creative choice, and a powerful force of living. It is a partnership with a Power greater than ourselves, a co-creatorship with God that allows us to be guided by God and yet take responsibility for our lives."[26]

Reflect on your personal beliefs about a higher power and what impact your beliefs have on your perceived stress. Are some aspects of your life that cause you stress out of your control? Do you believe that releasing control of these stressors and believing that a higher power is in control would result in greater peace for you?

"When you come to the edge of all the light you know, and are about to step off into the darkness of the unknown, faith is knowing one of two things will happen: There will be something solid to stand on or you will be taught how to fly." (As quoted by Barbara J. Winter)

150

Heaven is my father and Earth is my mother and even such a small creature as I find an intimate place in its midst. That which extends throughout the universe, I regard as my body and that which directs the universe, I regard as my nature. All people are my brothers and sisters and all things are my companions.

—*The Western Inscription, Chang Tsai, 11th century, China*

Connectedness As part of her doctoral dissertation, Dr. Judy Howden conducted extensive research on spirituality. She defined spirituality as "the dimension of one's being that is an integrating or unifying factor and that is manifested through unifying interconnectedness, purpose and meaning in life, innerness or inner resources, and transcendence." She described **connectedness** as "the feeling of relatedness or attachment to others, a sense of relationship to all of life, a feeling of harmony with self and others, and a feeling of oneness with the universe and/or a universal element or Universal Being."[27]

Connectedness implies that some aspect of humanity connects each of us with each other. We are one at a deeper level. Wayne Dyer accurately calls it the "uni-verse," the "one song" of which we are all a part. The practical application of this understanding becomes immediately apparent. If you are a part of me and I am a part of you, I will be much more likely to treat you in loving and friendly ways. If we are made "of the same stuff," as Deepak Chopra has said, why would we want to hurt or cause pain to ourselves? Recognizing our oneness invites us to be more loving and caring with all things and all people around us. Functioning in more loving rather than hating ways toward everyone and everything is stress-relieving.

If we are all connected at the spiritual level, we are all part of the same whole. The Indian poet, philosopher, and Nobel Prize winner Rabindranath Tagore described this connectedness beautifully when he created this poem:

> The same stream of life that runs through my veins night and day runs through the world and dances in rhythmic measures.
>
> It is the same life that shoots in joy through the dust of the earth in numberless blades of grass and breaks into tumultuous waves of leaves and flowers.
>
> It is the same life that is rocked in the ocean-cradle of birth and of death, in ebb and in flow.
>
> I feel my limbs are made glorious by the touch of this world of life. And my pride is from the life-throb of ages dancing in my blood this moment.

Realizing that all we see and can experience in our awareness is part of our own nature, an aspect of ourselves, helps us choose behaviors that tend to enhance rather than destroy everything around us, including the animal and plant kingdoms, as well as fellow human beings. Behind all of our varied ideologies, cultures, classes, and religions, we are brothers and sisters on this planet.

Do you experience connectedness as a feeling of harmony with yourself and others and a feeling of oneness with the universe? We tend not to give questions like this much thought as we go about our daily life, yet conscious attention can have a significant impact on our thoughts, choices, and contentment with life. Connectedness has to do with our connection to other human beings and also to our belief that we are part of a greater reality. Spiritually, knowing that you are part of something much larger than yourself, is comforting.

Compassion for Others   His Holiness the Dalai Lama said:

> Love, compassion, and tolerance are necessities, not luxuries. Without them, humanity cannot survive. If you have a particular faith or religion, that is good. But you can survive without it if you have love, compassion, and tolerance. The clear proof of a person's love of God is if that person genuinely shows love to fellow human beings.[28]

Because the spiritual dimension of health transcends the individual, it has the capacity to be a common bond between individuals. It rises above the individual and goes beyond the limits of the individual. With this common bond, we are motivated to share love, warmth, and compassion with other people. We choose to do unselfish and compassionate things for others. We are able to put someone else's life and interest before our own. This common bond also prompts us to follow a set of ethical principles, and to make a commitment to God or a higher power.[29] Two important qualities of compassion that have special relevance to stress management are forgiveness and altruism.

Forgiveness   It has been said that forgiveness is a gift you give to yourself, and to the people who love you. We can forgive out of compassion for others, and in the process we also receive great benefits.

In a series of studies of the Stanford Forgiveness Project, Dr. Fred Luskin studied forgiveness and relationships. He defined **forgiveness** as the experience of psychological peace that occurs when injured people transform their grievances against others.[30] This

Just like a sunbeam can't separate itself from the sun, and a wave can't separate itself from the ocean, we can't separate ourselves from one another. We are all part of a vast sea of love, one indivisible divine mind.

—Marianne Williamson

A human being is a part of the whole called by us "universe," a part limited in time and space. He experiences himself, his thoughts and feeling as something separated from the rest, a kind of optical delusion of his consciousness. This delusion is a kind of prison for us, restricting us to our personal desires and to affection for a few persons nearest to us. Our task must be to free ourselves from this prison by widening our circle of compassion to embrace all living creatures and the whole of nature in its beauty.

—Albert Einstein

Namaste The people of India have an interesting way of relating to their understanding of connectedness. When they greet and when they part, they hold their hands close together in prayer position, bow briefly, and say, "Namaste." **Namaste** means "I honor the place in you where the entire universe resides. I honor the place in you where lies your love, your light, your truth and your beauty. I honor the place in you, where … if you are in that place in you … and I am in that place in me … then there is only one of us."

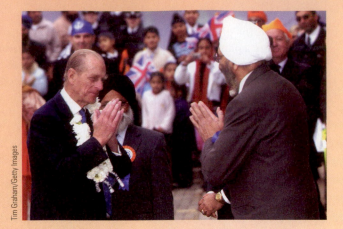

Tim Graham/Getty Images

Royal Namaste greeting.

transformation takes place by learning to take less personal offense, to attribute less blame to the offender, and to understand the personal harm that comes from unresolved anger.

Dr. Luskin and Dr. Carl Thoesen conducted a study at Stanford University in which they trained 55 college students to forgive someone who had hurt them. After 6 weeks, the students in the treatment group were significantly less angry, showed greater self-efficacy, were more hopeful, and showed greater emotional self-management than their peers in the control group. When they were tested 10 weeks later, they had maintained their improved mental health.

People who refuse to forgive harbor resentment, anger, and bitterness. This negative attitude is harmful both emotionally and physically, because the release of potent stress-related hormones causes our heart to pound, muscles to tense, and blood pressure to soar. Mentally replaying situations in which we felt wronged or misunderstood activates the stress response. "When people hold on to anger and past trauma so strongly that the stress response never goes away, they pay a toll in their physical and emotional well-being," says psychologist Ann Webster, director of the Mind/Body Cancer Program at the Mind/Body Medical Institute.[31]

Researcher Charlotte Witvliet of Hope College in Michigan found that when we mentally replay a hurtful memory or nurse a grudge against a person who mistreated or offended us, our body reacts with a stress response. Our brow muscles tense, sweating increases, heart rate and blood pressure rise, and other measures indicate that the nervous system is on high alert. If we imagine granting forgiveness instead—or simply picture how that person might have felt or what might have contributed to hurtful behavior—our physical stress indicators remain fairly steady. You can't change the past, but this study shows that changing how you think about past hurt can reduce its impact on you, and the resulting likelihood of stress-related illness.[32]

Psychotherapist Robin Casarjian says:

> Forgiveness is a relationship with life that frees the forgiver from the psychological bondage of chronic fear, hostility, anger, and unhealthy grief. Forgiveness is an attitude that implies that you are willing to accept responsibility for your perceptions, realizing that your perceptions are a choice and not an objective fact."[33]

Forgiveness is a choice not to let past grievances compromise our future by filling our mind with negative thoughts and emotions. It is a skill to be learned.

When you forgive someone, you make yourself, rather than the person who hurt you, responsible for your future happiness. When we learn to forgive by realizing that our perception is what allows another person to hurt us, and refusing to take offense from others' actions, the consequence is inner peace. This is powerful stress management.

The following list tells us what forgiveness is not:[34]

- Pretending everything is fine
- Stuffing away angry or hurt feelings

The Forgiveness Factor

Evolving research based on data from position emission tomography (PET) is showing that different parts of the brain are activated when we contemplate forgiveness rather than revenge or retaliation. Pietro Pietrini, M.D., Ph.D., in the Cognitive Neuroscience Section at the National Institute of Neurological Disorders and Stroke, is assessing the neurobiological response associated with forgiveness and unforgivingness. He is testing his hypothesis that forgiveness allows a person to overcome a situation that otherwise would be a major source of stress both mentally and neurobiologically. Forgiveness is thought to dramatically change the individual's biological homeostatic equilibrium.

Source: "Study of the Brain Functional Correlates of Forgiveness in Humans by Using Position Emission Tomography (PET)," by P. Pietrini, retrieved April 20, 2005, from www.forgiving.org

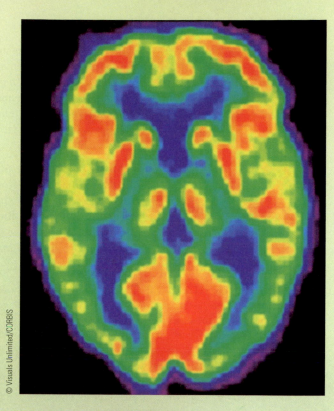

© Visuals Unlimited/CORBIS

Different parts of the brain are activated when we contemplate forgiveness rather than revenge or retaliation.

- Condoning hurtful behavior
- Necessarily reconciling or having contact with an offender
- Something you can be pressured to do
- Forgetting—you can picture a past hurt without dwelling in the emotions

Author Gerald Jampolsky indicates that if we want to have inner peace in our life, our single function should be forgiveness.

> Through selective forgetting, through taking off the tinted glasses that superimpose the fearful past upon the present, we can begin to know that the truth of Love is forever present and that by perceiving only Love, we can experience happiness. Forgiveness then becomes a process of letting go and overlooking whatever we thought other people may have done to us, or whatever we may think we have done to them.
>
> When we cherish grievances, we allow our mind to be fed by fear and we become imprisoned by these distortions. When we see our only function as forgiveness and are willing to practice it consistently by directing our minds to be forgiving, we will find ourselves released and set free. Forgiveness corrects the misperception that we are separate from each other and allows us to experience a sense of unity and "at-one-ment" with each other. The unforgiving mind sees itself as innocent and others as guilty. It thrives on conflict and on being right, and it sees inner peace as its enemy. It perceives everything as separate.[35]

Try this forgiveness exercise: Find a comfortable, quiet place to sit. Take a couple of deep, cleansing breaths. Imagine someone you feel resentment toward or who has hurt you. Start with something small. Invite that person into your heart, noticing any emotions that block his or her entrance. Silently say, "I forgive you," for whatever he or she may have done to hurt you. As you breathe and relax, forgive and let go of the resentment. After a few minutes, imagine letting the person depart, touched by your forgiveness and compassion. You can repeat the exercise with the image of asking someone you may have hurt to forgive you. See yourself thankfully accepting his or her forgiveness.[36]

Altruism

Imagine a world where people give of themselves simply because they want to. Not out of a sense of debt or because they want something in return. No ulterior motives. No guilt feelings. Just a desire to give for the sake of giving. Now instead of imagining this kind of world, do your part in making it happen. Make a charitable donation. Volunteer your time to improve your community. Give back to the world that gives so much to you. And if it happens to make you feel good, that's all right. Feeling good is the one ulterior motive that's acceptable.[37]

Altruism is the act of helping or giving to others without thought of self-benefit. Altruism enhances self-esteem, relieves physical and mental stress, and protects psychological well-being.[38] In the last chapter, you learned about altruism as a value. You learned how giving of ourselves benefits the giver and the receiver alike. Many colleges offer community service or service-learning courses to provide students with an opportunity to give to their community. Students who participate report increased self-esteem, a belief that they can make a difference, and a greater commitment to do more volunteer work.

Many people report that when they do something for someone else without seeking any external reward, they feel inwardly happier and more content. When we take our mind off our own troubles and problems as we try to help someone else with theirs, our difficulties seem to be less significant and our stress is reduced.

The Random Acts of Kindness movement started when Ann Herbert began promoting the idea of altruism. The idea spread, and one night as a college professor was listening to TV, the phrase "another random act of senseless violence" stuck in his mind. In a moment of inspiration, he decided to assign his human relations students an essay on random acts of "senseless kindness." Students were asked to do something out of the ordinary to help someone who wasn't expecting it, and then write about it. One student bought 30 blankets from the Salvation Army and took them to the homeless people who were living under a bridge near his home. Another pulled out of a parking place she had just pulled into and motions for a motorist who appeared to be frantically in a hurry to take her place. Then the kind student parked in the only other available parking place about a half-mile away. Challenge yourself to commit a random act of kindness today—and in the days to come. The possibilities are endless. Here are a few ideas:

- Write an anonymous thank-you note to an instructor.
- Pick out someone behind you in line at the movies and inform the ticket seller that you want to pay for that movie-goer's ticket. Make sure the person does not know who paid for the ticket.
- Ask a couple who has been married for over 25 years to share with you their five tips for a successful marriage.
- Buy a cold drink for your entire row at the baseball game.
- Ask an older person to tell you a story about his or her youth, such as his or her favorite song or how he met his spouse.
- Drop off a geranium plant and a thank-you note at your local fire station.

Sir John Templeton said, "Know that there is no power in the universe greater than love, and no act more important than loving. **Agape** is the unselfish love that gives of itself and expects nothing in return. It is the love that grows as you give it to others." Think about how much of the distress between people—and nations—could be eliminated if altruism were a guiding principle for behavior.[40]

In his book *The Ways and Power of Love*, Pitirim Sorokin said,

If unselfish love does not extend over the whole of mankind, if it is confined within one group—a given family, tribe, nation, race, religious denomination, political party, trade union, caste,

Once you begin to acknowledge random acts of kindness— both the ones you have received and the ones you have given— you can no longer believe that what you do does not matter.

—Dawna Markova

social class or any part of humanity—such an in-group altruism tends to generate an out-group antagonism.[41]

The rise in volunteer work worldwide indicates that people want to help others. Altruism can point the way to a new future, a future in which we are less focused on what we can get *from* others and more focused on what we can contribute *to* their lives. Altruism grows out of compassion for others.

Religious Behaviors and Meaningful Spiritual Rituals

The final quality of spiritual health relates to meaningful spiritual practices that we integrate into our lives. Author and psychiatrist Paul Tournier said he used to live a restless life, always racing the clock. But after he began to devote an hour a day to quiet reflection, devotional meditation, and prayer, he has been happier, healthier, and better able to distinguish between priorities, and has actually accomplished more.[42]

Dr. Kenneth Ferraro, a medical sociologist at Purdue University, examined 1,473 people to determine how their religious practice, or lack of it, had affected their health. Those who prayed regularly, read religious literature, attended church or synagogue, and considered themselves strong and active in their religious faith reported only half the health problems as nonpracticing people did.[43]

Author Anecdote   Random Acts of Kindness   Several years ago I read a little book called *Random Acts of Kindness*.[39] A random act of kindness (RAK) is a little, out-of-the-ordinary thing we do to help someone who wasn't expecting it. It is acting out of love and caring and expecting nothing in return. It feels good. You feel connected to humanity in a way that is hard to explain.

The idea of doing something for someone while expecting nothing in return was not a new idea to me—just an idea I needed to be reminded of. When I was a young girl, my mom frequently committed RAKs. Although she didn't call them "random acts of kindness," that's what they were. For instance, on May Day each year we made baskets filled with flowers and cookies and brightly colored homemade cards. The idea was to sneak up to neighbor's houses and leave a May basket at their door without getting caught. The recipients were not to know who delivered this gift. I still remember the excitement as Mom would wait in the car for my sisters, brother, and me to deliver the basket and race for the car without getting noticed.

Years later, I still remembered how good it felt to help others, so I assigned students in one of my classes to commit two or three RAKs, then report back to the class later in the semester. One student, Nik, related that he had become a RAK addict. He said it felt so good that he found himself planning and committing RAKs nearly every day. He had been planning a Halloween party and decided he could combine fun and altruism. He asked those he invited to the party to bring a couple of cans of food for the local food pantry. In addition, they went out in teams with a list of needed supplies prepared by the food pantry. They trick-or-treated for the food pantry and were amazed at the generous response. It was a win/win idea. The people giving the food felt good, the workers at the food pantry were inspired by the good works of the students, the recipients of food appreciated the support and food, and the students felt great about being able to help others in a time of need.

Another student paid for the coffee of the person behind her at the Starbucks drive-up window. When she returned the next day for her daily coffee, the person working at the drive-up window shared with her that the person she bought the coffee for the day prior also decided to pay for the coffee of the person behind him. The kindness spread.

—MH

Numerous studies have found lower rates of depression and less anxiety-related illness among those who are religiously committed. Non-churchgoers have been found to have a suicide rate four times higher than church regulars.[44] Spiritual rituals with a strong connection to peace include prayer and an appreciation of nature.

Prayer   The ritual of prayer has special relevance in stress reduction. Prayer—communication with a higher power—has meaning for many individuals. The most common form of spiritual ritual, prayer is practiced by religious and nonreligious individuals alike throughout the world.[45] Virtually every culture includes prayer in one form or another, especially during times of stress and at the end of life.[46]

Author, educator, and researcher Dr. Lyn Freeman specializes in the practices of relaxation, meditation, and imagery. Many clients have told her that prayer was the ultimate form of relaxation therapy for them. In prayer, they put their trust in a divine power, relax, let go of their fears, and experience great peace. She believes that relaxation is not the end product but, instead, part of the experience. She says:

> Spiritual healers often describe becoming still and entering into a deeply relaxed state as part of their healing practice. I hear this from Traditional Healers in Alaska all the time; they turn inward to "Speak to the Grandfather." Other spiritual practitioners or energy healers talk about "centering" themselves, turning inward, becoming relaxed and calm. Relaxation seems to be a part of all these disciplines."[47]

Prayer has powerful beneficial physiological and psychological effects as these studies demonstrate:

- In a national survey of family physicians, 94% stated that they believed personal prayer or other spiritual practices can aid medical treatment and improve healing.[48]

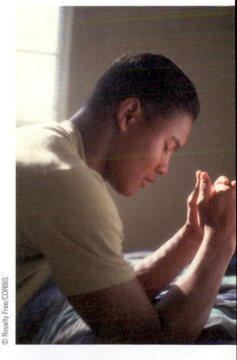

© Royalty Free/CORBIS

Virtually every culture includes some form of prayer as a meaningful spiritual ritual, especially during times of stress.

Prayer in the Coronary Care Unit

Over a 10-month period, a computer assigned 393 patients admitted to the coronary care unit at San Francisco General Hospital to either a group that was prayed for by home prayer groups (192 patients) or to a group that was not remembered in prayer (201 patients). The study was designed according to rigid criteria, the kind usually used in clinical studies in medicine. It was a randomized, double-blind experiment in which neither the patients nor the nurses and doctors knew the group to which the patients had been assigned.*

Researcher Byrd recruited various religious groups to pray for members of the designated prayed-for group. The prayer groups were given the first names of their patients, as well as a brief description of their diagnosis and condition. They were asked to pray each day but were given no instructions on how to pray. "Each person prayed for many different patients, but each patient in the experiment had between five and seven people praying for him or her," Byrd explained.

The results indicated that the prayed-for patients differed in several areas:

1. They were five times less likely than the unremembered group to require antibiotics.

2. Fewer members of the prayed-for group developed pneumonia or had cardiac arrests.

3. They were three times less likely to develop pulmonary edema.

4. None of the prayed-for group required endotracheal intubation, in which an artificial airway is inserted in the throat and attached to a mechanical ventilator, while 12 patients in the unremembered group required the support of a mechanical ventilator.

5. Fewer patients in the prayed-for group died (although this difference was not statistically significant).

If the technique being studied had been a new drug or a surgical procedure instead of prayer, it almost certainly would have been heralded as some sort of "breakthrough." Even some hardboiled skeptics agreed on the significance of Byrd's findings. Dr. William Nolan, who has written a book debunking faith healing, acknowledged, "It sounds like this study will stand up to scrutiny. . . . Maybe we doctors ought to write on our order sheets, 'Pray three times a day.' If it works, it works."**

Sources:
*"Positive Therapeutic Effects of Intercessory Prayer in a Coronary Care Unit Population," by R. Byrd, *Southern Medical Journal* (1988, July), *81*(7), 826–829.
**Cited in *Healing Words: The Power of Prayer and the Practice of Medicine,* by L. Dossey (San Francisco: HarperCollins Publishers).

FYI

Students and Prayer

According to the UCLA Higher Education Research Institute study, 69% of college students say they pray; 61% pray at least weekly, and 28% pray daily. They frequently pray for loved ones (68%), to express gratitude (59%), for forgiveness (58%), and for help in solving problems (58%).

Source: http://www.spirituality.ucla.edu/spirituality

At a certain point you say to the woods, to the sea, to the mountains, the world, "Now I am ready. Now I will stop and be wholly attentive." You empty yourself and wait, listening.

—Annie Dillard

- Research documented that among women who were about to undergo breast biopsies, those with the lowest stress hormone levels were those who used faith and prayer to cope with stress.[49]
- Lyn Freeman reported on the findings of numerous studies on the outcomes of prayer that prayer has modulated stress levels in the face of cardiovascular surgery, loss of spouse, and chronic and intractable pain. The intensity levels of pain, stress, distress, or impairment predicted how likely a patient was to turn to prayer as a source of coping.[50]
- Larry Dossey, a physician of internal medicine, has written extensively on the healing power of prayer. In his book, *Healing Words,* he reported on his research on the studies on prayer, stating that he found more than 100 different studies demonstrating that when a person prays for someone or something else, a real effect takes place for the person or object being prayed for.[51]

Can prayer heal? Providing scientific proof is a challenge at best. Can prayer bring peace? The evidence is strong that prayer—as well as other spiritual rituals such as meditation, spending time in nature, music, storytelling, and art—provides comfort for many.

Nature Spending time in nature can be a profound spiritual experience. The vivid sky at sunset, a shimmering waterfall, the majestic forest, a quiet stream—these manifestations of nature can remind us that we are part of something much greater than ourselves. Throughout history, most religious and cultural traditions have included a connection with nature. We discuss nature in more detail in Chapter 14, Creating a Healing Environment, but a mention is important here so we understand that spending time in nature is a meaningful spiritual practice for many.

Spending time in nature helps restore balance in our life and also deepens our connection with a higher power. Many people consider nature to be the most visible manifestation of the spirit.

Ecospirituality Ecospirituality is a relationship that an individual experiences personally with the environment. A spiritual view provides a context for living with the Earth and the universe. This relationship arises from a personal, inner experience and reflects an acquired state of inner harmony. Think about your experiences in being nurtured by nature. Also think

Nature-Centered Spirituality

Native Americans believe in the sacredness of special places. They believe that good health results from harmony and balance with the physical, social, and spiritual components of life. Native American religious traditions express a positive relationship with nature called *nature-centered spirituality*. This connection with nature is not limited to Native Americans. It is found in many other religious traditions worldwide.

Source: "Mother Earth: American Indian Beliefs and Practices in Childbearing," by V. Rose, *Midwifes Chronicle & Nursing Notes* (1993), *106*(1263), 104–107.

about your responsibilities to honor nature and the environment. What do you do to sustain the environment?

Two of the spiritual rituals that have special relevance in managing stress are prayer and an appreciation for nature. Think about other rituals that provide emotional and spiritual renewal in your daily life.

Now that you have learned about the five qualities of spiritual health, we will suggest an action plan for you. You will learn how to apply spirituality in your daily life to reduce stress and enhance wellness.

> **Author Anecdote** **Solo Time Is Renewal Time** Several years ago I started taking one day each season for what I call "solo time." For one day each spring, summer, fall, and winter I escape by myself for a day of solitude. I plan for the day and write it in my schedule book or it probably would not happen.
>
> Solitude is the experience of being by yourself without feeling lonely or alone. Invariably I end up in nature for my day of rest and rejuvenation. We live in the beautiful Black Hills of South Dakota, so I'm fortunate to enjoy hikes in the autumn, cross-country skiing in the winter, swimming in cool, clear lakes in the summer, and long, relaxing bike rides in the spring. But mostly on my solo days I walk, sit, think, listen, and *be*, instead of *do*. I can hardly put into words how these days of solitude restore my sense of balance. When was the last time you spent a day or two completely alone for the sole purpose of self-renewal?
>
> —MH

An Action Plan for Stress Management Through Spiritual Wellness

Surveys indicate that over 50% of students place strong importance on "integrating spirituality into my life." What about you? Where should you begin in your quest to manage stress through spiritual wellness? How do you put this knowledge into action? The challenge may seem daunting and overwhelming. Certain tools to reduce stress are very tangible: talking with friends, managing your money, and exercising more. But as you have learned in this chapter, there is another tool for helping you manage life challenges that can be just as beneficial—embracing your spirituality. Although wellness of spirit comes to a person in different ways and spiritual growth can take many paths, this growth starts with a single step:

1. Begin by defining what spirituality means to you.
2. Next, close your eyes and take a few minutes to reflect on some spiritual moments in your life—times when you were keenly aware of your spirituality. As clearly as you possibly can, reflect on these spiritual experiences.
3. Based on your definition of spirituality, reflect on how spirituality relates to stress in your life. Examine the values that guide your life. Do you see a relationship between your spiritual beliefs and the values you prioritized in Chapter 9? Spirituality determines values, and values determine actions. When our actions are consistent with our values and beliefs, the outcome is balance, peace, and fulfillment.

I go to nature to be soothed and healed, and to have my senses put in tune once more. (John Burroughs)

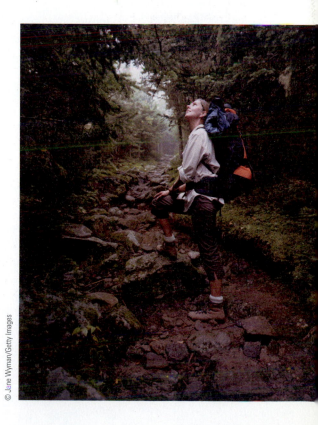

© Jane Wyman/Getty Images

4. Complete the Stress Management Lab, Spiritual Wellness Assessment & Response, at the end of the chapter to guide you in your action plan for stress management through spiritual wellness.

Conclusion

The path to spiritual health is not prescribed. The right way is the one that works for you. Based on your cultural beliefs, your experiences in life, and your values, only you can decide on the path that will lead to greater peace for you. Spiritual well-being is not an endpoint or a prescribed set of activities to accomplish on a one-time basis. Spiritual health involves a lifetime of deliberate choices and an intentional inner focus on matters of the spirit. Making choices that fulfill your purpose in life will bring the ultimate stress-relievers—peace, joy, and love—into your life. The overriding message is not to ignore the spiritual dimension. Peace comes from deliberate balance in body, mind, and spirit.

The intent of the chapter is not to support or promote any specific religious or spiritual perspective but, instead, for you to reflect on the role of spirituality and religion in your life. Commitment to a whole-person way of living prevents and relieves negative stress. The spiritual dimension of health acts as the force that unifies the other dimensions of health: intellectual, emotional, physical, and social.

At the beginning of this chapter, you learned that discovering the contemplative, spiritual life requires not so much a radical change in lifestyle as a shift in awareness, an inner change. Spirituality is the inner intention of our spiritual essence, rather than the outward circumstances of our lives. Take a minute to think about what this means for you. This inner stability enables you to be a self-fulfilling person despite all life's changes and challenges. You are able to find meaning, and therefore grow, from even the most difficult times in life. Spiritual health is the quality of existence in which you are at peace with yourself and in harmony with the environment.

The Hebrew language has a word, **shalom,** that cannot be translated fully into an English word. Shalom is more than wellness or wholeness. It can best be translated as "peace." Shalom involves the total person and the person's environment. To have shalom involves spirituality. Peace is an outcome of spiritual health.

Stress Relief Activity

The Guided Imagery—Inner Wisdom Relaxation Activity found at the Premium Website provides an opportunity to explore your spiritual nature through guided imagery.

10.1 Spiritual Wellness Assessment & Response

I. Spiritual Wellness Assessment

FIGURE 10.2 Spiritual Wellness Assessment

Instructions: In front of each item below, choose one of the following: S = I am doing *superior* in this area of my spiritual life   SS = I am doing *so-so* or okay in this area, but I could improve   NS = I *need strengthening* in this area (an area of growth for me)

___S___ I have a deeply held belief system or personal theology.
___S___ I have faith in a higher power.
___S___ My faith gives meaning to the experiences and relations in my life.
___SS___ Even during difficult times, I have a sense of hope and peace.
___NS___ My spiritual beliefs help me remain calm and strong during times of stress.
___NS___ I feel a connection to the people and the world around me.
___NS___ I am able to forgive people, even when I think they have wronged me.
___NS___ I seek time with nature and reflect on how nature contributes to my quality of life.
___SS___ I find comfort in the practice of spiritual rituals (prayer, meditation, music).
___NS___ I feel loved.
___SS___ I am able to express my love for others freely.
___SS___ I respect the diversity of spiritual expression and am tolerant of those whose beliefs differ from my own.
___SS___ I can clearly articulate the meaning and purpose of my life.
___S___ My inner strength is related to my belief in a higher power.
___S___ I take time to be of service to others and enjoy doing so.
___NS___ I feel a sense of harmony and inner peace.
___NS___ I think my life is balanced.
___NS___ I feel responsible and am actively involved in preserving the environment.
___SS___ I see myself as a person of worth and feel comfortable with my own strengths and limitations.
___S___ The way I live my life is a reflection of what I value most.

Source: *Stress Less: Four Weeks to More Abundant Living,* by M. Hesson (Nashville, TN: Abingdon Press, 1999).

II. Assessment Response Questions

The Spiritual Wellness Assessment has no right or wrong responses. It is intended to help you identify areas in which you may decide to do some spiritual growth work. Continue to practice your positive spiritual habits, while you look for new ways to grow spiritually. Reflect on your response to the statements in the assessment as you answer the following questions to help you with your spiritual growth:

1. What activities do you practice currently that help you feel spiritually healthy?

2. When all the surface layers of your life are peeled away, what do you believe makes up the core of your life—your purpose for being?

3. List two items from the Spiritual Wellness Assessment that you rated with an *S* and that you believe are most important for your spiritual well-being. Why are these items so important to you?

4. Of the items you rated *SS* or *NS*, which two do you think are most important for your spiritual growth?

5. What are three specific things you can do to grow spiritually for greater fulfillment and peace in your life?

Key Points

- Human spirituality is at the heart of stress management. People with a deep sense of spirituality view life differently than those who do not.
- Discovering the contemplative, spiritual life requires not so much a radical change in lifestyle as a shift in awareness.
- We each have a spiritual dimension, a quality that goes beyond religious affiliation that strives for inspiration, reverence, awe, meaning, and purpose even in those who do not believe in any God. The spiritual dimension seeks harmony with the universe, strives for answers about the infinite, and especially comes into focus as a sustaining power when the person faces emotional stress, physical illness, or death.
- Spirituality is a much broader concept than religiosity.
- Scientific methods are not always adequate for exploring concepts such as faith and spirituality.

- Five qualities of spiritual health are:
  (1) a sense of peace, meaning, and purpose in life
  (2) faith in God or a higher power, however you choose to define it
  (3) participation in religious behaviors or meaningful spiritual rituals
  (4) compassion for others
  (5) feeling connected to others and perceiving the self as part of something bigger
- Prayer is a ritual that can have special relevance in reducing stress.
- Appreciation of nature can be a spiritual experience.
- You can enhance spiritual health in many ways. Assessing your spiritual health and developing an individualized plan will help you make choices that bring peace.

Key Terms

spiritual dimension
spirituality
religiosity
placebo
spiritual

faith
connectedness
namaste
forgiveness
altruism

agape
ecospirituality
shalom

Discussion Time For Critical Thinking/Discussion Questions, please visit this book's Premium Website.

Notes

1. *Mind/Body Health* (3rd ed.), by K. Karren, B. Hafen, N. Lee Smith, and K. Frandsen (San Francisco: Benjamin Cummings, 2006).
2. http://wellness.uwsp.edu
3. *Discovering the Mystic Within . . . at the Beach*, by C. Smith, *The Anchorage* 4(2) (Nov. 2003).
4. "The Spirituality of Academic Physicians: An Ethnography of a Scripture-based Group in an Academic Medical Center," by C. Messikomer and W. De Craemer, *Academic Medicine* 77(6) (2002): 562–573.
5. *The Purpose Driven Life: What on Earth Am I Here For?* by Rick Warren (Grand Rapids, MI: Zondervan, 2002); *The Tao of Pooh,* by B. Hoff (New York: Dutton, 1982); *Handbook to Higher Consciousness*, by Ken Keyes (Coos Bay, OR: Living Love Center, 1975); *The Celestine Prophecy,* by J. Redfield (New York: Warner Books, 1993); *The Five People You Meet in Heaven,* by M. Albom (New York: Hyperion, 2003); *You Can Have It All,* by A. Patent (New York: Simon & Schuster, 1995).
6. *Sharing Spiritual Health: Health Exchange,* by D. Diaz (St. Louis: Mosby Publishing, 1994).
7. *Health Yourself: Ten Weeks to a Healthier Lifestyle* (2nd ed.), by M. Hesson (Spearfish, SD: Self-published.)
8. *Health Assessment and Promotion Strategies through the Life Span* (6th ed.), by R. Murray and J. Zentner (Stamford, CT: Appleton & Lange, 1997).
9. *Fundamentals of Nursing* (3rd ed.), by H. Harkreader, M. Hogan, M. Thobaben (Philadelphia: Elsevier/Saunders, 2007).
10. "Spiritual Well-being, Religiosity, Hope, Depression, and Other Mood States in Elderly People Coping with Cancer," by R. Fehring, J. Miller, and C. Shaw, *Oncology Nursing Forum* 24(4) (1997): 663–671.
11. UCLA Higher Education Research Institute, 2005. Retrieved from www.templeton.org.
12. "Spirituality and Healing," by L. Skokan and D. Bader, *Health Progress* 81(1) (2000): 1–8.
13. (2001). "Religious Involvement, Spirituality, and Medicine: Implications for Clinical Practice," by P. Mueller, D. Plevak, and T. Rummans, *Mayo Clinic Proceedings* 76(12) (2000): 1225–1235.
14. Empirical Research on Religion and Psychotherapeutic Processes and Outcomes: A 10-year Review and Research Prospectus," by E. Worthington et al., *Psychology Bulletin* 119(3) (1996): 448.

15. *Mosby's Complementary & Alternative Medicine: A Research-Based Approach* (3rd ed.), by L. Freeman (St. Louis: Mosby, 2009).

16. Freeman, *Mosby's Complementary & Alternative Medicine.*

17. Freeman, *Mosby's Complementary & Alternative Medicine.*

18. "Does Religious Attendance Prolong Survival?" by H. Koenig, J. Hays, D. Larson, L. George, et al., *Journal of Gerontology: Med Sciences 54A*(7) (1999): M370–M376.

19. "Should Physicians Prescribe Prayer for Health? Spiritual Aspects of Well-being Considered," by C. Marwick, *Journal of the American Medical Association 273* (May 24/31 1995): 1561.

20. "Spiritual Health: Definition and Theory," by S. Hawks, *Wellness Perspectives 10*(4) (Summer 1994): 3.

21. *Man's Search for Meaning* (revised), by Victor Frankl (New York: Pocket Books, 1984).

22. *The Best Alternative Medicine,* by Ken Pelletier (New York: Simon and Schuster, 2000).

23. *Life Maps: Conversations on the Journey of Faith*, by J. Fowler and S. Keen (Waco, TX: Word Books, 1985).

24. "The Surprise Key to Stress Management," by D. Nelson, *Vibrant Life 14*(5) (Sept–Oct 1998): 24.

25. "Health and the Spiritual Dimensions: Relationships and Implications for Professional Preparation Programs," by R. Banks, *Journal of School Health 50* (1980): 195–202.

26. *When God Becomes a Drug,* by L. Booth (East Rutherford, NJ: G.P. Putman, 1991).

27. "Development and Psychometric Characteristics of the Spirituality Assessment Scale," by J. W. Howden, unpublished doctoral dissertation, Texas Women's University, Denton.

28. "Love, Compassion and Tolerance," Dalai Lama, cited in *For the Love of God: New Writings by Spiritual and Psychological Leader,* by B. Shield and R. Carlson (San Rafael, CA: New World Library, 1990).

29. Karren, Hafen, Lee, and Frandsen, *Mind/Body Health.*

30. Pelletier, *The Best Alternative Medicine.*

31. In "Five for 2005: Five Reasons to Forgive," *Harvard Women's Health Watch 12*(5) (Jan. 2005).

32. "Embodied Forgiveness: Empirical Studies of Cognitive Emotional & Physical Dimensions of Forgiveness-Related Responses," by C. Witvliet, retrieved April 20, 2005 from www.forgiving.org.

33. Karren, Hafen, Lee, and Frandsen, *Mind/Body Health.*

34. "Five for 2005," note 31.

35. *Love Is Letting Go of Fear,* by G. Jampolsky (Berkeley, CA: Celestial Arts, 1979).

36. *Guided Meditations, Explorations and Healings,* by S. Levine (City: Anchor Books, 1991).

37. Retrieved December 31, 2004, http://www.altruism.org/altruism.

38. *An Invitation to Health 2009-2010 edition,* by D. Hales (Belmont, CA: Wadsworth/Cengage Learning, 2009).

39. *Random Acts of Kindness,* by A. Herbert and editors of Conari Press (Berkeley: Conari Press, 1993).

40. *Agape Love: A Tradition Found in Eight World Religions,* by J. Templeton (West Conshohocken, PA: Templeton Foundation Press, 1999).

41. *The Ways and Power of Love: Types, Factors, and Techniques of Moral Ttransformation,* by P. Sorokin (West Conshohocken, PA: Templeton Foundation Press, 2002).

42. "The Surprise Key to Stress Management," by D. Nelson, *Vibrant Life 14*(5) (Sept–Oct, 1998).

43. Nelson, "The Surprise Key to Stress Management."

44. Nelson, "The Surprise Key to Stress Management."

45. *Spirituality, Health, and Healing,* by C. Young and C. Koopsen (Thorofare, NJ: Slack Inc., 2005).

46. "Is There a Role for Prayer and Spirituality in Health Care?" by D. O'Hara, *Medical Clinics of North America 86*(1) (2002): 33–46.

47. Freeman, *Mosby's Complementary & Alternative Medicine.*

48. "Meditation and Prayer Facilitate Healing Hope, *HealthInform: Essential Information on Alternative Health Care 4*(1) (1999).

49. Pelletier, *The Best Alternative Medicine.*

50. Freeman, *Mosby's Complementary & Alternative Medicine.*

51. *Healing Words: The Power of Prayer and the Practice of Medicine,* by L. Dossey (San Francisco: HarperCollins Publishers, 1993).

Notes

11 Time and Life Management

■ No matter how much time I spend on my schoolwork, I can't seem to catch up. What can I do? ■ What is the best system to help me get organized so I can get the most important things done? ■ How can I find time to have some fun? All I do is work and study. ■ I'm a "go-with-the-flow" type person. A daily "to-do" list seems too rigid for me. Are other options available for managing time that fit my personality better? ■ I do most of my studying immediately before the tests. Does any evidence suggest that I would better spend my time spreading out my studying more?

Study of this chapter will enable you to:

1. Select a time management technique that will work for you.
2. Identify time wasters.
3. Prioritize to gain control of your time.
4. Overcome procrastination.
5. Reduce your stress by being more efficient and effective.

Dost thou love life, then do not squander time, for that is the stuff that life is made of.

—*Ben Franklin*

Students Share Their Experience "In planning out my day and arranging things in order of priority, I found that I was getting a lot more of the important things done and being controlled less by things that seemed urgent. I was more prepared when it came time to put out fires, and because my priorities were written down, I delegated many of the urgent things to others. My stress levels were much lower because I had a better idea of the things I wanted to get done. I seemed to accomplish a lot more in less time. I had more peaceful relaxation time because my other concerns were written and scheduled. Before, I normally laid in bed thinking about all the things I had to do the next day, but by making a list beforehand, I actually slept better and my day flowed better. When my life is organized, my comfort level rises. I'm happier and less of a grouch. I'm a better student, a better husband, and a better father. When I'm organized, I tend to get off track less and don't get upset over the small stuff."

—*Jeff S.*

* * *

"I'm a very organized person. I like to have things laid out so I can prioritize and plan. Prioritizing my time was a perfect assignment for that! It especially helped me keep my homework done. Being able to assign an A, B, or C helped me not to be so stressed about getting everything done at once, too! In respect to my time, I thought I efficiently used the little time I had. I always feel better when I get something done, and this was a no-fail way of being productive. I had my own version of time management, but after reading this chapter and practicing these ideas daily, I was able to lay things out better and become more familiar with prioritizing. I was able to use my time in a good way, and I still had some time left over to do something fun!"

—*Karen M.*

Time and Life Management

Time management is like a diet. We hope for the magic pill that will make our time management struggles magically disappear. But time management is about taking action. The perception that we don't have enough time is one of life's great stressors. Yet we all have exactly 60 minutes in every hour, 24 hours in every day, and 168 hours in every week. No one gets more, and no one gets less. So time management is really about managing our self and our life to do and have the things that are most important to us.

In this chapter you will learn some tools and techniques to reduce your stress by getting a grip on how you use your time. First we will explain three time management techniques. Then we will offer some tips on how to overcome procrastination and eliminate time wasters, which will put you on the path for finding balance in your daily life.

What Is Time Management?

We live our lives within the context of time. Time is the medium through which we live our lives. Development, maturation, learning, wisdom, and serenity are critically related to the passage of time. Time is an omnipresent factor in our lives.[1] How we choose to spend our time determines the level of satisfaction we experience.

Time is nothing more than the occurrence of events in sequence, one after another. Getting out of bed is an event; walking to answer the phone, getting into the car, and everything else we do in a day are events. Time is the occurrence of all of the events of our lives, one after another. Albert Einstein once said that time is what keeps one thing after another from all happening at the same time. **Management** is the art or manner of controlling. A working definition of **time management,** therefore, is the art or manner of controlling the sequence of events in our lives.

We live in deeds,
not years;
In thoughts, not
breaths; In feelings, not
in figures on a dial.
We should count time
by heart throbs.

—*Aristotle*

Time Pressure and Stress

Findings from a study conducted to examine the relationship between the use of time, subjectively perceived time pressure, life stress, mental health, and life satisfaction, using data from Canadian General Social Surveys and the Canadian National Population Health Survey, are as follows:

- The subjective sense of time pressure is grounded in objective reality. Those reporting higher levels of perceived time pressure carry heavier loads of paid and unpaid work and are limited in their access to leisure-time resources.
- Both low and excessive time pressures seem to correlate negatively with mental health.
- Life-cycle situations strongly affect respondents' sense of life satisfaction and emotional well-being. Employed married respondents in the 25-to-44 age group, and particularly the 45-to-64 age group, with or without children at home, reported the highest levels of emotional well-being, even though some of these groups are pressed for time.
- Unemployed people, students, and divorcees reported the lowest levels of life satisfaction.

In the above research, notice that both low and high time pressures can have a negative impact on mental health. People with a perceived sense of control over their time and their life reported less stress. This helps explain why the unemployed, students, and divorcees reported less satisfaction and control and greater stress.

Source: "Time Use, Time Pressure, Personal Stress, Mental Health, and Life Satisfaction from a Life Cycle Perspective," by J. Zuzanek, *Journal of Occupational Science* (1998), *5*, 26–39.

Time and Stress

Psychologists tell us that our stress levels are directly related to how much control we feel over events and situations in our life. To the extent that we feel like we have less control, we correspondingly experience more stress. Emotions associated with feeling out of control include distress and anxiety. When we feel in control of something, we typically experience the emotions of calmness, security, and inner peace. Time is one of those areas in life in which we often feel like we have lost control. Gaining some control over how we use our time is crucial to managing stress. Research has shown that time management has a positive impact on employees' mental health, and that this may be attributable primarily to enhanced feelings of control over time.[2]

Women and men rate themselves differently in terms of time management and stress levels. In one study, women were more likely to rate their time management skills as "above average," but they also were twice as likely as men to indicate that they felt frequently overwhelmed by all they had to do. According to Linda Sax, UCLA associate professor of education and director of the survey, women's greater tendency to feel overwhelmed may reflect the differences in how women and men spend their time. Perhaps as a function of their comparatively higher levels of involvement in potentially stress-buffering activities, men were more likely than women to perceive lower levels of stress and to rate their emotional health as above average. Men also were less likely than women to report that they felt frequently or occasionally depressed over the past year.[3] Based on a national survey of college freshmen, Figure 11.1 summarizes how men and women spend their time.

What about children? Are today's kids too busy? It seems the stress related to a perceived lack of time starts early. Adults might think that kids' lives are carefree and full of free time; however, a recent KidsHealth KidsPoll[4] shows that kids have quite a different opinion. Of the 882 kids ages 9 to 13 who were polled, 41% report feeling stressed most of the time or always because they have too much to do. Most agreed on one thing: 77% wish they had more free time.

Adults and children, college students and employees, women and men—many share the common perception that they are too busy. We feel stressed because we

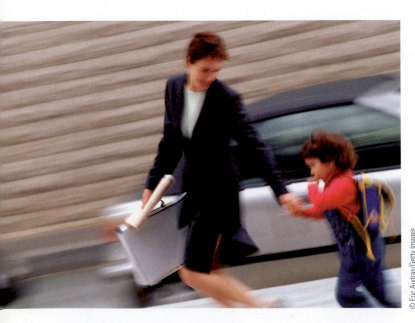

Today's kids feel rushed and stressed. They want more free time just to be kids.

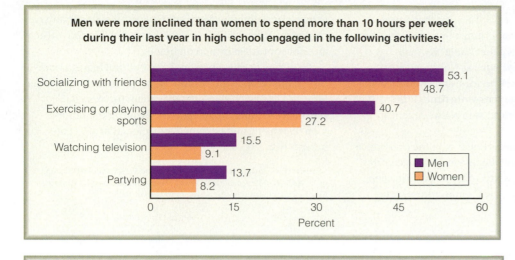

Men were more inclined than women to spend more than 10 hours per week during their last year in high school engaged in the following activities:

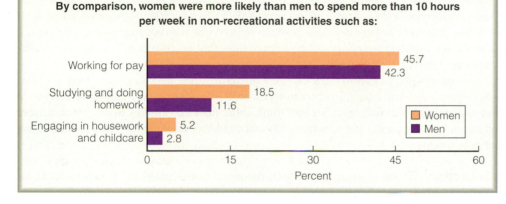

By comparison, women were more likely than men to spend more than 10 hours per week in non-recreational activities such as:

believe we have too much to do and not enough time to do it. So, how can we take control of our time to reduce our stress? Deliberate planning and time management techniques are the answer.

Planning for Control

Planning will help you get control of your time and your life. **Planning** is the act of bringing future events into the present so appropriate control can be applied. Once you master the skill of planning, it will free you from the underlying feeling that your life is out of control.

Why do we sometimes avoid planning? Maybe we think that planning inhibits our creativity, keeps us from going with the flow, takes too much time, or doesn't allow for interruptions and is restricting. Or maybe we have no idea how to plan in a way that makes any sense, or maybe we lack the discipline to develop and follow a plan.

Pareto's Law A principle that can help you in planning was developed by Vilfredo Pareto, an Italian economist and political sociologist who lived from 1848 to 1923. He devised the law of the "trivial many and the critical few," better known as **Pareto's law,** or the 80:20 rule. This rule says that, in many activities, 80% of the potential value can be achieved from just 20% of the effort, and that one can spend the remaining 80% of effort for relatively little return. Even though Pareto lived a century ago, his 80:20 rule, in its many forms, is accepted as almost universal truth.

The reverse is also true: Things that take up 80% of your time and resources will produce only 20% of your results. Let's say your term paper is due tomorrow, so the pressure is on. You plan to complete the assignment in 3 hours, and tonight is the night. You gather your assignment instructions and related materials, tell your friends to leave you alone, and turn on your computer. You hear the message, "You have mail," so you decide to check your messages. Half an hour later, you have replied to your messages and are determined to focus on your paper. You connect to the online library resources and start

> I get up every morning determined to both change the world and to have one hell of a good time. Sometimes, this makes planning the day difficult.
>
> —E.B. White
> (20th-century American writer)

What Time Is It?

Time is a theoretical construct laden with cultural value judgments. Anthropologist E.T. Hall identified societies as either being based on **monochromic time** (M-time), such as Northern and Western European, European American, and "westernized" cultures, or being based on **polychromic time** (P-time), such as Middle Eastern, Latin American, and Native American cultures.

M-time societies view time as linear with the preference being to do one thing at a time. People in M-time cultures tend to view time as a commodity, to be saved/lost, spent/wasted, or squandered/managed. P-time cultures tend to be cyclical and unscheduled, typically viewing time as a natural rhythm in which several things can happen at once and not controlled by human beings.

Exploring our own personal and cultural biases about time is important. Understanding the relationship between time and ethnicity, gender and age, can increase our sensitivity to different perspectives while at the same time increasing our awareness of factors that affect our perspective.

Source: "The Concept of Time: Its Cultural and Functional Implications," by A. MacRae, *American Occupational Therapy Association: Conference, Abstracts and Resources* (Bethesda, MD: Author, 1995).

with a search of key words. You scroll through some abstracts that might relate to your paper. You come across a link to an interesting Web site, which leads to another, and then another, and an hour later, you still have not written one word of your paper. You get the idea. Concentrating your efforts on the key activities that get results will increase your efficiency and decrease your stress.

The universality of Pareto's law can be a powerful guide for you in planning how you spend your time. You have the power to set the vital priorities that will mean the difference between failure, survival, and success. Think about how this applies to you. This chapter will help you determine the activities that will yield the most benefits in your achieving what you value.

Methods of Time Management   Of the many useful planning and time management methods, most begin by asking these four crucial questions:

1.   What are my highest priorities? (What is most important to me?)
2.   Of my priorities, which do I value the most?
3.   What can I do about my highest priorities in the days and weeks to come?
4.   When, during today or this week, will I do these things?

This chapter introduces you to three effective methods to help you answer these questions so you can take control of the events in your life.

1.   ABC123 Prioritized Planning
2.   Quadrant Planning
3.   Lifebalance

Because we are all different, no time management system works equally well for everyone. As you will observe, these three methods have similarities and differences. In reading them, you may find yourself attracted to one method more than the others. You also might find ways to modify the methods according to your own circumstances and preferences. Each has been found to be effective in helping people gain control over their lives and, as a result, significantly reduce their stress.

ABC123 Prioritized Planning

A simple, yet powerful method of managing the events of our lives involves moving beyond the traditional "to-do" list. Called the **ABC123 Prioritized Planning** method, it was introduced by Alan Lakein.[5] The focus of this method is to move from crisis management and putting out fires toward doing those things that are most important to us.

First, dedicate 15 minutes each day to thoughtful planning. This could be either at the beginning of the day or the evening prior to the next day. During the 15-minute daily planning, follow this three-phase procedure:

Phase I: Make a List   Make a list of everything you want to accomplish today. At this point, don't assign any value to anything on the list. Simply unload onto a piece of paper or a planner the things you want to and need to do today. At this point, it looks much like a traditional "to-do" list. This may be a long list. That is okay.

Phase II: Give a Value to Each Item on the List, Using ABC

Put an "A" next to each item on your list that *must* be done today. These are the vital things that are most important to you. "Important" is not the same as "urgent," and you must clarify the difference. Urgent items shout for immediate action. Many times these urgent things are not necessarily important but they have the appearance of having to be handled *right now.* Answering a telephone or checking an e-mail may seem urgent but often lacks relative importance.

Examples of "A" priority items might include studying for a test that will take place in 2 or 3 days, putting some gas in the car if you're running on empty, going to the gym to work out, taking your daughter to a movie, spending some quiet time meditating, or beginning research for a paper that is due in 3 weeks. These are all important items, though they may not be hollering at you to be done "right now." These important but not necessarily urgent items *must* get on your list as "A" items.

Next, place a "B" beside each item that should be done today. These are items with *some importance* to you. An example of a "B" item might be deciding on a topic for a paper that is due in 6 weeks, filling your car with gas when it still has a quarter of a tank left, or changing the water in the fish tank.

The items on your list that will get a "C" are the tasks that have *very little importance* to you. These items could be done but won't suffer at all if they are not. Examples of "C" items might be washing your car, going to a store to buy a shirt, reading the newspaper, or cleaning out the garage.

Mark shared in class that he realized he had let a "C" item replace an "A" item the day before. He said, "My three-year-old daughter, Annie, asked me to read her a bedtime story last night. I promised I would as soon as I finished reading the newspaper. When I finished the paper and went into Annie's room, I found her sound asleep. I felt a lump in my throat when I realized I had let something as unimportant as reading the paper come before spending some time with Annie at the end of the day."

The value you give items will change as the events in your life change. What was once a "C" item, such as cleaning the garage, might soon become a "B" item if you no longer can get your car into the garage. The level of importance of working on a research paper changes as the due date for the paper approaches. The key point is that you are the one who is evaluating the relative importance of each of the items on your list based on how you currently perceive them.

Phase III: Prioritize Again, Using 123

In Phase III of the planning process, give a numerical value to each item on the list based on its relative importance to you. First, move through the "A" items

Remember, spending your time on what is truly important can contribute to joy and happiness.

FYI Tyranny of the Urgent   We have a tendency to do the urgent things at the expense of the highly important things. For example, most people would agree that spending time developing a relationship is important. Spending quality time with a friend or a family member is vital to the relationship. Yet, the amount of time that parents spend talking to each other or their children is small in relation to the time they spend doing seemingly more urgent but far less important items of the day such as watching a favorite TV program or surfing the Internet. Charles Hummel, President of Barrington University, had this to say about the difference between the urgent and the important task:

> The important or vital task rarely must be done today or even this week. The urgent task calls for instant action. The momentary appeal of these tasks seems irresistible and they devour our energy. But in the light of time's perspective, their deceptive prominence fades. With a sense of loss, we recall the vital task we have pushed aside; we realize we have become slaves to the tyranny of the urgent.[6]

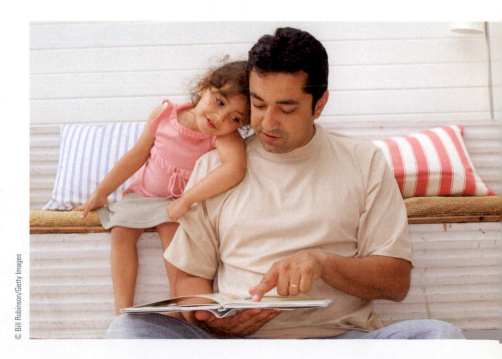

The Time of Your Life

A study was conducted to examine time-use patterns and related variables, including feelings about time use, time management, and academic achievement by traditional college students. In the study, 106 male and female students completed self-report questionnaires to measure their use of time (activities they engaged in during a typical 24-hour period) and feelings about their use of time (related to competence, value, enjoyment) for the activities they reported.

They also completed a Time Management Questionnaire that measured their attitudes, preferences for short-range planning, and preferences for long-range planning. Results of the study suggest that older students and those experiencing role overloads perceive themselves as less competent, and they value and enjoy their use of time less than younger students and those with fewer role demands. In addition, the use of time management was related to academic achievement.

Source: "Time Use, Time Management and Academic Achievement Among Occupational Therapy Students," by A. Henry, C. Costa, D. Ladd, C. Robertson, J. Rollins, and L. Roy, *Work: A Journal of Prevention, Assessment & Rehabilitation* (1996), *6*, 115–126.

and compare each one. Ask yourself which of these very important items is *the most important of all*. That item gets a "1" next to the "A" so it becomes "A1" on your list. Proceed through each of the As until you have given a ranking to each. Then proceed to the Bs, and then the Cs.

Table 11.1 is an example of how your planning list might appear after following through on each of the three phases. The action plan for the day would begin with the item that received the A1, followed by A2, and on through the A items. When the A items are completed, you proceed to B1, B2, and so on.

What you have just done is determine the order in which you will do the things you want to do based on their relative value to you. You are determining the sequence of the events of your day. You have begun to gain control of your day, because you have put your most important things first.

A word of warning if you want to make this work effectively: The human tendency is to skip the most valuable and important things (the "A" items on the list) and move to the items that are easier, more fun, or less demanding (the "B" and "C" items on the list). Doing this will have consequences. First, and most notably, many of your important items will turn into urgent items. If you put off working on the research paper until a couple days before it is due, you are in panic mode. The quality of your paper probably will suffer and you are less likely to enjoy working on your paper. This is called "putting out the fires." It is the urgency mode. Stress levels definitely increase when we operate in this mode.

The other consequence of doing the "B" and "C" items first and putting off the "A" items is inner chaos. As we discussed in Chapter 9, on values, when we do the things that are

TABLE 11.1 Example of Prioritized Daily Planning

ABC	Task List
B4	Schedule appointment for a haircut
A5	Get snacks for tonight's party
A3	Go to the gym to work out
C3	Check e-mail
B3	Send thank-you letter for last week's job interview
C4	Go to the mall to look for new jeans
C5	Play Nintendo with Eric
A2	Go to eye doctor appointment
A4	Meditate for 15 minutes
A1	Study for tomorrow's math test
B2	Study for next week's history test
C2	Make appointment with a counselor to decide on a major at school
B1	Call players on intramural team about next week's game
C1	Write a letter to parents

most important to us, we experience inner peace because what we do and what we value are aligned. When we don't do the things that are aligned with what we value, we lose our inner peace.

On most days you won't finish everything on your list. In fact, you rarely will. Classes, meetings, work obligations, and interruptions will interfere with your plan. The real value of the ABC123 system becomes clear when we do have periods of free time and so can choose among several activities. During those times in the day, we can go to the top of our list, our A1 item, and work from there.

This method of planning can be an effective way to get some control over the events of life, especially if you currently aren't doing anything to plan your days and frequently feel overwhelmed. By using the ABC123 method, you can gain back some of that control.

Tip: A simple adaptation of the ABC123 method is to start each day by making a list of the six most important things you want to accomplish that day. With careful thought, this one simple action can help relieve your stress and free your mind to focus on what is most important to you.

Quadrant Planning

The second method of time and life management, **Quadrant Planning,** is one of the most popular time management systems today. This method was developed by Stephen Covey and explained in his best-selling book, *The 7 Habits of Highly Effective People.*[7] Quadrant Planning relates to the habit of highly successful people called "First Things First."

First Things First   Quadrant Planning begins with a long-term approach to time management by inviting you to first answer some questions. The answers to these questions will guide you in your daily decisions. Covey believes that traditional time management methods don't bring peace and fulfillment because we don't put the most important things (first things) first. He compels us to assess what our first things are with some thoughtful questions:

- Are the things that are less important in your life receiving the most attention?
- Are too many good things getting in the way of your best?
- Are you making the tough decision to choose the best over the good?
- What activities, if you knew you did superbly and consistently, would have a significant positive impact on your life?
- How many people, on their deathbed, wish they had spent more time at the office?

We should ask ourselves first, "Am I doing the right things?" After we have answered this question, we can ask, "Am I doing things right?" When we do this, we begin to put our lives in a direction that is much more fulfilling and effective.

Urgency Versus Importance   The key to doing first things first is to distinguish again between the urgent and the important. We may be busy working as hard as we can only to find that at the end of the day, we feel unfulfilled. This is because we put the **urgent,** those things demanding our attention in the moment, before the **important,** the things that would make a difference in the long-term. Urgency seems to control our lives. The only way to truly master our time is to organize our schedule each day to spend most of our time doing things that are important but not necessarily urgent.

In the Activity Matrix, Figure 11.2, Quadrant 1 activities will demand our attention at times, but the point to remember is that if urgency is what is driving you, you may be missing the important things. Quadrant 2 activities, the important activities, should be our first things—the things on which we focus most of our time and energy.

Imagine a big jar sitting on a table, and next to the jar is a pile of rocks of varying sizes, including a few cups of sand that signify the smallest rocks. We want to put all the rocks in the jar. If we put the sand in first and then proceed to try to put the bigger rocks in after the sand has filled the jar, we will not have room for the big rocks. But if we put the big rocks into the jar first, we then can add the smaller rocks and even the sand.

Think of Quadrant 2 activities as the big rocks. If we don't plan those things first (putting first things first), they will not make it into our daily activities because we become so busy doing the less important, but often urgent things. When we plan the Quadrant 2

Advanced Planning and Preparation   Plan ahead. Take time to think ahead to future activities. Think about things that could go wrong, and deal with them in advance. For example, if you know you have an early appointment and won't have much time to get ready, take your shower and lay out your clothes the night before. Other examples of advanced planning include keeping the gas tank at least one-quarter full and having a well-stocked home emergency shelf of food staples.

FIGURE 11.2 Activity Matrix

Quadrant 1: Urgent and Important
- Crises
- Pressing problems
- Deadline-driven projects
- Urgent meetings
- Important things that we have procrastinated on

Quadrant 2: Important, Not Urgent
- Preparation
- Prevention
- Values clarification
- Planning
- Relationship building
- True recreation
- Empowerment

Quadrant 3: Urgent, But Not Important
- Interruptions, some phone calls
- Some mail, some reports
- Some meetings
- Many proximate, pressing matters
- Many popular activities

Quadrant 4: Not Urgent, Not Important
- Trivia
- Busywork
- Some phone calls
- Time wasters
- "Escape" activities

activities into our weeks and days, we find ourselves doing the most important things first. As a result, we enjoy inner peace, our self-esteem goes up, and we find ourselves being more productive.

Quadrant Planning in Action

To put the principles of Quadrant Planning into a time management action plan, follow these steps:

Step 1: Quadrant 2 Questions In our planning time, rather than starting by listing all of the "things to do," Covey suggests that we should *first* ask ourselves the more important questions. As we do this, we find ourselves doing more things that are in Quadrant 2 and, as a result, we live according to those most important things.

- What do I want to be, do, and contribute in my life?
- What three or four things are most important to me?
- What are my long-range goals?
- Which relationships are most important to me?
- What are my main responsibilities?
- What contributions would I like to make?
- What principles do I value?
- What feelings do I want to experience in life?
- How would I spend the coming week if I were to have only 6 months to live?

When we are thinking about the days and weeks ahead and what we will spend our time doing, we first answer these questions. The answers will guide our choices.

Step 2: Identify Roles To increase our feelings of order and balance and to help answer Quadrant 2 questions, we focus on our roles in life. Much pain can come from realizing that we are succeeding in one role at the expense of another. Too often we hear of people who are successful in their business life but encounter problems with their family life or their spiritual life. A holistic view of life involves a balance between the various dimensions of life, including the physical, social, intellectual, emotional, and spiritual. Our roles help us fulfill the needs of these dimensions and give us a sense of wholeness in quality of life. These roles may include family, personal, business, school, relationships, and community. List your roles, and then go back and ask the Quadrant 2 questions for each role.

Select Quadrant 2 goals for each role. Do this by asking the question: What is the most important thing I can do in this role today or this week to have the most positive impact in my life? For example, a mom might decide that the most important thing she can do in her relationship with one of her kids is to spend half an hour each night reading to him before he goes to bed. Perhaps only one goal per week is all that is necessary.

Step 3: Sharpen the Saw Covey recommends that we include in our planning a focus he calls "sharpening the saw." A man is feverishly sawing away at a tree with his handsaw.

A friend walks by and asks the man why he doesn't stop for a while and sharpen his saw so he can cut the tree more easily. The man cutting the tree replies that he can't stop to sharpen the saw because he is too busy sawing. Have you ever felt like you are continually busy, yet you are not accomplishing anything important? Taking time to sharpen your saw can dramatically affect the level of accomplishment you feel in your life. Instead of busily sawing with a dull saw, you are cutting down the trees.

There are things in life that we can do that, if we did them on a regular basis, would help us to sharpen our saw and allow us to do all the other things that we do with greater ease and effectiveness. As we plan, consider some of those saw-sharpening activities for each of our dimensions. For example, for the physical dimension, we might focus on activities such as getting regular aerobic exercise or eating a healthier diet. We also might strive to go to bed earlier and awaken earlier to get off to a good start. In the emotional dimension we might decide to meditate regularly. In the social dimension, we could plan to spend quality time with family and friends. In the spiritual dimension, we might read inspiring literature, participate in service-oriented projects, attend religious services, or pray more frequently. These examples have value in themselves, and they also help us do more easily and effectively all the other things we want or need to do.

Step 4: Evaluate—How Did I Do? **Integrity** is the ability to carry out a worthy decision after the emotion of making the decision has passed. When we are alone in our planning sessions, we tend to design our days and weeks according to our conscience and according to the things we decide are most important. The real challenge arises when we get to a moment of decision. As we proceed through the day according to our plan, someone invites us to do something that is far less important, though it may be enticing. The challenge is to keep first things first in this moment of choice. Are we going to sacrifice the best for the good in that moment? Or will we remain true to our plan and continue focusing on the best? Goethe said, "Things that matter most must never be at the mercy of things that matter least."

Part of our movement toward developing ourselves, reducing stress, and reaching our goals involves assessing what we have done to propel us toward each of these goals with integrity. Evaluation is the art of looking back and seeing what we did, how we did it, and if it worked to produce the results we intended. If it did, great! We can add to our pat on the back the question of how we can use that success to continue learning and growing. If we did not see the results we intended, what adjustments can we make to get results in the future?

Here are a few questions for evaluating ourselves as the days and weeks go by:

- What have I learned about myself?
- What goals have I achieved, and what empowered me to accomplish them?
- What goals did I not achieve, and what kept me from accomplishing them?
- What patterns of success or failure do I see in setting and achieving goals?
- Am I setting goals that are realistic but challenging?
- Am I dedicating sufficient time to the three or four things that matter most in my life?

Author Anecdote **It's about Time** When I worked as the director of a corporate health promotion program, one of the most common excuses I heard for not exercising was, "I don't have enough time." Yet, I couldn't help but notice that the most productive employees were those who made time to incorporate exercise into their daily routine. Rather than decreasing their productivity because of the time they spent exercising, their productivity actually increased. This could have been because the time they took to exercise relieved their stress, or increased their endorphins, or helped them think more clearly, or just plain made them feel better about themselves and their job. Whatever the reason, they were sharpening their saw.

—MH

WHAT ELSE

CAN I DO?

Regular Preventive Maintenance Like advanced planning, regular maintenance can go a long way to minimize daily stress. Regular preventive maintenance will make these things less likely to break down or fall apart at the worst possible moment, so when bad things do happen, the impact will not be as disastrous.

Here are a few examples of ways to keep your "important stuff" in top working order:

- Make backup copies of important papers and documents.
- Make regular backups of important items on your computer.
- Change dead or worn-out batteries in your smoke alarms, flashlights, and other necessary electrical appliances.
- Repair things that aren't working properly as soon as possible.
- Have your car serviced regularly.
- Change the filters in your home's heating and cooling system regularly.
- If your alarm clock, wallet, shoes, windshield wipers, or anything else is a constant aggravation, get it fixed or get a new one.

- What challenges did I encounter, and what were my responses?
- Did I take time to keep my saw sharp in the dimensions of my life?

In review, Quadrant Planning for time management includes:

1. Differentiating between what is urgent and what is important
2. Identifying roles in each dimension of life
3. Sharpening the saw
4. Evaluating our performance

You have to decide what your highest priorities are and then have the courage to say "no" to other things. You do this by having a bigger "yes" burning inside and leading your way. The end result is not the feeling that you have deprived yourself but, rather, a sense of satisfaction and accomplishment that you have concentrated on what you value.

Lifebalance

A third method of time management is called **Lifebalance.** Although this approach seems to be significantly different from the previous two approaches, it can be equally as effective in helping you organize your time to relieve stress.

Critics of traditional time management approaches contend that planning is too rigid and tends to dwell too much on doing and having, and not enough on being. These management approaches do not take into consideration our natural rhythms of life. It is as if we can stop to smell the roses only as we are running by them quickly to do something apparently more urgent. In the meantime, we miss life's important unplanned moments. If we have planned every minute of our day and if we do not cross off every planned action from our list, we feel like we have failed. These approaches, critics say, do not seem to allow for spontaneity, freedom, and going with the flow. To some, traditional approaches have an emptiness.

The Lifebalance approach to time and life management promotes a balance of purposeful planning and a healthy mix of going with the flow. In their book, *Lifebalance,*[8] authors Richard and Linda Eyre contend that we live too much of our lives out of balance. Unbalance results from bad habits—habits that emphasize work at the expense of family and personal growth, structure at the expense of spontaneity, or accomplishments at the expense of relationships (or vice versa on any of these). The result of this imbalance is what Thoreau called "lives of quiet desperation."

The search for a simpler, slower, more flexible, and more meaningful life has vanished in our culture with the constant search for *more, better,* and *different.* Contentment has been replaced by competition. Serenity has been replaced by speed. By contrast, balance implies a healthy combination of all that is important to us and letting our inner nature, rather than our environment and culture, dictate our speed and direction.

Some people are more comfortable with a lifestyle that takes things as they come and simply "show up" with whatever seems to unfold in their daily experience. To those who are vigorous planners, this approach seems frivolous and unproductive. How can people accomplish anything if they don't know where they are going? This follows the adage, "If you fail to plan, then you plan to fail." Again, we are reminded that time management is subjective.

The frustration many people feel with time management planners includes the following:[9]

- 95% of what is written in planners has to do with work, career, or finance, which creates an imbalance between work and family and personal needs.
- Planners cause us to live by lists, to act rather than respond. If we're not careful, our lists will control us rather than the other way around. We begin to view things that are not on our lists as irritations or distractions rather than as opportunities, and we begin to lose the critical balance between structure and spontaneity.

- Because they are problem-oriented and accomplishment-oriented, most planners direct their attention to things, on getting and on doing things, sometimes at the expense of people and giving and thinking, which results in an imbalance between achievements and relationships.

Taking an example from *Lifebalance*: Consider a typical businessman who uses a schedule book or a time organizer. If we analyze the contents, we will find three things: First, we find that more than 95% percent of his entries (lists, plans, appointments, reminders) have to do with work. It is hard to find anything relating to his family or to his own personal growth. Second, his planning leaves no time for spontaneity or flexibility. He prides himself on using every hour of the day, and he gets his kicks from checking off everything on his list. His motto is "act, don't react." He likes to say that people who are good planners don't like surprises, and he avoids them by allowing only the things on the list. Third, just as he makes no room on his schedule for spontaneity and surprises, he leaves precious little space for relationships. Planning and lists seem to deal much more with things than with people.[10]

Keys to Creating Balance

Keys to creating balance include simplifying, doing what really matters, sitting and thinking, and balancing structure with spontaneity.

Simplifying In theory, knowing what we value most and acting on the things we value is an obvious way to live. In practice, it is something quite different. We constantly are wishing we had more time for the really important things in life. When we sit down to plan using this type of balancing, rather than asking, "What do I have to do?" we ask questions such as, "What do I *choose* to do? or "What do I *want* to do?"

Unfortunately, day-to-day concerns occupy so much of our time that they tend to keep us from making time for these more important things. The essence of balancing the things we value is to simplify. We can develop the ability to simplify our days, and our lives, by regularly asking these four questions:

1. Will it matter in 10 years?
2. What do I need more of in my life?
3. What do I need less of?
4. How can I make this simpler?

The Fisherman As the story goes, a lone fisherman sat on the beach, his fishing pole planted in the sand. Along came a corporate executive on vacation. "Why don't you have two poles so you can catch more fish?" the executive asked. "Then what would I do?" asked the fisherman. "Then you could take the extra money, buy a boat, get nets and a crew, and catch even more fish." "Then what would I do?" asked the fisherman. "Then," said the executive, "you could move up to a fleet of large ships, go wholesale, and become very rich." "Then what would I do?" asked the fisherman. "Then you could do whatever you want!" shouted the executive. And the fisherman replied, "That's exactly what I'm doing right now!"

We can use this story to guide us in making decisions about what really matters in life. We work longer hours to pay for an expensive vacation so we can collapse. What if we just work less so we don't so desperately need to rest? We frantically work to increase our income so we can buy that big, expensive house only to find that we have to work even harder to maintain it. We can choose to simplify.

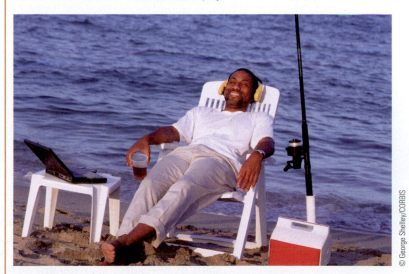

Simplifying your life can help you get in touch with what brings real peace.

© George Shelley/CORBIS

When we begin to ask these questions, we learn to say "no" more frequently to those things that aren't worth doing. Continually adding more things to our life has the effect of complicating and speeding up the pace of our life. Removing things from our life brings simplicity and freedom. The first step to balance our priorities is to simplify.

Doing What Really Matters The second aspect of balance, related to simplification, is to direct our priorities to three specific areas, then work to balance these areas. The three priorities common to everyone are:

1. *Family:* our relationships with family and friends
2. *Work/career/school:* all areas of our professional development
3. *Self:* development with our inner self and also the way we serve others, including activities with church and community groups

To create more balance in your life spend 5 minutes each day, before writing down any other plans or thinking about your schedule, deciding on the single most important thing you can do that day for family, professional development, and yourself. Imagine how many of your important goals you would accomplish if you were to focus on things that really matter.

Don't Just Do Something—Sit There! Planning our days involves a commitment to stop everything and spend at least 5 minutes stopping and doing nothing other than thinking. Before planning your schedule, give yourself some sit-down time each day to ask yourself the key questions mentioned previously.

In our solitude time, rather than asking, "What do I really want?" ask challenging, but perhaps more useful, questions such as: "What do I need?" "What do I need in my physical life?" "What do I need in my social life…my spiritual life…my intellectual and emotional life?" Get in the habit of asking yourself these questions daily—then choose the thing you need to do most and do it that day.

Balancing Attitude—Balancing Structure and Spontaneity Balancing our attitude involves considering both the destination and the journey. Our culture thrives on our reaching goals and enjoying the good feeling that comes with accomplishment. In doing this, we frequently tend to forget about the joy of the journey and the footsteps we take on the way to the goal, which are just as important as the goal itself.

The *Lifebalance* authors offer the comparison of the jets and the hot air balloons. The jets are the people who strive to arrive. People ride in jets to get where they are going as quickly as possible. People who dislike formal planning because of its inflexible structure say the jets lack spontaneity. People ride in hot air balloons for the sheer pleasure of riding in them. The hot air balloons are those who stop to smell the roses, who go with the flow of the wind wherever it might take them.

On our way to living our days in more fulfilling ways, we can have both—the balloon and the jet. The yin and the yang of the Taoist symbol, shown in Figure 11.3, imply that we are made up of both the jet and the hot air balloon. We feel drawn to both ways of being.

Antiplanning describes the attitude of setting goals and being firm about where we want to go but at the same time being flexible on how we are to get there. With our limited wisdom, we don't always know the best way to do something. If we remain open to opportunities rather than staying attached rigidly to what we have planned, we may find new directions, new opportunities, and sometimes even better

Author Anecdote Go with the Wind While on the Happy Trails bike ride through Iowa, I met a fascinating couple, Carter and Kaye. They related an experience that exemplifies hot air balloon living. They explained that every year they meet up with a group of friends at a predetermined location. After breakfast they get on their bicycles and ride in whatever direction the wind is blowing. They continue riding for several days with no specific destination in mind. The only plan is that the wind is always at their back. By remaining open to the spontaneity of discovering whatever lies around the next bend, they have experienced some amazing adventures that they never could have planned for.

—MH

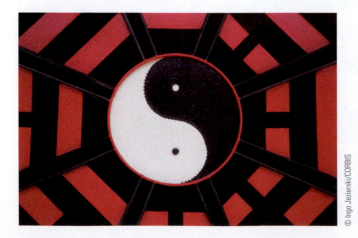

© Ingo Jezierski/CORBIS

FIGURE 11.3 Yin-Yang Symbol
The Taoist yin-yang symbolizing balance.

goals. Antiplanning shifts our focus to a simpler attitude of enjoying each step of the journey as much as the goal we will reach.

When do our best ideas come to us? Running around working frantically to get through the daily "to-do" list usually leaves no room for insights or ideas to pop into our awareness. Our best ideas come during times when our thinking has slowed and we aren't concentrating on anything in particular. Examples include when we are in the shower, daydreaming, sleeping in, taking a leisurely solo stroll, and driving. During these times we should have a pen or a recorder handy to catch fleeting ideas. Often these insights can completely change an entire day, or even an entire lifetime, in the direction of a more fulfilling and joyful experience. If we don't let the ideas through because of the busyness of our mind, we miss out on these best things.

Serendipity

Closely related to the Lifebalance approach to time management is the idea of serendipity. The English writer Hugh Walpole first coined the term **serendipity** to describe the quality that, through good fortune and sagacity, allows a person to discover something good while seeking something else. He came up with this word and definition after reading a Persian fable about the three princes of Serendipity.

The Three Princes of Serendipity

The story tells of three princes who went into the world to seek their fortune. None of them achieved what they were seeking, but they each got something else, something better. One found love, one found beauty, and the third found peace.

> These three men, while traveling through the world, rarely found the treasures they were looking for but continually ran into other treasures equally great or even greater which they were not seeking. In looking for one thing, they found something else, and it dawned on them that this was one of life's sly and wonderful tricks. When they realized this, they got an entirely new slant on life, and every day resulted in a new and thrilling experience.[11]

The essence of this principle is that the happenings you don't expect are actually the things that are supposed to happen. Other definitions for serendipity are:

- The capacity for making happy and unexpected discoveries by accident.
- The gift of finding valuable or agreeable things not sought after.[12]
- An unexpected discovery of something worthwhile during a search of an expected something worthwhile.[13]

The Keys to Serendipity Serendipity emphasizes that:

1. We need to be working toward something. We need to set some goal(s) for ourselves and be moving in the direction of the goal(s).
2. We need to be aware, to be alert, to be observing things to realize the so-called "happy accidents" that occur as we are on the way to our original goal. If we aren't tuning in to what is happening, we will miss things such as beauty, spontaneous moments, new and even better goals and directions, opportunities, and needs of others as they arise.

With serendipity, we can have both worlds—the jet and the hot air balloon. We can still set goals and work toward them. But the flexibility of serendipity allows us to be open

FYI

Gaining the Quality of Serendipity

- *Slow down.* Hurry tramples watchfulness and thoughtfulness. Smell the flowers, feel the sun, pause to breathe. Notice the needs of others and try to feel empathy. Sometimes, relaxing your pace can lengthen your stride.
- *Welcome surprises.* Anticipate them, look for them, expect them, and relish them. Surprises don't knock you off course; they reveal new destinations and new directions.
- *Enjoy the journey.* Look for and find joy today. Life is not a dress rehearsal.
- *Hold "Sunday Sessions."* On Sunday, look ahead to the next 6 days thinking about what matters, about priorities and opportunities. These sessions adjust and refine goals as new options appear and new capacities grow.
- *Simplify and set your own standards.* Trading time for things is usually a bad deal. Trying to impress others with the newest and costliest car, fashion, brand name, address, toy, or trend is often a losing proposition.
- *Make goals without plans.* Although goals are an indispensable part of serendipity, tight, detailed plans are not. Spend your Sunday Session and other "thought time" conceptualizing your goals and laying out a general road map toward them, but acknowledge that your actual route will be some combination of the schedule and the surprise.
- *Add playfulness and humor to each day.* Lighten up and allow yourself to make mistakes, to enjoy the more humorous parts of life, to laugh like a child.
- *Take risks and follow your feelings.* The dullness of our comfort zones lulls us into a false sense of security. Living fully involves taking risks and enjoying the surprises of what might come with the risks.

Source: *Serendipity of the Spirit*, by R. Eyre (Salt Lake City: Homebase Publishers, 1988), pp. 61–64.

to spontaneous events as they occur. We don't treat interruptions as annoyances but, instead, as opportunities to discover something good that might add to our joy and fulfillment. Richard Eyre summed up this idea with the following thoughts:

> Too much planning can make the actual experience of living almost anticlimactic. Too much thinking about a thing removes us from it. We become observers, analysts, spectators, or critics rather than participants. If we can approach life more as an experience which contains vast variety and infinite potential for surprise, we will find ourselves dealing less with "success" and "failure" and more with progress and growth. If we have to think about every detail of our lives, we ought to think about them after they have been lived (when we can learn from experience) not before and during (when the very thought may intercept or alter the experience).

> Approaching life as an experience makes us, moment-to-moment, more aware of what is happening and of what we are feeling—and less aware of what we plan to have happen or wish had happened. Thus we see opportunities we could never have planned and realize far more serendipity than we otherwise could. Goals can co-exist with experience—they can shine like beacons and allow us to see our experiences more clearly in their order and light.[14]

> Live your life each day as you would climb a mountain. An occasional glance toward the summit keeps the goal in mind, but many beautiful scenes are to be observed from each new vantage point. Climb slowly, steadily, enjoying each passing moment; and the view from the summit will serve as a fitting climax for the journey.
>
> —*Harold B. Melchart*

Applying Serendipity Knowing about serendipity and applying the principle in daily life are two very different things. Serendipity is not a common way of being for most people in our culture. We tend not to think and act this way. But we can learn to move in this more balanced direction. This activity can help get you started.

Split-Page Scheduling Start your planning time by drawing a line down the middle of your daily planning page. The left side of this page is for our traditional scheduling of activities and planning items to do that day. The right side of the page is left blank. We will fill this side, during the day or at the end of the day, with those unanticipated needs, unforeseen opportunities, and unexpected moments that come up during the day. These are the items we could not have planned for but turn out to be as valuable as, or more valuable than, the things we had planned. The left side gets the list, and the right side gets the day's serendipitous after-it-happens notes, such as a new acquaintance, a fresh idea, a child's question, an unexpected opportunity, a friend's need, a chance meeting, a beautiful sunset.

We have to be in pursuit of something (left side of the page), and we have to be aware, sensitive, and observant of those other things that we didn't plan for (right side of the page). The right side of the page reminds us to be playful, spontaneous, take risks, and be serendipitous.

With this type of flexibility automatically worked into our days, we create a new definition of a perfect day. A perfect day used to be one in which our high priorities, our "A" items, were checked off the list. Now a perfect day will still include that, but in addition, we jump the line to do the serendipitous things as well. Living in this more flowing and balanced way involves intentionally changing the way we function throughout the day. From the outside, we may not appear to be doing anything differently, but inside we manage things in vastly different ways.

Lifebalance and awareness of serendipity do not mean "no plan and no goals." The guiding principle is *be strong and fixed on the destination, but be creative and flexible on the route.*"[15]

The Lifebalance approach to time management is significantly different that the ABC123 and Quadrant Planning methods, yet all three methods can be effective in helping individuals accomplish their goals, manage their time, and relieve their stress. Next, let's look at a variety of tips on how to overcome procrastination and eliminate time wasters.

Procrastination

Procrastination is the avoidance of doing a task that needs to be accomplished. This can lead to feelings of guilt, inadequacy, depression, and self-doubt. Procrastination has a high potential for stressful consequences. It interferes with our academic, professional, and personal success.

Procrastinators Finish Last

In studies with students taking a health psychology course, researchers at Case Western Reserve University found that although procrastinating provided short-term benefits, including periods of low stress, the tendency to dawdle had long-term costs, including poorer health and lower grades. Early in the semester, the procrastinators reported less stress and fewer health problems than students who scored low on procrastination. By the end of the semester, however, procrastinators reported more health-related symptoms, more stress, and more visits to healthcare professionals than nonprocrastinators. They also were more likely to turn in their papers late and received significantly lower grades on term papers and exams.

Source: "Longitudinal Study of Procrastination, Performance, Stress, and Health: The Costs and Benefits of Dawdling," by D. Tice and R. Baumeister, *Psychological Science* (1997), *8*, 454–458.

Styles of Procrastination Psychologist Linda Sapadin identified six styles of procrastinators.[16] See if any of these sound like you.

1. *Perfectionists* fear that they can't complete tasks up to their expectations. They focus on details rather than overall objectives, and they fear making mistakes.
2. *Dreamers* have big goals but fail to translate their ideas into a plan for action. They contrast with perfectionists because dreamers don't get to the details.
3. *Worriers* focus on the worst-case scenario and see the problems rather than the solutions. They tend to avoid change and risk-taking.
4. *Crisis makers* wait until the pressure mounts to take action. By waiting until the last minute to complete a task, they create excitement from a temporary rush of adrenalin—and put their projects at risk.
5. *Defiers* resist new tasks and often don't follow through on what they promise to do. They avoid teamwork and are reluctant to make agreements.
6. *Overdoers* make the job harder than it needs to be and create extra work. They fail to set priorities and refuse to delegate.

Notice that the styles of procrastination are really just a collection of habits. Habits are learned, and they can be unlearned.

Tips for Overcoming the Procrastination Habit Here are some are tips for overcoming the procrastination habit:

Turn elephants into hors d'oeuvres. Cut a huge task into smaller chunks so it seems less enormous.[17] When you can't seem to get started on a project, try breaking it down into smaller tasks and do just one of the smaller tasks or set a timer and work on the big task for only 15 minutes. If you know that your 30-page term paper is due in one month, start today by picking your topic or writing a rough outline. By doing a little at a time, you won't feel so overwhelmed, and eventually you'll reach a point where you will want to finish.

Avoid cramming. Despite their best intentions, students often study in ways that encourage forgetting. In addition to studying in noisy places where attention is easily diverted and interference is maximized, they often try to memorize too much at one time by cramming the night before an exam.[18] The single most important key to improving grades may be **distributed study time**, which refers to spacing your learning periods with rest periods between sessions. Cramming is called **massed study** because the time spent learning is massed into long, unbroken intervals. A comparison of 63 separate studies found that distributed study produced superior memory and learning compared to massed study.[19]

> Nothing is so fatiguing as the eternal hanging on of an uncompleted task.
> —William James

FYI

Cramming Research shows that most students do most of their studying right before the test. Although an intensive review before a quiz or exam does help, you are not likely to do well in college courses if this is your major method of studying. One of the clearest findings in psychology is that spaced practice is a much more efficient way than massed practice to study and learn. Just as you wouldn't wait until the night before a big basketball game to begin practicing your freethrows, you shouldn't wait until the night before an exam to begin studying.

Source: "Measuring Study Time Distribution: Implications for Designing Computer-based Courses, Behavior Research Methods, Instruments, & Computers," by R. Taraban, W. Maki, and K. Rynearson, Behavior Research Methods, *Instruments & Computers*, (1999), *31*, 263–269.

Manage your time zappers. A significant deterrent to successful time management is the **time zapper,** something that takes time away from what is more important. Probably the most significant time zapper is television viewing.

Television viewing is a time zapper because it steals time that we could be spending on things that are more important. Imagine what you could accomplish if you were to spend those 4 hours working on more productive things such as learning a foreign language or how to play a new instrument or even doing homework. Time zappers include driving from place to place, videogames, unnecessary meetings, excess socializing, oversleeping, talking on the phone, surfing the net, and worrying. You probably can think of many other things that would fall into the category of time zappers.

The best way to manage time zappers is by *planning.* This chapter has suggested several excellent ways to do this. When you decide what the order of your activities will be through the day and you follow through with discipline while maintaining appropriate flexibility, you will have an easier time saying "no" to the things that waste so much of your time.

Work hardest during your "best times" of the day. Most of us can identify 2 or 3 hours during the day when we are most productive. Are you a "morning person," a "night owl," or do you do your finest work in late afternoon? During these times we usually have the most energy and are the most creative. Try to schedule your time so your most important activities can be done during these "best times" of the day.

Keep an activity log. Just as a nutrition log is a record of everything you eat over a period of time, an activity log allows you to see what you do with your time. Without modifying your behavior, record everything you do, as you do it, from the moment you awaken until you go to bed. Every time you move from one activity, say eating breakfast, to watching the morning news, to the time you spend getting dressed, make a note of the time in your time log. After doing this for a few days, look carefully at what your log tells you about how you spend your time. You may be surprised at how much time you spend doing things that might be considered a waste of time or have little value for you or anyone else.

Choose to refuse. Learn to say "no" to the unimportant or less important things. Most of us have difficulty saying "no," but this becomes easier when we focus on our goals. You have to be convinced that you and your priorities are important. Before you agree to undertake any additional tasks, ask yourself if those tasks or activities will lead you in the direction of your goals and priorities. Saying "no" to extra projects, social activities, and invitations you know you don't have the time or energy for can prevent a lot of unnecessary worry, guilt, and wasted emotional energy down the road.

Try delegating. Rethink the old saying, "If you want something done right, you have to do it yourself." If some things don't require your personal attention, delegate them to someone else.

Author Anecdote

A Waste of Time

We don't need to completely eliminate time wasters, but frequently they take up so much of our time that little is left for us to do the important things that have higher priority for us. One day while we were discussing this principle in class, a student in the back of the room raised his hand and proudly declared that he had played a videogame for 24 hours straight. He took only brief breaks as needed, then quickly resumed his videogame marathon. When I asked him how he felt about that, he mentioned that the time went quickly and it was an enjoyable experience. He did mention that it probably was not time well spent, though. The rest of us in the class agreed.

—MO

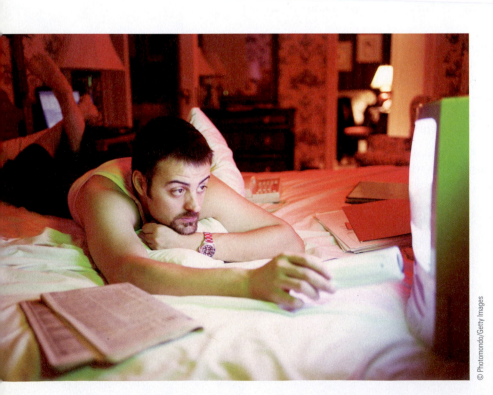

Do you ever watch TV as a means of procrastination to avoid doing something? Watching television is one of the most common ways we waste time.

Establish levels of acceptable perfection. It is human nature to want to do our best on every task. We have difficulty sometimes submitting work that may not reflect our best performance. Frequently, though, some things we do don't necessarily require anything approaching perfection. When this is the case, complete the task at an appropriate level, depending upon the importance of the item. E-mails sent to a friend do not require perfect grammar and perfect spelling. Take a realistic look at similar tasks and determine which can be your "good" work and which should be your "best."

Do the most difficult or most unpleasant tasks first. Once you have the tough tasks out of the way, you are freer to enjoy other tasks that are more pleasant and fun. The most unpleasant tasks usually are the ones that rank more highly on our priorities list. When we do those first, we earn the satisfaction and inner peace that comes from doing those things.

Use "wasted" time. Time we spend sitting in the doctor's office or waiting for an oil change can be useful downtime. Read a novel, take some deep breaths, or practice visualization. You can even use these times to write in a journal.

Enjoy the process. Ask yourself how you can do the task *and* have fun in the process. Maybe you can do your homework with your best friend or go to a place with a stunning view of nature and do your homework there. If you know that something has to be done but is unpleasant to even think about, ask yourself how you can add something enjoyable to the process. Maybe you somehow can make it a game or competition with someone else.

Reward yourself. Even for small successes, celebrate the achievement of goals. Promise yourself a reward for completing each task, or finishing the entire task. Then keep your promise to yourself and indulge in your reward. Doing so will help you maintain the necessary balance between work and play. As time management author Ann McGee-Cooper says, "If we learn to balance excellence in work with excellence in play, fun, and relaxation, our lives become happier, healthier, and a great deal more creative."[19]

Let some things go undone. Follow the advice of Lin Yu Tang, 20th-century essayist and philosopher, who said, "Besides the noble art of getting things done, there is the more noble art of leaving things undone. The wisdom of life consists in the elimination of nonessentials." Let it be okay not to finish some things, and even not to do some things that are on your list. An incomplete list has only the meaning you give to it. It doesn't mean you are not being effective, and it certainly doesn't mean you are a failure. You decide what can be left undone, and you can allow yourself to be okay with that.

Author Anecdote 92 Is Still an A Greg was one of those students who wasn't satisfied with any grade less than an "A." Not only that, but he felt like a failure if he didn't receive every single point on every single assignment. A grade of 95 left him asking, "How did I fail to achieve 100?"

As an assignment in my health promotion class, the students set a goal and developed a contract for improving health in an area of their choosing. Greg decided to work on stress management. He realized that his drive for perfectionism was driving him into a state of constant stress. As one of his interventions, Greg came up with the creative idea of posting notes everywhere—in his car, at his desk, in his notebook—with the simple message, "92 is still an A." Gradually, this simple reminder to himself allowed Greg to put things in perspective and realize that he didn't have to be perfect at everything. He still could accomplish his goal of earning an "A" in class, but with much less self-induced pressure.

—*MH*

Conclusion

In the final analysis, how you spend your time, and what events you participate in every moment of each day, is your choice.

You say that you *have to* be in a class at a specific time, or you *must* be at work during a specific time period. No life requirement says you *have to* be there. Although not showing up to work has consequences, you still have a choice. The point is that we decide what we do with the 24 hours of our day, or 168 hours of our week.

As you make those choices, don't mistake activity for achievement. Take time to pause from time to time and remind yourself of where you are going and how you want to get there. Henry David Thoreau once said, "It is not enough to be busy; so are the ants. The question is, what are we busy about?"

In this chapter you learned three time management systems. All are designed to help you gain more control of your life and thereby reduce your stress and enhance your well-being. You will find that planning sets you free. Experiment with these systems, and determine which has the most appeal to you and your current circumstances.

We introduced a new way of looking at time, called serendipity, as a way to have both the stability of working toward the destination and the freedom to enjoy the journey along the way. You also learned tips for overcoming procrastination and eliminating time zappers. You can reduce your stress by focusing on the things that matter. In the end, time management is really more about managing yourself and your life than it is about managing time. You replace "I don't have enough time" with "I have plenty of time for what matters to me."

LAB

11.1 Time Log

PURPOSE The purpose of this activity is to first, determine exactly how you spend your time and second, analyze how you can spend your time more effectively.

DIRECTIONS

I.   For 3 or 4 consecutive days, including at least one weekend day, keep track of how you spend your 24 hours. Write down each activity and account for every minute of your day, including the time you spend sleeping. Keep a journal or notebook with you throughout the day so you can immediately write down the following in your time log:

   1. Date
   2. Time of day
   3. The time spend doing the activity
   4. What you are doing

II. Once you have completed your time log for 3 or 4 days, analyze how you can use your time more effectively.

   1. What is your most productive time of the day?
   2. What are your biggest time zappers?
   3. Review the styles of procrastination content in this chapter. Do you see evidence of any of these procrastination styles when you review your time log? If so, what style most clearly describes you?
   4. What is one specific thing you can do to more effectively manage your time?
   5. What is the most important new insight you gained from completing this lab?

Key Points

- Planning is the act of bringing future events into the present to help you determine how you spend your time.
- Pareto's law holds that 80% of the potential value can be achieved from 20% of the effort.
- ABC123 Prioritized Planning is a time management system that enables us to prioritize the most important activities in our day.
- Quadrant Planning starts with a long-term approach to time management by guiding us to put first things first and determine what is important versus what is urgent.

- Lifebalance is an approach to time and life management that blends planning and spontaneity.
- Serendipity is part of Lifebalance and allows a person to discover something good while seeking something else.
- Procrastination is a habit that interferes with effective time management.
- Activity should not be mistaken for achievement.
- Time management is more about managing ourself than about managing time.

Key Terms

time
management
time management
planning
Pareto's law
monochromic time
polychromic time

ABC123 Prioritized Planning
Quadrant Planning
urgent
important
integrity
lifebalance

antiplanning
serendipity
procrastination
distributed study
massed study
time zapper

Discussion Time For Critical Thinking/Discussion Questions, please visit this book's Premium Website.

Notes

1. "Time and the Body: Re-embodying Time in Disability," by W. Seymour and W. Bunrayong, *Journal of Occupational Science 9* (2002): 135–142.
2. "Preventing Short-Term Strain Through Time Management Coping," by D. Lang, *Work & Stress 6* (1992): 169–176; *Time Management: Test of a Process Model*, by T. Macan, *Journal of Applied Psychology 79* (1994): 381–391.
3. http://www.gseis.ucla.edu
4. HExtra—American Association for Health Education, Vol. 31, No. 2, Summer 2006. KidsPoll survey—nahec.org/KidsPoll.
5. *How To Get Control of Your Time and Your Life,* by A. Lakein (New York: Signet Book/New American Library, 1973).
6. *Time Management: An Introduction to the Franklin System*, by R. Winwood (Salt Lake City: Franklin International Institute, 1990).
7. *The 7 Habits of Highly Effective People*, by S. Covey (New York: Simon & Schuster, 1989).
8. *Lifebalance: Bringing Harmony to Your Everyday Life,* by R. Eyre and L. Eyre (New York: Ballantine Books, 1987).
9. Eyre and Eyre, *Lifebalance*, p. 105.
10. Eyre and Eyre, *Lifebalance*, pp. 42–43.
11. *The World of Serendipity,* by M. Bach (Marina del Rey, CA: Devorss and Co., 1970).
12. *Webster's New Collegiate Dictionary* (Chicago: G & C Merriam Co., 1967), p. 791; also found at the Merriam-Webster Dictionary Web site: http://www.m-w.com/
13. Bach, *The World of Serendipity*, p. 22.
14. *Serendipity of the Spirit*, by R. Eyre. (Salt Lake City: Homebase Publishers, 1988).
15. Eyre, *Lifebalance*, pp. 65–66.
16. *It's About Time—The Six Styles of Procrastination and How To Overcome Them*, by L. Sapadin (New York: Penguin, 1997).
17. *An Invitation to Health*, by D. Hales (Belmont, CA: Wadsworth/Thomson Learning, 2003).
18. *Psychology in Action* (7th ed.), by K. Huffman (Hoboken, NJ: John Wiley & Sons, 2004).
19. "A Meta-Analytic Review of the Distribution of Practice Effect: Now You See It, Now You Don't," by J. Donovan and D. Radosevich, *Journal of Applied Psychology 84* (1999): 795–805.
20. *Time Management for Unmanageable People*, by A. McGee-Cooper (Dallas: Ann McGee-Cooper & Assoc, 1983).

12 Money Matters

■ My money seems to disappear. I would like to know where my money is going and maybe even plan a budget, but I have no idea how to start. Is there a simple way to budget my money so I can get the things I really want and stop feeling constantly stressed about running out of money? ■ Everyone I know is stressed about money. What can I do to deal with my growing credit card debt? ■ My dad tells me I should start saving while I'm young. Even if I could save a little, it doesn't seem like it would be enough to make a difference. If I could save $5 a day, how much would I have in 10 years? ■ In Puerto Rico the people seem happy, even though most of them live in poor conditions. How does having money relate to being happy and feeling satisfied with life?

Study of this chapter will enable you to:

1. Explain the ABCs of money management.
2. Create and implement a plan for financial fitness.
3. Set financial goals to reduce money-related stress.
4. Discuss how doodads and credit cards contribute to financial stress.
5. Investigate what the research says about the relationship between money and satisfaction in life.

I've got all the money I'll ever need, if I die by four o'clock.

—*Henny Youngman*

© Joson/zefa/CORBIS

Sami's Story One day when I was a freshman, my friends and I decided to take off for the mall. It had been a tough week at school, and I needed something to make me feel better. I had plans to buy a new CD, but when I got ready to pay, my credit card was denied. I could have died from embarrassment! That had never happened to me before. I had acquired three credit cards since I started college, and it suddenly hit me that I was in way over my head.

The first time I applied for a credit card was on my first day on campus. Some guys with clipboards were signing people up—and giving away t-shirts. I liked the idea of being old enough to have my own credit card and promised myself that I would use it only for emergencies. It didn't take long for the first "emergency" to come along. My car clunked out, and it cost me nearly $200 to get a hose replaced. Before I knew it, I had maxed out the $1000 credit card limit. When I couldn't make even the minimum payments, I used another credit card to get cash to make the payments.

I honestly don't know where the money went, but I knew I needed help. I went to the counseling center on campus, and the counselor helped me set up a budget, but even now, 3 years later, I still have a bad credit history.

Money Matters

DVDs, a new car, a nice apartment, a digital camera, new clothes, a cell phone—we face temptations to spend money every day. These are the things we *want*, but what about the things we *need* to survive in college? Tuition, books, computer, food, a safe place to live, and transportation to classes—these are just some of the many expenses we have to juggle to be a successful student.

Money is a leading source of stress for Americans, according to a 2007 survey by the American Psychological Association. In the survey, 73% of the respondents cited money as a significant source of stress in their lives. More than three out of every four American families are in debt, according to the Federal Reserve's Survey of Consumer Finances. Not surprising, an American Psychological Association study revealed that debt-related stress was 14% higher in 2008 than in 2004. Living above your means is a tremendous burden. The true cost of debt and financial problems isn't just the interest rate you're paying to Visa or Mastercard. The true cost is the toll that it's taking on your life and your relationships.

This chapter relates to one of the most common stressors around the world—not enough money. And though money truly won't make you happy, lack of money is one of life's great stressors. The bottom line is that money matters! In this chapter you will complete a series of exercises to start you on the road to financial fitness. You will learn how to manage your money so you can reduce your stress now and for years to come. We will also investigate the relationship between money and satisfaction in life. You might be surprised at what the research shows.

What is required to get your finances in shape? Just as we would like to have a strong, fit body without having to exercise regularly, we would prefer to have healthy finances without having to expend any effort. In the real world of college students, though, chances are slim that you will gain financial fitness without exercising some healthy habits to get you there.

Financial pressure ranks high in the list of stressors facing college students. Studies show that the majority of college students experience stress because of various academic commitments, financial pressures, and the lack of time management skills.[1] Financial problems rank up there along with poor grades as the major reason for dropping out of college.

So while the college years are often a time of getting out of shape financially, you will be relieved to know that you can undertake some specific financial exercises to help you develop financial fitness. The ABCs of money management can get you started.

FYI

There's a Reason "Loan" Sounds Like "Moan"
Paying for college is a major expense. More than half of recent college graduates report owing between $10,000 and $40,000 in student loans, with an average debt of $20,000.

Source: "College Grads, Student Loans, and Job Hunting," by J. Kim, *Wall Street Journal*, September 2, 2003

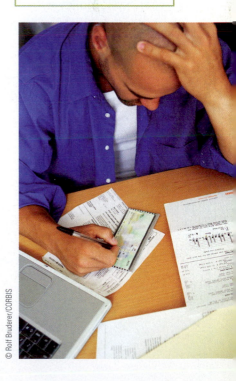

© Rolf Bruderer/CORBIS

Financial pressure ranks high in the list of stressors facing college students.

Financial Worries Top Stressor List; Young Adults Most Stressed

ATLANTA—October 2, 2008 /PRNewswire/—Americans are feeling more stress today than they did six months ago, according to a new national stress study. The survey of 1,000 men and women, ages 18 and older, revealed that 47% of respondents currently feel more stress than they did six months ago. And no surprise, **the # 1 source of stress reported is personal finance concerns**, the top response for almost half (49%) of those surveyed. Surprisingly, international unrest, the war, and the presidential election were reported significantly lower as primary causes of stress, registering only 2% each. The stress survey focused primarily on American's self-reported sources of stress and methods for coping with stress.

Young and Stressed, Older and Mellower

Young people report higher levels of stress than their older counterparts. Nearly six in ten respondents, in the 35–44 years of age category, reported high or very high levels of stress (58%), while less than one quarter (23%) of respondents in the 55-plus age group reported experiencing the same upper levels of stress. The youngest age group surveyed, those 18-24 years of age, registered the highest response (64%) indicating they are more stressed now than 6 months ago.

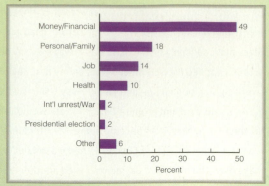

FIGURE 12.1 Sources of Stress.
Of the following, which would you say is the biggest source of stress for you?

Source	Percent
Money/Financial	49
Personal/Family	18
Job	14
Health	10
Int'l unrest/War	2
Presidential election	2
Other	6

Source: https://prnewswire.com/mnr/fboothresearch/35279/ ATLANTA - October 2, 2008/PRNewswire/

Americans Adapt New Age Approaches for Handling Stress

When asked about stress coping strategies, more respondents cited "meditation and breathing techniques" (28%) than the more traditional approach of "taking a vacation" (25%), which may also point to economic factors—which can turn vacationing into as much a source of stress as a stress reliever. On a healthy note, "exercise" tops the list of reported methods for tackling stress.

Source: https://prnewswire.com/mnr/fboothresearch/35279/

The ABCs of Money Management

> We are obsessed with money. Yet we don't take money seriously enough.
> —*Jacob Needleman*

Management is necessary when there are many demands upon your finite amount of money, as is the case for most college students. Practicing the ABCs of money management can put you in control of your money instead of your money in control of you. The ABCs refer to **A**ssessment, **B**udget, and **C**ontrol.

Assessment   Assessment means looking at where you are right now and evaluating how you got there. Assessment includes both awareness and analysis. All change starts with awareness of what has to change. So you should begin by becoming more aware of your current spending habits as associated with the thoughts and emotions linked to spending. Lab 12.1 at the end of the chapter can guide you through the assessment.

EXERCISE 1: Current Spending Habits

> To get started, keep track of what you spend for one week. Write down every penny you spend, and what you spend it on, each day for a week. This will give you a clearer picture of where your money is going. For now, don't worry about your monthly expenses. Simply record your daily spending for a full week, including the weekend. Write down each item immediately so you don't forget.
>
> Don't forget to keep track of how much you spend on pleasure and enjoyment. You might be amazed to find out how much you spend on movies, alcohol, coffee, CDs, or cigarettes.

Thoughts and Emotions Linked to Money   In addition to allowing us to pay for the things we need, we sometimes use money to address our emotional needs. Assessment entails more than merely tracking where our money goes; it also is done to figure out *why* we spend money. We may believe that money can buy us pleasure, friendship, power, and happiness. We have to be careful not to let money become a substitute for emotional needs that we would be better off addressing in other ways.

Think carefully about how this money–emotion connection relates to you. Have you ever gone out and bought something expensive when you were sad or lonely, as a way to try to feel better? Or maybe you felt a real sense of power and importance when you picked up the dinner tab for four of your friends. Although we may get temporary pleasure from impulse buying and spending, those feelings of pleasure quickly turn into feelings of stress. If we don't feel regret the next day, we probably will when the credit card bill arrives!

Tip: As a way to deal with stress, people sometimes use shopping much like eating. When people spend money in an attempt to feel better, they are using shopping as a stress management tool. Shopping is not inherently problematic, but when it is used as a quick and temporary emotional fix, it may lead to higher stress levels from overspending and incurring debt. Take time to make a list of what you need before you go shopping, and stick to the list to avoid emotional shopping.

FYI **What Matters Most** Members of the Financial Planning Association responding to a *USA Today* poll ranked establishing goals, paying yourself first, and sticking to a budget as the three most valuable steps people can take to improve their financial lives.

Source: "Financial Diet Tip #1: Carve Up Your Expenses," by M. Fetterman, *USA Today*, April 22, 2005, 1B.

As you track your spending for Exercise 1, analyze the thoughts and emotions attached to your spending. Begin to notice how often issues of stress and money are related. Did you head to the mall when you were bored? Was going to the movies a way to escape from studying? These things are not necessarily good or bad. The point of this exercise is to help you get in touch with the thoughts and feelings linked to spending so you can make conscious decisions about what is most important to you in relieving stress over both the short-term and long-term.

EXERCISE 2: Money and Emotions

Budget Once the assessment is complete, you can move to the "B" of money management—budgeting. "Budget" is not a dirty word, even though the word has negative connotations for many. It is sort of like the word "diet" in that both create a sense of deprivation. A **budget** is just a plan you develop to manage your money so you can have what is most important to you and accomplish your financial goals. It is a road map to get you where you want to go. If more money is going out than is coming in, no matter how much money that is, you are creating a potential stressor. A budget can guide you in eliminating the stressor.

Tip: If you don't like the word "budget," call it a "cash-flow plan" or a "money tally"—whatever works for you. "Cash-flow plan" has a positive ring, reminding you that cash actually flows both in and out.

The budgeting process starts by first writing your financial goals, and then developing a plan to accomplish those goals. Many people go through life not really thinking much about their financial goals. The first step in creating a successful budget is to develop your goals and write them down so you can see what you want with your money. After graduation you may want to reassess and set goals for the future, but for now, write your financial goals with an emphasis on your college years. Include both short-term and long-term goals for your years as a student.

Tip: In doing this, you are much more likely to accomplish SMART goals. **SMART goals** are **S**pecific, **M**easurable, **A**ction-oriented, **R**ealistic, and **T**ime-based. For example, you might set as a goal: "I will work 20 hours per week as a work-study student to pay for my room and board for spring semester." To say, "I want more money by the end of the semester" is meaningless. This is no time to be wishy-washy. The more specific you are in your goals, the more likely you are to succeed.

Here are some examples of short- and long-term financial goals to get you thinking:

- I will pay myself first by using direct-deposit to put 5% of my paycheck immediately into a savings account.
- I will spend a maximum of 10% of my paycheck on entertainment.
- I will graduate from college with no debt.

EXERCISE 3: Financial Goals

(Continued)

Once you have written your financial goals, look back to Exercise 1, where you recorded everything you spent for a week. Take a red pen and cross out all the expenditures that were unnecessary and did not contribute to your recently written financial goals.

EXERCISE 4: Income and Expenditures

To get an idea of your income and expenditures, begin by calculating what you expect your income to be over the academic year. Add up all sources of money, including from your work, financial aid, and money from your family. Next determine your expenses for the year. Think about tuition, room and board, books, car, and any miscellaneous expenses.[2] Take a broad look at what is coming in and what is going out. What does this tell you about your balance of income and expenditures?

Now you are ready to develop a budget. The key to developing a budget is to make it as easy as possible. If you make it too complicated, you won't do it. The only things you need are a legal pad and a pencil. If you'd rather work on the computer, financial software such as Quicken or Microsoft Money can be a good way to view your financial picture. Remember, this is *your* plan.

EXERCISE 5: Develop Your Budget

You can develop your own budget in many ways. One simple, yet effective method follows these steps:[3]

1. Get your checkbook, credit card statements, or other records of expenditures. (See Exercise 4.)
2. Make a column for each category of spending—for example: tuition, food, rent, entertainment, car expenses.
3. List each purchase as best you can under the proper column. Round to the nearest dollar.
4. Total each column.
5. Add all the column totals together.
6. Compare this amount with your income.
7. Make adjustments where necessary.

Step 7, "Make adjustments where necessary," is where we often need help. How do we do this? And what is necessary? This is where we start to take control of our income and expenditures. You can do this in many ways, as you will learn in the C step, Control, of the ABCs of money management.

Control Now that you can clearly see the money coming in and the money going out, you can begin to make informed choices on how to balance your financial picture to accomplish your financial goals and, as a result, experience less stress and more satisfaction.

One of the things you will notice from your budget is that you have some fixed expenses, such as tuition and car payments, and you have some flexible expenses, such as going out to eat or buying a new shirt. Many people find that a budget helps them daily with these flexible expenses that require frequent decision making.

This is a good time to differentiate between what you want and what you truly need, as the two are easily confused. How many pairs of jeans do you need? How many CDs or DVDs do you need? Do you really need a cell phone? Even though you don't always see it this way, you do have choices in both income and expenditures. The key to financial success is to understand that your budget does not mean simply recording your income and expenses but, in addition, consciously deciding how you will manage your money.

In the remainder of this chapter, you will gain information and receive practical tips to guide you in making adjustments so you can take control of your money. By decreasing your expenditures and increasing your income, you can take control in many ways. Although everyone's situation is different, some common factors can leave us feeling out of control in managing our money.

Stress Busting Behavior: Money Management Checklist

The ABCs of money management require action. Check the box if you've completed the exercise.

☐ Recorded your current spending habits

☐ Assessed the thoughts and emotions attached to your spending

☐ Developed your personal financial goals

☐ Calculated your expected income and expenditures for the year

☐ Developed your budget

Completing each step provides you with valuable information toward financial freedom.

Doodads and Credit Cards

Two areas of financial management that deserve extra attention because they so frequently leave us feeling out of control and contribute to financial stress are doodads and credit cards.

Doodads Author Robert Kiyosaki[4] defines **doodads** as expenses, often unnecessary or unexpected, that take money out of your pocket. Doodads are small but steady expenses that can drain away our cash. Author David Bach[5] calls this the **latte factor.** The latte factor is a metaphor for where you are spending money on little things that you could cut back on without changing your lifestyle. He explains what happens when we spend $3.50 a day to buy a latte (or any other small, nonessential purchase).

Beware of the Latte Factor

A latte a day = $3.50

A latte a day for a week = $24.50

A latte a day for a month = $105

A latte a day for a year = $1,277.50

A latte a day for a decade = $12,775

A latte a day for 30 years = $38,325

The latte factor illustrates how we spend money without realizing how it adds up. Just think! The money you spend in one year on a daily $3.50 latte, or similar item, could buy a new computer; the money you spend in 10 years could buy a new car or a trip around the world. So whether it is beer, or bottled water, or newspapers you never read, or a drink and a candy bar during breaks, think carefully about whether the purchase is worth it to you. We waste a lot of money by not thinking carefully about the purchases we make.

EXERCISE 6: Doodads Do Add Up

Take a few minutes to think of one doodad—a small but steady expense that drains your cash—that is part of your routine. Maybe you can't walk by the bookstore without going in and buying a paperback or two, or maybe you eat lunch at the student union every day when you could pack a lunch instead. Maybe you smoke a pack of cigarettes a day. Maybe you pay a $2 charge every time you use the ATM or $1.50 every time you dial 411 to get a phone number. Maybe you pay for many more minutes on your cell phone than you really need. Once you have identified your doodad, determine its cost. Calculate what you would save in a month if you were to eliminate the doodad. Then calculate the total savings for a year, 5 years, and 10 years. What could you do with that money in 10 years?

To carry the latte factor a step further, Bach illustrates the power of saving by explaining what would happen if you were to put the money you would have spent on a latte to work for you by investing the money.[6]

(Continued)

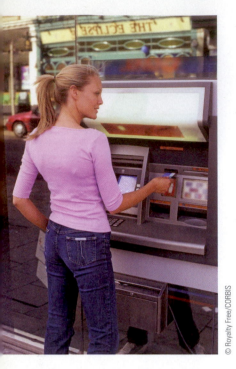

24/7 easy access to money can contribute to impulse buying and overspending.

The Strength of Saving

$3.50 per latte $\times$ 7 days a week = $24.50

If you were to invest $24.50 a week and earn a 10% annual rate of return, you would wind up with:

1 year	$ 1,339
2 years	$ 2,818
5 years	$ 8,257
10 years	$ 21,870
15 years	$ 44,314
30 years	$ 242,916

In these days of lower interest rates, 10% may be a little high, but you get the point. Saving money may be the last thing on your mind when you are in college, but you can easily see how saving even a small amount on a regular basis can help tremendously in achieving your financial goals and, as a result, bring you financial peace of mind.

Strategies for Saving Some strategies for saving include the following:

- Eliminate a doodad and deposit the money into savings.
- Pay yourself first. Put a portion of every check into your savings account before you pay your other bills. Make this automatic so the amount you set is automatically moved from checking into savings.
- Empty all your loose change into a big can and deposit it into savings when the can is full.
- Put your tax refund into your savings account.
- Save one hour a day of your income. For instance, if you make $10 an hour and work for 8 hours a day, have $10 automatically moved from your checking account to your savings account for every day you work.

Eliminating doodads can go a long way toward improving your peace of mind. The intent is not to eliminate the special things that bring pleasure to life but, instead, to thoughtfully analyze where you are spending your money to determine if the costs are worth the benefits. If going out with the guys every Wednesday for a soda and burger is something you look forward to all week, you will want to find a way to work that into your budget. But if you find that nearly every night you are putting three bucks into the vending machines for a soda and a snack, mostly because you need a break from studying, you might want to explore other options.

Credit Cards Doodads are not the only money-drainers. Credit cards can be an especially subtle way to accumulate debt.

Once upon a time, a frog jumped into a pot of hot water. Feeling the intense heat, it immediately jumped out and saved its life. But another frog jumped into a pot of cool water sitting on a burner over low heat. One degree at a time the temperature increased, but the frog became accustomed to it, stayed in the pot, and eventually was boiled.

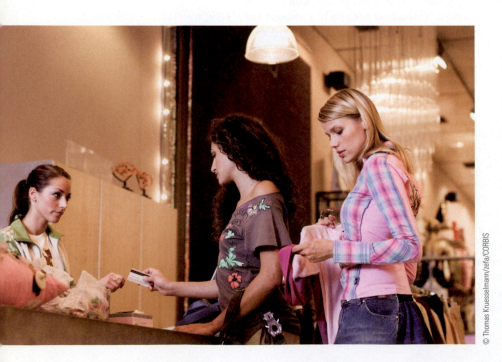

Credit cards make it easy to buy lots of stuff, but stuff doesn't equal happiness.

The moral of this story is that gradual, hardly perceptible changes can do us in—like our slow but steadily increasing credit card debt. We become accustomed to the gradually increasing credit card debt until one day we open our credit card bill and wake up to the realization that we are in way over our head and see no way out. As Sami testified in the opening vignette, credit card debt can haunt a person for years to come.

Somehow, when you charge your purchases to a credit card, it doesn't seem like you are spending real money. Financial advisors estimate that we would spend about 20% less by switching to cash-only payments. Believe it or not, people used to get along just fine without credit cards!

Tips for Managing Credit What can you do to avoid becoming buried under credit card debt? Here are some suggestions that might work for you:

- Use credit cards only for emergencies or carefully planned-in-advance purchases.
- If you must use a credit card, make every effort to pay off the full balance each month.
- Limit yourself to one credit card. Do you really need the free t-shirt or clock radio that credit card companies are giving away to get you to sign up?
- Remember that credit is *debt*, not supplementary income.
- Don't pay just the minimum payment each month. Paying even $20 or $25 more than the minimum can save you thousands of dollars over time.
- Try to get a credit card with a lower interest rate.
- Learn to defer gratification. Avoid impulse buying by making your money or credit card hard to obtain. Leave your credit card home or take only a predetermined amount of money with you when you go out.
- Wrap your credit card and secure it with tape when you carry it with you. The mere act of unwrapping it might allow you time to reconsider if you really need to make this purchase.
- Limit the amount you allow yourself to put on your card every month.
- Be aware that student credit card deals aren't always your best bet. Students with a limited credit history are considered credit risks so although you may get the card, you'll probably have a high interest rate.
- Rather than a credit card, use a debit card so the money will come out of your checking account immediately. That way, you can't spend more than you have.

Our friend Anne shares this additional tip:

When my husband started his first job after college, he wisely realized that he could go wild with his credit card if he didn't put up some kind of roadblock to using it easily. So he hid it in a book at home. The title of the book? *Irrational Man*.

Author Anecdote Interest Rates on a Home Mortgage The power of searching for a better interest rate became glaringly obvious to me when we became home buyers. This principle holds true, though on a much smaller scale, with credit cards. When we moved into our home, we had a mortgage interest rate of 8.64%. If we would have paid off the house in 30 years, we would have paid $370,302 in interest alone.

Three years later we refinanced the home. The balance had not decreased much, but this time we got an interest rate of 4.875%. If we pay the loan off in 15 years (rather than 30), we will pay only $71,024 in interest. By paying a little more principle each month and dropping the interest rate by slightly more than 4%, we will end up saving just under $300,000 on our home! That's stress reduction!

—MO

Although credit cards have the potential for creating financial havoc, they also can serve a valuable function if they are used carefully. Make a list of the pros and cons of having a credit card. Then reflect on whether the pros outweigh the cons. If you decide a credit card is valuable to you, what conditions would help you control your use of credit?

Your list might look something like this:

Pros:

- Establish a good credit rating so if in the future I want to buy something big, like a house or a car, I will be able to secure a loan.
- A credit card could save the day if a true emergency arises and I need money fast.
- Some credit cards include insurance for the items I purchase.

(Continued)

EXERCISE 7: Pros and Cons of Credit Cards

- A credit card might come in handy so I don't always have to carry cash.
- For some purchases—such as airline tickets—it is more convenient to pay with a credit card.

Cons:

- I might spend more money with a credit card because it doesn't seem like real money.
- Interest rates can be high, so if I can't pay off the balance, I might end up throwing away my money on interest.
- The fine print on the credit card agreement can be impossible to understand. I may not know what I am getting into.
- If I can't keep up on my payments, I can mess up my credit rating for 7 years (or more).

Managing your use of credit cards can go a long way toward reducing financial stress. Conversely, getting and using credit without a plan is like riding a bike without brakes full-speed ahead down a steep slope. The rush of the wind on your face may feel great, but you'd better brace yourself for the crash that's coming when you reach the bottom.

Additional Tips for Managing Your Money

What else can you do to manage your money wisely? Students in several classes were asked to list strategies they have found effective to prevent or reduce financial stress. Here is their advice:

- Look for activities that don't involve money, such as working out or playing intramural sports.
- Make a budget!
- Put away 3% of every paycheck for emergencies, no matter how big or small your check is.
- Carpool to save money and help the environment—or better yet, walk or ride your bike.
- Take advantage of free or low-cost activities on campus, such as discount movies, sports events, and activities associated with free food.
- Eat in the cafeteria or cook at home. Eating out is expensive.
- Have your paycheck automatically deposited to the bank.
- Talk to the counselors and find out about scholarships. Many scholarships don't get used because students don't apply.
- Don't buy a new car!
- Have only one credit card, and use it only for emergencies and gas.
- Save on groceries by always shopping with a list of items you need and never shopping when you're hungry.
- Avoid buying on impulse and ending up purchasing things you don't need by never spending more than $75 on anything without taking 24 hours to think about it. This allows time to decide rationally whether the purchase is really necessary.
- Do laundry at your parents' house.
- Always go out with people who say they will buy.

Learning to control spending is not easy in this time of instant gratification, but the pay-off in reduced stress and financial management is worth the control. Applying the ABCs of money management can give you control over your spending habits and reduce your financial distress, but as you will learn in the next section, there is more to the topic of money and stress than just learning how to budget.

Can Money Make You Happy?

We have heard warnings such as, "There's more to life than money" and "Money can't buy you love." The well-known verse, "The love of money is the root of all evil," prompts us to explore the issue of how money impacts our life and our stress. Money is a good thing and a necessity to get what we need, but money also can contribute to stress, put a strain on relationships, and have other negative consequences.

> Better is bread with a happy heart than wealth with vexation.
>
> —Amenemope (11th century)

Can Money Make Us Happy?

What has the science of positive psychology discovered about what makes us happy? More than you might imagine—including what *does not* increase our level of happiness. Research has shown that once your basic needs are met, additional income does little to raise your sense of satisfaction with life.

How happy are we?

Would you say you are happy…?	most or all of the time	some of the time	not very often
Under $35,000 a year	68%	24%	7%
$35,000 to $49,999	81%	14%	5%
$50,000 to $99,999	85%	13%	2%
Over $100,000 a year	88%	11%	1%
U.S. total	78%	16%	5%

This *Time* poll was conducted by telephone Dec. 13–14, 2004, among 1,009 adult Americans, by SRBI Public Affairs.

Source: "The New Science of Happiness," by C. Wallis, *Time* 165(3), Jan. 17, 2005, A2.

What do we know about the relationships between money, satisfaction in life, and stress? Now that we have examined the practicalities of money management, we can benefit from exploring some philosophical issues. We need to understand that the source of much stress is not just money itself but, rather, the value we give to money. Stress-relieving money management may be just as much about managing our mind as about managing our money.

If we track American life since the end of World War II, we find that inflation-adjusted income per American has almost tripled. New houses have doubled in size. We have more clothes, requiring closets the size of our grandparents' bedrooms, and so many vehicles and toys that a two-car garage is no longer sufficient. Surely in this life of plenty, we must be much happier than our ancestors were half a century ago. Not so, according to polls taken periodically since the 1950s by the National Opinion Research Center. In the 1950s, about one-third of Americans described themselves as "very happy," and the percentage remains almost exactly the same today.[7]

Many people mistakenly believe that more money means more happiness. The *Time* poll found that happiness tended to increase as income rose to $50,000 a year. After that, more income did not have a dramatic effect.

An increasing body of social science and psychological research has shown no significant relationship between how much money a person earns and whether that person feels good about life. Edward Diener, a psychologist at the University of Illinois, interviewed members of the Forbes 400, the richest Americans, and found these very rich people to be only a tiny bit happier than the public as a whole.[8]

Affluenza A millionaire was asked, "How much money would it take to make you content?" He replied, "Just a little bit more." No matter how much money we make, it seems we always want just a little more.

We live in a culture that encourages consumerism and overspending. This ongoing battle with consumerism can lead to a dangerous trap—living beyond our means. The more we make, the more we spend. This never-ending desire to acquire has been given a name: **affluenza.** Affluenza describes the disease-like epidemic that is causing our society to have more and more material possessions and to spend money we don't have, resulting in growing debt. We confuse the "have-to-haves" with the "want-to-haves."

As with the millionaire, we always want just a little bit more. The more we have, the more we have to insure and maintain. It is like running on a treadmill when you have to run faster and faster just to stay in the same place. As Leo Buscaglia pertinently said, "The more you have, the more you have to worry about."

Reference Anxiety—Keeping Up with the Joneses The phenomenon in play here seems to be what sociologists call **reference anxiety,** in which people judge their possessions

FYI **Who Wants to Be a Millionaire?** Have you always dreamed of winning the lottery? Surely then all your troubles would be over. A study of lottery winners found that they did not wind up significantly happier than a control group.

Source: "The New Science of Happiness," by C. Wallis, *Time*, 165(3), Jan. 17, 2005, A2.

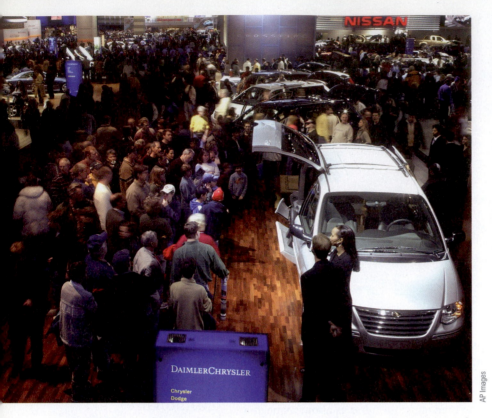

in comparison with others, not based on what they need. If your friend has a newer, more expensive car than yours, even though your car works just fine and gets you where you need to go, you may experience reference anxiety from comparing what you have with what others have.[9]

Some financial distress is of our own making. When we are fixated on always getting more, we fail to appreciate and be grateful for what we have. We can look around and invariably see someone else who seems to have more—and when we gauge our happiness on that comparison, we end up chasing money rather than meaning. The outcome is stress, frustration, and dissatisfaction with what we have. Money no longer provides a sense of well-being, even when we have more than an adequate amount to meet our needs.

In nations with high levels of income equality, such as the Scandinavian countries, well-being is reported to be higher than in nations with unequal wealth distribution such as the United States, where the gap is widening between the wealthy, the middle class, and the poor.[10] Because wealth is so visible in today's society, it triggers dissatisfaction and results in wanting more.

Affluenza, the never-ending desire to acquire, is a source of great stress. Happiness and peace are not dependent on possessions. More "stuff" does not make us happier.

> It is the preoccupation with possession, more than anything else, that prevents men from living freely and nobly.
>
> —Bertrand Russell

Benjamin Franklin said, "Who is rich? He that is content. Who is that? Nobody."

It is sad to think that we can be financially wealthy and yet emotionally bankrupt. We can spend most of our waking hours away from the people we love and working in jobs that we find boring and unfulfilling. Why not do everything in our power to find a job that is nourishing to our checkbook as well as our mind and soul? Increasingly, people are expressing the desire to find meaningful life work. Many want to make a contribution rather than merely working for a living.

The point is, of course, that money can't make us happy. If we believe this to be true, we don't act like it. We spend most of our time and energy pursuing money and the things that money can buy at the expense of activities that create real life fulfillment, such as nurturing relationships with friends and family and helping others. Some people even lose their health in the quest for money and, ironically, once they have lost their health, most would pay anything to have it back.

Money and Relationships Money is a source of stress in many relationships. It is not just the perceived shortage of money that causes stress in relationships, but also the time we spend making money rather than being with family and friends, as well as disagreements on how money should be used. Respondents in one survey said that managing their finances is the biggest strain on their relationships. Figure 12.2 depicts complaints of respondents with financial issues.

What we find is that money management is really mind management. Once our basic needs are met, the money, or lack of it, is not necessarily what causes us stress. How we think about money is what determines the role it plays in our well-being. We determine the value we give to money and, as a result, either the satisfaction or distress it produces.

The Research Highlight helps us understand that fear of debt is powerful. Being poor can indeed contribute to stress and unhappiness. Sociologists in Europe and the United States have found that the

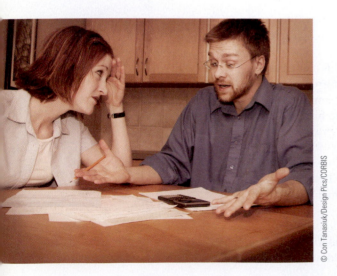

Managing finances is a major stressor on relationships.

The Haves and the Have-Nots

An international survey of college students in the mid-1990s compared national differences in positivity (positive feelings) and subjective well-being. Relatively poor Puerto Rico, Colombia, and Spain ranked as the three most cheerful locales. These results are surprising if we equate money and material possessions with high spirits. The results are not so surprising if you look at cultural norms that support the premise that Latin Americans are happier because they tend to look at the sunny side of life and believe life in general to be good.

Source: "It's a Glad, Sad, Mad World," by W. Kirn, N. Mustarfa, & E. Coady, *Time, 165*(3), A65.

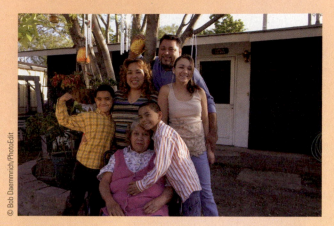

Cultural norms in some populations support the intention of looking at the sunny side of life and believing life, in general, is good, regardless of material possessions.

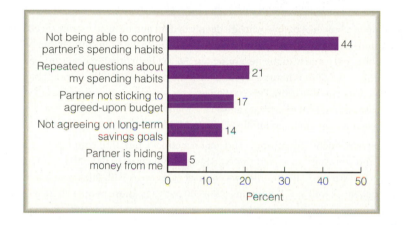

FIGURE 12.2 Complaints of Tightwads and Spendthrifts

Source: "Money and Relationships," by D. Haralson and S. Parker, *USA Today*, March 15, 2005.

poor are more often unhappy in part because of the never-ending frustration and stress of poverty. But worth considering is the repeated finding that after people reach a certain level of income, happiness and money don't seem to have much relationship to each other. Placing too much value on money can be a source of unnecessary fear and distress.

Putting It All Together—What the Experts Say

Dave Ramsey, the well-known financial guru, was asked this very important question, "What is the most important financial principle?" This was his reply:

"The Dave Ramsey Show" and my company, the Lampo Group, have become very well known for teaching people how to get out of debt, save money, and get on a budget. All of us on staff here are very thankful for the response we've had to these concepts, but another financial concept is the hinge on which the door of successful personal finance swings. I have only begun to realize the full significance of this concept during the last year or so. When you understand this concept, all the other concepts work, and until you implement it, none of them will work. When you stick this concept deep in your soul, it becomes easy to save money and even have money to invest. Getting out of debt happens quickly once you learn how to apply this concept in your life. Budgeting is made easier, and your marriage or relationships regarding money are freed up and made smooth. This is the most important financial concept.

Contentment. That's right, contentment. Contentment brings peace. Not apathy. Not the deadhead fog of Prozac or Valium. Only contentment brings peace. We live in the most marketing-focused society in the history of the world. The very essence of marketing is to disturb

Graduates Fear Debt More Than Terrorism

The Partnership for Public Service conducted a survey of 805 randomly sampled college seniors in the class of 2005. This class of students, referred to as "The 9/11 Generation" began their 4-year academic journey just days before the attack of 9/11. The survey report provides a view of how the war on terror has shaped these students' views.

The data reveal that fully 30% of graduating seniors do not think the war on terror will ever be over, and another 27% expect it will go on beyond their lifetime. That means that more than half of graduating seniors do not expect to live to see the end of the war against terrorism. Despite thinking that terrorism is an inevitable part of their lives, their greatest fears are going into debt (32%) and being unemployed (31% percent). Fewer than one in seven say their greatest fear is more terrorism.

Source: http://www.ourpublicservice.org

your peace. We say things to ourselves like, "I'll be happy when I get that boat," or "I'll be happy when I get that china cabinet," or "I'll be happy when I get that house." Or, or, or, or!!!

NOT TRUE. Happiness is sold to us as an event or a thing, and consequently, our finances have suffered. *Fun* can be bought with money; happiness cannot.

We live among a bunch of people who are deeply in debt and have no money saved because their emotions were tricked. Just like drug addicts, people have been conned into believing that happiness will come with the next purchase. So, Daddy works hundreds of overtime hours and Mommy works 40-plus hours a week … all in the name of STUFF. You probably think I am writing about someone else, but I'm not. I am writing about you. I know because I suffer from the same disease, but I am recovering and so are many of you. The human spirit was not created to attain peace, contentment, or fulfillment by gathering more stuff.

You *can* get out of debt, save money, and get on a budget, but until your intellect forces your emotions and your spirit to accept that STUFF does not equal CONTENTMENT, your finances will always feel stressed. At our office we counsel every week with folks who are making $25,000 per year as well as folks making $250,000 per year. These people share a common problem: they all suffer from some level of "stuffitis," the worship of stuff. Change your focus and change your life for the better."[11]

Author Anecdote

How Money Changes People

I was watching a television show about child actors and where they are today as young adults. The program presented story after story of how life had taken a turn for the worse when opportunities faded for these child actors. In most cases, relationships with family and friends were strained. One young woman in her 20s said, "I just wanted my dad to be my dad, not my manager. He told me if he couldn't be my manager, he wouldn't be my dad."

A young man made a simple, yet profound statement in saying, "Money changes people." He described how he had completely severed his relationship with his parents because he believed they cared only about the money he generated. Some cases had even ended up in court with parents suing children or children suing parents—and it all revolved around money.

Although you may have trouble relating to the problem of too much money and who gets it when you are only trying to pay the rent, stories like this do give rise to questions about the value we put on money. A student in class shared her sadness that she had not spoken to her brother, her only sibling, in more than 5 years because of a disagreement about who should get what after their parents had been killed in a car accident. Another student said that his older brother cut off all contact with their parents because they would not lend him money for a down payment on a house.

Don't lose sight of the important message that money can't buy love or happiness. When money becomes a priority over people and relationships, it can become the source of great stress and sadness. It is up to you to decide.

—MH

Conclusion

Even though changing how you spend and save money can be challenging, it can bring a lifetime of financial freedom. You have to be flexible, however, and give yourself some time to get it right. In any case, you deserve the financial peace of mind that comes with managing your money so you can have the things that are most important to you. The ABCs of money management can guide you in developing a plan that will help relieve financial stress. Think of a budget not as giving up what you want but, instead, getting what is really most important to you. Evaluating how issues including doodads, the use of credit, and savings impact your financial status will give you the information you need to make informed decisions about your money.

Using money involves more than just earning and spending it. Money often is connected to feelings and wealth mistakenly is believed to represent the road to happiness. Not having adequate money can and does contribute to stress, but money in and of itself does not assure happiness. Happiness and satisfaction with life are more about good health, supportive relationships, and finding meaning in life than about accumulating more money. Talking about money is sort of like talking about religion. It is a highly personal topic. The key to reducing financial stress and finding contentment is to assess what is most important to you and then implement a plan to achieve it.

Money is neither good nor bad. It is simply a tool, just as a pencil is a tool. Robert Kiyosaki writes:

> A pencil can be used to write a beautiful letter or a memo firing someone from a job. While a pencil is designed to write with, it can also be used as a lethal weapon to stab a person in the eye. The thing that makes the difference isn't the object, but the motives of the person holding the pencil—or handling the money."[12]

12.1 Spending Habits and Emotions

PURPOSE The purpose of this activity is to provide you with an opportunity to track your spending habits, to increase awareness of emotions that influence spending, and to plan your financial goals.

DIRECTIONS For one week, track your spending. At the end of the week, go back and review your log, answer the reflection questions, and use this learning to plan financial goals.

I.   Track your spending.

Include the following information in your spending log for each purchase you make:

1. Day, date, and time
2. Place
3. Amount spent
4. What you purchased
5. Whether your purchase was a 'want' or a 'need' (Ask yourself this question, "Is this purchase something I truly need or is it something I would just like to have?")
6. The emotions associated with the purchase (Were you happy, depressed, lonely, or bored?)

Try not to change your spending habits during the week you complete the log. Let this serve as a record of your normal spending habits.

II. Analyze your spending

After you have completed your spending log for one week, review your log and respond to these reflection questions:

1. Do you notice any patterns to your spending behaviors? For example, do you spend more money when you are with certain people or at certain times of the day?
2. What do you notice about your emotions related to spending?
3. Are there any purchases that you made this week that you now regret making?
4. Do your spending habits contribute to your stress? If so, how and what changes can you make to help you reduce financial stress?
5. What are two new insights you gained from completing this activity?

III. Plan for the future

Using the SMART format, write two personal financial goals.

Key Points

- Financial pressure ranks high on the list of stressors facing college students.
- Practicing the ABCs—assessment, budget, and control—of money management can put you in charge of your money.
- A budget is a plan to manage your money so you can have what is most important to you and accomplish your financial goals.
- Financial goals can guide you in getting what you want financially.
- Money allows us to pay for the things we need, and it also can be used to address emotional needs.
- The latte factor is a metaphor for spending money on little things that you could cut back on without changing your lifestyle.

- Two areas of financial management that deserve extra attention because they so frequently contribute to financial stress are doodads and credit cards.
- Saving even a small amount of money regularly can contribute to financial freedom.
- The source of much stress is not just money itself but, rather, the value we give to money. It may be just as much about managing our mind as about managing our money.
- Money does not necessarily equate to happiness, but a lack of money to meet basic needs can contribute to the stress of poverty.

Key Terms

budget

SMART goals

doodads

latte factor

affluenza

reference anxiety

Discussion Time For Critical Thinking/Discussion Questions, please visit this book's Premium Website.

Notes

1. "Academic Stress of College Students: Comparison of Student and Faculty Perceptions," by R. Misra, *College Student Journal 21* (2000): 1–10.
2. In *Psychology of Money Management*, by R. Boyum, retrieved 2004 from http://www.campusblues.com.
3. http://frugalliving.about.com.
4. *Rich Dad, Poor Dad*, by R. Kiyosaki (Paradise Valley, AZ: TechPress, 1998).
5. *The Finish Rich Workbook: Creating a Personalized Plan for a Richer Future*, by D. Bach (New York: Broadway Books, 2003).
6. Bach, *The Finish Rich Workbook*.
7. "The Real Truth about Money," by G. Easterbrook, *Time 165*(3) Jan. 17, 2005, A32.
8. Easterbrook, "The Real Truth about Money."
9. Easterbrook, "The Real Truth about Money."
10. Easterbrook, "The Real Truth about Money."
11. http://wealthcoach.daveramsey.com/index.cfm?event=dspFAQ#q1
12. *If You Want to be Rich and Happy Don't go to School*, by R. Kiyosaki (Fairfield, CT: Aslan Publishing, 1993).

13 Social Support, Relationships, and Communication

■ Do men and women communicate differently? ■ My boyfriend just doesn't understand me. What can I do to get him to really listen to what I am saying? ■ When I ask my girlfriend what's wrong and she says "nothing," I believe her. Why is it that she means something else, and what can we do to communicate better? ■ I just transferred to a new school and I don't have any friends here. Everyone seems to have their cliques, and I don't fit in. I'm stressed and lonely. What can I do?

STUDENT OBJECTIVES

Study of this chapter will enable you to:

1. Describe the connection between social support and stress.
2. Describe the types of social support.
3. Explain how effective listening is the key to healthy communication.
4. Explain the importance of touch as a form of nonverbal communication.
5. Discuss how men and women may handle stress differently.
6. Identify the styles of conflict management.

Our need for each other is not an obstacle to overcome, but a virtue to be celebrated.

—Robert F. Allen

Matt's Story Living an active lifestyle over the course of my college years has placed me in a multitude of stressful situations with a wide variety of stressors. Whether it has been stress from time constraints, money, family, or school, stress has been a regular occurrence in my life. But I can easily pinpoint the most stressful time in my life.

One year ago I learned that my dad had a lump in his lung. Doctors told my dad, a 35-year smoker, that he likely had lung cancer. While we awaited the test results, I found it difficult to concentrate on school. Trying to come to terms with the likelihood that I would be losing my dad had an effect on every moment of my life. In the end, my prayers were answered and after some serious surgeries, my dad is recovering.

Looking back on this stressful situation, I used a variety of methods to help cope with the stress. One way was through God. I began to pray more often, in more places. Another was through nature. I searched for answers by engaging in many hikes in solitude. These helped a lot. I exercised more than usual and talked to family and friends.

The most important thing that I learned from the entire situation was to love, and to spend as much time as possible with those who matter to me. If I could offer advice on the situation, I would tell people to be proactive rather than reactive to help reduce stress. I would have been less stressed if I had been able to be at my dad's bedside with more memories of spending good times with him. Sitting next to him in the hospital, regretting not spending more time with him, was something I hope to never experience again. After enduring this near miss, I will be more prepared in the future for a death in the family. I now spend more time with my family and the people I love. I believe this proactive approach to reducing stress will pay off someday. I was given a second chance with my dad, and I won't forget it.

Social Support, Relationships, and Communication

Friends are good medicine, especially when it comes to preventing stress. Social support and close relationships are known to go hand-in-hand with good health, and studies indicate that loneliness has the opposite effect. Supportive relationships can serve as a shield to protect us from potential distress and well may be one of the most important ways to prevent stress. Close, rewarding relationships can provide a powerful emotional lift to boost your self-esteem and happiness and ultimately contribute to overall health and well-being.

In Chapter 1 you learned that social health is one of the dimensions of health. The focus of this chapter is on providing you with information and skills to grow in the social dimension. We will investigate how a social support system and healthy relationships can provide a buffer for stress. Because communication is essential to a healthy relationship, you will learn about communication skills, including empathic listening. Finally, you will learn how to manage conflict, which is a source of stress in many relationships. The outcome is healthier, less stressful relationships and an improved quality of life.

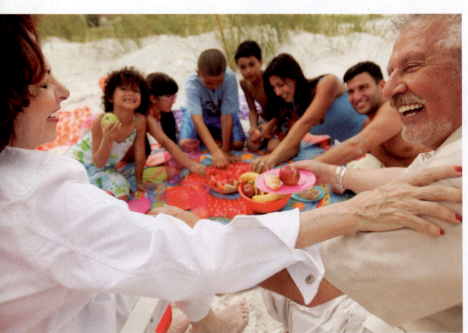

© Tim Pannell/CORBIS

Healthy relationships play a role in helping buffer the effects of stress.

Don't Worry, Be Happy University of Illinois researchers Ed Diener and Martin Seligman specifically looked at happiness in a study they conducted with 222 undergraduates. Diener and Seligman compared the upper 10% of students who consistently rated themselves as "very happy" people with those who rated themselves as "average" and "very unhappy" people. The very happy people were highly social and had stronger romantic and other social relationships than less happy groups. The very happy people were more extroverted, more agreeable, and less neurotic. The results indicated that the most salient characteristics shared by the 10% of students with the highest levels of happiness and the fewest signs of depression were their strong ties to friends and family and commitment to spending time with them. One might infer that good social relationships are, like food and thermoregulation, universally important to human mood. "Word needs to spread," concludes researcher Ed Diener. "It is important to work on social skills, close interpersonal ties, and social support in order to be happy."

Source: "Very Happy People," by E. Diener and M. Seligman, *Psychological Science, 13*(1), January 2002, pp. 81–84, cited in "The New Science of Happiness," by C. Wallis, *Time, 165*(3), Jan. 17, 2005, A2.

Social Support

We are social animals. People crave human connections. Even the most reclusive of us has relationships of one kind or another. In our time of widespread stratification and separation, we still are constantly communicating and developing support systems.

Social support has been described as the individual's knowledge or belief that he or she is cared for and loved, belongs to a network of communication, and has a mutual obligation with others in the network.[1] The social support system is made up of all the people who help meet financial, personal, physical, and emotional needs. Social support is belonging, being accepted, feeling loved, and being needed.

Benefits from social support come from feeling supported and also from our ability to give caring support to others. Much like the penguins, the balance between our willingness to support others and our willingness to be supported is what results in healthy relationships.

> No man is an island, entire of itself; every man is a piece of the continent, a part of the main.
> —*John Donne*

Types of Social Support J. S. House[2] and other researchers[3] distinguished between different types of social support including:

1. **Instrumental** (or tangible) **support,** such as giving assistance through money, use of a car, or a place to stay.
2. **Emotional support,** which includes building esteem, emotional comfort, love, trust, concern, and listening.
3. **Informational support,** which consists of giving advice, suggestions, directives, and other information.
4. **Appraisal support,** which provides affirmation, feedback, and information for self-evaluation.

To whom do you turn for support? Think about a time when you really needed support from someone. What type of support did you need, and who offered it? What type of support best helps you manage stress at this stage of your life? Social support can come from friends, family

FYI You've Got a Friend Humans need each other. We aren't the only creatures that need social support, as this story illustrates:

* * *

Penguins spend their lives battling some of the harshest weather on the planet—ice, snow, wind, and brutal cold. Left alone in these conditions, they surely would perish. Huddling in masses called scrums, the penguins take turns standing on the edge, using their bodies to shelter the others. When an outside penguin begins to grow weary, it is folded gently into the inner warmth and comfort of the scrum and another penguin takes its place. It is both their strength as protector and their willingness to be protected that allows them to survive.

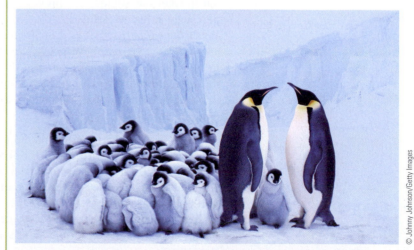
© Johnny Johnson/Getty Images

Penguins spend much of their life battling harsh conditions. Their willingness to support and protect each other helps them survive.

Source: "Kailo: An Organizational Case Study," by K. Putnam, in *The Spirit and Science of Holistic Health*, edited by J. Robison and K. Carrier (Bloomington, IN: AuthorHouse).

members, teachers, members of your religious congregation, members of clubs and school organizations, and so on. The people who make up your social support system are the ones with whom you spend time and to whom you could turn in times of need.

Stress Busting Behavior: Social Support Network

Write down the names of the people you turn to for each type of social support. Briefly describe what they do to provide you with support and think about how this support helps reduce your stress. Recognizing and acknowledging the people who provide support is an important step toward experiencing their support.

☐ **Instrumental or tangible support**

  People that support me:

  What they do:

☐ **Emotional support**

  People that support me:

  What they do:

☐ **Informational support**

  People that support me:

  What they do:

☐ **Appraisal support**

  People that support me:

  What they do:

Social Support and Stress It doesn't take a scientific study to show that surrounding yourself with supportive family, friends, and co-workers can have a positive effect on your physical and emotional well-being, but there is plenty of research to confirm it. Research has shown that social support provides a buffer for stress in these ways:[4]

- *When the support is received at the point of appraisal of a potential threat.* An example is when a person is told that she is to be a guest speaker at an important upcoming meeting. Speaking in front of a large group of people can be stressful, but if the potential speaker has someone to provide advice and support prior to the event, it can be perceived as less stressful.
- *When the support serves as a buffer against the potentially unpleasant effects experienced during the coping phase of a stressful situation, that is, when the person is trying to recover from a stressful experience.* Examples are the times when a person has gone through a painful divorce, failed a class, or been turned down for a job. The sting of that unpleasant event may be cushioned by a close friend who is available to turn to for support and comfort.

Whether the social support is offered prior to, during, or after a stressful event, the support can have a positive effect on the person who is experiencing the stress. Indirectly, having a support system can contribute to an overall sense of happiness. This belief that life is good creates a more optimistic approach to life so a person does not perceive many things as stressful in the first place. A strong social support network can be critical to help you through the stress of tough times, whether you had a bad day at school or a year filled with loss or chronic illness. It is never too soon to cultivate these healthy relationships.

Social Support and Health Early evidence for the influence of social support on health came from an epidemiologic study conducted on residents of Alameda County in California. Individuals 30 to 69 years of age were surveyed in 1965 on their physical, mental, and social well-being, as well as their health-related habits such as exercise and use of

Supportive Relationships: More Is Better

Sheldon Cohen, professor of psychology and researcher at Carnegie Mellon University, studied the effects of psychological stress and social support on immunity and susceptibility to infectious disease. His work shows that those having more types of social relationships, including family but also neighbors, friends, workmates, and members of religious and social groups, were less likely to develop a cold when exposed to a rhinovirus. Those who had one to three types of social relationships were more than four times as likely to develop a cold than those with six or more types of social relationships. Network diversity—receiving support from different networks of people (church, school organizations, family)—was a more important determinant of susceptibility than the total number of people in one's social network.

Source: "Social Support, Stress, and the Common Cold," by S. Persons (A Summary of a Presentation), Office of Behavioral and Social Sciences Research, *NIH Record* (National Institute of Health), Dec. 2, 1997.

---

cigarettes and alcohol. They also were asked about their social networks, such as marital status, number of close friends and relatives, church membership, and affiliation with other organizations. Over the years, death certificates were monitored to assess their mortality rates and follow-up surveys were conducted on survivors to assess their health status.[5]

As expected, the study found a strong association between certain unhealthy behaviors and higher mortality rates. More surprising, the study also found that individuals' health status and risk of dying were strongly associated with the extent and nature of their social network. This association remained true even after taking unhealthy behaviors into consideration. Throughout the socioeconomic spectrum, the mortality rates of men and women with few social contacts were two to three times higher than those with many social connections.

Many more recent studies have supported the conclusions of the Alameda County study. Absence of social support has been related to an increase in coronary heart disease, complications in pregnancy and birth, suicide, and other unhealthy outcomes. In a study of breast cancer survivors, women who joined a support group after surgery lived twice as long as those who didn't.[6] Married men are documented to live longer than single men. The positive effects of social support on the immune system provide more evidence that a support system can alleviate the major stressor of poor health.

One of the best examples of how the information on the relationship between social support and health is being applied clinically is Dr. Dean Ornish's work on reversing heart disease. For more than 20 years, he has shown that modifying one's lifestyle can cause blockages in the coronary arteries to regress. His program includes a low-fat diet, exercise, yoga, and meditation components. But what Ornish believes is the most important part of his program has to do with "transcending that isolation that I think really is the root cause of so many of the self-destructive behaviors and emotional stress, which in turn are such major contributors to so many of the illnesses of which so many people suffer."[7] Regarding heart disease, Ornish views isolation as a risk factor that is as important as high cholesterol levels or obesity.

Tip: Think about the culture you grew up in and to what extent it valued and supported social support. Did your family have close, supportive friends as you were growing up? Were relationships with extended family part of your childhood? Did family and friends participate in important events in your life?

Social support means having the support of people you trust and can talk to, those you feel a close connection with, and those you share both the good times and the bad with. Why social support should have such a broad and consistent effect on health is not fully understood. Researchers

A strong and diverse social support system helps buffer the negative impact of stress.

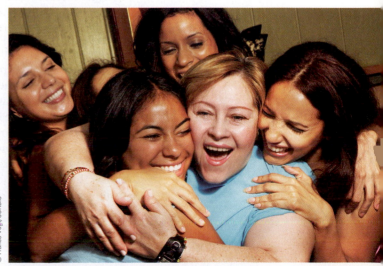

© Franco Vogt/CORBIS

The Roseto Effect

Over many years, a study was conducted in Roseto, Pennsylvania, a close-knit community of religious immigrants from southern Italy. Researchers interested in the lifestyle of the community residents followed their health status and rates of death for years. They found that the residents of Roseto had average incidences of exercise, cigarette smoking, obesity, high blood pressure, and stress. Their diets were higher than the average American diet in fat and cholesterol. The researchers were surprised to learn, then, that the men in Roseto had only about one-sixth the incidence of heart disease and death from heart disease as random population groups in the United States. Rates for the women of Roseto were even better.

The researchers concluded that the protective factor was the strong sense of community and strong social ties between the residents. One of the researchers, Stewart Wolf, said:

More than any other town we studied, Roseto's social structure reflected old-world values and traditions. There was a remarkable cohesiveness and sense of unconditional support within the community. Family ties were very strong. What impressed us most was the attitude toward the elderly. No one was ever abandoned.

Over the years, as the younger generation began changing and the social cohesiveness of the community began to weaken, the heart disease rates in Roseto climbed to levels comparable to those in the surrounding communities. The researchers theorized that social connectedness was the buffering factor against heart disease.

Source: Quoted information is from "People Who Need People Are the Healthiest People: The Importance of Relationships," by B. Hafen and K. Frandsen, in *Mind/Body Health* (2nd ed.), edited by K. Karren, B. Hafen, N. Lee, and K. Frandsen (San Francisco: Benjamin Cummings, 2002).

FYI

Family Rituals

David Palmiter, clinical psychologist expert in counseling children and families, thinks family rituals are one of the most powerful prophylactic measures that parents can bring to bear when there are significant stressors. Because it says to a kid, "Planes may be crashing into buildings, kids may be shooting kids in schools, everybody is worrying about their finances, but we still have pizza night, or we still go to the synagogue." It doesn't matter what you fill in the blank with as long as it involves a consistent ritual including quality family time together.

Source: *Stressed About Money? The Kids Might Be Too*, by Lindsay Lyon, U. S. News & World Report, October 27, 2008.

hypothesize that social support probably acts in part through its ability to buffer stress. The comfort and support provided by a friend or family member reduces the intensity of events that could seem threatening. As a result, a person is protected from diseases caused by stress. A strong and diverse social support system can help to maintain good health and reduce the impact of disease.

Relationships

Social support systems are composed of a web of relationships. During his lifetime, author and educator Leo Buscaglia, who wrote and lectured extensively about love and relationships, said this about relationships:

There is no being or becoming without relationships. From the beginning, we grow to sense the need and importance of relatedness. We human beings have the longest period of dependency of any living creature. At birth, in total helplessness, we engage in our first coupling, mother–child, and from that time on, the more sophisticated our lives become, the more interrelated we become. In a sense, we spend our entire existence weaving one relationship into another until we've created, like the web of a spider, a complete pattern.[8]

Relationships play an important role in determining whether the young adult and college years are satisfying and positive or lonely and stressful. Going off to college is a time of developing new friendships, dating, forming intimate relationships, and often falling in love and choosing a life partner. With the independence of moving from home, relationships with family and siblings can change significantly. Throughout life, the close relationships we develop and maintain are integral in shaping who we become and how we deal with life.

Tip: Map out your current social relationships. Earlier in the chapter you determined who you go to for different types of social support. Now consider each person that makes up your network of relationships. Remember that not all relationships are supportive. Consider the positive and negative aspects of each of your relationships. Does the relationship give you energy or drain you of energy? Does the person help relieve your stress or contribute to increased stress?

Man is but a network of relationships, and these alone matter to him.

—Antoine de St. Exupery

Sources of Stress in Relationships

Stress often involves our relationships with other people. We argue, fight, and worry when things aren't going well with the important people in our lives. Social psychologist Pamela Jackson studies the effect of stressful life events on mental health. She reports that relationships may pose one of the greatest challenges for emotional development, especially during adolescence and the young adult years, simply because people can offer or deny us their friendship. Forming relationships with others increases the possibility of being rejected.[9]

You would do well to choose friends around whom you can be yourself. To constantly try to be someone you're not, to try to live up to someone else's expectations or standards of how you should or shouldn't be, can be stressful. A wise person once said, "A true friend is someone who thinks you're a good egg even though he knows you're slightly cracked."

The way we interact with those around us can have a potent effect on the stress we feel. The relationships we have with others may even reflect the relationship we have with ourself. In their research on college students, psychologists at the University of Texas found that if students were lacking in self-esteem, their relationships suffered. Students with a low opinion of themselves tended to seek out relationships with people who were critical and rejecting. The friends, roommates, dates, and other people they chose to associate with confirmed their low opinion of their own worth.[10]

Despite the potential for stress in close personal relationships, it is becoming increasingly clear that long, healthy lives depend on strengthening our bonds with others. A full and rewarding social life can nourish the mind, the emotions, and the spirit, and good physical health depends as much on these aspects of our self as it does on a strong, well-functioning body.[11]

If results of a *Time* magazine poll conducted by telephone among more than 1,000 adult Americans are an indication, most people find happiness in family connections and friendships. The findings of their poll are presented in Figure 13.1.

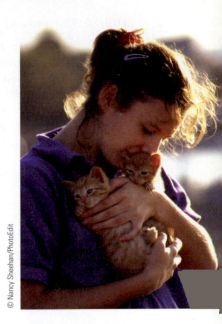

As most pet-lovers know, stress-relieving, loving relationships are not limited to humans.

© Nancy Sheehan/PhotoEdit

Relationships with Pets

Relationships with Pets As most pet-lovers know, stress-relieving, loving relationships are not limited to humans. Note from the *Time* poll that playing with pets ranks higher than exercising, eating, or having sex as a way to improve mood. Sometimes pets are better than people for improving our mood. Research shows that owning a pet, which constitutes a giving and receiving relationship, has long-term health benefits. Pet owners have longer lives and fewer symptoms of stress than those who do not own pets. When you are stroking a kitten or running with a dog, you are a lot less likely to feel tense or stressed. This is a form of social interaction with no pressure to meet anyone's expectations.

Pet therapy has been useful in dealing with emotional problems in people of all ages and situations. Elderly people are given pets to curb loneliness and take their mind off their own conditions. People who are depressed are given pets for the same reasons. Kids enjoy pets as a way to learn to serve and care for another life. Across the life span, pets give you love and are a source of stress-relieving comfort.

Relationships in Marriage If pets provide more comfort than a spouse and if, according to the *Time* happiness poll, only 9% ranked the spouse as a source of greatest happiness, these people might turn to Gotmann's Love Lab for some help. John Gottman, a clinical psychologist and professor of psychology at the University of Washington, has been studying conflict in relationships. In his physiology lab, nicknamed the Love Lab, Gottman observes how people behave within relationships. The research suggests that

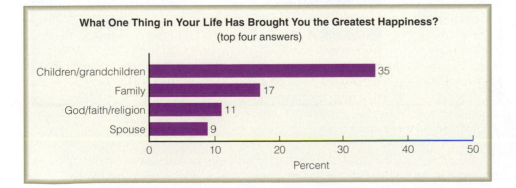

What One Thing in Your Life Has Brought You the Greatest Happiness?
(top four answers)

	Percent
Children/grandchildren	35
Family	17
God/faith/religion	11
Spouse	9

FIGURE 13.1 What Makes Us Happy? *(Continued)*

Source: "The New Science of Happiness," by C. Wallis. *Time 165*(3), Jan. 17, 2005, A2

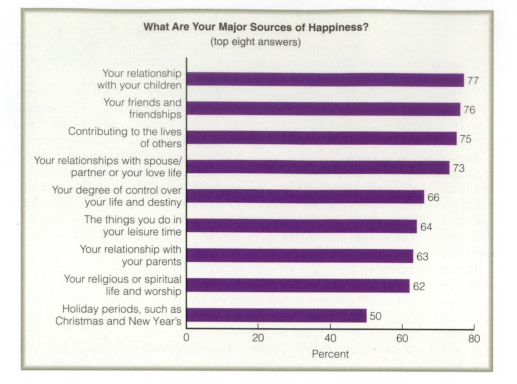

What Are Your Major Sources of Happiness?
(top eight answers)

Source	Percent
Your relationship with your children	77
Your friends and friendships	76
Contributing to the lives of others	75
Your relationships with spouse/partner or your love life	73
Your degree of control over your life and destiny	66
The things you do in your leisure time	64
Your relationship with your parents	63
Your religious or spiritual life and worship	62
Holiday periods, such as Christmas and New Year's	50

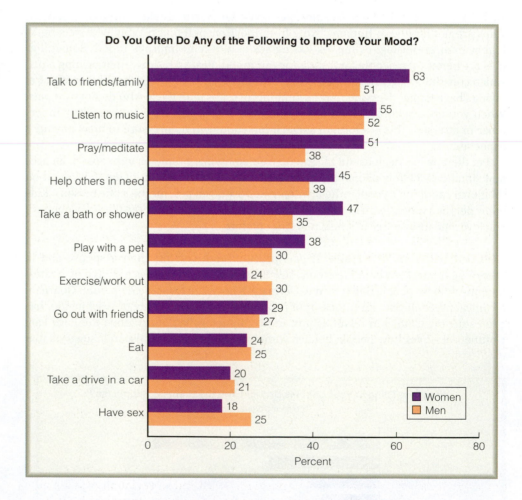

Do You Often Do Any of the Following to Improve Your Mood?

	Women	Men
Talk to friends/family	63	51
Listen to music	55	52
Pray/meditate	51	38
Help others in need	45	39
Take a bath or shower	47	35
Play with a pet	38	30
Exercise/work out	24	30
Go out with friends	29	27
Eat	24	25
Take a drive in a car	20	21
Have sex	18	25

The Truth about Cats and Dogs—Pets Comfort College Students

Can social support cross species? When you are stressed out, do you turn to Lassie for comfort? A new study shows that pets may be a source of stress relief for college students.

The study included 241 students, mainly freshmen, and 100 adults age 30 and older living in the same area, but not affiliated with the college. When asked why they had pets, companionship was the most common reason for people of all ages; those people said they would be lonely without their pet. The second most common reason was that their pet helps keep them active. And the third most common reason was that their pet helps them "get through hard times."

College students were more likely than the older participants to say their pet helps them get through hard times. That may be because college freshmen are in a transitional period and haven't yet built their social network and resources for coping, note the researchers, who included Sara Staats, PhD, professor emeritus of psychology at Ohio State University.

According to Staats, "College is a very stressful environment for students and sometimes they can feel isolated or overwhelmed with the change. Many feel their pets will help them get through these difficult and stressful situations, and many more say that without their pet, they would feel lonely."*

A second study from *Psychosomatic Medicine* found that pets are better than people at calming their stressed owners, in part because they are nonjudgmental. In this study, 240 married couples were given stressful tasks to do: mental arithmetic or keeping their hand in ice water for 2 minutes. People who had pets nearby before and during the tests had lower heart rates and lower blood pressure. They completed the arithmetic tests with fewer errors. And their heart rate and blood pressure returned to normal faster after the ice-water test.

Non-pet owners, by comparison, didn't perform as well—demonstrating more stress and more mistakes even when they were alone or when their spouse or a friend was nearby. This was despite the encouragement to have spouses and friends lend support during both experiments. When asked whether the stress-inducing tasks were "challenging" or "threatening," the pet owners were more inclined to say they were challenging.

The findings suggest that pets can buffer reactions to acute stress as well as reduce the perception of stress. The researchers also suggest that the study participants may have perceived their spouse or friend as judgmental of their performance, which increased their stress levels. Pets were not seen as judgmental. Recall the old saying, "A dog is a man's best friend."**

Sources:
*WebMD Health News, Dec. 26, 2008—By Miranda Hitti from Staats, S. *Society and Animals*, vol 16: pp 279–291. News release, Ohio State University.
**"Cardiovascular Reactivity and the Presence of Pets, Friends, and Spouses: The Truth About Cats and Dogs," by K. Allen, J. Blascovich, and W. Mendes, *Psychosomatic Medicine* (Sept/Oct 2002), 64(5), 727–739.

even though disagreements are not pleasant, they are necessary to some extent in all good marriages. But, although Gottman found that conflict is common in relationships, he also found that only 31% of conflicts get resolved over the course of a marriage. The other 69% continue as unsolved problems.[12]

John Gottman and his research partner, Robert Levenson, developed a model that can predict the likelihood of marital bliss with more than 90% accuracy.[13] They found that couples who have successful marriage unions maintain the *five-to-one ratio:* Stable relationships have five times as many positive factors—love, affection, interest in one another, humor, and support—as negative factors. Maintaining a consistent balance of five loving or kind events for every instance of anger, contempt, or complaints keeps a marriage relationship healthy. Success is based on more positive factors than negative factors.

The research suggests that people should first select a mate with whom inevitable annoyances can be managed and then learn how to manage the conflicts. The couple must realize that not all of their problems will be solved. The key to success or failure in a relationship is how the couple handles the inevitable differences that arise in any situation.

Love and Relationships

In his best-selling book, *The Five Love Languages,* Gary Chapman explains that people have a need to feel loved and that relationships are nurtured when we understand how to give and receive love.[14] When this need is not met, the relationship will suffer no matter how committed the partnership. Just as we need gas to keep our cars running, people who have empty "love tanks" will feel unloved or unappreciated.

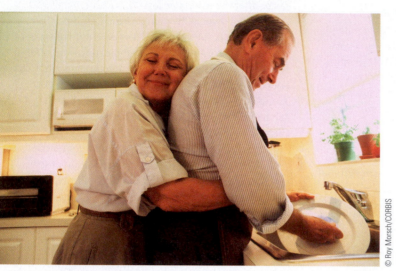
Chapman discusses how to keep the love tank full to nurture a healthy and successful relationship. The key to a flourishing relationship is to figure out what your partner needs to feel most loved and then do it. Chapman suggests that people express love and receive love in different ways, which he calls "love languages" and proposes five love languages—words of affirmation, quality time, gifts, acts of service, and physical touch.

Words of Affirmation People like to be complimented. Compliments boost our confidence and self-esteem. Words of affirmation can be offered through verbal compliments such as, "You look great today" or, "Thank you for taking out the garbage." Verbal compliments that communicate love and appreciation are important. Another form of words of affirmation is to encourage partners to pursue their dreams even though they may feel insecure about the journey.

Quality Time Quality time means giving someone your undivided attention. It means not having a discussion while you watch TV or merely being in the same house with your mate at the same time. It means taking a walk together or having a talk without interruption. Quality time means doing something wholeheartedly with your partner that he or she wants to do but you are less enthusiastic about, such as going to the symphony or the ballet, or going on a picnic. Chapman states, "A central aspect of quality time is togetherness. I do not mean proximity.... Togetherness has to do with focused attention."[15] You can spend quality time with a partner by simply being "alone together" without outside distractions, engaging in quality conversation with a balance of talking and listening, and finding activities that both of you thoroughly enjoy.

Receiving Gifts Gifts are visual symbols of love. Gift giving is less about the cost of the gift and more about the intention of giving out of love. Whether gifts are made or purchased, they are visible signs of love that will have an impact on those who receive them.

Acts of Service Acts of service are those things you do for your partner that you know they would like you to do. Acts of service require thought, planning, time, effort, and energy. If they are done with a positive attitude, they are expressions of love. Acts of service may involve departing from the typical "husband" and "wife" stereotypes that many people have grown up with. An individual whose love language consists of acts of service will feel loved if the partner helps with things such as cooking, cleaning, yard work, or house maintenance no matter what role the partner believes he or she should play in the relationship.

Physical Touch Physical touch is a common expression of love. Hugging, kissing, and holding hands are familiar ways to express emotion. Some may consider physical touch as their love language because sex is such an important part of their relationship. But sex is only a small part of physical touch and is not necessarily a love language. Physical touch can be used to express many forms of emotion.

Hugging, Kissing Lower Stress Hormones

Couples who spend more time hugging and kissing have lower levels of stress hormones in their bodies, new research suggests. A Swiss study has found proof that intimacy improves psychological health—but you need to have a close relationship, preferably a marriage, to benefit. Researchers from the University of Zurich in Switzerland studied 51 German couples, most of whom were married, and found that those who reported more physical contact, from holding hands to sexual intercourse, had lower levels of the stress hormone, cortisol, in their saliva. Cortisol is responsible for several stress-related changes in the body and is secreted in higher levels during the body's fight-or-flight response to stress.

The finding, reported in the journal *Psychosomatic Medicine*, found that couples who reported more problems at work had the biggest drop in levels of the hormone through intimacy. Lead author Dr. Beate Ditzen said intimacy was thought to improve hormone levels simply by boosting mood. But she stressed that couples should not race to express more intimacy as such, but rather find things to do together that create positive feelings for both partners. According to Dr. Ditzen, "Intimacy means different things for different couples. This means that there is no specific behavior that couples should show in everyday life. Rather, all kinds of behavior which couples themselves would consider intimate...might be beneficial."

Source: Psychosomatic Medicine, reported at http://au.news.yahoo.com/a/-/latest/5141547/hugging-kissing-lower-stress-hormones/, 11-12-2008.

Determining Your Love Language After looking at these five different types of love languages, how do you determine which is your primary love language? Author Chapman suggests that you ask yourself these questions:[16]

1. What does your partner do or fail to do that hurts you most deeply? The opposite of what hurts you most is probably your love language.
2. What have you most often requested of your partner? The thing you have requested most often is likely the thing that would make you feel the most loved.
3. In what way do you express love to your partner regularly? Your method of expressing love may be an indication of what also would make *you* feel loved.
4. Think back to a time in your life when you felt totally and completely loved. Which of the love languages were you receiving at that time?

Once you have determined your preferred love language(s) (you probably have more than one), pass along this important information to the person with whom you have a deep relationship. If you don't let your partner know, chances are that your love tank won't get filled. To enhance your relationship even more, find out your partner's love language so you can fill his or her love tank as well. In so doing, your relationship will flourish and continue to grow and develop.

Tip: If you are in a loving relationship with someone, what do you think his or her primary love language is? Make and carry out a plan to do something out of the ordinary to express your love in the language that is most important to your partner.

Communication

One of the most important qualities for a relationship to survive and thrive is effective communication. Relationships develop through communication. If we were unable to communicate, there would be no relationships. Author and educator Leo Buscaglia[17] suggests that the most important quality of a working relationship is communication. In order of importance, here are the qualities that support a working relationship:

1. Communication
2. Affection
3. Compassion/forgiveness
4. Honesty
5. Acceptance
6. Dependability
7. Sense of humor
8. Romance (including sex)
9. Patience
10. Freedom

These desirable features of a good relationship all have an element of communication. According to Buscaglia, the qualities believed to be most destructive to a loving, growing, mature relationship are:

1. Lack of communication
2. Selfishness
3. Dishonesty
4. Jealousy
5. Lack of trust

Communication happens in a variety of ways. We receive one-way communication through television, Internet, iPod, radio, and a variety of other media. Two-way communication happens when we talk with each other face to face, by phone, e-mail, or chat room. Communication occurs both verbally and nonverbally. Communication involves both the sender and the receiver of information. Listening and touch are especially relevant due to the impact they can have on stress related to communication.

Communication between people is not always entirely clear. The sender may not deliver the message with the precise meaning intended. The person receiving the message does not always capture the precise meaning the sender of the message meant to give. The message always has room for interpretation. The imperfection of communication is frequently a source of stress and frustration.

Listening Communication takes place from the day we are born. Communication may even be happening between the mother and the child while the unborn baby resides inside the womb. We learn to speak while we are very young. As we get older, we learn how to read and write. During our earliest years we learn to observe others. We learn about body language and the silent nonverbal communication. Also from our very first days, we learn to listen. Of these modes of communication, there is some agreement that listening is the facet of communication for which we receive the least amount of training.

Listening is not the same as hearing. Lack of listening skills seems to be one of the biggest barriers to effective communication and a source of great stress. Stephen Covey stated, "The single most important principle in the field of interpersonal relations is this: Seek first to understand, then to be understood. Most people listen, not with the intent to understand, but with the intent to reply."[18] Herein lies the problem and the cause of so much avoidable stress.

Autobiographical Listening We tend to listen in the way that Covey calls **autobiographical listening.** In this type of listening, we listen from the perspective of our own experience. We can listen autobiographically in four ways:

1. We *evaluate.* Evaluation is a form of judgment that can be either positive or negative. Evaluation is a method of viewing a situation according to *our* past experience, and we may not necessarily see the entire picture from the other person's situation and perspective.
2. We *probe.* In probing, we attempt to dig out information. Probing seems as if we are seeking to understand, but the questions we ask come from our past experience, not from the other person's point of view. The person may not be ready to reveal the information yet. When we probe, we are trying to pull information out of the other person at *our* pace rather than his or hers.
3. We *advise or tell.* In advising, we are prescribing a course of action. Unfortunately, the person may not be ready for a definite course, or the advice might be inappropriate if the advisor does not yet know all the pertinent information. Often we mean well, but advice almost always comes from our own experience and biases, which may be completely wrong for the other person.
4. We *interpret.* Interpreting means explaining the behavior of another person in terms of *our* motives. This might have the effect of making the other individuals feel that they are not responsible for their actions. They may feel manipulated or insulted.

In short, autobiographical listening can result in a lack of clear communication and the speaker's not feeling heard.

Empathic Listening Few of us routinely practice empathic listening, the most advanced form of listening. **Empathic listening** is active listening with the intention and commitment of truly understanding the other before seeking to be understood. Learning how to listen more effectively is a skill that involves focusing on what the other person is saying rather than what we are going to say next. Covey believes that empathic listening is the key to better communication, leading to better understanding, and, as a result, leading to better relationships.[19] At the root of many relationship problems is the feeling that "my partner doesn't understand me." When we actively try to understand other people, respecting their frame of reference and uniqueness, we give them the freedom to say what they really think and feel. This affirms them and fosters the relationship.

When we listen empathically, we are doing our best to express the other person's point of view better than they do. We are trying to listen to more than the words the other person is saying. We are striving to discern what he or she is feeling. Empathic listening has four stages:

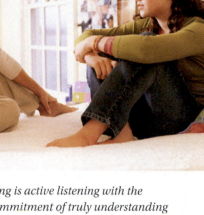
© Ryan McVay/Getty Images

Empathic listening is active listening with the intention and commitment of truly understanding the other before seeking to be understood.

Stage 1: Mimic content of communication. Simply repeat exactly what is said. For example, if someone says: "I enjoy this class, but I don't feel challenged," you would say, "You like this class, but you don't feel it challenges you." To mimic, just listen and repeat what is said. At this stage you aren't focusing on feelings.

Stage 2: Rephrase the content. Put the other person's meaning in your own words. This takes more thought or mental processing than merely mimicking the content. For example, if the other person says: "It really sucks that I got a D on my last test, because the grade I get in this class can ruin my overall GPA." To rephrase the content, you might respond by saying, "You're very concerned that your GPA will suffer because you're getting a low grade in this class."

Stage 3: Reflect feeling. Listen and look to the nature of the emotion behind the communication, observing things such as facial expression, body language, and voice (tone, intensity, volume). For example, someone might say, "I talked with my professor about how I might be able to improve my grade. She got mad and jumped all over me about how poorly I had done during the semester and said I didn't deserve any leniency." Reflecting the emotional content, you could say, "You're upset and frustrated and feel completely misunderstood."

Stage 4: Rephrase the content and reflect the feeling. Combine Stages 2 and 3 by putting both the other's verbal meaning and emotional content in your own words. Using the example in Stage 3, you might say, "It bothers you when you get reprimanded for seeking information." Remember—you are not agreeing or disagreeing. You are only trying to reflect back to the other person your understanding of how he or she *feels*.

Empathic listening is not appropriate in all circumstances. It is most effective when the interaction has a strong emotional component, when we are not sure that we understand, and when we are not sure the other person feels confident that we understand. We do not have to listen empathically when the conversation deals primarily with facts or logic. For example, if you were talking about who won the World Series last year or where you are going to eat later today, listening empathically probably would be counterproductive. The moment that the speaker becomes emotional, empathic listening becomes the more appropriate way to listen. Assess carefully to determine if what initially seems to be a non-emotional issue actually may be charged with emotion, as the author anecdote demonstrates.

Author Anecdote **Why Didn't You Just Say So?** When we were having a class discussion about empathic listening, Joe raised his hand and said, "Sure, it sounds easy, but sometimes I have no clue what my girlfriend will get emotional about. This happened just last Friday when I met up with Cassie after class and asked her if she wanted to go to Greg's house to watch the NBA playoffs. It seemed like a non-emotional issue to me. Cassie said she didn't care, so I thought she really didn't care. Was I ever wrong! Later that night we had a huge fight because she said I never consider her feelings about what she wants to do."

We had a lively class discussion when I asked the class to apply the stages of empathic listening to Joe's situation. One student, Deb, said, "If you had done even Stage 1, I bet you would have found out that Cassie really did care. By listening carefully to her and repeating, 'You don't care?' when Cassie first replied, I think she would have talked more about what she wanted to do with you and you could have prevented the fight from ever happening."

—MH

Tip: Practice applying each stage of empathic listening to Joe's situation. Role-play in class to see how empathic listening can open up communication and change the outcome for the better.

The important component of empathic listening is not the technique you are using but, rather, the attitude you project. Communicating an attitude of caring and a true desire to understand creates the possibility for developing the relationship further.

Here are some tips for becoming a better listener:

- *Listen more, talk less.* You can't get to the root of the problem if you're doing all the talking. Listening sends the important message to the other person that he or she is worth listening to.
- *Suspend judgment.* You may agree or disagree with the other person. When you are seeking understanding, you aren't concerned with right or wrong.
- *Look for the interesting aspects of the other person.* Ask the other person questions that will elicit more thought-provoking answers. Enjoy learning about this person.
- *Avoid giving advice.* What may be right for you may be completely wrong for someone else. As much as you want to help solve his or her problem, you might be doing more harm than good by trying.
- *Allow moments of silence.* Don't fear the silent pauses. Sometimes people have to think about what they are really feeling. If they aren't allowed room to speak because you are filling in the gap, they may not take the opportunity to let the real feeling come to the surface.
- *Listen with your eyes and your heart as much as your ears.* Pay attention to body language, voice tone, how rapidly the other person speaks, and other nonverbal signals.
- *Use appropriate body signals.* Let the other person know you are interested by your own nonverbal signals (facing the other person, using eye contact) and verbal signals ("yes…uh-huh…I see").

Empathic listening is an important tool to facilitate clear communication. Using the techniques of effective communication can reduce stress and enhance the quality of relationships.

Just Listen

Why won't you just listen?
That's all I ask of you.
I don't need to hear what you think about what I say.
I don't need you to think of something clever to comfort me.
I just need you to listen.
So when I say, "I need to talk," that's what I mean.
I just want to tell you something.
You will have your turn later to talk, but for now, just listen to me.
I don't need your clever advice, for if that's what I wanted, I would write to Dear Abby.
You don't understand that I just want you to listen, nothing more.
You not talking, and just hearing what I have to say…
It is worth more to me than any advice you could ever give.
Me just listening to myself say[ing] my problem out loud can help me solve it sometimes.
And if I do need your advice, I will ask.
But until I do ask for your advice, just listen.
So please, oh please, don't try to solve my problems for me,
Just listen.

—*Anonymous*

Touch   Touch is a form of nonverbal communication. It can convey powerful messages.

Nonverbal Communication   Much of what we communicate in relationships relates not to words but to actions. You may have heard the adage, "Your actions speak so loudly that I can't hear a word you're saying." Touch as a form of nonverbal communication has been found to be especially powerful in influencing stress. We may communicate more with our touch than with our words.

"Touch is one of the most valuable forms of communication we have," says Stanley Jones, professor of communication at Colorado University at Boulder. Over the years, Jones

Hold My Hand

An interesting study presented at a meeting of the American Psychosomatic Society explored the effects of social support in relation to stress. The researchers showed that a brief hug and 10 minutes of handholding with a romantic partner greatly reduce the harmful physical effects of stress. According to Karen Grewen, one of the principal researchers in the study, loving contact before a tough day at work could carry over and protect a person throughout the remainder of the day.

In the study, 100 adults with spouses or long-term partners were asked to hold hands while viewing a pleasant 10-minute video, and then asked to hug for 20 seconds.

Another group of 85 rested quietly without their partners. Then all participants spoke about a recent event that made them angry or stressed. Blood pressure soared in the no-contact group. Their systolic (upper) reading jumped 24 points, more than double the rise for the huggers, and their diastolic (lower) reading also rose significantly. Heart rate increased 10 beats a minute for those without contact compared with 5 beats a minute for the huggers.

Source: *Recent Warm Physical Contact with Partner is Related to Lower Cardiovascular Reactivity to Stress*, by B. Anderson, K. Grewen, and K. Light, address given at 61st annual scientific meeting of American Psychosomatic Society, 2003.

---

has identified 16 meanings of touch. "We don't touch enough, and people know it—at least subconsciously. That's why we found that people will actually sneak touches to get their quota," Jones says.[20] Even things such as asking someone to rub suntan lotion on your back or touching the hand of the cashier when you pay can be ways to experience touch. Touch deprivation may explain why massage has undergone a real boom in recent years.

According to Elaine Yarbrough, president of the Yarbrough Group business communication company, touching varies from region to region within the United States. Among her findings, she reported that the South touches more than the North. Generally the East Coast isn't a "touching region," but some populations—such as the Jewish communities—are more touch-oriented. The West, says Yarbrough, is too diverse to say one way or the other.[21]

Touch is one of the ultimate expressions of caring relationships. A substantial body of research in both animals and humans supports the fact that caring touch is necessary for emotional health. A classic study found that when young monkeys are deprived of touch, they grow up with a variety of emotional abnormalities that lead them to be aggressive and incapable of exhibiting warmth and affection toward their offspring.[22]

In Touch with Touch Waitresses who touch their customers get better tips than waitresses who don't.

Source: "The Big Deal with Feel," by D. McPherson, *Coloradan*, Sept. 2003.

211 Communication

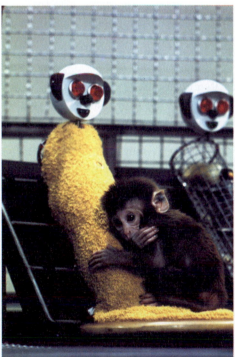

A classic study found that when young monkeys are deprived of touch, they grow up with a variety of emotional abnormalities that lead them to be aggressive and incapable of exhibiting warmth and affection toward their offspring.

© Martin Rogers/Stock Boston, LLC 115

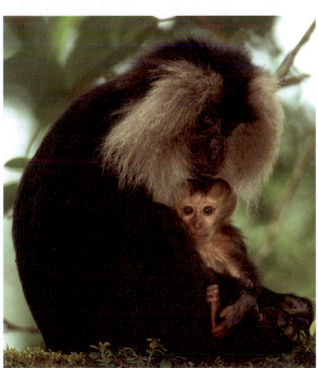

Loving relationship between mother and baby monkey. Safe and secure babies become healthy adults.

© Frans Lanting/CORBIS

Reach Out and Touch

Someone
Studies suggest humans are "hard-wired" to thrive as social animals, says Tiffany Field of the Touch Research Institute at the University of Miami Medical School. Field's research shows that touch lowers output of cortisol, a stress hormone. When cortisol dips, two "feel good" brain chemicals, serotonin and dopamine, surge.

U.S. couples aren't very "touchy-feely" in public, Field says. Her studies in U.S. and Parisian cafes found that French couples spent about three times as much time touching as Americans did. Comforting physical contact is out of favor among friends and co-workers because of the legal climate, she says. "If you happen to touch someone at the fax machine, you run the risk of being sued."

Source: "Hugs Warm the Heart, and May Protect It," by Marilyn Elias, retrieved December 31, 2004 from http://www.usatoday.com/news/health/2003-03-09-hug-usat_x.htm.

Could something as simple as a pat on the back, shaking a hand, or a gentle hug make a difference? Through the sense of touch, messages from the external environment come to the attention of the body and mind. Touch can make that message positive by reinforcing our perceived sense of social support. Don't underestimate touch as a powerful form of communication.

Men and Women—Different Can Be Good In communication and relationships, males and females generally differ. In Chapter 3 you learned about the research on the "tend and befriend" response. Studies have found that males are more likely to prepare to fight or flee when encountering a stressor and females are more likely to "tend to" and protect their loved ones and seek social support from other trusted females (befriend). Some evidence indicates that we learn these responses at an early age. Boys report that they have fewer people they feel comfortable in turning to for support than girls do. Rather than turning to friends for support, boys are more likely to turn to exercising, watching TV, and spending time on the computer as a means of coping.[23]

Dr. John Gray is an expert in the field of communications and author of the best-seller *Men Are from Mars, Women Are from Venus.* In working with scores of people who were struggling with relationship problems, he found some interesting differences between men and women and how they deal with stress. Based on his experience, Gray believes that when women are stressed, they tend to feel a need to talk about their feelings. Women may be less concerned with finding solutions than with feeling relief by expressing their concerns and feeling understood.[24]

By contrast, he found that when men get upset, they are less likely to talk about their concerns. Men tend to think about the problem, mulling it over to find a solution. If they can't find a solution, they are likely to do something to forget the problem, such as read the news, watch a football game, or mow the lawn. By disengaging the mind from the problems of the day, they can gradually relax. If a man's stress is really high, he gets involved with something even more challenging, such as racing a car, competing in a contest, or climbing a mountain."[25]

Although Gray's idea about how men and women deal with stress and how they prefer to be treated when they are stressed is a generalization, the point he makes throughout his book is that people respond to love in different ways and if we don't treat others lovingly in the way that resonates with them, the loving gesture will not be perceived as such.

Men and women may communicate differently and may deal with stress differently. What is important, though, is to be aware that people do not see things the same, nor do they require the same responses to feel listened to and supported. The key is to respect and appreciate the differences in each person. Despite our best efforts, we cannot avoid conflict in relationships, but we can take measures to alleviate the associated stress.

Managing Conflict

Inevitably, anyone involved in a relationship will face conflict. **Conflict** has been defined as an expressed struggle between at least two independent parties who perceive incompatible goals, scarce rewards, and interference from the other party in achieving their goals.[26] When the conflict can be described in a clear, concise way, the parties stand a better chance of solving a problem before it becomes unsolvable or destructive.

No two people perceive the world in the same way. Gender, ethnicity, and culture are significant influencers on how individuals view their own world. Too often, we mistakenly believe that one individual understands exactly what another person is thinking and feeling.

Perception is individual. For this reason, even people who have pledged their love to each other have disagreements. Conflicts can be found everywhere—in personal lives at home, at school, in the workplace, and among groups in our society. Most relationships are not intimate and personal. Of all communication, 90% involves sharing *impersonal* information in the course of managing daily life.[27] No matter where conflict arises, or whom it is with, the tensions must be faced and managed.

Frequently, conflict is associated with stressful outcomes such as aggression, anger, damaged relationships, violence, and even wars. But conflict can be constructive. Confronting disagreements through productive communication can lead to positive growth and improvement. Conflict is not an enemy. Differences of opinions present an opportunity to consider solutions that otherwise would not be examined or explored. Relationships can be strengthened by sharing feelings and concerns. Conversely relationships can be destroyed by prolonged conflict unless the parties agree to resolve points of contention in a constructive manner.[28] The key to whether the outcomes will be constructive or destructive is how the conflict is managed.

Expressing your view in a clear, bold manner can open communication. **Assertiveness,** or assertion, means standing up for personal rights and expressing thoughts, feelings, and beliefs in direct, honest, and appropriate ways that do not violate another person's rights. Assertiveness is constructive when facing differences and conflicts with others.

Styles of Conflict Resolution

According to the Thomas-Kilman Mode Instrument,[29] conflict can be handled through five different styles of conflict resolution. Different situations and different people require different techniques. Too often, individuals get stuck using a limited number of techniques and applying them inappropriately to resolve conflict. Although there is not a right or wrong style, it is helpful to rank either high or low the importance of the individual's needs or goals involved in the conflict, then apply the appropriate style of conflict resolution at the right time.

Turtle

1. Avoidance style of conflict resolution

    The avoidance style is unassertive and uncooperative. When individuals do not pursue their own concerns or those of the other person, they do not address the conflict but, rather, sidestep, postpone, or simply withdraw. Turtles prefer to hide and ignore conflict rather than resolve it. Common characteristics of someone using the Turtle style of conflict management are these:

    - Is nonconfrontational
    - Denies issues that are a problem
    - Is highly dependent without inner direction
    - May postpone conflict or avoid it at all costs
    - Moves away, leaves, loses

It is appropriate to use the avoidance approach:

- When the stakes aren't that high and you don't have anything to lose; when the issue is trivial
- When you don't have time to deal with it; when more important issues are pressing
- When the context isn't suitable; it isn't the right time or place
- When you see no chance of getting your concerns met
- When you would have to deal with an angry, hotheaded person
- When you are totally unprepared, taken by surprise, and need time to think and collect information
- When you are too emotionally involved and the others around you can solve the conflict more successfully.

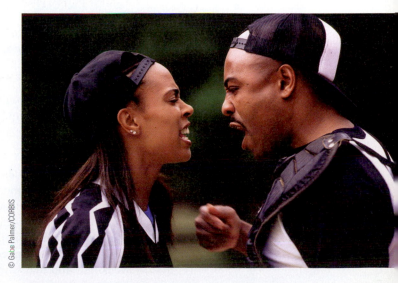
© Gabe Palmer/CORBIS

Learning to manage conflict is vital for preventing unnecessary stress.

Avoidance in action: Stephanie recently lost her job and was concerned about whether she would have enough money for next semester's tuition. Her friend Megan had called her three times during the same day wanting to know if she should try to line up a date for Stephanie for the coming weekend. Stephanie felt she had more important things to worry about than dating, so she didn't answer the phone or return Megan's messages.

Teddy
Bear

2. Accommodating style of conflict resolution

The accommodating style is unassertive and cooperative. This is the opposite of competing. When accommodating, an individual neglects his or her own concerns to satisfy the concerns of the other person. This mode has an element of self-sacrifice. The emphasis of this "teddy bear" style of managing conflict is on human relationships. Common characteristics of a person using the Teddy Bear style of conflict management are these:

- Is agreeable, nonassertive
- Cooperates even at expense of personal goals
- Yields; moves toward the other person; friendly

It is appropriate to use the accommodating approach:

- When the issue is not so important to you but it is to the other person
- When maintaining the relationship outweighs other considerations
- When you discover that you are wrong
- When continued competition would be detrimental; you know you can't win
- When preserving harmony without disruption is most important; it's not the right time

Accommodating in action: David and his college roommate disagreed over where in their room to place the new desk the dormitory provided. David prefers to study in the library. He realizes this is not as important to him as it seems to be for his roommate. He accommodates his college roommate and lets him make the decision.

Shark

3. Competing style of conflict resolution

The competing style is aggressive and uncooperative. An individual pursues his or her own concerns at the other person's expense. This is a power-oriented mode in which the person uses whatever power seems appropriate to win his or her position. Common characteristics of someone using the Shark style of conflict management are these:

- Uses power, position, personality, or status to get one's own way
- Commonly reflects a mindset of academics, athletics, and the law
- Is assertive and aggressive
- Is forceful, moving against others

It is appropriate to use the competition approach:

- When you know you're right
- When you need a quick decision
- When you meet a steamroller type of person and you need to stand up for your own rights

Competing in action: At the end of the semester, Brooke was overloaded with homework. Her mother kept calling and leaving messages. She wanted Brooke to be sure to come home for her birthday, which happened to be in the middle of finals week. Brooke feared that her mother wouldn't take *no* for an answer, but she understood the importance of finishing her homework before going home on the weekend. She called her mom and said, "Mother, I'm not coming home this weekend, and that's final! I'll hang up the phone if you refuse to take *no* for an answer."

Fox

4. Compromising style of conflict resolution

    Compromising is an intermediate position between assertiveness and cooperative-ness. Its objective is to find some expedient, mutually acceptable solution that partially satisfies both parties. It falls in a middle group between competing and accommodating. Compromise gives up more than competing but less than accommodating. Common characteristics of someone using the Fox style of conflict management are these:

    - Is assertive but cooperative
    - Tries to bargain, compromise, and split the difference

    It is appropriate to use the compromising approach:

    - When the goals are moderately important and not worth using more assertive modes
    - When people of equal status are equally committed
    - To reach temporary settlement on complex issues
    - To reach expedient solutions on important issues
    - As a back-up mode when competition or collaboration don't work

    Compromising in action: Karla, a university freshman, eagerly made plans for her family to visit her on campus the coming weekend. Just as the family was ready to leave, her father was called into work unexpectedly. Karla was disappointed but suggested to the rest of the family that they still come and leave Dad at home for the weekend.

Owl

5. Collaborating style of conflict resolution

    The collaborating style is both assertive and cooperative. It is the opposite of avoid-ing. Collaboration involves an attempt to work with the other person to find some solution that fully satisfies the concerns of both persons. It includes identifying the underlying concerns of the two individuals and finding an alternative that meets both sets of concerns. The common term for this type of conflict resolution is *win–win*. This way of resolving conflicts is usually the most satisfying to all parties involved with the least residual negative feelings. Common characteristics of someone using the Owl style of conflict management are these:

    - Is highly respectful for mutual benefit
    - Recognizes the needs and mutual benefit of both parties
    - Strives for a win–win situation or recognizes the abilities and expertise of all
    - Integrates; works toward the solution with others

    It is appropriate to use the collaboration approach:

    - When others' lives are involved
    - When you don't want to have full responsibility
    - When a high level of trust is present
    - When you want to gain commitment from others
    - When you need to work through hard feelings or animosity

Collaborating in action: John and Melanie were making plans for a June wedding. They eagerly anticipated their honeymoon until they discovered what each other wanted. John thought they would spend time in Montana at an exclusive ranch near a river where he could spend his days fishing. Melanie had dreamed for years about a honeymoon on the beach in Hawaii. She wanted to bathe in the sunshine during the daytime and enjoy the nightlife at the end of the day. They soon realized they were faced with a conflict.

Each person set aside his or her desires to listen to what the other person wanted. Knowing that Montana and Hawaii were distant from each other, John and Melanie researched other places where they could spend their honeymoon.

After a beautiful June wedding, John and Melanie enjoyed their honeymoon in Florida, where John went deep-sea fishing and Melanie basked in the sunshine during the day. They both enjoyed Florida's nightlife.

Understanding the appropriate ways to resolve conflicts can make an enormous differ-ence in the stress that we feel. Relationships invariably contain emotions that can run the gamut from ecstasy and joy to heartache and suffering. By applying appropriate solutions to conflicts, we can remain on the more positive end of the emotional roller-coaster that accompanies relationships.

Conclusion

Social support engenders a sense of belonging, feeling accepted and loved, and being needed. Our support systems consist of a network of relationships. From the moment we are born, bonding with our parents starts us down a path of personal relationships that shape our experience of trust and confidence in dealing with life. Supportive, healthy relationships with other people can help protect against stress and are essential for physical, emotional, and social health. Compelling evidence supports the findings that social support can even help us live longer.

Effective communication skills are essential for developing and maintaining relationships. Empathic listening is especially important in communicating a message that you care and truly desire to understand what the other person is saying.

Despite our best intentions, conflict and stress are inevitable in relationships. Understanding conflict-resolution styles can help you determine the best approach for dealing with various conflicts when they arise.

Take Matt's advice from the opening vignette by being proactive in your relationships. Spend time with the people you care about. Be deliberate in nurturing your relationships using the information in this chapter, and the benefits will be yours.

> It's not enough to have lived. We should be determined to live for something. May I suggest that it be creating joy for others, sharing what we have for the betterment of personkind, bringing hope to the lost and love to the lonely.
>
> —Leo F. Buscaglia

LAB

13.1 Empathic Listening

PURPOSE The purpose of this activity is to give you an opportunity to practice empathic listening. Use this listening opportunity when another person is talking about an emotional issue, rather than about something mundane or an event that contains no emotional intensity. Do not tell the person that you are intentionally listening to practice being empathic. For approximately 30 minutes, simply focus all of your listening energy on listening for the single purpose of understanding. After you have finished, respond to the following questions. Be as thorough with your responses as possible.

1. Describe the situation: Who was involved? What was the main topic of conversation?

2. Describe how you noticed yourself vacillating between listening empathically and listening autobiographically.

3. Describe how the person you were talking with responded to you when you listened with empathy.

4. Describe how easy or difficult you found that it was to listen empathically for that long.

Key Points

- Supportive relationships can serve as a shield to protect us from potential distress and may well be one of the most important ways to prevent stress.
- Social support has been described as a network of relationships that engender a feeling of being cared for and loved. Those in social relationships have a mutual obligation to each other's well-being.

- Types of social support include instrumental support, emotional support, informational support, and appraisal support.
- Effective communication is one of the most important qualities for a relationship to survive and thrive.

- Empathic listening is active listening with the intention and commitment of truly understanding the other person before seeking to be understood oneself.
- Touch is an important form of nonverbal communication.
- Men and women may have different ways of wanting to feel loved. Understanding the most effective ways to love and care for your friends and loved ones improves the

likelihood that you can help when they are feeling low and need support.
- Conflict can be constructive. Confronting disagreements through productive communication can lead to positive growth, change, and improved relationships.
- Five styles of conflict resolution are avoiding, accommodating, competing, compromising, and collaborating.

Key Terms

social support

instrumental support

emotional support

informational support

appraisal support

autobiographical listening

empathic listening

conflict

assertiveness

Discussion Time For Critical Thinking/Discussion Questions, please visit this book's Premium Website.

Notes

1. "Social Support as a Moderator of Life Stress," by S. Cobb, *Psychosomatic Medicine, 38*, 300–314.
2. *Work, Stress and Social Support*, by J. S. House (Reading, MA: Addison-Wesley, 1981).
3. "Social Support and Its Relation to Health: A Critical Evaluation," by J. Jung, in *Basic and Applied Social Psychology 17*(1) (1984): 31–38; "Social Support and Psychological Disorder: A Review," by R. L. Leavy, *Journal of Community Psychology 11* (1983): 3–21.
4. "Stress, Social Support and the Buffering Hypothesis," by S. Cohen and T. A. Wills. *Psychological Bulletin 98* (1985): 310–357.
5. *Health and Ways of Living: The Alameda County Study*, by L. Berkman and L. Breslow (New York: Oxford Press, 1983).
6. *Introduction to Public Health* (2nd edition), by M. Schneider (Gaithersburg, MD: Aspen Publishers, 2006).
7. *The Spirit and Science of Holistic Health,* by J. Robison and K. Carrier (Bloomington, IN: AuthorHouse, 2004).
8. *Loving Each Other: The Challenge of Human Relationships,* by L. Buscaglia (New York: Ballantine Books, 1984).
9. *College Students and Stress,* by S. Williams. Retrieved December 31, 2004 from http://www.homepages.indiana.edu/101201/text/stress.html.
10. Socialization Patterns of Depressed and Non-Depressed College Students," by W. Swann, et al., *Journal of Abnormal Psychology 104* (1992).
11. *Good Relationships are Good Medicine,* by B. Powell (Emmaus, PA: Rodale Press, 1987).
12. *Why Marriages Succeed or Fail*, by J. Gottman (New York: Simon and Schuster, 1994).
13. Gottman, *Why Marriages Fail.*
14. *The Five Love Languages: How To Express Heartfelt Commitment to Your Mate*, by G. Chapman (Northfield Publishing, Chicago, 1995).
15. Chapman, *The Five Love Languages.*
16. Chapman, *The Five Love Languages.*
17. Buscaglia, *Loving Each Other.*
18. *The Seven Habits of Highly Effective People: Audio Learning System Application Workbook*, by S. R. Covey (Provo UT: Covey Leadership Center, 1991).
19. Covey, *The Seven Habits of Highly Effective People.*
20. Cited in "The Big Deal with Feel," by D. McPherson, *Coloradan* (Sept 2003).
21. *The Spirit and Science of Holistic Health,* by J. Robison and K. Carrier (Bloomington, IN: AuthorHouse, 2004).
22. McPherson, "The Big Deal with Feel."
23. "Coping with Stress," *Washington Post Health,* September 8, 1998, p. 5.
24. *Men Are from Mars, Women Are from Venus*, by J. Gray (New York: HarperCollins Publishers, 1992).
25. Gray, *Men Are from Mars, Women Are from Venus.*
26. *Collaborative Negotiation,* by J. L. Hocker and W. W. Wilmot (Los Angeles: Roxbury Publishing, 1997).
27. *The Communication Process: Impersonal and Interpersonal*, by K. M. Galvin and C. A. Wilkinson (Los Angeles: Roxbury Publishing, 2000).
28. *Access to Health*, by R. J. Donatelle and L. G. Davis (Needham, MA: Pearson Education Co, 2007).
29. Retrieved December 31, 2004 from http://www.training.itcilio.it/delta/managinegodl/Preactivity/THOMAS-KILMANConflictQuestionnnaire.doc.

14 Creating a Healing Environment

■ My friend said she read a book on *feng shui* to give her ideas on how to arrange the furniture in her new apartment. What is *feng shui* anyway? ■ When I walk into my neighbor's living room, I seem to relax. Something about that place helps me unwind. Do things like color, plants, and light really make a difference in how we feel? ■ Is it my imagination, or do I feel more stressed and frustrated in hot weather? ■ If all this new technology is supposed to help me have more time to relax, why do I feel busier than ever?

Study of this chapter will enable you to:

1. Define what is meant by a "healing environment."
2. Describe the role of color, light, smells, air, noise, and temperature in creating a healing environment.
3. Describe the role of the aesthetic qualities of surroundings in creating a healing environment.
4. Explain how a healing environment helps to prevent stress.
5. Evaluate your personal level of technostress.
6. Explain how technology can be managed to prevent stress.

I go to nature to be soothed and healed, and to have my senses put in tune once more.
—*John Burroughs*

© Reuters/CORBIS

Home, Sweet Home Joe comes home from classes and throws his jacket on top of the pile on the floor. His dark, cold apartment smells like cigarette smoke and greasy French fries from last night's dinner. Joe just wants to plop down on the couch and relax for a few minutes, but he hasn't checked his e-mail all day and the light on his answering machine is flashing. Technology is calling him, and he can't resist the urge.

An hour later, after checking his phone messages and e-mails, Joe gives up on any hope for a nap. He has to get busy and finish his term paper, but first he has to find his notes, which are buried somewhere on the kitchen table under old newspapers and pizza coupons. After a couple minutes of searching, his cell phone rings. It's his boss asking him to come in to work early because someone called in sick at the last minute. He really needs Joe's help. Joe feels his stress level rising.

Creating a Healing Environment

Imagine this scenario: You have studied hard but still feel stressed and nervous as you walk across campus to take your math test. You walk into your classroom and immediately begin to relax. The quiet, comfortable room is filled with natural light and painted in a soothing color. The chairs are designed ergonomically for comfort and support and are arranged in an appealing manner. Headphones are attached to each chair so you can choose a relaxing melody from a long list of music, or maybe you prefer listening to the sounds of nature to block out distracting noises while you take the exam. You breathe in the subtle scent of lavender and feel yourself relaxing with each breath. Does this sound anything like your classrooms? Or do you find that the settings where you take tests add to the stress that you are already feeling? How does our environment affect stress and what can we do about it?

Stress and the Environment

In the broadest sense, **environment** encompasses everything both internal and external to an individual. An **environmental stressor** is some aspect of our environment that we perceive as annoying, distracting, uncomfortable, or stressful. In this chapter we will explore facets of the external environment, particularly physical surroundings, that may contribute to stress. We will highlight some of the common environmental stressors and investigate ways to create a more healing, relaxing environment.

Types of Environmental Stressors Some environmental stressors—such as the Indonesian tsunami and the terrorist attack on the World Trade Center—make the headlines. Other environmental stressors—such as the constant hum of machines and the clutter of too much stuff—are more subtle. Environmental stressors typically include:

Air pollution	Insects
Noise	Tobacco smoke
Overcrowding	Poor ergonomics
Disasters (natural and manmade)	Furniture arrangement
Climate conditions	Room clutter
Lighting	Room temperature
Room colors	

All of these external environmental conditions can play a role in our levels of comfort or discomfort.

Individual Perceptions Environments are more than merely locations. They contain memories, experiences, energy, and meaning.[1] Like all stressors, environmental stressors are different for each of us. One person may perceive going to a rock concert and sitting in front of the speakers as pleasurable and relaxing. To another person, this would be one of the most stressful experiences imaginable. Perception is the important component of whether an environmental factor is stressful. Sometimes perception is based on past experience.

Learned Response and the Environment Imagine this: Your heart is pounding, your stomach is in a knot, and you can hardly breathe. You've arrived at the dentist's office! **Learned response theory** helps explain why we might feel stressed in certain environments. When we associate a specific environment with something painful in that environment, the two get linked. When this happens, we might perceive the environment itself as unpleasant. Simply being in an environment that we associate in our mind with discomfort or pain can elicit the stress response, even when that environment poses no pain or danger.

Dentists often are well aware of the learned response and go to great efforts to alter patients' perception of the environment in a way that helps them relax. Relaxing music, entertaining movies, plants, comfortable chairs, and artwork—all can help create an environment that is conducive to relaxation. (Of course, advanced pain relief doesn't hurt either!)

Say a woman who has morning sickness during the early stages of her pregnancy shops often in a certain mall. Repeated exposure to the mall combined with her morning sickness may trigger the unpleasant response of feeling sick each time she goes to the mall in the future. Under normal conditions, a shopping mall would not cause this response, but when one condition is paired with another and pain or discomfort is involved, the first becomes a trigger for a response of discomfort.

Think about aspects of your environment that trigger the stress response. To prevent and manage stress, environmental stressors have to be managed. Only you can decide how best to do that based on your individual preferences and experiences.

Managing Environmental Stressors Many people do not even notice the effects of the environment on them. They become accustomed to living and working in buildings that lack natural lighting, have windows that cannot be opened to let in fresh air, and are painted in cold colors. Their house may have been built on a tiny lot with no open space and no room for trees, wildlife, or even grass. Individuals living in Western society may live a "disconnected" existence. This disconnect from the natural world can leave people feeling estranged and unfulfilled. They may feel stressed and seek artificial substitutes for natural experiences.[2]

By taking a proactive approach toward environmental stressors, you may be able to reduce or eliminate stressors from your environment. If you can't eliminate the stressor, try to remove yourself from the environment or adapt and think differently so you do not perceive the stressor as painful or uncomfortable. Some stressors in the environment are not in our control, but creating a calming, healing environment in our home and surroundings is usually within our control.

A Healing Environment

A **healing environment** is one in which individuals are supported and nurtured, in which they feel calm, and in which health and well-being are promoted. Healing environments play a vital role in maintaining a healthy lifestyle and are just as important as eating properly, exercising regularly, practicing proper healthcare, and having meaningful relationships and support systems. Healing environments promote a sense of relaxation and peace, and they help to vitalize senses that may have been dulled.[3] The remainder of this chapter informs you about elements of the physical environment that can promote a sense of peace and productivity.

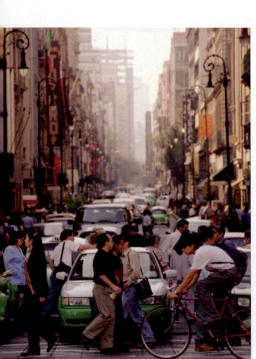

© Keith Dannemiller/CORBIS

The physical environment surrounding you each day has an impact on stress. Is your environment healing and relaxing or hectic and stressful?

Healing Color

Color has been an important part of healing for thousands of years. The ancient Egyptians ascribed healing powers to various colors. The culture of India assigns colors and specific meaning to the 12 chakras, or energy centers of the body. Archeologists have found that ancient temples were oriented in such a way that light shining through various openings created prisms of light that shone in special chambers used for healing the sick.

Source: *Spirituality, Health, and Healing,* by C. Young and C. Koopsen (Thorofare, NJ: Slack Incorporated, 2005).

Some components of a healing environment are color, light, smell, air, noise, temperature, and the aesthetic quality of your surroundings. Healing environments engage all five senses and can be created in work and personal settings. As we discuss each of the components, think about your physical surroundings and what you can do to make your environment a healing, peaceful setting.

Nature does not hurry, yet everything is accomplished.

—*Lao tsu*

Color

Studies suggest that the different colors can raise or lower your stress and energy level. Some people associate the color red with feelings of anger or hostility and blue with feeling depressed.[4] The use of color to promote health and healing is an emerging area of study, with a premise that different colors affect moods and behaviors.

The physiological and psychological effects of color are well documented. Color affects heart rates, brainwave activity, respiration, and muscle tension. Color has meaning to most people, and lack of color can be a source of stress. Color can make a space feel restful, cheerful, stimulating, or irritating.[5]

Chromotherapy is a specific discipline that uses colors to treat individuals who have certain disorders.[6] Here are some findings related to the use of color:[7]

- Warmer colors, such as peach, soft yellows, and coral, can stimulate the appetite and encourage alertness, creativity, and socialization; these colors are useful in areas such as dining rooms and meeting spaces.
- Blues, greens, violets, and other cool colors are useful in areas designed to be restful, spiritual, contemplative, and quiet, such as bedrooms and meditation areas.
- The primary colors—red, yellow, and blue—and strong patterns are pleasing at first but can be overstimulating and may contribute to fatigue.
- Green symbolizes growth, healing, spirituality, and peace, and has been used to reduce tension and nervousness.
- The brain requires constant stimulation. Monotonous color schemes contribute to sensory deprivation, disorganization of brain function, deterioration of intelligence, and an inability to concentrate. These colors slow the healing process and are perceived as "institutional."
- Color affects an individual's perception of time, size, weight, and volume. For example, warm color schemes are better in rooms where pleasant activities, such as dining or recreation, take place, because the activity seems to last longer. In rooms where monotonous tasks are performed, a cool color scheme can make time pass more quickly.

Tip: Create your study and working environments in colors that are pleasing to you. Some colors, such as dark blue and violet, are known to be more relaxing, and other colors, such as red and orange, can have the opposite effect. Color preferences are highly individualistic, however, so you should choose colors that work for you. If you live in a dorm or an apartment where you are not permitted to paint, hang a large piece of material, such as a blanket or a rug, on the wall.

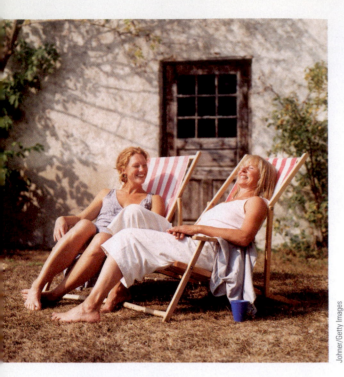
Johner/Getty Images

Natural sunlight contributes to health and healing.

Light

Light is a form of electromagnetic energy that can have both positive and negative effects on living organisms.[8] The differences between natural and artificial light are significant when health is concerned. The importance of natural sunlight to healing has been explored in a number of strong studies including the following:[9]

- Depressed patients in a psychiatric unit recovered faster in rooms that had brighter lights.
- Increased exposure to daylight had a uniformly positive and statistically significant effect on student performance as evidenced by better test scores.
- Increased daytime exposure to light had an impact on the quality of nighttime sleep in hospitalized and healthy youth alike.

Shorter periods of daylight, as occur naturally in the winter, have been shown to trigger **seasonal affective disorder** (SAD). According to the National Mental Health Association, "SAD is a mood disorder associated with depression episodes and related to seasonal variations of light."[10] Symptoms include depression, irritability, and fatigue. **Melatonin,** a sleep-related hormone, is secreted in increased levels in the dark by a part of the brain called the **pineal gland.** Melatonin may help our bodies know when to go to sleep and when to wake up. Artificial light is believed to suppress the normal nocturnal production of melatonin. Regular exposure to full-spectrum lighting has been demonstrated to improve SAD by increasing the amount of melatonin produced in the brain.[11]

Ultraviolet light can do the following:[12]

- Increase protein metabolism
- Lessen fatigue
- Stimulate white blood cell production
- Increase the release of endorphins
- Lower blood pressure
- Elevate mood
- Promote emotional well-being

> The best remedy for those who are afraid, lonely, or unhappy is to go outside, somewhere where they can be quiet, alone with the heavens, nature, and God. Because only then does one feel that all is as it should be and that God wishes to see people happy, amidst the simple beauty of nature.
>
> —*Anne Frank*

Natural daylight is believed to be best for health, yet many people live and work in environments lit by fluorescent lighting. Full-spectrum fluorescent lamps have been designed as an alternative to traditional fluorescent lighting. They mimic the spectral qualities of daylight and provide health-promoting effects similar to those of natural light. The premise is that because life evolved around daylight, optimal physiological functioning will continue under this type of light.[13]

Although natural light has many health benefits, you might want to control the amount of direct sunlight when you work indoors, to protect your eyes. Use blinds and curtains to create indirect light.

Tip: Spend time outdoors in natural light. Indoors, take advantage of windows for the natural light and the view. Use lighting to draw the eye toward positive, mood-enhancing artwork or views.

> Smell is a potent wizard that transports us across a thousand miles and all the years we have lived.
>
> —*Helen Keller*

Smells and Air

Smell can play a role in managing stress. What smells do you associate with relaxed, happy times in your life? Maybe it is the smell of homemade bread, or your grandpa's aftershave lotion. Or maybe it is the pine smell of a Christmas tree, the smell of an ocean breeze, or the smell of a campfire. Smells also can be associated with negative memories.

Smell is analyzed in the limbic part of the brain, an area associated with emotions. It is not surprising, then, that an aroma can affect how we feel. Smell is acutely retained in

Common Scents

Some elderly people in Europe associate lavender with death. Lavender bags were used to keep linen sweet-smelling and moth-free. However, if a person was bedridden with an illness, the lavender smell could become a signal of impending death. As the person became sicker, the linen was changed more frequently, and the smell of lavender became more prevalent. Lavender has undergone a tremendous revival with aromatherapy, and it appears to be universally enjoyed by people less than 60 years of age. However, the association with death may explain why older Europeans do not respond similarly to lavender.

Source: *Mosby's Complementary & Alternative Medicine: A Research-Based Approach* (3rd ed.), by L. Freeman (St. Louis: Mosby, 2009).

memory, even more than sounds or visual images, and frequently is associated with an experience.[14] This is a form of learned memory in which the reaction to an odor has been learned through experience. The reaction may be happiness, or it may be fear, depending on the original experience.

A student related in class that even many years later, he felt stressed and nauseated every time he smelled a certain perfume. He associated the scent with a sixth-grade teacher around whom he frequently felt dumb and embarrassed. The response to smells is individual.

Aromatherapy

Studies have shown that **aromatherapy,** the therapeutic use of essential oils, can lower stress levels. Smelling the essential oils sends a direct message to your brain via your olfactory nerves, where they affect the endocrine and hormonal systems via the hypothalamus. Odors have an effect on our emotional states because they hook into the emotional or primitive parts of our brains such as the limbic system.[15]

Technically, aromatherapy involves the use of essential oils, not just the use of smell. As a word of caution, many so-called aromatherapy products on the market contain synthetic aromas. Synthetic aromas have dubious therapeutic effects, and the long-term effects are unknown. Safe, effective use of essential oils requires knowledge of the sometimes powerful effects and proper administration of the oil.

Inhalation is one of the simplest and fastest methods of introducing essential oils into the body. Years of research have proven the efficacy of many of the essential oils and have shown their measurable physiological and psychological effects. Aromatherapy has been used to relieve pain, enhance relaxation and relieve stress, relax tense muscles, soften dry skin, and enhance immunity. The most common uses are to relieve stress and anxiety, chronic pain, depression, and insomnia.[16]

Aromatherapy is used routinely by midwives in many countries, and increasingly in the United States, to reduce anxiety and pain during childbirth. An analysis of 8,058 women who received aromatherapy during labor indicated that more than 50% of mothers found aromatherapy helpful for relaxation.[17]

Most essential oils from plants and flowers have the potential to reduce stress. Certain essential oils, such as lavender, rose, neroli, and petitgrain, are well known for this characteristic.[18] Jasmine and rosemary have been found to increase beta waves in the brain and result in a more alert state, and lavender increases the brain's alpha waves, thereby promoting relaxation.[19]

Air Quality

We do not want to forget the benefits of good, clean, fresh air. A good deep breath of fresh air can clear the mind and calm the body. A study of student performance found that students in classrooms with operable windows progressed 7% to 8% faster on standard tests in 1 year than students in rooms with fixed windows.[20]

Tip: Spend as much of your work or study time as possible in fresh air. If the weather allows, open the windows. If this is not possible, or

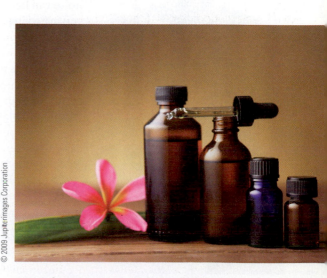

Aromatherapy uses essential oils to lower stress levels.

The Nose Knows Magnetic resonance imaging (MRI) is frequently perceived as stressful because it usually involves lying still in a small tube-like machine for a period of time. In a study designed to investigate the effect of using aroma to reduce distress during the administration of MRIs, a pleasant smell was found to reduce the patients' stress and enhance their coping ability. Via a small tube inserted into their nostrils, 57 participants received either heliotropin (a vanilla-like scent) or plain air. Patients who received the heliotropin reported 64% less anxiety than the patients who received plain air.*

Source: *Redd, W., & Manne, S. (1995). Using aroma to reduce distress during magnetic resonance imaging. In Gilbert, A., *Compendium of Olfactory Research 1982–1994*. New York: Olfactory Research Fund. *Mosby's Complementary & Alternative Medicine: A Research-Based Approach (3rd ed.)*, by L. Freeman (St Louis: Mosby, 2009).

FYI

Indoor Pollution The Environmental Protection Agency (EPA) has estimated that indoor air pollution is one of the top five environmental risks to public health. The EPA stated that indoor air pollutants can cause eye, nose, and throat irritation; headaches; loss of coordination; nausea; cancer; and damage to the liver, kidneys, and central nervous system. Indoor air may contain more pollutants, and often at higher concentrations, than outdoor air.

Source: "Healing Spaces: Elements of Environmental Design That Make an Impact on Health," by M. Schweitzer, L. Gilpin, and S. Frampton, *Journal of Alternative and Complementary Medicine 10*(1) (2004), pp. S71–83.

if pollution levels are unfavorable, make sure ventilation is adequate or the room has air filters to clean the air. If the air is dry, introduce plants, which give off fresh oxygen and help to absorb air pollutants. They also add to the visual appeal of the environment.

Tip: Reduce exposure to tobacco smoke. Smoking is banned in many areas, but if you find yourself in a place where tobacco smoke isn't banned, take action to reduce your exposure by getting as far away as possible from the smoke or using an air purifier to help remove the smoke. Smoke can irritate the eyes, and consistent exposure to tobacco smoke is known to cause respiratory problems, especially in people who already have respiratory concerns such as asthma.

Tip: When creating a healing environment, remember that pleasant odors, flower arrangements, and plants can reduce stress, absorb odors, and help clean the air.

Noise

We are surrounded by hundreds of potentially stressful sounds every day. Noise from machinery and industrial plants; road, rail, and air traffic; business and community services; construction; domestic activities; and leisure activities make noise one of our most pervasive pollutants.[21]

Loud noises cause hearing loss in an estimated 10 million Americans every year, and noise can harm more than our ears. Stress from noise can come from the TV blaring while you are trying to read, the non-stop talker sitting next to you in the library, your neighbor mowing the yard while you are trying to nap in the hammock, or the party going on next door while you are trying to sleep. Noise can raise blood pressure, increase heart rate, and cause muscle tension.[22] Sounds a lot like the stress response, doesn't it?

Noise is measured in **decibels.** Decibels (dB) range from about 20 in a quiet rural area, to 50–70 dB in towns during the daytime, to 90 dB or more in noisy factories and discotheques, to higher than 120 dB near a jet aircraft takeoff.[23] Prolonged exposure to sounds over 85 decibels or brief exposure to louder sounds can damage hearing. Research indicates that even low noise levels of 40–58 decibels can worsen health outcomes in hospitalized patients.[24] Figure 14.1 illustrates decibel levels.

To recognize if a sound is loud enough to damage your ears, you should know both the loudness level (decibels) and the length of exposure to the sound. In general, the louder the noise, the less time required to cause hearing loss. According to the National Institute for Occupational Safety and Health, the maximum exposure time at 85 dB is 8 hours.

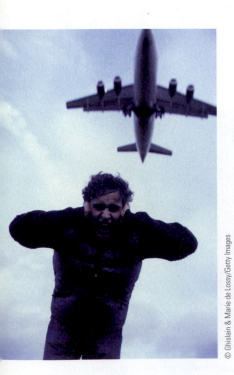

© Ghislain & Marie de Lossy/Getty Images

We are surrounded by hundreds of potentially stressful sounds every day.

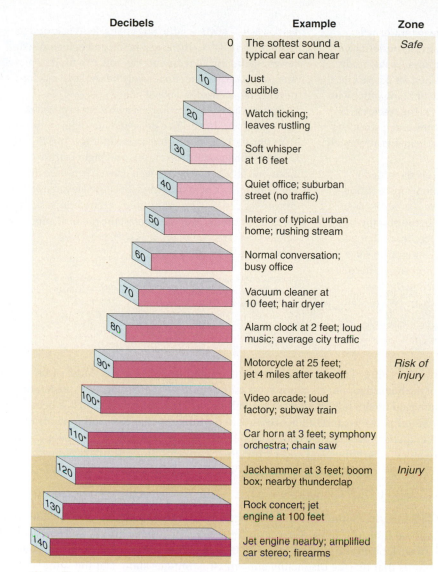

Decibels	Example	Zone
0	The softest sound a typical ear can hear	Safe
10	Just audible	
20	Watch ticking; leaves rustling	
30	Soft whisper at 16 feet	
40	Quiet office; suburban street (no traffic)	
50	Interior of typical urban home; rushing stream	
60	Normal conversation; busy office	
70	Vacuum cleaner at 10 feet; hair dryer	
80	Alarm clock at 2 feet; loud music; average city traffic	
90*	Motorcycle at 25 feet; jet 4 miles after takeoff	Risk of injury
100*	Video arcade; loud factory; subway train	
110*	Car horn at 3 feet; symphony orchestra; chain saw	
120	Jackhammer at 3 feet; boom box; nearby thunderclap	Injury
130	Rock concert; jet engine at 100 feet	
140	Jet engine nearby; amplified car stereo; firearms	

*Note: The maximum exposure allowed on the job by federal law, in hours per day, is as follows: 90 decibels—8 hours; 100 decibels—2 hours; 110 decibels—$1/_2$ hour.

FIGURE 14.1 Loud and Louder

An Invitation to Health 2009–2010 Edition, by D. Hales (Belmont, CA; Wadsworth/Cengage Learning, 2009). Used by permission.

At 110 dB, the maximum exposure time is 1 minute and 29 seconds. If you must be exposed to noise, it is best to limit the exposure time and/or wear hearing protection.

Perceived Noisiness One person's noise is another person's music. The subjectivity of noise makes it difficult to determine how much noise pollution is too much, especially as it relates to psychological distress. What is noise to one person can be appreciated sound to another, as this story illustrates:

A woman was visiting her elderly father-in-law. When they sat in his backyard and tried to visit, she found the neighbor's loud music to be irritating and was sure this would be stressful to her father-in-law. Finally, when her stress level had risen to the point at which she decided to say something, she said, "Dad, how can you stand that noise? It must be so annoying to you!" The elderly gentleman replied, "Not at all. I'm just thankful I can still hear the music."[25]

Noise becomes a stressor when we appraise it as annoying or subjectively determine it to be stressful because it interferes with our ability to concentrate, function, or relax. **Perceived noisiness** is the term describing the subjective assessment of noise that combines the decibel level and the context in which a noise occurs. Perceived noisiness actually may be a better predictor than loudness of adverse reaction to sound.[26] For instance, you actually might enjoy listening to your roommate play his drums when you're sitting around the dorm in the evening. It is another matter all together when he decides to practice at 8 o'clock in the morning!

FYI

What Did You Say? An estimated 5.2 million young Americans between the ages of 6 and 19 have permanent damage to the hair cells within the ear as a result of exposure to damaging noise levels. These hair cells play a vital role in the ability to hear sounds at varying decibel levels.

Source: "Noise-induced Hearing Loss: Common Condition Easily Prevented," *Facts of Life: Issue Briefing for Health Reporters* 6(5) (2001).

Quiet Down

A research team at Cornell University headed by Professor G. W. Evans undertook a study of stress and noise from open offices. In this study, 40 female clerical workers were examined for 3 hours in one of two situations: (1) a quiet office or (2) an office with typical open-office, low-intensity noise. The researchers measured levels of stress hormones, how much stress the participants reported, and how the participants attempted to work and complete tasks.

Although some stress hormone levels remained unchanged, urinary levels of the hormone epinephrine—which the adrenal glands release in the classic "fight-or-flight" stress reaction—were elevated in the employees who were exposed to typical office noise. Those in the typically noisy office also made fewer attempts to solve a difficult task (an unsolvable puzzle), indicating a decrease in motivation. Further, workers exposed to the low-level noise made fewer ergonomic adjustments to their workspaces—such as adjusting chairs, footrests, or document holders—than the group in the quiet office. Making fewer ergonomic adjustments can lead to a fixed or perhaps inappropriate posture, increasing the workers' risk for developing a musculoskeletal injury.

Interestingly, the employees who were exposed to the typical low-level office noise did not report more stress than the workers in the quiet surroundings. This finding suggests that higher stress levels and higher stress hormone levels may occur even when people are not consciously aware of the stress. Because elevated stress hormones can worsen many medical conditions such as high blood pressure and diabetes, the medical effects of this stress may be as great as with perceived psychological stress.

Source: "Stress and Open Office Noise," by G. W. Evans, *Journal of Applied Psychology, 85*(5) (2000): 779–783; http://stress.about.com/cs/workplacestress/a/aa040901.htm

Effects of Noise Environmental noise is related to stress levels. Most of us are not aware of the hazardous effects of noise, yet many studies have associated exposure to noise with increased health risk and decreased well-being. High-volume sound has been linked to high blood pressure and other stress-related problems that can lead to heart disease, insomnia, anxiety, headaches, colitis, and ulcers. Noise frays the nerves; people tend to be more anxious, irritable, and angry when their ears are constantly barraged with sound. Researchers speculate that noise, especially if it stresses the mother, may even be hazardous to their unborn babies.[27]

Relaxing Sound Sound can be soothing. A plethora of tapes and CDs provide soothing sounds to help you relax. Typical of these types of sounds are cascading waterfalls, the ocean surf, birds chirping, or the wind blowing. This **white noise** helps to drown out other sounds that may be distracting and stressful. Studies show that the sounds of running water and music can stimulate the production of endorphins and lower heart rates.[28] In Chapter 24 you will learn about music as a popular and effective stress reducer.

Tip: Try to reduce or eliminate background noise. Turn off the TV, radio, and other sources of extra sound when possible. Find ways to spend time in silence. If there are low-level noises in the background, select some peaceful music to cover it up. If noise comes from neighbors, communicate to them about this distracter in a pleasant, yet assertive way. Ask them to turn down the music or decrease the volume of noise in general.

> I pray thee, good Mercutio, let's retire;
> The day is hot, the Capulets abroad,
> And, if we meet, we shall not 'scape
> a brawl, For now, these hot days, is the mad blood stirring.
> —William Shakespeare, *Romeo and Juliet,* Act 3, Scene 1

Temperature

In the final minutes of the National Hockey League game, one player nails another with an unprovoked, injury-causing blow. The newspaper described the event as happening "in the *heat* of the moment." What impact does temperature have on our level of stress and on environmental factors such as violence and aggression?

Some of the most conclusive evidence relates to hot temperatures and aggression. The **heat hypothesis** states that hot temperatures can increase aggressive motives and behaviors. The **heat effect** is the observed result of higher rates of aggression by people who are hot relative to people who are cooler.[29]

Notwithstanding alternative explanations, studies using a variety of methods

FYI

Hot-Headed
There are about 2.6% more murders and assaults in the United States during the summer than other seasons of the year. Hot summers produce a bigger increase in violence than cooler summers. Violence rates are higher in hotter years than in cooler years.

Source: "Temperature and Aggression," by C. Anderson, K. Anderson, N. Dorr, K. DeNeve, and M. Flanagan, in *Advances in Experimental Social Psychology,* edited by M. Zanna), 2000, 32, 63–133.

Cool Down

Data consistently show that violent-crime rates are higher in the South than in other regions of the United States.* Is this because the South is hotter, or could alternative explanations be possible? Pause for a minute and think critically of other possible explanations for this association between heat and crime in the South.

One alternative explanation to the heat hypothesis is that, for some reason, a culture of violence developed in the U.S. South, and that this cultural difference remains today. But claims that Southern culture accounts for high violent-crime rates in hotter regions are contradicted by an analysis of crime rates in 260 U.S. cities. This analysis concluded that hotter cities were more violent than cooler cities even after city-to-city differences in "Southern-ness," population size, and socioeconomic status were statistically controlled, casting doubt on the claim that a Southern culture of violence is the sole or primary cause of higher violent crime in hotter U.S. cities.**

Think about how temperature affects you. Evidence supports the premise that heat-induced discomfort makes people cranky and lowers their tolerance level, resulting in angry feelings. An accidental bump in a hot and crowded bar can lead to the trading of insults, punches, and bullets.†

Sources:
*"Temperature and Aggression: Ubiquitous Effects of Heat on Occurrence of Human Violence," by C. Anderson, *Psychological Bulletin 106* (1989): 74–96.
**"Heat and Violence," by C. Anderson, *Current Directions in Psychological Science 10*(1) (February 2001): 33–38.
†"Temperature and Aggression," by C. Anderson, K. Anderson, N. Dorr, K. DeNeve, and M. Flanagan. In M. Zanna (Ed.), *Advances in Experimental Social Psychology* Vol. 32. (New York: Academic Press, 2000), pp. 63–133.

consistently support the heat hypothesis. Hot temperatures increase aggression by directly increasing feelings of hostility and indirectly increasing aggressive thoughts. Better climate control in many settings, including prisons, schools, and the workplace, may reduce stress and tension and the resulting aggression-related problems.[30]

Results from the following studies support the link between temperature and behavior:

- Baseball pitchers are more likely to hit batters with a pitched ball on hot days than on cool days.[31]
- Rates of violent crime increased during the hottest times of the year and were higher in regions with hotter climates.[32]
- A classic study in Phoenix, Arizona, found that aggressive horn honking increased at hotter temperatures, but only for drivers without air-conditioned cars.[33]
- In a field experiment in which Dutch police officers performed a simulated burglary scenario under hot or comfortable conditions, the officers operating in hot conditions reported more threatening impressions of the suspect and were more likely to draw their weapons and shoot the suspect (with laser training weapons), relative to officers in cool conditions.[34]

Tip: Are you a "hotter the better"-type person, or does the heat make you irritable and short-tempered? We are genetically programmed to handle heat differently, so you will have to assess the temperature conditions that optimize your productivity and comfort levels. Whenever possible, be deliberate in altering your environment to create these optimal conditions.

Aesthetic Quality of Surroundings

In addition to color, light, smells, air, noise, and temperature, what elements of your surroundings can you consider to help you create a comfortable, healing environment? *Feng shui,* nature, and organizing and simplifying your environment can bring an appealing, aesthetic quality to your surroundings.

Feng Shui *Feng shui* (pronounced "phung schway") is the ancient Chinese study of the natural environment. It is based on the belief that physical and emotional well-being is influenced strongly by our immediate environment. It is used to determine the most favorable location for

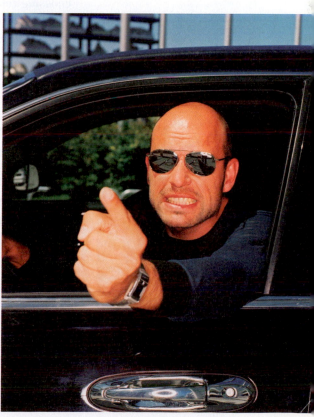

© Creasource/CORBIS

In the heat of the moment. The heat hypothesis states that hot temperatures can increase aggressive motives and behaviors.

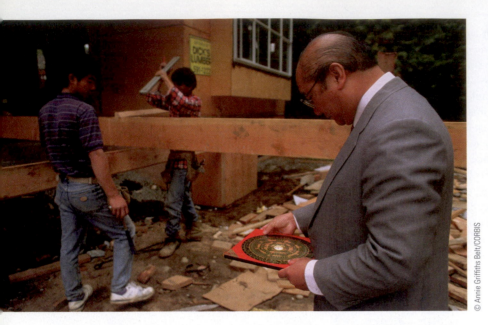

A feng shui *consultant uses a special compass, called a* lo-pan, *to determine the energy characteristics at a construction site.*

people and things in a given environment. *Feng shui* is used to promote an optimally productive and harmonious environment that supports the people in that environment.[35]

Practitioners of feng shui use a special compass, called a **lo-pan**, to determine the energy characteristics of a building or room. The layout of spaces and arrangement of furniture is said to affect the energy flow. The idea is to balance the energy so it will have a positive effect. Good *chi*, or energy flow, is believed to have a strong impact on the health and peace of mind of occupants.

Details such as where to hang a mirror, how a door should open, and where to put a red or green plant or flower are believed to be capable of redirecting energy and enhancing the flow of energy within a house.[36] Some general guidelines are the following:[37]

- Provide direct views to entrances so as not to have people's backs to doorways.
- Avoid arranging furniture so that people sit in the direct line of the doorway. This reportedly puts the person directly in the rush of *chi*, with resulting negative effects on health and productivity.
- Use warm lighting, as opposed to glaring fluorescent lighting. Overly bright light is believed to irritate people and result in headaches.

Although many people have no awareness of the idea of energy flow, the principles of *feng shui* are gaining in popularity across the United States. *Feng shui* consultants guide architects in positioning and arranging buildings such as hospitals and office buildings, as well as rooms within the buildings. Interior designers apply *feng shui* principles in arranging furniture, using plants and other living things, placing mirrors and pictures, and choosing colors. Even though the underlying principle of *feng shui*—living in harmony with nature—is sound ecologically, to determine empirically the effectiveness of *feng shui* may be impossible.

Tip: Make your home a place of sanctuary. Leave school and work activities at school or work. When you come home, listen to music, exercise, or sit peacefully to make a positive transition. Take off your watch; select a specific place in your home that is a sanctuary from stress. In this place practice relaxation exercises, read pleasant books, plan, and organize. Don't pay bills, watch television, or deal with conflicts in this place. Devote a time and space for hobbies. This will give you a sense of control and a release from the frenzied pressures of work and school. Decorate a place in your home for items—plaques, trophies, certificates, and awards—that recognize your accomplishments. This will give you a sense of pride in accomplishment, remind you of your strengths and capabilities, and motivate you to continue doing your best toward achieving your goals and objectives.

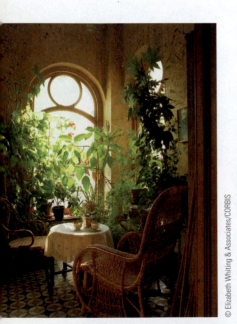

What can you do to incorporate the healing qualities of nature into your daily life?

Nature Any discussion on the effect of environment on stress would be incomplete without including the impact of nature. Stichler reports, "Human beings are intimately connected to planet Earth. They share the planet with every other living organism and they are just one strand in the complex web of life. When they live a disconnected existence, they become unhealthy, unbalanced, and unhappy. Yet, when they are in a healing environment, they know it. They feel welcome, balanced, relaxed, reassured, and stimulated."[38]

Many of us have experienced the stress-relieving benefits of a relaxing walk on the beach or a hike through the country, but what about when we spend our days indoors? Do you go from your home to your car, to school or work, to the grocery store, and back home again with barely a moment's exposure to fresh air and nature? What can you do to incorporate the healing qualities of nature into your surroundings? Here are some suggestions for bringing nature into your daily life:

- *Indoor and outdoor garden:* Research shows that plants, and even a view of plants, lower people's stress levels, lower blood pressure, reduce muscle tension, and contribute significantly to healing.[39] If you can't have an outdoor garden, create an indoor garden with an arrangement of plants.
- *Bring nature indoors:* Even in the middle of the largest city, you can create an indoor environment that brings you in touch with nature. Rocks, leaves, flowers, seashells, pinecones, pieces of wood—you can use whatever appeals to you to create a nature oasis in your home.
- *View of nature:* Arrange your home and office to get maximum enjoyment from the view. At home, place your recliner next to the window for a relaxing view. Employees with a window view of nature report less stress, better health status, and higher job satisfaction.[40]

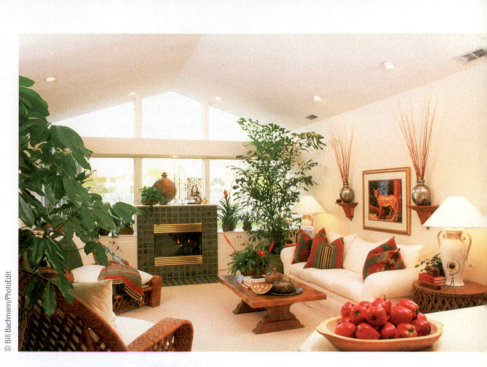

Create a relaxing oasis in your home.

- *Artwork:* If you don't actually have a window view of nature, consider artwork depicting relaxing nature scenes.
- *Light and fresh air:* As we discussed earlier, use natural light and fresh air to help relieve stress and create a feeling of being in nature, even indoors.

Tip: Put an aquarium in the room where you feel the most stress. Many hospitals and medical offices have aquariums to reduce stress and create a calming atmosphere for their patients. You can create the same peaceful environment at home. Place an aquarium where you study or work—unless, of course, an aquarium is just another distraction for you.

As you read the Culture Connection—Healing Places, reflect on how the description of the ancient Greek healing place compares to hospitals—our modern-day places of healing. Which is more conducive to providing a calming, stress-relieving, healing environment?

Organizing and Simplifying

Creating a simple, uncluttered environment can reduce your stress. In the search for happiness, many people turn to *things.* We all know deep down that life is about more than having the latest fashions, the best toys, the newest car, or the biggest house, yet we often fill our lives with more stuff. Eliminate the useless clutter from your life.

Tip: Remove clutter in your work or study environment. Look around the room and decide which things are really important to you and which things you can toss or recycle. Be honest with yourself. Ask yourself if you actually will read that magazine on the coffee table or if you will finish the craft project you started 3 months ago. Similarly, assess your furniture. Decide what you really need, and get rid of unnecessary items that are making your room feel crowded.

Tip: Take a look at the areas in which you work, study, and live, and then organize these areas so you don't waste time trying to find things. Do you ever waste time looking for your keys, purse, billfold, glasses, or books? Put things away so you can easily find them rather than spending stressful moments searching. And, with a little organization, you can reduce the clutter that can be distracting when you are trying to concentrate.

Tip: Plan an "organization day" at least once a month. Use that day to sort through the stack of unread mail, clean off your desk, toss the month-old food from the fridge, throw away old newspapers, clean your car, organize your closets, and whatever else helps you feel more in control of your environment.

Any intelligent fool can make things bigger, more complex, and more violent. It takes a touch of genius—and a lot of courage—to move in the opposite direction.

—*Albert Einstein*

Healing Places

The ancient Greeks worshipped the god of healing by building healing temples within cypress groves near the ocean. They faced the ocean and took advantage of the sea breezes and the sun. Patients at the temples used libraries, gardens, baths, theaters, gymnasiums, and special sleep rooms to heal. They took part in activities specially designed to restore their natural body rhythms, and thereby achieve harmony between their body and their mind. The ancient Egyptians decorated their healing places with murals because they believed the murals helped patients maintain their interest in life.

Source: *Spirituality, Health, and Healing,* by C. Young and C. Koopsen (Thorofare, NJ: Slack Incorporated, 2005).

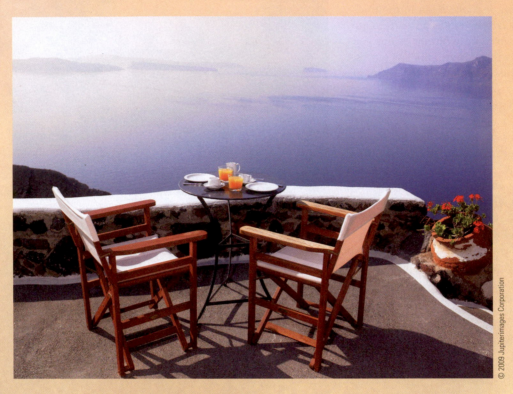

© 2009 Jupiterimages Corporation

Healing places bring harmony to body, mind, and spirit.

Ergonomics

Employers are becoming increasingly aware of the impact of the physical environment on their employees. An entire area of study has evolved to explore aspects of the environment that affect employee well-being and productivity. **Ergonomics** is the study of individual workers and the tasks they perform, for the purpose of designing appropriate living and working environments. Many companies hire a person trained specifically to assess the ergonomics of work areas.

The major goals of ergonomics are (1) to make work safer, and (2) to enhance worker and worksite well-being. Much of the ergonomic research can be applied to the home environment as well.

Tip: Design your computer workstation and arrange your office furniture so you don't struggle with tension and pain from bad posture, eyestrain, back pain, or other symptoms of poor ergonomics. Your computer monitor and keyboard should be in a place where neither leads to discomfort from continued use. If you notice strain or muscle tension, make adjustments.

Tip: Reduce eyestrain from spending hours working at your computer by looking away from the screen regularly. The small muscles of the eyes become tight and have to be stretched, just like other muscles in the body. You can do this by taking a few seconds from time to time to look at objects at varying distances.

Technology and the Environment

In Greek mythology, Sisyphus was an evil king who was condemned to Hades. His eternal punishment was to roll a big rock to the top of a mountain, only to have it always roll down again in an unending cycle. A similar version of this punishment is experienced every day by people who find their e-mail boxes at work forever full.[41]

Although a discussion of technology in this chapter may seem out of place, the impact of technology on our environment is becoming increasingly significant. We would have difficulty imagining a world without computers. These technological aids have contributed enormously to the productivity and efficiency of workers and opened communication between homes throughout the country and abroad. Computers and other technology, however, also have introduced new sources and symptoms of stress that we could not have imagined a few years ago.

Many people feel overwhelmed, frustrated, and irritated at the seemingly never-ending flood of new technology. During the past decade, technology has invaded our homes, our cars, our movie theaters, our grocery stores, our jobs, and literally every place in our lives. Every innovation—from cell phones to e-mail, from faxes to Websites—demands new skills, speedier reaction times, creativity on call 24 hours a day. Technology keeps coming at us, and we are told that we must adapt or fall behind. No wonder 85% of us are hesitant or outright resistant to technology![42]

Technostress If you have ever had the ATM machine at the bank gobble up your card; if you have tried in vain to turn on the water in an airport bathroom where the faucet has been replaced by a sensor; if you have felt absolutely helpless when your computer goes down; if your Palm Pilot malfunctions, leaving you with no idea about when you are supposed to be where; you may be a victim of **technostress.** These feelings of dependence, incompetence, anxiety, and frustration

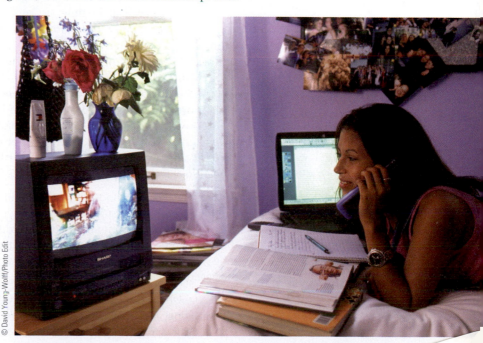

We live in an environment where we are surrounded by technology. Computers and other technology have introduced new sources and symptoms of stress that we could not have imagined a few years ago.

© David Young-Wolff/Photo Edit

FIGURE 14.2 Are You a Victim of Technosis?

Source: *TechnoStress: Coping with Technology @WORK@HOME@PLAY.*, by M. Weil and L. Rosen (New York: John Wiley & Sons, 1998) © M. Weil and L. Rosen. Used with permission.

Yes	No	
Yes	No	Do you feel stressed if you haven't checked your voice or e-mail within the last 12 hours?
Yes	No	Do you think you can't cook a meal without technological gadgets?
Yes	No	Do you become upset when you can't find an ATM for quick cash?
Yes	No	Do you have difficulty writing unless you are sitting in front of your computer?
Yes	No	Do you have a hard time determining when you are finished researching a topic on the Internet?
Yes	No	Do you feel less adequate than your highly technologized peers?
Yes	No	Do you rely on pre-programmed systems to contact others?

describe what top authorities on the psychology of technology, Michelle Weil and Larry Rosen, call technostress.

Regardless of our level of technological expertise, technostress, they assert, affects every aspect of our lives, whether we're at work, at home, or at play. Weil and Rosen assert that the growing dependence on technology affects us negatively. We count on our machines to do so much that when something goes wrong with our technology, we are thrown into a tailspin.

> People allow themselves to be sucked into this technological abyss, and in doing so they become more machine-oriented and less sensitive to their own needs and the needs of others. Some people become so immersed in technology that they risk losing their own identity, a condition called **technosis**."[43]

To see if you are afflicted with technosis, take the quiz in Figure 14.2. If you answer "yes" to any of these questions, you may be suffering from technosis. Victims of technosis develop an attachment to technology. It grows slowly, but before people know it, they have lost sight of where they end and technology begins. Symptoms of technosis include overdoing work and never feeling finished, believing faster is better, and not knowing how to function successfully without technology.

Technology and Stress Several issues relate to how technology may contribute to a stressful environment:

- *Alienation and isolation* of people from each other—so many ways to communicate, so little communication. Today's faceless forms of communication go against the basic human need to connect in person. Obsession with the emerging technology may lead to a loss of capacity to feel and relate to others.
- *Blurring the boundaries* from the intrusion of computers and technology at work and home. Telecommuting and home-based business are blurring the boundaries between work and downtime. Cell phones, pagers, Palm Pilots, and e-mail can leave you feeling like you are on call all the time.
- *Information overload and multitasking madness.* We may feel overwhelmed, like we have never completed a task successfully. There is always more information "out there." How do we cope with the onslaught of information and frantic pace of our technological world?
- *Higher expectations* as computers and constantly changing software create demands for more efficiency and expectations of higher productivity. The pressure to produce more work faster becomes a stressful condition.
- *Pressure to keep up* with "mine is bigger than yours." How do we deal with "machine machismo" when people are "flexing their RAM" as a way of competing in today's high-tech society?[44]

Weil and Rosen propose a pro-humanity, rather than an anti-technology, approach. Technology is here to stay, so rather than presenting a negative view of technology, the intent is to encourage us to move forward with an uplifting, inspiring look at ways to master the Information Age. The outcome is to help us perform better at work, spend more quality time with our families, and experience the wonder of technology without the technostress. Suggestions include the following:

- Recognize that there is more technology than you will ever want or be able to use. With technology, like magazine subscriptions, you get to select what you want and use only what works for you. It's okay to leave the rest alone.

FYI

Turning Off and Dropping Out
According to authors Weil and Rosen, many people are choosing to rid themselves of computers, answering machines, and other electronic gadgets for a simpler life. The frustrations and fears of living in a digital world have led to the emergence of anti-technology groups such as the Lead Pencil Club and Neo-Luddites.

Source: *Technostress: Coping with Technology @WORK @HOME @PLAY*, by M. Weil and L. Rosen (New York: John Wiley & Sons, 1998).

- Understand that the way technology is implemented in most businesses almost guarantees technostress. In their "12-phase people-centric training model," Weil and Rosen encourage corporations to provide ample time for "free play" with any new technology to ensure success.
- Just because technology is capable of doing multiple jobs at the same time does not mean that we are. "Multitasking madness" is hitting us all as we attempt to juggle more and more. It is interfering with our sleep at night and our concentration and memory by day.
- At home, family members are in their own "techno-cocoons," each hooked up to a different techno-gadget. Create family rules for technological use to avoid this isolating trend.[45]

Although technology can, and frequently does, work for us, the hopes and promises that technology would make life easier and allow more time for relaxation and rejuvenation have not come to fruition. The problem is that sometimes we become trapped and end up working for the technology. Carefully evaluate how and when you use technology. We can live well with technology and without technostress. Create an environment where you control the technology rather than the technology controlling you.

Conclusion

A healing environment starts with you. Many aspects of your surroundings can contribute to creating a relaxing, stress-reducing environment. Think about how you can use the factors of color, noise, smells, light, and nature to create a healing environment. Think about how you manage technology. Create an environment that contributes to your sense of peace and control in a sometimes chaotic world. The peace you create at home will spread to your community and beyond.

The impact of our environment on our health and well-being is profound. Sometimes we just need to step back and assess our environment and how it is affecting us. We live in a world where so much seems out of our control. Ours is a world in which:

- A tsunami kills nearly 200,000 people and leaves 1.5 million homeless
- Terrorist attacks have become daily news
- According to the FBI, domestic violence claims the lives of four women each day[46]

Yet we also live in a world where individuals make a difference; where people donate millions of dollars to help the tsunami victims in Asia and the victims of Hurricane Katrina in the United States; where young men and women take pride in defending their country; and where volunteers spend countless hours coming to the aid of strangers who need help. We should not underestimate the difference one person can make in creating a healing environment.

Some of what happens is out of our control, but not everything. We can start at the individual level to create healing environments. Creating healing environments in our homes, our communities, our nation, and around the entire planet will be necessary if we are to fully experience deep and enduring well-being. This Chinese proverb sums it up best:

If there is light in the soul, there will be beauty in the person.

If there is beauty in the person, there will be harmony in the house.

If there is harmony in the house, there will be order in the nation.

If there is order in the nation, there will be peace in the world.

14.1 How Healing Is Your Environment?

PURPOSE The purpose of this activity is to increase your awareness of your environment. Do this activity in a place where you spend considerable time, such as your dorm room or home. Evaluate your environment by responding to the following:

1. Location you are assessing:

2. Describe the environment in as much detail as possible including color, light, smells, air, noise, and temperature. Also include the aesthetic quality of the setting as described in your textbook.

3. What aspects of the environment do you find to be relaxing? Why?

4. What aspects of the environment do you find to be stressful? Why?

5. What are three things you would or could do to make this environment more relaxing and healing?

Key Points

- An environmental stressor is some aspect of our environment that we perceive as annoying, distracting, uncomfortable, or stressful.
- Environments are more than locations. They contain memories, experiences, energy, and meaning.
- Perception is a significant component in whether an environmental factor is stressful to individuals.
- A healing environment is one that supports and nurtures individuals, one in which they feel calm, and one that promotes health and well-being.
- Studies suggest that different colors can raise or lower your stress and energy level.
- Regular exposure to full-spectrum lighting has been demonstrated to improve seasonal affective disorder by increasing the amount of melatonin produced in the brain.
- Smell is analyzed in the limbic part of the brain, an area associated with emotions.
- Aromatherapy, the therapeutic use of essential oils, can lower stress levels.

- Noise is among the most pervasive and destructive environmental pollutant.
- Perceived noisiness describes the subjective assessment of noise that combines the decibel level and the context in which a noise occurs. Perceived noisiness may be a better predictor than loudness of adverse reactions to sound.
- According to the heat hypothesis, hot temperatures can increase aggressive motives and behaviors. The heat effect is the observation of higher rates of aggression in people who are hot compared to people who are cooler.
- *Feng shui,* the ancient Chinese study of the natural environment, is based on the belief that physical and emotional well-being is strongly influenced by our immediate environment.
- Ergonomics is the study of individual workers, and the tasks they perform, for the purpose of designing appropriate living and working environments.
- Technostress describes feelings of dependence, incompetence, anxiety, and frustration related to technology.

Key Terms

environment
environmental stressor
learned response theory
healing environment
chromotherapy
seasonal affective disorder
melatonin

pineal gland
aromatherapy
decibels
perceived noisiness
white noise
heat hypothesis
heat effect

feng shui
lo-pan
chi
ergonomics
technostress
technosis

Notes

1. *The Meaning of Everyday Occupation,* by B. Hasselkus (Thorofare, NJ: Slack Incorporated, 2002).

2. *Spirituality, Health, and Healing,* by C. Young and C. Koopsen (Thorofare, NJ: Slack Incorporated, 2005).

3. "A Quiet Place: A Healing Environment," by B. Spalding, *Support for Learning 16*(2) (2001): 69–73.

4. *Understanding Your Health* (10th ed.), by W. Payne, D. Hahn, and E. Mauer (New York: McGraw-Hill, 2009).

5. Young and Koopsen, *Spirituality, Health, and Healing.*

6. "Designing Humanistic Critical Care Environments," by D. Fontaine, L. Briggs, and B. Pope-Smith, *Critical Care Quarterly 24*(3) (2001): 21–34.

7. Young and Koopsen, *Spirituality, Health, and Healing.*

8. Fontaine, et al., "Designing Humanistic Critical Care Environments."

9. "Healing Spaces: Elements of Environmental Design That Make an Impact on Health," by M. Schweitzer, L. Gilpin, and S. Frampton, *The Journal of Alternative and Complementary Medicine, 10,* Supp. 1 (2004): pp. S71–83.

10. http://www.nmha.org

11. Schweitzer, et al., "Healing Spaces."

12. "Creating Healing Environments in Critical Care Units," by J. Stichler, *Critical Care Nurse Quarterly, 24*(3) (2001): 1–20.

13. Young and Koopsen, *Spirituality, Health, and Healing.*

14. Young and Koopsen, *Spirituality, Health, and Healing.*

15. *Understanding Your Health* (10th ed.), by W. Payne, D. Hahn, and E. Mauer (New York: McGraw-Hill, 2009).

16. *Mosby's Complementary & Alternative Medicine: A Research-Based Approach* (3rd ed.), by L. Freeman (St. Louis: Mosby, 2009).

17. "An Investigation into the Use of Aromatherapy in Intrapartum Midwifery Practice," by E. Burns, et al., *Journal of Alternative and Complementary Medicine 6*(2) (2000): 141.

18. Freeman, *Mosby's Complementary & Alternative Medicine.*

19. Fontaine, et al.."Designing Humanistic Critical Care Environments."

20. "Windows and Classrooms," by L. Heschong, *The Journal of Alternative and Complementary Medicine, 10,* Supp. 1 (2004): S71–83.

21. Noise Clearinghouse (2003). http://www.nonoise.org/aboutno.htm.

22. *Office Work Can Be Dangerous to Your Health,* by J. Stellman, and M. Henifen (New York: Pantheon, 1983).

23. *Community Noise,* by B. Berglund and T. Lindvall (Geneva: World Health Organization, 1995).

24. Schweitzer, et al., "Healing Spaces."

25. *Stress Less: Four Weeks to More Abundant Living,* by M. Hesson (Nashville: Abingdon Press, 1999).

26. *Community Noise,* by B. Berglund and T. Thomas Lindvall (Geneva: World Health Organization, 1995).

27. *An Invitation to Health 2009-2010 Edition* by D. Hales (Belmont, CA: Wadsworth/Cengage Learning, 2009).

28. *Design Details for Health,* by C. Leibrock (New York: John Wiley & Sons, 2000).

29. "Heat and Violence," by C. Anderson, *Current Directions in Psychological Science 10*(1) (February, 2001): 33–38.

30. Anderson, "Heat and Violence."

31. "Temper and Temperature on the Diamond: The Heat-Aggression Relationship in Major League Baseball," by A. Reifman, R. Larrick, and S. Fein, *Personality and Social Psychology Bulletin 17* (1991): 580–585.

32. "Temperature and Aggression: Ubiquitous Effects of Heat on Occurrence of Human Violence," by C. Anderson, *Psychological Bulletin 106* (1989): 74–96.

33. "Ambient Temperature and Horn-Honking: A Field Study of the Heat/Aggression Relationship," by D. Kenrick and S. MacFarlane, *Environment and Behavior 18* (1984): 179–191.

34. "Aggression of Police Officers as a Function of Temperature: An Experiment with the Fire Arms Training System," by A. Vrij, J. van der Steen, and L. Koppelaar, *Journal of Community and Applied Social Psychology 4* (1994): 365–370.

35. Schweitzer, et al., "Healing Spaces."

36. *Feng Shui,* by R. Cottrek, (2002), http://www.skeptic.com.

37. Schweitzer, et al., "Healing Spaces."

38. Stichler, "Creating Healing Environments in Critical Care Units."

39. "Grow with It: The Role of Plants in Health Care Facilities," by M. Gilhooley and C. Rice, *Medical Group Management Association Connexion 2*(17) (2002): 17–18.

40. "Windows in the Workplace: Sunlight, View, and Occupational Stress," by P. Leather, M. Pyrgas, D. Beale, and C. Lawrence, *Environmental Behavior 30* (1997): 739–762.

41. http://www.softpanorama.org/index.shtml

42. *TechnoStress: Coping With Technology@WORK@HOME@PLAY,* by M. Weil and L. Rosen (New York: John Wiley & Sons, 1998).

43. Weil and Rosen, *TechnoStress: Coping With Technology@WORK@HOME@PLAY.*

44. Weil and Rosen, *TechnoStress: Coping With Technology@WORK@HOME@PLAY.*

45. Weil and Rosen, *TechnoStress: Coping With Technology@WORK@HOME@PLAY.*

46. "Violence Against Women: A National Crime Victimization Survey Report" (Washington, DC: U.S. Department of Justice, January 1994).

15 Healthy Lifestyles

■ What kind of exercise is best to help reduce stress? ■ Should I take vitamins when I am stressed? ■ Could stress have anything to do with the extra fat I have accumulated since I started college? ■ When I get stressed, I can't sleep, and when I can't sleep, my stress level rises. It feels like a vicious cycle. What can I do to ease my stress so I can sleep better? How do I figure out how much sleep I need? ■ Since I started college, I've been drinking more. I know drinking isn't good for me, but it helps me relax. If I give up drinking, what can I do to help me deal with the stress of college?

Study of this chapter will enable you to:

1. Explain the health and stress-relieving benefits of a balanced exercise program.
2. Describe the components of a healthy diet.
3. Explain the impact of stress on nutritional needs and body fat.
4. Explain the relationship between stress and eating disorders.
5. Assess the amount of sleep you require.
6. Explain unhealthy coping strategies, including the negative effects of tobacco, alcohol, and drugs.
7. Incorporate healthy lifestyle habits into your life to reduce and eliminate stress.

When health is absent, wisdom cannot reveal itself, art cannot manifest, strength cannot fight, wealth becomes useless, and intelligence cannot be applied.

—*Herophilus*

Jason's Story In the first month of college, I drank more than I did all during high school. It started out as just a way to relax and socialize with my buddies. After the first week of classes, I felt so stressed I thought I would explode. Some guys in my dorm invited me to a kegger that weekend, and we had a blast. Even though I felt rotten the next day, drinking helped me forget—for at least a little while—all the pressures of school. After I joined a fraternity, my drinking increased to the point where I was having several beers most nights. I started to realize that alcohol was adding to my stress, not reducing it, but I didn't seem to have the motivation to change.

I don't know where I would have ended up if I hadn't met Sonya. What I noticed first about her was how much fun she was. She didn't drink but still seemed to always be having fun. She really liked to do things, and I got caught up in her excitement for living. We went biking and hiking. Sonya would pack a picnic lunch and we would spend hours at the lake just talking and relaxing. I never thought I'd see the day, but she even talked me into running a 5K to raise money for the women's shelter. I finally caught on to the idea that I didn't need to drink to relax and have fun.

Healthy Lifestyles

Traditional students entering college have greater freedom to choose their lifestyles than ever before. This transitional period from leaving home to starting a new phase of life at college is an opportune time to establish healthy lifestyle habits. Exercise, nutrition, sleep, and avoiding unhealthy habits are key components of a healthy lifestyle.

Stress is known to influence health through its direct physiological effect and also through its indirect effect via altered health behaviors.[1] Maintaining a healthy lifestyle includes avoiding activities that people sometimes believe will help them relax or cope with the stress they feel, but which actually increase stress by contributing to a decline in health. These activities include drinking, smoking, and using drugs, which are not effective in managing stress over the long term.

Taking care of your body is an important stress-prevention strategy. This chapter focuses on the physical dimension of health. A strong, healthy body is more resilient, more able to adapt, and less likely to incur the negative effects of stress at the mental, emotional, physical, social, and spiritual levels.

Exercise

The benefits of a regular, balanced exercise program are well known and significant. It is one of the key components of a healthy lifestyle. Exercise can also help you prevent and manage stress. Numerous studies have shown that exercise reduces anxiety, muscle tension, and blood pressure—three measures of stress.

Exercise as a Stress Buffer Exercise is one of the most powerful stress buffers for a variety of reasons. To understand why exercise is beneficial in reducing stress, recall the discussion about the stress response in Chapter 3. When we sense danger, the body automatically gears up for activity—fight or flee. Therefore, exercise is a way of following through on that message by using our fighting and running muscles.

By participating in activities that use our fighting and running muscles, the body uses excess blood sugar; muscles use the stress hormones adrenalin and cortisol; and other circulating fats in the bloodstream are used for energy. The body goes through

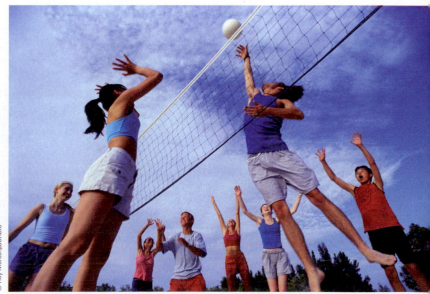

Exercise is a great stress reliever. It turns off the stress response and activates the relaxation response.

© Roy Morsch/CORBIS

Looking Good, Feeling Great

A review of research evaluating the relationship between exercise, physical activity, and physical and mental health supports the evidence that regular exercise has a beneficial influence on much more than just the physical dimension. Exercise helps us feel better emotionally, and it helps us function more effectively in our daily activities. Regular activity improves our general levels of health and well-being and overall quality of life. This is true of every population that has been studied, including both genders, a variety of ethnic groups, and across the life span.* Exercise seems to be the magic pill that enhances every dimension of a person's life.

Only 10 minutes of moderate exercise can improve overall mood, as well as increase vigor and decrease fatigue. Why does this happen? A number of theories have been proposed, including the release of "feel-good" brain chemicals such as endorphins and serotonin; a reduction in the stress hormone cortisol; increased self-esteem resulting from better body image and weight control; and even the muscle relaxation resulting from raised body temperature. Also, those who "exercise away" bad feelings are less likely to turn to smoking, overeating, or alcohol, which can feed cycles of tension and depression.**

Sources:
*"Exercise and Well-Being: A Review of Mental and Physical Health Benefits Associated with Physical Activity," by F. Penedo and J. Dahn, in *Current Opinions in Psychiatry*, *18*(2): 189–193.
**"Attitude Adjustment," by L. Shelton, *Natural Health, 34*(3).

a process similar to the stress response—a period of arousal and hyperstimulation followed by a period of exhaustion and rest.

Noted fitness expert Covert Bailey describes how regular exercise over time decreases the amount of adrenalin and cortisol released during other stressful times:

> Extensive studies on rats and baboons have shown that when they are exposed to mild but repeated stress such as cold, shock treatment, restraint, intermittent loud noises, or aerobic exercise, there is a big change in the stress responses. They get tough, able to handle the stress better.
>
> And they handle it better in two ways. First, if the stress is something with which they are familiar, they produce smaller amounts of stress hormones. It's as if their bodies say, "Ho hum. We're used to that stress. We don't have to get in a snit over it." Second, if the stressful situation is novel, something they haven't previously experienced, they produce more stress hormones than normal. Their bodies gear up better than usual with the stress. Additionally, after the stress is over, their bodies are able to get rid of the no-longer-needed hormones faster.[2]

Other Benefits of Exercise Exercise can make you feel better by improving your mood, reducing your anxiety, and increasing your energy. Exercise generates the natural release from the brain of the mood-lifting hormones called endorphins. These "feel-good" hormones act the same way the chemical morphine acts in the body, only without the negative side effects. Exercise also can give you a sense of accomplishment and boost your confidence. Exercise increases the flow of blood to the brain, which results in improved concentration and alertness and helps you to think more clearly. Thoreau said, "The moment my feet begin to move, my thoughts begin to flow." Many people find that they do their best thinking while exercising.

Tip: Instead of cramming for the 15 minutes immediately before an exam, take a brisk walk around the block or run up and down the stairs a few times. This will help you relax, increase blood flow to the brain, and help you think more clearly.

Physical conditioning also offers important protection. Individuals whose heart, lungs, and skeletal muscles are conditioned by exercise can withstand cardiovascular and respiratory effects of the alarm stage of stress better than those who lead a sedentary life.[3] Regular exercise conditions us to become stronger and able to adapt to daily pressures more readily. Stress impedes optimum functioning of the immune system. Because exercise relieves stress, a physically fit person does not

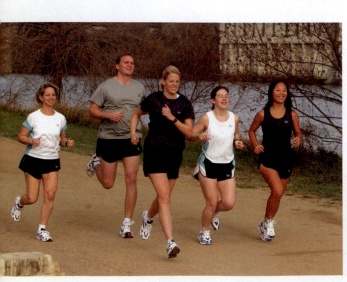

© Bob Daemmrich/PhotoEdit

Exercise contributes to a sense that we can take control of our life and health.

get sick as often as one who has a weaker immune system. A physically fit person has greater endurance, and as a result is less likely to feel fatigued at the end of a long day.

One more benefit of exercise related to stress management involves the component of *control*. As mentioned, the more a person feels in control of a situation, the less stress he or she is likely to feel. When we work out, we are participating in an activity over which we usually have a lot of control.

Components of Physical Fitness For optimal results, exercise should be regular and balance the following components of physical fitness:

1. **Cardiorespiratory fitness:** the ability of the heart, lungs, and blood vessels to process and transport oxygen required by muscle cells so they can meet the demands of prolonged physical activity. Cardiorespiratory fitness is produced by physical activity that requires continuous, repetitive movements, such as jogging, swimming, and biking.

2. **Muscle fitness:** muscle strength and endurance. **Muscle strength** is the ability of skeletal muscle to engage in work and relates to the force that a muscle can exert. **Muscle endurance** is the ability of muscles to function over time and is supported by the respiratory and circulatory systems. Weight-lifting exercises can improve muscle fitness.

3. **Flexibility:** the ability of joints to move freely through a full range of motion. Stretching exercises are effective to maintain and improve flexibility. These exercises are especially effective for relieving stress-induced muscle tension. Chapter 22 will introduce you to a wide variety of yoga poses to help you increase flexibility.

    Tip: Stretching exercises are effective in promoting relaxation. If you do a lot of sitting or repetitive activity, take frequent stretch breaks. This can get your blood flowing, relieve muscle tension, and help you return to your work better able to focus on the task at hand.

4. **Body composition:** makeup of the body in terms of fat tissue in relation to lean body tissue (muscle, bone, organs). Knowing your ratio of body fat to fat-free weight is especially important given the national increase in obesity and related health problems. The same types of activity that improve cardiovascular fitness are effective for improving body composition. Typically, for body composition benefits, these exercises are done at a lower intensity but longer duration. You will learn later in the chapter that stress has an effect on body fat, which makes these exercises especially important for individuals with high-stress levels.

Which Exercise Is Best? Which is the best exercise to help you reduce stress? The easy answer is *any exercise that you enjoy, that is healthy, and that you will do.* Cardiorespiratory exercises such as jogging, bicycling, rowing, hiking, brisk walking, or playing in some higher-intensity sports such as racquetball and volleyball are especially effective for bringing about post-exercise relaxation. Workout routines including aerobics classes or kickboxing, which use both fighting and running actions, are ideal stress-reducing activities. Whatever exercise you choose, do it and enjoy all the benefits!

Equally important is what you want to accomplish from your exercise. Do you want to relieve built-up tension or get energized? Do you want to slow down and relax, or do you want to work off some anger? Choose the activity you need at the time to transform your mood. Restorative exercises like those explained in Table 15.1 are especially helpful because they aid in physical and mental relaxation.

But remember, too much of a good thing can be harmful to your health. Over-exercising can become a stressor to the body and may lead to several problems including overuse injury, muscle strain, and joint pain. It is even possible to become addicted to exercise to the point where the enjoyment is replaced by physical decline, irritability, and depression. Approaching

FIGURE 15.1 Student Snapshot—How Active Are College Students?

An Invitation to Health 2009–2010 Edition by D. Hales (Belmont, CA: Wadsworth/Cengage Learning, 2009). Used by permission.

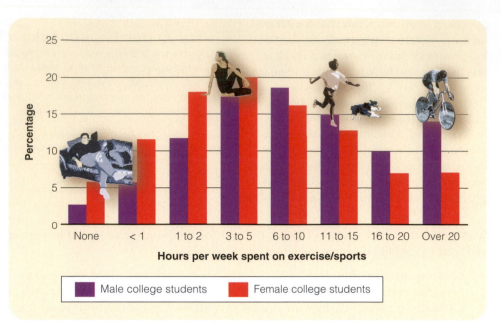

Hours per week spent on exercise/sports

◼ Male college students ◼ Female college students

Couch Potatoes in the Making

According to the U.S. Department of Health and Human Services, the highest rate of decline in physical activity occurs in the early adulthood period between 18 and 24 years of age.*

Students report a decline in physical health over the first three years of college. Between 2004 and 2007, the percent of students who engaged in exercise or sports for more than 5 hours per week declined by nearly half (from 52.0 to 28.8).**

Sources: *Healthy People 2010: Understanding and Improving Health* (2nd ed.) (Washington, DC: U.S. Department of Health and Human Services, 2000). ***Spirituality in Higher Education—A National Study of College Students* http://spirituality.ucla.edu/news, 2007.

exercise as a highly competitive activity can also defeat the stress-relieving benefits. Keep in mind that exercise should be enjoyable. When it becomes an addiction or a way of avoiding other things in your life, then you can be fairly certain you aren't doing it for the right reasons and you're not as likely to reap the benefits of consistent and appropriate exercise.

Sticking with Exercise Three factors help people start and stick with an exercise routine:

1. *Enjoyment.* Select activities you enjoy. Exercising just because someone says it is good for you may cause more stress than it relieves. Go for a jog, lift weights, dance, or do whatever you choose to get moving. Even gardening, mowing the lawn, and housework can be beneficial.
2. *Convenience.* Walking is such a good option. Cost and time barriers can prevent you from participating in certain exercise programs that involve driving to a location and

TABLE 15.1 What Mood Are You In?[4]

Mood	Moves That Work
Your mood is low and you are feeling dejected, listless, apathetic.	Move for at least 10 to 30 minutes at mild to moderate intensity. Focus on your body, not your brain, until you can feel yourself regain vitality. Take a mindful walk to expand your senses. Listen to music that invigorates you and lets you express your emotions; move or dance to it. Walk the dog. Swing your arms vigorously front and back. Make faces expressing different emotions. Practice smiling.
You are bored and tired and you feel lazy and exhausted.	Rev up your heart rate. Engage in moderate aerobic activity for at least 10 to 30 minutes as an energy booster and pick-me-up. Take a brisk walk or jog (don't stroll). Skate, bicycle, use the elliptical machine, or perform any other cardio activity that you can comfortably sustain.
You are nervous and hyperactive and feel wound up and overstimulated.	Relax and slow down your breathing and heart rate. Engage for 10 to 60 minutes (or as long as it takes) in any repetitive activity that will calm you. Practice yoga, tai chi, or take a long, slow stroll. Swim laps.
You are restless and complaining and feel irritable and short-tempered.	You have excess energy to burn, so work out hard. Engage in exercise that will focus your attention for at least 20 to 40 minutes. Lift weights, punch a punching bag, or jump rope. Run sprint/jog intervals by interspersing 30 to 60 seconds at high intensity with 2 to 3 minutes at moderate intensity. Play racquetball, and hit the ball as hard as you can.

paying for a class. But if all you have to do is put on your shoes and sweats and walk out your door to immediately begin exercising, you are more likely to do it. Having weights or exercise videos at home can also make it easier to get started.

3. *Social support.* Although some people like to exercise alone, many find that combining exercise with social activity, such as intramural basketball or tennis, increases their enjoyment and helps them stick with it. Walking with a couple of friends who are counting on you to be there can increase your motivation and make your exercise time more enjoyable.

Take a few minutes to think about what type of exercise would be most beneficial to you. Develop a plan for incorporating activity into your life. Consider a regular exercise routine as well as exercises you can incorporate on an "as needed" basis—for example, a brisk walk around the block prior to your next stressful test. When you have been working at the computer for hours, do push-ups and stretch, rather than taking a junk food break. A balanced exercise program, along with a healthy diet, is integral to both a healthy lifestyle and a stress management program.

Nutrition

"I can't eat a bite when I'm stressed." "When I'm stressed, I eat like a horse." Stress can initiate altered eating behaviors from one end of a continuum to the other, which creates some unique nutritional needs. We differ in how stress affects us nutritionally. Food is the fuel that feeds our body. When we overeat, don't eat enough, don't eat often enough, or select unhealthy foods, the body does not have the proper fuel it needs to run efficiently. The results are fatigue, low energy, and an overall decline in the ability to deal with stress.

A Healthy Diet Healthful eating is an important component of the prescription for optimum health and well-being. A well-nourished body is best prepared for dealing with the stressors of life. The best nutritional preparation for stress is a varied and balanced diet. Two tools to guide healthy eating are the *Dietary Guidelines for Americans* and *MyPyramid*. The **Dietary Guidelines for Americans** provides science-based advice to promote health and reduce the risk of major chronic diseases through diet and physical activity. A complete description of the guidelines can be found at www.healthierus.gov/dietaryguidelines.

The *Food Guide Pyramid*, a widely recognized nutrition education tool, translates nutritional recommendations into the kinds and amounts of food to eat each day. The original Pyramid has been replaced by *MyPyramid* and can be found at www.mypyramid.gov.

Nutrition and Stress Nutrition experts recommend a foundation of fresh fruits, fresh vegetables, whole grains, and legumes. Moderate amounts of protein and dairy foods are also included in a healthy diet. The body gets energy from three sources: carbohydrates, fats, and proteins. During stress, we draw upon all three of these energy fuels in increased quantities. Therefore, we should maintain a balance of nutrients from these sources. Although a varied and balanced diet provides the foundation for healthy nutrition, stress places some additional nutritional demands on the body.

Even though you need a balanced diet that includes foods from all the food groups, fruits, vegetables, legumes, and whole grains are especially important. Complex carbohydrates are an ideal anti-stress food because they boost the brain's level of the mood-enhancing chemical **serotonin.** Good sources include broccoli, potatoes, corn, cabbage, spinach, whole-grain breads and pastas, and cereals. Leafy vegetables, whole grains, nuts, and seeds also are rich in other important nutrients.[5]

Fresh Fruits and Vegetables Many of the vitamins and minerals we need are found in a variety of fruits and vegetables. They contain thousands of plant chemicals, including antioxidants, immune-system boosters, and enzymes. A rule of thumb is to eat a variety of different colors of fruits and vegetables.

Legumes Legumes should be a regular part of our daily diet. These include all peas, beans, chickpeas, soybeans, peanuts, and lentils. Legumes are high in fiber and are loaded with important nutrients.

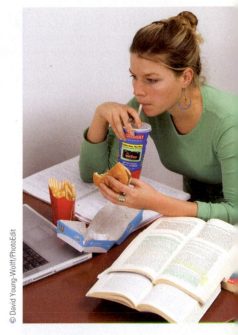

© David Young-Wolff/PhotoEdit

"When I'm stressed I can't stop eating." "When I'm stressed I can't eat a thing." We differ in how stress affects us nutritionally.

Do I Need a Vitamin?

Because some people seem unable to eat when they are stressed, and because the body requires extra quantities of some nutrients during stress, many nutritionists recommend taking a vitamin–mineral supplement to prepare for stressful times. Megadoses aren't necessary, merely amounts comparable to the **Recommended Dietary Allowances (RDA),** the daily amount of a nutrient considered adequate to meet the known nutrient needs of almost 98% of all healthy people in the United States. Supplements, of course, do not take the place of eating a balanced diet.

Cut Sugar, Cut Stress According to research by psychologist Richard Surwit, some evidence indicates that managing stress can help to control diabetes, especially type 2 diabetes. He found that high stress levels raise stress hormones in the body and then increase the amount of glucose in the blood. Surwit found that teaching diabetics how to relax was helpful to them. Biofeedback and muscle relaxation techniques resulted in better control of their diabetes. The subjects also were taught how to deal more realistically with stress by using reason to fight off fearful thoughts.

Source: "Cut Stress. Cut Sugar," by M. Carmichael, *Finance CustomWire*, Sept. 30, 2004.

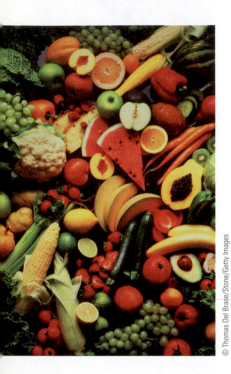

Fruits and vegetables are part of a healthy, balanced diet.

© Thomas Del Brase/Stone/Getty Images

Whole Grains White bread has been processed so completely that nearly all of its nutritional value has been removed. All that is left is the equivalent of simple sugars. Enriched flour has some of the nutrients added back, but it is still deficient compared to 100% whole wheat. The same is true of white rice and other processed grains. Whole grains retain more of their original nutrients than highly processed grains. Whole grains also tend to have more fiber, which slows glucose absorption and is valuable in maintaining good colon health.

Whole grains are important to a healthy diet in part because of how they relate to blood sugar levels. The **glycemic index** is a measure of foods and how quickly they convert into blood sugar. Foods that enter the bloodstream quickly have a higher glycemic index. The result of high glycemic index foods, such as simple sugars, is that the blood sugar level increases rapidly. The body responds by secreting insulin, which results in a decline in blood sugar level. This fluctuation can leave you feeling low on energy and less able to mentally and physically combat stress. Lower glycemic index foods, including whole grains, result in a more stable blood sugar level and, as a result, a more stable mood and energy level.

Drinking Water Several variables—climate, activity level, and intake of caffeine or alcohol, among others—affect the amount of water you need. Common side effects of stress that increase the body's demands for water include dry mouth, increased respiration, and increased perspiration. Low water levels in the body can affect our moods and perceptions dramatically. A decrease in the body's water level of as little as 1% to 3% can make us feel agitated and irritable. A 3% to 5% drop can cause headaches, weakness, and fatigue. A drop of more than 5% can result in hospitalization. We often fail to recognize that the cause of our sluggishness and headaches may be mild dehydration. Nutritionists recommend drinking enough water so your urine is light yellow or clear, not dark in color.

Tip: Carry a bottle of water with you throughout the day. At home, put a full pitcher of water in the refrigerator every morning, and be sure it is empty by bedtime. Squeeze a few drops of lemon into the water to give it a more pleasant taste and to neutralize chlorine.

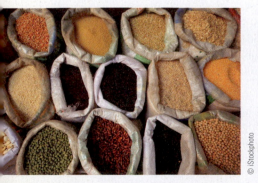

Legumes are high in fiber and are loaded with important nutrients.

© iStockphoto

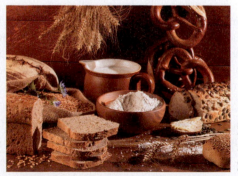

Whole grains are important to a healthy diet.

© Bon Appetit/Alamy

What to Limit or Avoid in Your Diet For optimum health and stress management, limit your intake of caffeine, fats, sugars, and especially soft drinks.

Caffeine Caffeine is the most widely used psychoactive (mind-affecting) drug in the world. Coffee, the caffeine source of choice, is enjoyed by approximately 80% of Americans. Consumption of energy drinks such as Red Bull and Rockstar has more than doubled in the last three years, especially among young people.[6] Caffeine is the main ingredient in these drinks with doses sometimes high enough to cause physical and psychological complications, including disrupted sleep, exaggerated stress response, heart palpitations, and increased risk of high blood pressure.[7]

Caffeine is known to increase stress hormones, which may persist long after drinking a cup of coffee or a soft drink.[8] Caffeine is a stimulant that in excessive amounts can lead to restlessness or nervousness (the "jitters"), as well as a racing heartbeat, tremors, sleep disturbances, and nausea. You also may feel anxious or even depressed if you consume large amounts of caffeine. For most people, moderate caffeine intake does not cause serious health risks; however, caffeine is addictive, and withdrawal symptoms can include headache, restlessness, and irritability when caffeine consumption is halted suddenly. Therefore, you should gradually reduce or eliminate the amount of caffeine you consume in a day.

Trans Fatty Acids Foods that contain hydrogenated or partially hydrogenated oil—trans fatty acids—should be avoided as much as possible. Consuming these and saturated fats results in an increase of plaque deposits in blood vessels. This can lead to blood vessel diseases including heart disease and stroke. Foods containing a lot of hydrogenated fat include margarine, pastries, crackers, cookies, and some cereals.

Soft Drinks A typical soft drink contains about 12 teaspoons of sugar. Many soft drinks contain caffeine and, frequently, other substances that are of no nutritional value to the body. Soft drinks have a high glycemic index. The carbonation also tends to inhibit absorption of essential minerals. Many people have replaced water with sugar and caffeine-filled or artificially sweetened soft drinks as their beverage of choice. Soft drinks with artificial flavoring such as aspartame tend to increase the craving of sugar throughout the day, with unhealthy consequences.

Overeating Consider these numbers from the Centers for Disease Control:

16.4—Pounds of food eaten per week by the average American in 1970
18.2—Pounds of food eaten per week in 2006
2 X—Growth in percentage of obese adults from 1970 to 2007

Digesting food requires a lot of energy. Recall how you feel after you have eaten a large meal. Most people say they feel tired and lethargic. Let's examine why this happens: Your stomach is about the size of two fists. Now consider the amount of food an individual consumes eating a typical super-sized meal, or eating seconds or thirds. This amount is far larger than a normal-sized stomach is designed to handle. Consider further that all this food is taken into the mouth, is subjected to a few obligatory chews, and then gets sent down into the stomach to be broken down further. The stomach's job is to transform those large amounts of food into microscopic portions to go to the small intestines, where they are absorbed into the bloodstream through tiny capillaries. A tremendous amount of work is necessary to convert a large hamburger into a tiny element to be used for energy or some other process in the body. No wonder we are tired after eating a large, heavy meal!

Overeating, probably more than any other factor, has contributed to the obesity epidemic in the United States. Obesity is a source of great stress for many.

Stress and Healthy Weight

Obesity has become a national epidemic and a leading cause of morbidity and mortality. Stress plays a unique role in the accumulation of excess body fat. Three factors help explain the role stress plays in contributing to obesity: eating to cope, unused glucose, and the cortisol connection.

Overeating leads to obesity, a source of great stress.

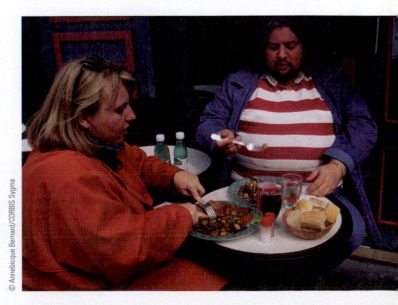

FYI

Hidden Sugars

Be on the lookout for hidden sugars. A can of soda has about 12 teaspoons of sugar; low-fat fruit yogurt has 7 teaspoons of sugar; and a tablespoon of catsup contains a teaspoon of sugar.

FYI

The Growing Epidemic

As of 1997, 46% of family food expenditures were spent on meals outside the home, with 34% of the total food dollars spent on fast foods. The typical fast food burger weighed about an ounce in 1957 compared to 6 ounces in 1997. It is not surprising to learn that from 1976 to 2000, obesity increased from 14.4% to 30.9% of the U.S. population.

Source: "How'd I Get So Fat?" by A. Krueger *AARP*, January/February, 2005.

Comfort Food

Do we eat more in response to a stressor, like an exam? Researchers studied changes in eating in response to a real-life stressor, in a field study using students awaiting an exam. The students were each given a pager, which beeped 10 times a day at random intervals. Upon each signal, the participants rated their emotional state and motivation to eat. If they had eaten since the last signal, they reported their perceived reason for eating.

Compared to the control subjects, the students awaiting an exam reported higher emotional stress and an increased tendency to eat to distract themselves from stress. The results indicate that regulating emotion through eating is experienced in a student population during stress under real-life conditions. The use of distraction techniques helped students manage their stress-related eating.

Source: "The Perceived Function of Eating Is Changed During Examination Stress: A Field Study," by M. Macht, C. Haupt, and H. Ellgring, *Eating Behavior* 6(2): 109–112.

Eating to Cope—The Food/Mood Connection

First, some people respond to stress by overeating. Emotional eating is often mindless and unrelated to hunger. Some eat more because they gulp down meals too quickly. Others reach for snacks to calm their nerves and comfort themselves. We do not know why stress drives some people to eat more, but this clearly happens. These people use food as a coping mechanism to help them feel better temporarily. One theory being investigated is the connection between eating certain foods and the release of substances in the brain that are experienced as soothing. For example, the consumption of carbohydrates is linked to changes in neurotransmitter levels.

Downing a bag of M&Ms while you study for a test will not reduce your stress, and actually will more than likely increase your stress. A whole box of Twinkies may taste good but it will result in added anxiety in the long run. When we eat, our body releases a chemical called **dopamine,** which makes us feel good and can help offset the emotional pain we may be feeling from our stressful day. But food does not address the problem, nor does it help reduce stress levels. Avoid using food as a stress reliever by learning coping skills, such as exercise, meditation, or listening to music, that do not rely on food as a source of comfort.

Over-eating and unhealthy eating at night is especially problematic. Pamela Peeke, a physician trained in nutrition and author of *Body-for-Life for Women,* offers the following advice to deal with nighttime eating in response to stress:

> Nighttime appetite is very strongly associated with stress. Many people, especially women, hold on to their stresses all day and then come home and implode. They let it all go, feeling too overwhelmed to stick with their healthy eating regimen. I'd recommend doing a stress inventory, and then start learning to become more stress-resilient. Also make sure to eat a balance of smart foods every three to four hours to stave off a large evening hunger and appetite. And don't forget daily cardio and twice-weekly weight training.[9]

Unused Glucose

Second, when the body calls upon the fight-or-flight response, it draws glucose from stored glycogen and fat. In preparation for action, a flood of nutrients, enzymes, and hormones moves into the bloodstream and toward target organs. The liver increases sugar levels (glucose) into the bloodstream; the fat stores release fat to be used as energy or to be converted into blood sugar; and the liver releases cholesterol into the bloodstream to be used as additional energy. The outcome is that glycogen stores are depleted but the glucose that was released was not used for energy. When glucose is not used for physical activity, it is stored as fat. This helps explain why exercise is effective in reducing excess body fat.

Also, as you learned earlier in this chapter, the body responds to an increase in glucose by secreting insulin. In response to

---

Author Anecdote **The Stress Diet** As director of a corporate health promotion program, one of my responsibilities was to teach Healthy Body Weight classes. One day while discussing the relationship between stress and overeating, one of the class participants said he would like to share his typical stress diet. It went like this:

Breakfast—1 cup of coffee, ½ cup bran cereal with skim milk

Lunch—½ cup cottage cheese, 1 small apple

Mid-afternoon snack—1 Oreo cookie

Supper—Large pepperoni pizza, 3 pieces of garlic bread, large glass of pop, rest of the bag of Oreo cookies

Evening snack—½ gallon of rocky road ice cream—covered with hot fudge and nuts

We all laughed because we could truly relate. We start the day with such good intentions, and then . . .

—MH

insulin, blood glucose levels fall, resulting in hunger and low energy. The end result may be the individual eats excess calories.

The Cortisol Connection Third, activation of the stress response results in massive secretion of the stress hormone cortisol. One of the jobs of cortisol is to store energy. The body knows that when it encounters threatening circumstances, food may not be available immediately, so it stores energy as fat. One result of the continued secretion of cortisol is that the body stores fat in the arteries and the abdomen. This increases the risk for an unhealthy cardiovascular system.

Too much or too little cortisol can alter blood sugar levels and metabolism, ultimately causing increased appetite and weight gain, according to Shawn Talbott, author of *The Cortisol Connection*.[10] To get cortisol back to healthier levels, he suggests changing the high-stress, low-sleep, no-exercise cycle that frequently accompanies high cortisol levels.

Eating to cope, unused glucose, and the cortisol connection help explain how stress affects body weight, and especially body fat. The cycle of high stress response can contribute to weight gain. Additional weight on the body is unhealthy and stressful for many reasons.

Eating Disorders

Obesity is not the only issue related to stress and body weight. Eating disorders are increasing at an alarming rate. Eating disorders such as anorexia, bulimia, and binge eating are accompanied by extreme emotions, attitudes, and behaviors surrounding weight and food issues. The accompanying emotional and physical problems can have life-threatening consequences for females and males alike, although it is much more prevalent in females. Research has highlighted the association between perceived stress and eating disorders such as binge eating. For example, women who binge may perceive their stressors as more intense and emotionally disruptive than women who do not binge.[11]

The number of women seeking treatment for eating disorders has risen alarmingly. Cynthia Bulik, co-author of *Runaway Eating*, maintains that growing numbers of women engage in unhealthy eating behaviors to "run away" from emotional and stress-related problems. She defines **runaway eating** as the consistent use of food and food-related behaviors, such as purging or exercising excessively, to deal with unpleasant feelings and the sense that these feelings are out of control. Although the driving forces behind runaway eating and clinically defined disorders such as anorexia and bulimia are the same, the symptoms are not as severe or frequent for a runaway eater.[12]

Warning signs include alternating between severely restricting one's diet and eating large quantities of food, regularly performing exhausting exercise routines to burn off calories, and having at least one out-of-control binge in the last year. People with runaway eating often are desperate for tools to help with their problematic eating behaviors. But because they "fly beneath the radar" of the healthcare system, they usually are on their own.[13]

Several theorists have hypothesized that stressful situations may trigger abnormal eating and even eating disorders in people who are predisposed. A study to assess whether a stressful situation would reveal associations between perfectionism, low self-esteem, worry, and body mass index and measures of eating disorder symptoms in female high school students found that stress may stimulate behaviors related to eating disorders in predisposed individuals.[4]

Types of Eating Disorders The three most widely recognized eating disorders are anorexia, bulimia, and binge eating. Comprehensive coverage of these eating disorders is beyond the scope and intent of this book; however, awareness of some of the symptoms and contributing factors may facilitate early diagnosis and prompt treatment. The connection with stress and the potential impact of these disorders make them too important to ignore.

Anorexia **Anorexia** is characterized by self-starvation and excessive weight loss. Symptoms include:

- Refusal to maintain body weight at or above a minimally normal weight for height, body type, age, and activity level
- Intense fear of weight gain or being "fat"
- Feeling "fat" or overweight despite dramatic weight loss
- Loss of menstrual periods
- Extreme concern with body weight and shape

Bulimia **Bulimia** is characterized by a secretive cycle of binge eating followed by purging. The person with bulimia eats large amounts of food in short periods of time, then gets rid of the food and calories through vomiting, laxative abuse, or over-exercising. Symptoms include:

- Repeated episodes of binge eating and purging
- Feeling out of control during a binge and eating beyond the point of comfortable fullness
- Purging after a binge, typically by self-induced vomiting, abuse of laxatives, diet pills and/or diuretics, excessive exercise, or fasting
- Frequent dieting
- Extreme concern with body weight and shape

Binge Eating Disorder (also known as compulsive overeating) **Binge eating disorder** is characterized primarily by periods of uncontrolled, impulsive, or continuous eating beyond the point of feeling comfortably full. Although no purging is involved, the binge eater may fast sporadically or diet repetitively, and often feels shame or self-hatred after a binge. People who overeat compulsively may struggle with anxiety, depression, and loneliness, which can contribute to their unhealthy episodes of binge eating. Body weight may vary from normal to mild, moderate, or severe obesity.[15]

Causes of Eating Disorders   Although eating disorders may begin with a preoccupation with food and weight, they most often are about much more than food. Eating disorders are complex conditions that arise from a combination of long-standing behavioral, emotional, psychological, interpersonal, and social factors. Scientists and researchers are still learning about the underlying causes of these emotionally and physically damaging conditions.

   People with eating disorders often use food and the control of food in an attempt to compensate for feelings and emotions that otherwise may seem overwhelming. For some people, dieting, binge eating, and purging begin as a way to cope with painful emotions and to feel in control of one's life, but ultimately these behaviors will damage a person's physical and emotional health, self-esteem, and sense of competence and control.

Factors That Can Contribute to Eating Disorders

Psychological Factors

- Low self-esteem
- Feelings of inadequacy or lack of control in life
- Depression, anxiety, anger, or loneliness

Interpersonal Factors

- Troubled family and personal relationships
- Difficulty expressing emotions and feelings
- History of being teased or ridiculed based on size or weight
- History of physical or sexual abuse

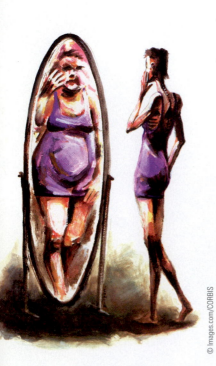

A distorted body image can result in eating disorders like anorexia and bulimia. These disorders have a profound impact on quality of life.

Social Factors

- Cultural pressures that glorify "thin" and place value on the "perfect body"
- Narrow definitions of beauty that apply to only women and men of specific body weights and shapes
- Cultural norms that value people on the basis of physical appearance and not inner qualities and strengths

Other Factors Scientists are still researching possible biochemical or biological causes of eating disorders. In some individuals with eating disorders, certain chemicals in the brain that control hunger, appetite, and digestion have been found to be out of balance. The exact meaning and implications of these imbalances remains under investigation.

Eating disorders are complex conditions that can arise from a variety of potential causes. Once begun, however, they can create a self-perpetuating cycle of physical and emotional destruction. All eating disorders require professional help.[16]

Clearly, stress has an impact on a wide range of factors related to eating and nutrition. Therefore, you should take time to carefully analyze your eating habits. Pay special attention to emotional factors associated with food and eating. Eating well is foundational to good health and positive stress management.

Sleep

In our busy world, getting a good night's sleep isn't as easy as it used to be. In 2001, 38% of people got 8 or more hours of sleep a night on weekdays. In 2005, that rate dropped to 26%.[17] Getting adequate sleep is vital to maintaining good health and reducing stress. Insufficient sleep is a prominent stressor and is responsible for a host of problems. Some people have difficulty going to sleep quickly, and others have difficulty staying asleep during the night. A good night's sleep is one in which you are fast asleep within a few minutes after your head hits the pillow, and the next thing you know, it is morning and you wake up feeling refreshed and alert.

It is easy to understand why it is difficult to fall asleep when we are stressed. The fight-or-flight response is one of arousal and activity—not rest. As we lay in bed trying to fall asleep, we simultaneously give ourselves messages that we should be on the alert for some potential threat—thinking over all the things that we must do tomorrow or all the problems we faced earlier today—which automatically initiates the stress response. Consequently, we remain awake and alert.

The hyperarousal caused by stress can upset the balance between sleep and wakefulness by altering the chemical and physiological balance. Stress and sleep affect each other. Stress is often a contributing factor to sleep problems, and insufficient sleep contributes to stress.

How Much Sleep Do You Need? There is no right amount of sleep for everyone. Some people function fine with 6 hours of sleep, and others can't function optimally with less than 9 hours. Most people need 7 to 8 hours of sleep each night.

Tip: To find out how much sleep is right for you, try this experiment: For four days in a row, go to sleep at about the same time each night. During this time, avoid unusual or excessive activities, such as too much exercise, drinking alcohol, or taking medication. Allow yourself to awaken naturally each morning without an alarm. Each morning write down the time and calculate the amount of time you slept. Calculate the average amount of sleep you get per night by adding each night's sleep time, and then divide by the number of nights. This will give you a fairly good indication of the amount of sleep that is appropriate for your mind and body.

Suggestions for Improving Sleep Once we reduce our stress levels, we usually find that sleep occurs naturally and effortlessly. Here are a few suggestions for improving sleep:

- Go to bed at the same time each day.
- Get up at the same time each day.

Sleep and Stress

Princeton Survey Research Associates conducted a survey of 1,250 adults investigating the relationship between stress levels and amount of sleep. The results showed that adults who sleep 6 or fewer hours each night are significantly more likely than those who get more sleep to feel great stress every day. By contrast, only 14% of adults who sleep 7 to 8 hours each night feel stress daily.

Source: "To Reduce Stress, Hit the Hay," by N. T. Kate, *American Demographics 16*(9): 14–15.

FYI

Sleep-Deprived

A poll by the National Sleep Foundation found that 75% of adults frequently have a symptom of a sleep problem such as frequent waking during the night or snoring. According to the report, only about half of respondents are able to say on most nights, "I had a good night's sleep." Results from the 2005 survey indicate that more adults are experiencing sleep problems regularly. A large majority (75%) report having had at least one symptom of a sleep problem a few nights a week or more within the past year. This continues an upward trend in the prevalence of sleep problems since 1999 (see figure below). For the purposes of the Sleep in America poll, symptoms of a sleep problem were defined as: having difficulty falling asleep, waking a lot during the night, waking up too early and not being able to get back to sleep, waking up feeling unrefreshed, snoring, unpleasant feelings in the legs (Restless Leg Syndrome), and/or experiencing pauses in breathing.

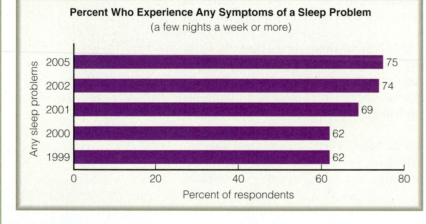

Percent Who Experience Any Symptoms of a Sleep Problem
(a few nights a week or more)

Year	Percent
2005	75
2002	74
2001	69
2000	62
1999	62

Any sleep problems — Percent of respondents

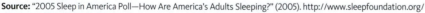

Source: "2005 Sleep in America Poll—How Are America's Adults Sleeping?" (2005). http://www.sleepfoundation.org/

- Get regular exercise each day. Evidence indicates that regular exercise—including stretching and aerobic exercise—improves restful sleep. It may be best to avoid vigorous exercise within 3–4 hours before bedtime.
- Get regular exposure to outdoor or bright lights, especially in the late afternoon.
- Keep the temperature in your bedroom comfortably cool. Have extra blankets if you get too cold.
- Be sure to have a quiet bedroom when you're sleeping.
- Keep the bedroom dark enough to facilitate sleep.
- Use your bed only for sleep and sex.
- Do a relaxation exercise just before going to sleep.
- Start winding down 2 hours before bedtime. This amount of time allows the brain to wind down and decrease its activity so the sleep systems can take over.

Do *not* do the following activities:

- Consume caffeine in the evening (coffee, tea with caffeine, energy drinks, sodas).
- Watch television in bed.
- Use alcohol to help you sleep. Alcohol has been found to disrupt the sleep cycle in some individuals.
- Go to bed too hungry or too full.
- Take another person's sleeping pills.
- Take over-the-counter sleeping pills without your doctor's knowledge. Tolerance can develop rapidly with some medications.
- Try to force yourself to sleep. This only makes your mind and body more alert.
- Sleep with your pets or children.

If you lie in bed awake for more than 20 to 30 minutes, get up and go to a different room, participate in a quiet activity, such as reading, then return to bed when you feel sleepy.[18]

A good night's sleep, regular exercise, and a healthy, balanced diet are all vital components of a healthy lifestyle and essential ingredients for your successful stress management plan. But it is not just what you do that is important; equally important are behaviors to avoid.

CULTURE CONNECTION

Risky Business

Researchers have shown that many college students engage in various risky behaviors, including alcohol use, tobacco, use, physical inactivity, and unhealthy eating practices. The failure of college students to engage in healthier lifestyle practices is not unique to the United States.* Researchers surveyed university students from 13 European countries in 1990 regarding smoking, physical exercise, fruit and fat intake, and beliefs about the importance of behaviors to health. They repeated the study in 2000 and found that the prevalence of smoking had increased and consumption of fruit had significantly decreased during this period, while physical exercise and fat intake remained stable.

*"Predictors of Health Behaviors in College Students," by D. Von Ah, S. Ebert, A. Ngamvitroj, N. Park, and D. Kang, *Journal of Advanced Nursing* 48(5) (2004): 463–474.

Source:
"Trends in Smoking, Diet, Physical Exercise, and Attitudes Toward Health in European University Students from 13 Countries, 1990–2000," by A. Steptoe, D. Phil, J. Wardle, W. Cui, F. Bellisle, A. Zotti, R. Baranyai, and R. Sanderman, *Preventive Medicine 35* (2002): 97–104.

Lifestyle Behaviors to Avoid

In our culture, chemicals are a common choice for combating stress. The next time you are watching a movie that portrays people who are stressed to the max, notice what they do. You may hear something like, "I could use a stiff drink." Another common option is to make a beeline to the medicine cabinet for the most powerful magic bullet they can find (usually in the form of a tranquilizer). Others reach for a cigarette as a means to relax—an ineffective means of long-term stress management, which contributes to the stress of declining health.

Tobacco An individual with a high stress level is approximately 15 times as likely to be a smoker as a person with low stress. About half of smokers identify workplace stress as a key factor in their smoking.[19] Inability to cope with stress has long been associated with risky health behaviors such as smoking in adolescents and young adults. Many young smokers justify smoking as a means of dealing with their stress.[20]

Nicotine is a dangerous and highly addictive stimulant. The effects of nicotine mimic those of the stress response in many ways, among them:

An individual with a high stress level is approximately 15 times more likely to be a smoker than a person with low stress.

- An increase in heart rate
- Increase in blood pressure
- Increase in output of blood cholesterol
- Decrease in size of blood vessels (especially dangerous when this happens to arteries in the heart or brain)
- Increase in blood clotting

If the result of tobacco use can be a heart attack or a stroke, why do people frequently "have a smoke" when they are feeling stressed? While smoking, the person may get an immediate "buzz" from the nicotine that feels better than the pain of the stress. Smoking also is a familiar behavior that results in a feeling of their being in control—even though the nicotine is what is really in control. By going outside in the fresh air or to a designated smoking area, the smoker escapes whatever is causing the stress. Another reason a person might feel more relaxed by smoking is that smoking results in breathing differently—inhaling more deeply, for example—and deep breathing can be relaxing. Whatever the reason people choose to smoke, it is an unhealthy and ineffective way to manage stress because of the harmful long-term effects.

FYI

Smoker Stats

According to government data, about one in three people in the United States currently smokes. Each year, smoking claims more than 400,000 lives in the United States. That is more deaths from smoking than AIDS, alcohol, drug abuse, car crashes, murders, suicides, and fires combined!

The good news is that more young people in the United States are deciding not to smoke. Cigarette smoking has declined in young adults between the ages of 18 and 25. The number of young people becoming daily smokers has dropped by a third.

Source: http://www.cdc.gov/tobacco. "HHS Report Shows Drug Use Rates Stable, Youth Tobacco Use Declines," *Medical Letter on the CDC & FDA*, Oct. 21, 2001.

Drinking and Race

In her book *An Invitation to Health*, Dianne Hales has compiled an insightful summary recognizing racial and ethnic differences in factors related to drinking.

* * *

The African American community. Overall, African Americans consume less alcohol per person than whites, yet twice as many African Americans die of cirrhosis of the liver each year.

The Hispanic community. The various Hispanic cultures tend to discourage drinking by women but encourage heavy drinking by men as part of machismo, or feelings of manhood. Hispanic men have higher rates of alcohol use and abuse than the general population, yet few enter treatment programs. This may be attributed to lack of information, language barriers, and the cultural values that discourage males from sharing personal information and the conviction that families should solve problems themselves.

The Native American community. Native Americans have three times the rate of the general population in alcohol-related injury and illness. Both a biological predisposition and socioeconomic conditions may contribute to alcohol abuse in this population. Certainly, not all Native Americans drink, yet in some tribes, 10.5 out of every 1,000 newborns have fetal alcohol syndrome, compared with 1 to 3 out of 1,000 in the general population.

The Asian American community. Asian Americans tend to drink very little or not at all. This may relate to cultural values and to inborn physiological reactions to alcohol that result in facial flushing, rapid heart rate, lowered blood pressure, nausea, and other unpleasant symptoms. A very high percentage of women of all Asian American nationalities abstain completely.

Source: *An Invitation to Health* 2009–2010 Edition by D. Hales (Belmont, CA: Wadsworth/Cengage Learning, 2009).

Men More Than Twice as Likely as Women to Develop Alcohol Dependence

Men have more than a 1 in 5 lifetime risk of developing alcohol abuse or dependence according to Marc A. Schuckit, MD, from the University of California, San Diego. Genetic factors account for about 40% to 60% of the risk for alcohol-use disorders, and environmental factors, such as alcohol availability, attitudes toward drinking, peer pressure, stress levels, coping strategies, and drinking laws, account for the rest of the risk, he added. As many as 80% of alcohol-dependent individuals are also regular smokers, which could either reflect an overlapping genetic predisposition or use of the second drug to deal with effects of the first drug.

The good news is that while there is a widespread public perception that treatment for alcohol abuse is ineffective, the majority of patients—both men and women—do well after therapy, according to Dr. Schuckit's recent *Lancet* article.

Source: *Lancet.* Published online January 23, 2009.

Alcohol

Much has been written about alcohol abuse in college populations. Excessive alcohol consumption is a widespread problem on many college campuses, as students away from home for the first time may feel overwhelmed and insecure. Many turn to alcohol as a means to let loose and feel accepted, as Jason's story related in our opening vignette. Students sometimes use alcohol as a form of self-medication to temporarily ease feelings of pain or stress.

Adolescents frequently use alcohol prior to and during the early college years. Drinking by adolescents and young adults is influenced by some unique factors: The adolescent's brain is unique and differs from that of both younger individuals and adults in ways that predispose adolescents to behave in certain ways, increasing their sensitivity to stressors and their propensity to initiate alcohol use.[21]

Alcohol consumption on college campuses has been linked to where students live on campus and what they perceive as the norm for acceptable drinking. Studies have found that stress-related drinking is common especially in competitive academic environments where students turn to alcohol to reduce their anxiety and pressure to perform. Athletes have higher drinking rates than nonathletes.[22] Fraternity members are among the heaviest drinkers, with the highest incidence of heavy drinking and binge drinking.[23]

The association between drinking and stress is complicated because both drinking behavior and an individual's response to stress are determined by multiple genetic and environmental factors. Many factors determine whether an

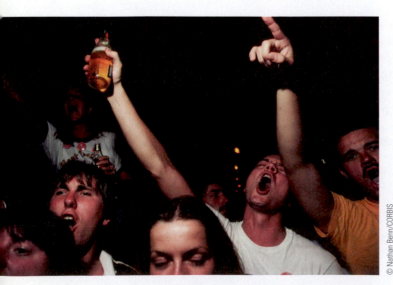

© Nathan Benn/CORBIS

Stress-related drinking is common especially in competitive academic environments where students turn to alcohol to try to reduce their anxiety and pressure to perform.

Stress and the Alcoholic

Researchers studied a group of men who completed inpatient alcoholism treatment and later experienced severe and prolonged psychosocial stress prior to and independent of any alcohol use. The researchers found that subjects who relapsed experienced twice as much severe and prolonged stress before their return to drinking as those who remained abstinent.

In this study, severe psychosocial stress was related to relapse in alcoholic males who expected alcohol to reduce their stress. Those most vulnerable to stress-related relapse scored low on measure of coping skills, self-efficacy, and social support. Stress-related relapse was highest among those who had less confidence in their ability to resist drinking and among those who relied on drinkers for social support.

Although many factors can influence a return to drinking, the researchers concluded that stress may exert its greatest influence on the initial consumption of alcohol after a period of abstinence.

Source: "Stress, Vulnerability, and Adult Alcohol Relapse," by S. Brown, P. Vik, T. Patterson, I. Grant, and M. Schuckit, *Journal of Studies on Alcohol,* 56(5) (1995): 538–545.

individual will turn to alcohol as a means of coping with life's challenges. Racial and ethnic variables may play a part.

Studies indicate that people drink as a means of coping with economic stress, job stress, and marital problems, often in the absence of social support, and that the more severe and chronic the stressor, the greater the alcohol consumption.[24] Whether an individual will drink in response to stress, however, seems to depend on many factors, including possible genetic determinants of drinking in response to stress, an individual's usual drinking behavior, one's expectations regarding the effect of alcohol on stress, the intensity and type of stressor, the individual's sense of control over the stressor, the range of one's responses to cope with the perceived stress, and the availability of social support to buffer the effects of stress.[25]

Although most people drink because they think it will help them reduce stress, more than one or two drinks per day can lead to many problems, including alcoholism, liver diseases, various cancers, and many types of accidents. Drinking also is associated with other unhealthy behaviors such as smoking, sexual aggression, and violence.

If you need help to reduce your drinking, support is available. Student health and counseling services are prepared to assist you. Excessive alcohol consumption is an unhealthy, ineffective strategy for preventing stress. This book is filled with more adaptive, healthy ways of coping with stress.

Drugs We live in a society in which many people turn to drugs as an answer to problems. Choosing drugs and alcohol as a way of coping with stress is an unhealthy choice, with many negative consequences. Because of the prevalence of two drugs—tobacco and

Stress Busting Behavior: Healthy Choices

Check those items that are currently part of your regular routine. Underline the item that you think has the greatest positive impact on your ability to manage your stress. Circle the item that you need to work on the most.

- ☐ Cardiorespiratory exercise
- ☐ Muscle fitness exercise
- ☐ Flexibility exercise
- ☐ Body composition exercise
- ☐ Eating a balanced diet from a variety of healthy foods
- ☐ Avoiding excessive caffeine
- ☐ Maintaining a healthy weight
- ☐ Avoiding eating to cope with stress
- ☐ Getting 7 to 8 hours of sleep
- ☐ Abstaining from tobacco products
- ☐ Avoiding use of alcohol to cope with stress
- ☐ Not using drugs to cope with stress

Stress and Drug Addiction

Stress may be one of the most powerful triggers for relapse in addicted individuals even after long periods of abstinence from abused substances. This is one of the conclusions of an extensive report published by the National Institute on Drug Abuse of the National Institute of Health on the relationship between stress and drug use and abuse. The report suggests several more conclusions on how stress may affect drug use.

- Individuals exposed to stress are more likely to abuse alcohol and other drugs or undergo relapse.
- High stress was found to predict continued drug use.

- In animals not previously exposed to illicit substances, stressors increased vulnerability for self-administration of drugs.
- Among drug-free cocaine abusers in treatment, exposure to personal stress situations led to consistent and significant increases in the craving for cocaine, along with activation of emotional stress and a physiological stress response.
- Stress induces relapse to heroin, cocaine, alcohol, and nicotine self-administration in animal studies. There is a strong relationship between stress coping resources and the ability to sustain abstinence.

Source: http://www.nida.nih.gov

FYI

Only 3% of Americans Follow a Healthy Lifestyle

Growing research shows that following a healthy lifestyle has substantial health benefits. Many public health messages emphasize the importance of adopting healthy lifestyle habits. But when it comes to healthy living, Americans have a long way to go. The results of one study found that only 3% of Americans follow all four key healthy lifestyle habits: not smoking, maintaining a healthy body weight, consuming five or more fruits and vegetables per day, and exercising at least moderately for 30 minutes or more at least 5 days per week.

Source: "Healthy Lifestyle Characteristics Among Adults in the United States, 2000," by M. Reeves and A. Rafferty, in *Archives of Internal Medicine* 165(8) (2005): 854–857.

alcohol—in college students, we focused in this chapter on these two, and their impact on stress. Although alcohol is the number-one drug of abuse among college students, marijuana is the most commonly used illegal drug.[26] Some students turn to a plethora of additional drugs, both legal and illegal, in a quest to find peace of mind.

Illegal drugs are unhealthy and ineffective for reducing stress. The results can be deceptive because some drugs create a cycle of dependence by masking the symptoms of stress, which results in temporarily feeling better. Nevertheless, drugs do not eliminate the cause of the stress and must be avoided. Fortunately, there are better tools than mind-numbing chemicals to reduce stress. Compelling research, along with strong anecdotal evidence of individual successes, demonstrates that certain stress-management techniques work powerfully and immediately to effectively reduce stress.

Occasionally, prescription or over-the-counter drugs are required, but these must be used with care. When people turn to tranquilizers to relax, they run the risk of becoming dependent and incurring the side effects that often accompany drug use. Your healthcare provider can help you determine if you need medication.

Putting It All Together

Understanding that making healthy choices and living a healthy lifestyle is fundamental to well-being is not a new idea to most of us. Still, it is an idea of which we need to be reminded frequently. The key is the difference between *knowing* and *doing*.

Now that you have read this chapter, take time to carefully reflect on your daily choices. Pay attention to both the healthy and the unhealthy ways you choose to deal with stress. Decide how you can integrate more healthy choices into your routine and eliminate unhealthy choices.

Author Anecdote ### The Power of Prevention

As a nurse for many years, I've seen the stress and suffering caused by poor lifestyle choices. We live in a society that favors quick-fixes to our health over the slow, steady prevention approach. We've become conditioned to the idea that regardless of what we do to ourselves, someone in the healthcare system will "fix" us. Once we are "broken," we will pay dearly to have our health back, yet we often fail to realize that we are frequently the cause of our ill health in the first place. We know that physical inactivity and a negative lifestyle poses a serious threat to our health and well-being, yet many continue to make unhealthy daily choices. When we look for the quick-fix—the pill, the drug, or the treatment that will fix us after we have neglected to do our part—we fail to fully grasp the importance of our own responsibility in making healthy choices.

The good news is that it is in our control to make daily choices that lead to better health and enjoyment of life. Our lifestyle and daily behaviors are by far the most significant factors in preventing stress and promoting health. We tend to greatly underestimate the importance of daily habits including regular exercise, a balanced diet, and adequate sleep, as well as the need to avoid unhealthy habits such as drinking and smoking. Think about your typical day—what you do from the time you wake up in the morning until you go to sleep at night. The many small choices and behaviors we make day in and day out determine to a large extent how healthy we are and how well we deal with stress. Best of all, a healthy lifestyle is your decision to make.

—MH

Conclusion

This chapter is about preventing stress through healthy lifestyle choices. Exercising, eating right, getting adequate sleep, and avoiding unhealthy behaviors are the foundations for good health. Think about how you can use the information in this chapter to feel better and more in control of your stress. Even small changes, consistent and over time, can yield great results.

15.1 The Power of Exercise to Reduce Stress

PURPOSE The purpose of this activity is to help you see the benefits of including exercise as part of a healthy lifestyle to help you reduce stress. Exercise, especially slightly higher intensity exercise like jogging or playing racquetball, follows through on the message to move that is inherent in the fight-or-flight response.

DIRECTIONS Exercise using any activity that will keep your heart rate elevated for 30 to 60 minutes. Do this activity at a time when you are feeling very high levels of stress such as just before or after an important test or after you've been in a heated argument with someone. During this time of extreme stress, instead of watching TV, sitting and dwelling on the event, or grabbing a beer, move. Do something with enough intensity that you get out of breath and find yourself sweating.

After you are finished, notice the change in how you feel. Certainly, the stressor hasn't changed, but you have followed through on the message you have been giving yourself to fight or run (fight-or-flight response) and you can now approach the situation in a more calm and level-headed way. Respond to these statements:

1. Describe the cause of your stress.

2. How did you feel before you started exercising?

3. What exercise or activity did you select?

4. Describe how you felt physically, emotionally, and mentally at the conclusion of your exercise session.

5. Explain in your own words how exercise works to manage stress.

Key Points

- Lifestyle habits have a significant impact on our ability to prevent and manage stress.
- Exercise is one of our most powerful stress buffers for a variety of reasons.
- An exercise program should be balanced, for cardiorespiratory fitness, optimum body composition, muscle fitness, and flexibility.
- The best nutritional preparation for stress is a varied and balanced diet. The *Dietary Guidelines for Americans* and *MyPyramid* provide science-based guidance for nutritional health.
- Three factors that help explain how stress contributes to obesity are: eating to cope, unused glucose, and the cortisol connection.

- Eating disorders—anorexia, bulimia, and binge eating disorder—have a clear connection to perceived stress and control.
- Getting adequate sleep is essential to maintaining good health and reducing stress.
- To maintain a healthy lifestyle, people should avoid activities such as tobacco, alcohol, and drug use, which they sometimes believe erroneously will help them relax or cope with stress.
- Two drugs that are especially prevalent among college students are alcohol and tobacco.
- Whether to adhere to a healthy lifestyle is your choice to make.

Key Terms

cardiorespiratory fitness
muscle fitness
muscle strength
muscle endurance
flexibility
body composition

Dietary Guidelines for Americans
Recommended Dietary Allowances
(RDA)
serotonin
glycemic index

dopamine
runaway eating
anorexia
bulimia
binge eating disorder

Discussion Time For Critical Thinking/Discussion Questions, please visit this book's Premium Website.

Notes

1. "Predictors of Health Behaviors in College Students," by D. Von Ah, S. Ebert, A. Ngamvitroj, N. Park, and D. Kang, *Journal of Advanced Nursing* 48(5) (2004): 463–474.

2. *Smart Exercise: Burning Fat, Getting Fit*, by C. Bailey (Boston: Houghton Mifflin Company, 1994).

3. *Health Assessment and Promotion Strategies Through the Lifespan* (6th ed.), by R. Murray and J. Zentner (Stamford, CT: Appleton & Lange, 1997).

4. "Attitude Adjustment," by L. Shelton, *Natural Health* 34(3) (Mar. 2004).

5. *An Invitation to Health* 2009-2010 Edition by D. Hales (Belmont, CA: Wadsworth/Cengage Learning, 2009).

6. "Sales of Energy Drinks Top $3 Billion—But at What Cost?," by S. Worcester, *Clinical Psychiatric News*, Vol. 35, No. 3, March 2007, p. 42.

7. "The Problem with Energy Drinks," *MMR*, Vol. 24, No. 1, January 8, 2007, p. 73.

8. "Caffeine Affects Cardiovascular and Neuroendocrine Activation at Work and at Home," by J. D. Lane, C. F. Pieper, B. G. Phillips-Bute, J. E. Bryant, and C. M. Kuhn, *Psychosomatic Medicine* 64(4) (2002 Jul–Aug): 595–603.

9. "Take a Stress Inventory for Diet Success," by P. Peeke, *USA Today,* 5D (2005, May 9).

10. *The Cortisol Connection: Why Stress Makes You Fat and Ruins Your Health—and What You Can Do About It*, by S. Talbott (Alameda, CA: Hunter House, 2002).

11. "The Role of Daily Hassles in Binge Eating," by J. Crowther, J. Sanftner, D. Bonifazi, and K. Shepherd, *International Journal of Eating Disorders* 29 (2001): 449–454.

12. "Women Binge to Relieve Stress," Newsview section, *USA Today Magazine 133*(2719) (2005, April).

13. Newsview, "Women Binge to Relieve Stress."

14. "The Role of Stress in the Association Between Low Self-Esteem, Perfectionism, and Worry, and Eating Disorders," by S. Sassaroli and G. Ruggiero, *International Journal of Eating Disorders* 37(2) (2005): 135–141.

15. http://www.nationaleatingdisorders.org

16. http://www.nationaleatingdisorders.org

17. http://www.sleepfoundation.org

18. "Sleep Hygiene for Patients," by D. St. John (2000), http://www.vh.org/adult/patient/psychiatry/sleephygiene/index.html.

19. Hales, *An Invitation to Health.*

20. "Personality, Stress and the Decision to Commence Cigarette Smoking in Adolescence," by D. Byrne, A. Byrne, and M. Reinhart, *Journal of Psychosomatic Research* 39(1) (1995): 53–62.

21. "The Adolescent Brain and the College Drinker: Biological Basis of Propensity to Use and Misuse Alcohol," by L. Spear, *Journal of Studies on Alcohol,* supplement no. 14 (2002): 71–81.

22. "Comparison of Patterns of Alcohol Use Between High School and College Athletes and Nonathletes," by K. Hildebran and D. Johnson, *Research Quarterly for Exercise and Sport 72* (March 2001).

23. Hales, *An Invitation to Stress.*

24. "Stress and Alcohol Interaction: An Update of Human Research," by L. Pohorecky, *Alcoholism: Clinical and Experimental Research* 15(3) (1991): 438–459.

25. "Alcohol Alert," *National Institute on Alcohol Abuse and Alcoholism,* No. 32 PH 363, April 1996.

26. "Binge Drinking Among Undergraduate College Students in the United States: Implications for Other Substance Use," by S. Jones, et al., *Journal of American College Health 50*(1) (July 2001): 33.

16 Introduction to Relaxation

■ What is relaxation and how is it different from simply unwinding in front of the television set to enjoy some rest? ■ What should I do if I try one of the relaxation exercises in the following chapters and it doesn't help me relax or feel any better? ■ How can I get the most out of a relaxation technique?

Study of this chapter will enable you to:

1. Define and explain what relaxation is.
2. Identify the benefits of relaxation.
3. Explain the tips for a successful relaxation experience.
4. Experience the benefits of the Power Nap.

But, of course, the instant I try to make myself relax, true relaxation vanishes, and in its place is a strange phenomenon called trying to relax. Relaxation happens only when allowed, never as a result of trying or making.

—W. Tim Gallway

The Power Nap Experience I love this exercise! Before I started the Power Nap for the first time, I was feeling really tensed up from the day. I felt good, but I felt really tired and ready to go to bed. I wasn't quite as relaxed as I wanted to be. So the Power Nap was a great opportunity for me to calm myself down before bed. I was a little apprehensive about the ordeal; I wondered what it would be like. During the Power Nap session, I felt so relaxed. It was surprising for me to feel this relaxed. I was glad that I was able to experience the Power Nap because I had no idea how relaxed I could be. I was actually only focusing on one thing at once, not a million things. It was so surprising that I actually started laughing! After the Power Nap exercise, I dropped right into bed and slept so well! I don't think I have slept that well in a long time. The whole night was relatively undisturbed. I woke up easily, which was so awesome because lately it has been *SO HARD* for me to wake up! I think I'll be doing this every night. —*Nikki R.*

The first time I did the Power Nap exercise was when I was exhausted, and my kids had just gone down for a nap. I was tired by mid-week; however, I had a million and one things that needed to be done. Therefore, I was not going to take a two-hour nap. To say the least, I was exhausted. I started the exercise. My whole body seemed to fall asleep except I was conscious of what was going on. As I continued the exercise, my body was numb. It was a totally awesome feeling. After I finished the exercise, I felt like I had just taken a nap. However, I didn't have the groggy yawning feeling of being awakened from a long nap. I began to do the things that needed to be done around the house. About an hour later, I never even noticed that I had been tired earlier in the day. I felt recharged. I fell asleep easily that night because I had not napped so long in the day. The second time I did the Power Nap exercise was after getting home from work at 11 o'clock at night. I was thoroughly drained of all energy. After I was done with the exercise, I felt like a zombie. I walked straight into my bedroom and melted into my bed. I didn't have a problem falling asleep and slept exceptionally well. When my children woke me at 7 o'clock the next morning, I wasn't tired or ornery. I was ready for the day! It's amazing what those 10 minutes can do for your body and mind. I'm delighted with this exercise! —*April L.*

Introduction to Relaxation

If we could manage stress by managing our thoughts and actions in the ways we have described thus far, the book could end here. We would have solved the problem of too much stress. In the real world, however, despite our best efforts to prevent stress, it happens. The stress response turns on automatically, and we find ourselves with the classic symptoms of stress. If you are living a typical modern-day life, stress is unavoidable. Therefore, we need tools that we can call upon immediately to turn off the stress response and, consequently, avoid the health problems associated with chronic stress.

Part III covered a variety of stress prevention strategies, with an emphasis on changing the way we think about potential stressors or by reducing or eliminating the number of stressors in our lives. But what do you do when this is not possible? In Part IV you will learn ways to reduce stress and tension through techniques that put your body into a relaxed state. These techniques work primarily on the mental and physical dimensions. As you will learn, cognitive relaxation techniques, such as guided imagery, autogenics, and meditation, have a powerful effect on reducing stress at the mental level. When you relax the mind, the body relaxes as well. Physical techniques, such as massage, progressive relaxation, and yoga, alter the body's physiology. These physical methods can diminish stress by turning tension into relaxation. Used together, the mental and physical relaxation techniques produce immediate and effective relaxation.

> Stress is inner biofeedback, signaling you that frequencies are fighting within your system. The purpose of stress isn't to hurt you, but to let you know it's time to go back to the heart and start loving.
>
> —*Sara Paddison*

FYI

Stress Balls to the Rescue You have probably come across at least one of the many stress-relief products touted as the answer to your stress troubles. It might have been in the form of a relaxation candle or a special scented pillow. Maybe it was tension-reducing tea—drink a cup and all your cares will disappear.

Do these stress-relief products work? The answer is: It depends. Some products, such as the soft, squeezable stress balls, actually might help reduce muscle tension in a manner similar to progressive muscle relaxation. Others, such as the relaxation candles, most likely won't work alone, but in conjunction with soaking in a warm bubble bath, they might help. But don't expect any magic cures or secret potions. Most of the stress products probably won't hurt, and some will help, especially if combined with a stress reduction exercise.

Understanding Relaxation

The *Oxford Dictionary of English* defines relaxation as 1: the state of being free from tension and anxiety; 2: the restoration of equilibrium following disturbance. Within the health literature, relaxation is described as "a state of relative freedom from both anxiety and skeletal muscle tension."[2] Herbert Benson, author of the *Relaxation Response*, defines relaxation as "a state of decreased psychophysiological arousal: a calming state."[3] For purposes of this text, we will define **relaxation** as the process of effectively moving the mind/body from the stress response to the relaxation response.

True relaxation requires commitment and action. This might sound like a contradiction but, fortunately, the kind of action involved in stress management is the kind that produces pleasant, positive results. The purpose of relaxation techniques is to directly activate parasympathetic nervous system activity. Relaxation exercises turn off the stress response and at the same time produce an increase in mental alertness and mental abilities. These exercises also tend to increase physical energy.

Relaxation as defined in this chapter is not the same thing as watching television, reading a good book, or even viewing a sunset. It also is not the same thing as daydreaming or letting the mind wander aimlessly. These things are easy to do, and they are pleasant and enjoyable, but they aren't designed to activate the relaxation response. Relaxation isn't even the same as sleeping or napping. The stress response can be activated even when you sleep—as anyone who sleeps with a teeth-grinding bed partner will attest. The relaxed state is the opposite of the stressed state; therefore, a person typically cannot be both stressed and relaxed at the same time.

In Part IV of this book, you will discover a wide assortment of relaxation techniques that you can immediately include in your busy days to help reduce stress. As you begin to practice and experiment with them, here are a couple of important points to keep in mind:

- *Not every relaxation technique works the same for everyone.* There is some variability in which methods work best for each person. Experiment with the different methods to discover which techniques are most effective for you. Soon you will find that some of the exercises relax you and restore your energy and others do not have a noticeable effect on you.
- *You should try each method several times.* With regular practice, the positive effects of relaxation carry over into daily activities. As sure as the weight lifter gets stronger with

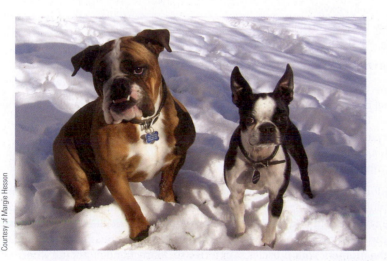

Courtesy of Margie Hesson

Jango and Wedge.

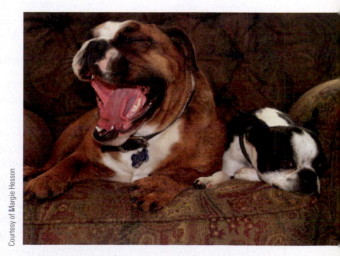

Courtesy of Margie Hesson

For Jango and Wedge total relaxation comes naturally.

Curbing Late Night Hunger Through Relaxation

Regularly practicing relaxation may be an important component of treatment for the condition known as Nighttime Eating Syndrome (NES). NES is characterized by a lack of appetite in the morning, consumption of 50% or more of daily food intake after 6:00 p.m., and difficulty falling and/or staying asleep. NES has been associated with stress and with poor results at attempts to lose weight.

Researchers randomly assigned subjects to either a relaxation group (each practicing 20 minutes of progressive relaxation each day) or a control group (each quietly sat for the same amount of time each day). After practicing these exercises daily for a week, the subjects who practiced the relaxation exercise exhibited lowered stress, anxiety, fatigue, anger, and depression. The results indicated that 20 minutes of the muscle relaxation exercise significantly reduced stress, anxiety, and salivary cortisol immediately after each session. Progressive relaxation also was associated with significantly higher morning and lower afternoon and evening ratings of hunger, and a trend toward both more breakfast and less nighttime eating. It follows that relaxation exercises may have a positive effect on preventing obesity.

Source: "Night Eating Syndrome: Effects of Brief Relaxation Training on Stress, Mood, Hunger, and Eating Patterns," by F. A. Pawlow, P. M. O'Neil, and R. J. Malcolm, *International Journal of Obesity, 27*(8), 970–979.

regular practice, the regular practice of relaxation exercises produces profound and noticeable results. We find ourselves calmer and more composed, less easily irritated, and feeling better generally. When that happens, the benefits spill over into other areas of life. Relationships may improve, we enjoy our days more, and life in general seems to be better. These are natural byproducts of regular practice. We simply need to practice and watch for the results.

Some of the methods of relaxation found in the following chapters may be familiar to you, and others are new and may seem unusual, yet each has been found to be effective. Approach each new technique with an open, inquisitive mind, and see which ones work for you. Several of the relaxation exercises also are found under the audio files at the Premium Website.

Benefits of Relaxation

Why relax? With so many things to do, it's easy to put off taking time to relax each day. But in doing so, you miss out on the health benefits of relaxation. According to experts at the Mayo Clinic,[4] relaxation can improve how your body responds to stress by:

- Slowing your heart rate, which translates into less work for your heart
- Reducing your blood pressure
- Slowing your breathing rate
- Reducing the need for oxygen
- Increasing blood flow to the major muscles
- Lessening muscle tension

After practicing relaxation skills, you may experience the following benefits:

- Fewer symptoms of illness, such as headaches, nausea, diarrhea, and pain
- Fewer emotional responses such as anger, crying, anxiety, apprehension, and frustration
- More energy
- Improved concentration
- Better ability to handle problems
- More efficiency in daily activities

Relaxation produces many health benefits. As you learn to relax, you will become more aware of muscle tension and other physical sensations caused by the stress response. In time, you may even notice your body's reaction before you take mental note of your stress. Once you know how the stress response feels, you can make a conscious effort to switch to relaxation mode the moment your muscles start to tense. Many benefits accrue when we move from physical and psychological arousal to relaxation.

Getting Started

As you are learning new relaxation methods, these suggestions can help make your experience more pleasant and effective. Once you are more experienced, you may find you can get results nearly anywhere at any time, but while you are learning, these suggestions can prove to be helpful:

- Give yourself a minimum of 10 to 20 minutes each day to practice a relaxation activity. Twice a day for 30 minutes may yield even better results. Just like getting regular exercise and eating a healthy diet, practicing relaxation exercises is an important component of a healthy lifestyle.
- Seclude yourself where you will not be interrupted. This is especially important when you are learning a new technique.
- Minimize background noises. Turn off the telephone, your cell phone, and any device that might have an alarm.
- Practice the relaxation techniques during the times of the day recommended for each one. Some are done more appropriately in the morning, and others have a more positive effect in the afternoon or immediately before going to sleep. With practice, you will find what works best for you.
- Don't be in a hurry to end the relaxation exercise. If you hurry to finish a relaxation exercise, it will feel much the same as you feel when you awaken from a deep sleep to a ringing telephone. Hurrying to end a relaxation exercise is disruptive and can leave you feeling off balance for the rest of the day, so at the end of your session take several minutes to return to normal waking consciousness. Hurrying to finish can spoil all the work you do resting and restoring your mind and body during a relaxation exercise.
- Approach each exercise without expectations. The best attitude is one of openness to whatever results you experience. As you practice, say to yourself, "I will take what I get. If I get nothing, that's what I get . . . and that's okay. If I get some deep rest and relaxation, that's what I get as well. It's also okay if I feel rejuvenated and energized." Trying too hard to make the exercise work will counteract the desired effects.
- Regardless of how unusual any of these exercises might seem to you, they have been found to be effective in turning off the stress response and restoring balance. If you notice yourself resisting an exercise because it seems too odd, simply acknowledge the thought and continue with an open, inquisitive mind. Don't let the unusual nature of the exercise prevent you from experiencing it fully.
- Don't judge a relaxation technique based only on what happens while you are doing it. The most important aspect of a relaxation exercise is not necessarily what happens while you are doing it but how you feel *after you have completed the exercise.* You may feel incredible during the activity; you might also find that your mind is moving a million miles a minute; or you may be quite physically involved, as is the case with progressive relaxation. The real effects of doing the exercise may occur later when you return to the activities of your day feeling more balanced, alert, relaxed, refreshed, or energized.
- Science has not yet fully explained why some relaxation exercises work so well. Autogenics and meditation are good examples. Science has not yet figured out why the simple repetition of a word produces such deep and profound rest, but deep relaxation happens even without full understanding. The woman who goes to the gym to lift weights to make her body stronger may have no idea why her muscles get bigger when she lifts heavy weights for many repetitions. But that may not matter to her. Lifting weights produces the results she is seeking. Similarly, with relaxation exercises, it is not always necessary to understand why the process works to enjoy the positive benefits.

Relaxation Sensations

Individuals may experience a variety of sensations while practicing relaxation exercises. A few that have been reported are:

Tingling
Warmth
Coolness
Floating

Swirling

Spinning

Heaviness

A pleasant numbness or seeming inability to move a part of the body

More pronounced heartbeat

Distortions in your sense of time (you may perceive time moving extremely fast or slow—usually fast)

Lightheadedness

These sensations typically feel pleasant and are natural responses to the body turning off the stress response and restoring balance to the body systems. They are indications that you are doing the exercises correctly. You have achieved deep relaxation. When you experience any of these sensations, simply go with them and observe what happens. Don't resist them. Your thoughts, when you notice anything unusual, should sound like, "Hmm, that's interesting." Don't add any more thoughts about the sensations. When you are doing the activity correctly, whatever happens while you are relaxing is entirely appropriate for you. While these sensations may never or rarely happen to you, if they do, just allow the sensations to happen freely.

Use Good Judgment

As always, use your good judgment when starting a new activity. Each of us is unique, so normal, safe recommendations may need to be altered depending on your individual situation. Consult with your physician if you have any concerns or questions about the safety of a technique. For example, pregnant women may want to consult with their healthcare provider prior to starting yoga. If you have a breathing or sleep disorder, you may need to alter some techniques.

Regularly practicing the relaxation techniques outlined here may reduce or even eliminate poor health conditions associated with stress. Regular practice of relaxation techniques, including meditation, is known to decrease high blood pressure,[5] cardiovascular disease,[6] and other chronic diseases.[7] As a result, some people may take more medication than is necessary as their stress-related conditions lessen. Therefore, you should consult with your physician from time to time to determine the appropriate amounts of medication as your stress-related symptoms decrease.

Time for a Nap—A Power Nap

The first relaxation technique we will introduce is the **Power Nap.** It combines elements of several relaxation exercises, including deep breathing, mindfulness, and yoga, to relax and rejuvenate body and mind. This is not a "nap" in the traditional sense of the word, but rather a specific technique to induce physical and mental relaxation. Power Nap is an appropriate name for this relaxation technique because it is so immediately powerful in restoring balance and homeostasis.

Benefits and Background The benefits of this relaxation technique, more than just about any other, include an immediate increase in energy, an increase in ability to focus, and a general feeling of rejuvenation. If you do the Power Nap just prior to bedtime, it can result in falling asleep quickly and remaining asleep throughout the night in a deeply restful sleep. The Power Nap, along with some of the other relaxation techniques you will learn, produces the seemingly contradictory effects of increasing energy and vitality if you return to daily activities or inducing peaceful sleep if used before going to bed.

How the Power Nap Works for Relaxation The Power Nap works so efficiently because of the position of the body during the exercise. When you do the Power Nap, you place yourself into a position that immediately relaxes the upper and lower back and shoulders, along with the neck, jaw, eyes, and other facial muscles. Another benefit of this body position is that it redistributes the flow of blood to the upper parts of the body. In doing so, oxygen and important nutrients move rapidly to the brain. By

Stress Relief Activity

Practice the Power Nap Relaxation Technique found in the Premium Website audio files.

contrast, standing or sitting in an upright position all day causes the blood to pool, because of gravity, in the lower parts of the torso and legs. The Power Nap helps balance this out.

How to Do the Power Nap

The Power Nap is simple to do. All that is required is a soft floor, chair, couch, or bed, and some privacy so you will not be interrupted. Figure 16.1 demonstrates the body position for the Power Nap.

These 10 easy steps will guide you through the Power Nap:

1. Place your body so your thighs are in a mostly vertical position, your knees are at a 90-degree angle, and your calves are horizontal on the chair or bed.
2. Close your eyes and begin by extending your arms up over your head, reaching as high as you can. With your arms straight, try to let the backs of your hands touch the floor above your head. Extend your arms as long and straight as possible and feel the comfortable stretch in your back as you do this. After several deep, full breaths, place your hands on your abdomen with your elbows touching the floor.
3. Notice the up-and-down movement of your abdomen as you breathe in and out. To enhance this focus, place one hand on your chest while keeping the other hand on your abdomen. For a few minutes, focus directly on your breathing. When you inhale, only your abdomen hand should be moving. Try to make your chest hand remain completely still as you inhale. Make a special effort to focus on breathing with your abdomen and not your chest.
4. After a few minutes of concentrating on your breathing and feeling yourself getting into the rhythm of this deeper, slower breathing, experiment with your hands to see where they feel most comfortable. You may either keep both hands on your abdomen or let them drop off to your sides. You may prefer having your palms up or palms down. Find the most comfortable position for you.
5. As you continue breathing slowly and deeply, bring your attention to your shoulders. Allow your shoulders to release into the floor. Turn off all tension by consciously releasing and letting go of any need to keep the muscles in your shoulders in the tightened state. Keep your shoulders wide and open, but do not pinch your shoulder blades together. Visualize your shoulders like butter melting into the floor. Each time you exhale, allow your shoulders to feel a little more relaxed, a little looser, a little limper.
6. Return your attention to your breathing and notice how your breathing has become even more slow and effortless. Next, bring attention to your face. Move through each set of muscles from your jaw through the middle of your face, your eyes, and into your forehead, and consciously relax all of those muscles. Consciously feel all of your facial muscles just release and let go.
7. Return to your breathing. Focus on deep, effortless breathing once again. If your mind wanders to other things, gently return it to your breathing.
8. After about 10 or 15 minutes of this exercise, slowly begin to return to normal consciousness. Begin to return to full alertness by moving your hands and fingers. Next, move your arms and neck as if you are looking from side to side around the room. Take your time and don't be in a

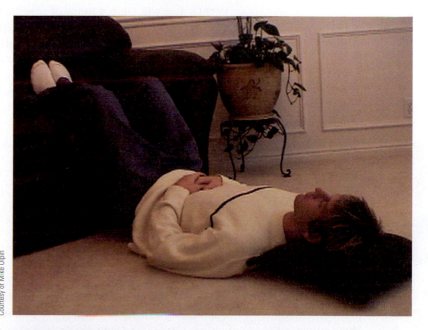

Courtesy of Mike Olpin

FIGURE 16.1 The Power Nap

Power Nap is an appropriate name for this relaxation technique because it is so immediately powerful in restoring balance and homeostasis.

hurry to return to sitting or standing. If you do this too quickly, you may become dizzy or feel sluggish after finishing.

9. Carefully lift your feet up off of the chair, bring your knees to your chest, and then roll to one side so you are lying in the fetal position. Spend a moment or two in this position.

10. Then, when you feel ready, bring yourself up into a seated position while still on the floor. After about a minute, you will be ready to return to daily activities with renewed energy and vitality.

Adding the Power Nap to Your Daily Routine The two "best times" during the day to do the Power Nap are:

1. Late afternoon after your day's activities and before evening activities.
2. Just before falling asleep:

    *   Complete your normal bedtime routine.
    *   Make the Power Nap the last thing that you do before your head hits the pillow and you close your eyes.
    *   Once you have finished this relaxation exercise, slip into bed and easily fall asleep.

Conclusion

Relaxation is the mind/body process of effectively moving from the stress response to the relaxation response. Benefits accrue when we move from physical and psychological arousal to relaxation. The purpose of relaxation techniques is to directly activate the calming parasympathetic nervous system activity. A number of suggestions can maximize outcomes when you incorporate relaxation techniques into your daily life.

   The Power Nap is a simple, yet powerful technique to activate the relaxation response. It combines the elements of deep breathing, mindfulness, and yoga. In the chapters in Part IV, you will learn a range of specific methods for eliciting the relaxation response. These strategies range from the simple, such as breathing deeply while repeating "let go," to approaches such as yoga and meditation, which can take more time to fully master. Some of the techniques focus to a greater extent on quieting the mind while others focus more on relaxing the body. You will have the opportunity to experience the techniques and decide which ones to incorporate into your life. Each time you participate in one of the relaxation techniques, think of it as taking a mini-vacation from stress.

Stress Relief Activities

Visit the Premium Website audio files to explore a variety of relaxation activities and techniques.

LAB

16.1 The Power Nap

PURPOSE To allow you to practice deep relaxation using the Power Nap.

DIRECTIONS Prepare your environment for relaxation. Follow along with the Power Nap instructions found in the Premium Website audio files. Practice this technique at least 2 times according to the instructions on the audio file. At least once, do it immediately before you sleep at night. Make sure it is the last thing you do before sleep. Do it at times when you will not be disturbed. Allow approximately 15 minutes to complete the exercise.

(Continued)

After completing Power Nap, respond to the questions below. Describe primarily how you were feeling in relation to your stress levels.

Afternoon:

1. How did you feel before the exercise?

2. What was your experience during the exercise?

3. How did you feel immediately after the exercise?

4. How did you feel several hours after completing the exercise?

Right before sleeping at night:

1. How did you feel before the exercise?

2. How quickly did you fall asleep?

3. How did you sleep, and how refreshed did you feel when you awakened the following morning?

4. How did this differ from a typical night's sleep?

Classroom experience (if applicable):

1. How did you feel before the exercise?

2. What was your experience during the exercise?

3. How did you feel immediately after the exercise?

4. How did you feel several hours after completing the exercise?

Summary   After you have practiced the exercise and described your experiences, include a brief review of what you liked and/or did not like about this technique. Compare this technique to some of the others you have practiced. Would this be a relaxation technique you would consider using on a regular basis for stress management? Why or why not?

Key Points

- Whereas cognitive techniques help stop the stress response from activating, physical techniques help to reduce stress by altering the physiological impact of stress.
- The purpose of relaxation techniques is to activate the parasympathetic nervous system.

- Specific suggestions can help you maximize the benefits of your relaxation experience.
- The Power Nap is a simple, yet powerful technique for relaxation.

Key Terms

relaxation   Power Nap

Discussion Time   For Critical Thinking/Discussion Questions, please visit this book's Premium Website.

Notes

1. *The Inner Game of Tennis,* by W. T. Gallway (New York: Random House, 1974).
2. *Pain: Clinical Manual for Nursing,* by M. McCaffery and A. Beebe (St. Louis: CV Mosby, 1989).
3. *The Relaxation Response,* by H. Benson (New York: Avon Books, 1975).
4. http://www.mayoclinic.com
5. "Effects of Education and Relaxation Training with Essential Hypertension Patients," by R. Lagrone, T. Jeffrey, and C. Ferguson, *Journal of Clinical Psychology* 44(2)(1988): 271–278.
6. "Impact of the Transcendental Meditation Program on Mortality in Older African Americans with Hypertension—Eight Year Follow Up," by V. A. Barnes, R. H. Schneider, C. N. Alexander, et al., *Journal of Social Behavior & Personality* 17(1) (2005): 201–217.
7. "Meditation's Impact on Chronic Illness," by R. Bonadonna, *Holistic Nursing Practice* 17(6) (2003): 309–320.

17 Take a Breath

■ I have heard that deep breathing is one of the best ways to relax. How does this work? ■ Is abdominal breathing more effective for relaxation than chest breathing?

Study of this chapter will enable you to:

1. Explain the benefits of breathing for relaxation.
2. Differentiate between several breathing techniques to facilitate relaxation.
3. Experience the benefits of breathing for relaxation.
4. Determine the breathing techniques that are most effective for you.

All things share the same breath—the beast, the tree, the man ... the air shares its spirit with all the life it supports.

—*Chief Seattle*

265

REAL PEOPLE, REAL STORIES

Breathing Works Before I began the Simple Diaphragmatic Breathing exercise for the first time, I was stressed out over an assignment for another class that I didn't understand. During the exercise I noticed a tension in my shoulders, and as the exercise continued, I felt the tension slowly reduce until it was gone. After the exercise, I felt energized and ready to attack the assignment again. This time I had a better understanding of the things in the assignment that I didn't understand before, and I got a better score on the quiz.

The second time that I did the exercise was just before bed. I had a day that was stressful as usual, and during this exercise I felt my body relax until I was ready to sleep. After I ended the exercise, I went right to sleep. Usually I toss and turn until I get comfortable, and then I fall asleep, but I went to sleep much faster using this exercise.

—*Alicia B.*

* * *

The Restful Breathing exercise was extremely relaxing and relieving. I felt both exhilarated and relaxed at the same time. Before the exercise, I was feeling tired from a long day, yet ready for another relaxation technique. It was amazing how easily I was able to feel the energy come into my body from simple, deep breathing. I noticed how my breath got deeper and more relaxed with each count down to zero. It was so awesome! Immediately afterward, I went to bed, and slept well all night. I was up late that night, yet I woke up feeling great. It was an awesome technique.

When I did the exercise the second time, it felt as though my breaths got even deeper and more relaxed. I found that I was able to fully concentrate on one thing. The second time was easier than the first time, when it was difficult to keep my mind from wandering. Because I was able to fully concentrate on the air going in and out of my lungs, the second time was more natural. Before the exercise, I was grouchy and tired, yet I didn't have the desire to be totally relaxed. But I did it anyway, and I was glad I did! Afterward, I felt energized and happier. About an hour later I still felt good. Things didn't bother me as much as they had earlier in the day.

—*Chad R.*

Take a Breath

The rhythm of the breath continues from our first moments of life to our last. Although we take the breath for granted, breath is life! Breathing represents an important point of contact between mind and body, as respiration occupies a unique interaction between the voluntary and involuntary nervous systems. Shallow and irregular breathing reinforces stress and can have negative physical consequences. Deep breathing, however, induces relaxation and promotes circulation.[1]

Adults normally breathe at the rate of 12 to 16 breaths per minute and inhale an average of 16,000 quarts of air each day. When nothing is done to restrict breathing, it will happen naturally and fully. Yet, in our busy lives, we continually inhibit our natural breathing patterns in many ways, including habitual patterns of emotional stress. Conscious relaxation breathing relieves stress, allowing a return to natural, uninhibited breathing.

Background

For centuries, breathing exercises have been an integral part of mental, physical, and spiritual development in Asia and India. Deep breathing continues to be an essential component of ancient Eastern practices such as yoga and tai chi chuan. Breathing techniques are part of a philosophical system that emphasizes balance and wholeness for achieving health.

How Breathing Works

The primary purpose of breathing is to supply the body with oxygen and to remove excess carbon dioxide. The body's ability to produce energy and to complete the various metabolic processes depends upon sufficient and efficient use of oxygen. Oxygen is necessary to help us repair and regenerate our bodies. An average human breath contains about 10 sextillion or 10^{22} atoms.[2] If any tissues in the body, including the heart and the brain, are deprived of oxygen for more than a few minutes, severe damage can result.

The two basic ways of breathing are:

1. **abdominal breathing,** also called **diaphragmatic breathing**
2. **chest breathing,** or **thoracic breathing.**

Normal breathing usually combines these two. Chest breathing is relatively shallow. The chest expands and the shoulders rise as the lungs take in air. Abdominal breathing is deeper. Jon Kabat-Zinn gives us some background on the anatomy and physiology of breathing:

> The **diaphragm** is a large, umbrella-shaped sheet of muscle that is attached all around the lower edges of the rib cage. It separates the contents of the chest (the heart and lungs and great blood vessels) from the contents of the abdomen (the stomach, liver, intestines). When it contracts, it tightens and draws downward because it is anchored all along the rim of the rib cage. This downward movement increases the volume of the chest cavity, in which the lungs are located on either side of the heart. The increased volume in the chest produces a decrease in the air pressure in the lungs. Because of the decreased pressure inside the lungs, air from outside the body, which is at a higher pressure, flows into the lungs to equalize the pressure. This is the **inbreath.**

> After the diaphragm contracts, it goes through a relaxation. As the diaphragm muscle relaxes, it gets looser and returns to its original position higher up in the chest, thereby decreasing the volume of the chest cavity. This increases the pressure in the chest, which forces the air in the lungs out through the nose (and mouth if it is open). This is the **outbreath.** So in all breathing, the air is drawn into the lungs as the diaphragm contracts and lowers, and it is expelled as the diaphragm relaxes and comes back up.

> Now suppose the muscles that form the wall of your belly (the abdomen) are tight rather than relaxed when the diaphragm is contracting. As the diaphragm pushes down on the stomach, the liver, and the other abdominal organs, it will meet resistance and will not be able to descend very far. Your breathing will tend to be shallow and rather high up in the chest.

> In abdominal or diaphragmatic breathing, the idea is to relax your belly as much as you can. Then, as the breath comes in, the belly expands slightly (on its own) in an outward direction as the diaphragm pushes down on the contents of the abdomen from above.[3]

In summary, abdominal diaphragmatic breathing involves inhalations that cause the diaphragm to contract and move down, drawing air into the lungs. When air moves down into the lungs at the lower levels, the abdomen tends to distend slightly. On exhalation, the diaphragm relaxes and moves upward and the abdomen moves back in.

Thoracic or chest breathing is frequently a signal that the fight-or-flight response is activated, even to the point of holding the breath or exhaling incompletely. Breathing thoracically can cause symptoms such as shortness of breath and tightness in the chest.[4] People who have chronic stress tend to breathe either with their chest almost exclusively, or with both their abdomen and chest simultaneously.

People who breathe primarily from the chest move only about 500 cubic centimeters of air in and out with each breath. A full abdominal breath moves 8 to 10 times that volume.[5] The exchange of oxygen from the lungs into the bloodstream is far greater in the lower portion of the lungs when a person is in an upright position and is breathing abdominally.[6] Breathing abdominally helps bring air into the lower lobes of the lungs, resulting in an increase in beneficial oxygenation throughout the various cells and systems of the body. If you watch the breathing of a young baby at rest, you will notice that the baby breathes abdominally. The abdomen moves in and out. The chest doesn't move at all. We are born as abdominal breathers. It is our natural way of breathing.

Benefits of Relaxation Breathing

Because stress and anxiety are major factors contributing to many problems in society, researchers are examining ways to effectively deal with these problems. Research on stress-reduction programs, however, sometimes overlooks the body's natural coping and defense mechanisms. The natural breathing process shows great promise as a coping technique for common anxiety and stress. Breathing techniques allow the mind and body time to slow down, energize, and develop harmony and tranquility.[7]

Deep, meditative breathing can have a significant effect on your physical and mental state. "Breathing may be the master function of the body, affecting all others," writes Andrew Weil, M.D. "How we breathe both reflects the state of the nervous system and influences the state of the nervous system."[8]

Slow, rhythmic breathing can turn an anxious mental state into a state of relative tranquility and release the body from many other adverse effects of anxiety. Adjusting our breathing back to its natural way of deep and slow breathing sends an instant message to the autonomic nervous system that there is no threat and the body can return to homeostasis. Breathing techniques induce relaxation and activate the calming parasympathetic branch of the autonomic nervous system.

When breathing is restricted, cells throughout the body do not receive an adequate supply of oxygen. When this happens, symptoms include drowsiness, irritability, and headache. One of the reasons exercise is so beneficial is that it forces you to breathe deeply and fully, thereby replenishing your supply of oxygen.

Practicing proper breathing techniques is one of the most vital healing techniques we have at our disposal, as a treatment for respiratory disease and also to reduce the anxiety associated with psychosomatic illness.[9] Breathing in a slow or regular manner or sitting in an upright posture helps to decelerate the heart rate, whereas slouching or breathing shallowly and quickly tends to accelerate it.[10]

When the body returns to a more balanced state, turning off the fight-or-flight response, the body comes into a balance in which the body can cure its maladies associated with stress. Studies have shown that deep abdominal breathing is effective in reducing levels of stress[11] and coping with stressful situations[12] including test anxiety,[13] and also in reducing blood pressure.[14]

Breathing techniques have been shown to be effective for a range of stress-producing conditions, from dealing with the pain of childbirth to alleviating hot flashes in menopausal women. For years, conscious breathing practices have been taught in childbirth preparation classes. Anxiety intensifies pain, and breathing consciously helps to relieve tension and anxiety and reduce pain.[15]

And while most of you may not be all that interested in hot flashes, some research in this area helps us understand the power of deep breathing on physiology. Hot flashes are the most common symptom women experience during menopause. Of the 2,500 participants in the Massachusetts Women's Health Study, 75% reported having had hot flashes during menopause.[16] Research shows that breathing exercises can

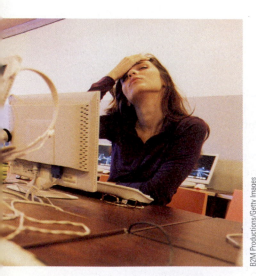

Take a breath—deep breathing can make the computer less stressful.

B2M Productions/Getty Images

Using Breathing Techniques to Ease Test Anxiety

A meta-analysis of 78 published studies on reduction of test anxiety in college students over a 13-year period concluded that simple relaxation is as helpful as more complex and time-consuming treatments.[*] One of the most basic relaxation techniques available to individuals is breathing. Breathing techniques for stress and anxiety reduction are simple to learn, can be used in multiple settings, and do not depend on educational trends and funding. They show promise for coping with the test-related stress and anxiety that are becoming prevalent in today's student environment.[**]

Typically, test anxiety is defined as extreme emotional arousal in testing situations. Teaching students natural, slow breathing can help them relax, energize, and acquire an inner sense of peace and tranquility. Normal breathing also lowers stress and anxiety, thereby increasing attention/concentration and allowing improved performance. Stress and anxiety reduction can result in improved academic achievement, as reflected in higher test scores.[†]

By mastering breathing techniques, students can control the effects of situational anxiety, thereby achieving a heightened state of awareness; increase their concentration; and become less easily distracted. These benefits from controlled natural breathing allow for optimal performance and maximal achievement on tests and essentially enhance the overall quality of life.

Breathing techniques are used optimally before and during tests to clear the mind, relax the body, and maintain the body's biochemical balance. During test breaks, students can use these nonintrusive techniques to relax while energizing themselves for the next portion of the test. Once students have learned these techniques, they can implement them whenever and wherever they encounter stressful and anxiety-provoking situations.[††]

Sources:
[*]"Meta-Analysis of Outcome Research in Reducing Test Anxiety: Interventions, Rigor, and Inertia," by A. A. Dole (paper presented at Annual Meeting of American Educational Research Association, Montreal, Quebec) (ERIC Document Reproduction Service No. ED 392 120).
[**]"Test Anxiety? Try a Stick of Gum," by E. L. Wilmore (ERIC Document Reproduction Service No. ED 231 844).
[†]"Standardized Test Preparation," by N. Duke and R. Ritchart, in *Instructor*, *107*(3), 89–91.
[††]"Using Breathing Techniques to Ease Test Anxiety," by L. Wilkinson, W. Buboltz, & E. Seemann, in *Guidance & Counseling*, *16*(3), 76–81.

relieve hot flashes—no small benefit to the masses of baby boomers entering menopause. Researcher Robert Freedman of Wayne State University reports in the *American Journal of Obstetrics and Gynecology*, "In three of our studies, slow, controlled deep breathing cut the frequency of hot flashes by about half." In his most recent trial, 24 women suffering at least five hot flashes a day were randomly assigned to practice either paced breathing or brainwave biofeedback. The number of hot flashes fell by half in the breathing group but didn't budge in those doing biofeedback.[17] So, deep breathing includes positive effects for both the body and the mind. The breathing techniques presented in this chapter will focus on relaxation breathing.

Breathing and Relaxation

Earlier, we assessed our breathing to see how many breaths we take in a minute. We also assessed whether we breathe more from our abdomen or from our chest. Refer back to those two assessments from Chapter 2. Among the wide variety of factors that affect respiratory rate—such as activity levels, anxiety levels, and disease states—your respiratory rate at rest can be a good indication of your state of relaxation.

Chest breathers with higher respiration rates are more likely to function with the stress response activated. Because the autonomic nervous system initiates the stress response, you may be unaware of this quicker, shallower breathing as a function of the stress response. Awareness of our current breathing is an important first step toward using this powerful tool to activate the parasympathetic nervous system, and thereby immediately feel more relaxed.

Nearly every stress management technique that is devised specifically to reduce sympathetic nervous activity includes a breathing component. As we will see in subsequent chapters, abdominal breathing is used with the significant relaxation techniques in this text, including progressive muscular relaxation, autogenic training, mental imagery, and yoga. It was also included as an important component of the Power Nap in Chapter 16.

FYI

Breathing Break Here's what happens when you flick on your iMac: "Your breathing rate goes up 30%, your blinking rate goes way down, and you tend to tighten your arms and shoulders without knowing it," says Erik Peper, Ph.D., director of the Institute for Holistic Healing at San Francisco State University. Sounds like some deep breathing might make the computer a little less stressful.

Source: "One hundred ways to reclaim your life," by S. Calechman, *Men's Health*, (2004, July/Aug.), p. 190.

How to Do Relaxation Breathing

Breathing exercises require no special equipment. They may be done lying down or sitting in a comfortable chair. Distractions should be kept to a minimum, in a room that is quiet and conducive to relaxation. Breathing exercises are best done with the eyes closed. Any time of the day is appropriate, but breathing exercises can be particularly beneficial in the afternoon or just before going to sleep. Often, relaxing breathing exercises are especially effective in helping one fall asleep.

Because some breathing techniques alter brainwave activity, avoid doing relaxing breathing exercises while driving or operating heavy machinery. If you are feeling stress and notice yourself breathing primarily into the chest only, however, adjust your breathing from chest breathing to deeper abdominal breathing. You can do this anytime, anywhere.

Experiment with the breathing exercises that follow. Try them several times to see which ones have the most value for you. Go to the Premium Website Stress Relief audio file to find the relaxation exercise called Restful Breathing. Using this exercise on the audio file, you can experience deep rest and relaxation with the help of a guide to take you through the process.

Breathing Exercises

Diaphragmatic breathing exercises are probably the easiest type of relaxation exercises to learn. Although these have many adaptations, they usually involve bringing attention to the inhalation and exhalation of the breath, sometimes holding the breath briefly, or varying the duration of the inhalation or the exhalation.

Simple Diaphragmatic Breathing You can immediately practice abdominal breathing by placing one hand on the stomach, approximately over the navel, and the other on the lower part of the sternum just over the heart. Then by noticing which hand is moving more—the upper or the lower hand—during inhalation and exhalation, you can make adjustments. By making the hand over the stomach move out with the inhalation and in with the exhalation, while the top hand remains still, the exercise of **simple diaphragmatic breathing** begins. For added benefit, repeat "I am" with each inhalation and "relaxed" with each exhalation. Follow these steps:

1. Sit comfortably and quietly
2. Tell yourself that you are going to use the next 5, 10, or 20 minutes to re-balance, to heal, to relax yourself.
3. Surrender the weight of your body, allowing the chair, or floor, to support you.
4. Close your eyes, gently cutting out visual stimulation and distraction.
5. As you inhale, repeat to yourself: "I AM"
6. As you exhale, say ... "RELAXED."
7. Continue to breathe normally not trying to change it in any way. Just watch it happening and continue to repeat: "I AM" with inhalation; ... "RELAXED" with exhalation.
8. As your mind begins to wander, gently bring it back to the awareness of your breath and your statement "I AM—RELAXED." Be compassionate and loving with your "leaping frog" mind, which wants to be anywhere but here.
9. Continue doing this for as long as you have established.
10. To conclude, discontinue the phrase and slowly stretch your hands and feet, your arms and legs, then your whole body.
11. Open your eyes a sliver at a time—like the sun coming up in the morning.
12. Continue on your way.[18]

Reduced Respirations Technique An easy and effective technique for controlling breathing and reducing stress is the **reduced respirations technique,** which works by reducing your breathing rate to as low as 4 to 5 breaths per minute.[19]

1. Take a deep, slow breath, drawing in through the nose and out through the mouth, which should be closed when inhaling. Inhaling and exhaling should take about six seconds each.
2. Place one hand over the diaphragm area of the abdomen and continue drawing long, slow, deep breaths using the same method. Aim to reduce breathing to 6-7 breaths per minute.

3. While breathing deeply through the nose, the hand should move up and down as the chest wall expands and contracts with lung inflation and deflation. Shoulders should remain stationary.
4. Continue this exercise for several minutes once you have achieved the desired breathing rate.

Restful Breathing A simple and effective type of focused breathing is called **restful breathing.** You may practice restful breathing in a seated position or lying down. The beauty of this technique is that you can do it whenever you think of it. It merely takes a moment to turn your attention to your breathing and consciously change which part of your torso is doing the work—the upper chest area or the lower abdominal area. You can experience the benefits any time, any place. You can use restful breathing while preparing for an upcoming athletic event, interviewing for a job, preparing to take a test, or waiting to speak in front of a group of people.

1. Begin restful breathing by focusing directly on your breath as it goes in and comes back out. This may be done with the eyes open or closed. Don't try to change anything about your breathing initially, just tune in to the rhythmic in and out pattern of your breathing. Keep your attention on your breathing.
2. When your mind wanders and distracting thoughts arise, let them pass, and return your focus to your breath. You may want to place your hands on your abdomen to increase your focus of abdominal breathing.
3. After a few minutes of attentive breathing, begin to change your breathing pattern by allowing your breath to go down as deep as possible into the lowest parts of your lungs. When you do this, your abdomen will naturally move outward. Notice your hands, which are resting on your abdomen, moving out as you breathe in. Notice your hands moving back in as you exhale.
4. To help you maintain your focus on this deep, slow breathing, use the counting method. Start counting at 20 (or whatever number you choose) and count backward to zero. When you inhale, silently say "twenty." When you exhale, mentally say the word "relax." Inhale again and say "nineteen." On the next exhalation, say "relax." Continue down this way until you reach zero.
5. If you notice your mind starting to wander—and it very likely will—gently bring yourself back to the counting. Your breathing will naturally become more slow and deep as you do this. You also can consciously make your breathing more slow and deep just by focusing on that mode of breathing.

You may increase the effect by taking little breaks between the inhale and exhale. As you inhale, say the word "twenty," then hold your breath for 3 or 4 seconds before you slowly exhale. Once all the air is expelled, pause briefly before your next inhalation.

If you are one of those people who struggle to fall asleep at night, this technique is especially powerful for alleviating sleeping problems. If you are in bed and notice yourself struggling to drift off, simply begin focusing on your breath and counting down. People who use this method find it almost universally successful at helping them nod off quickly, and remain asleep for the entire night.

This may seem like a strange exercise if you are unaccustomed to this mode of breathing, but with regular practice you will find that you will return to this natural way of breathing more and more during the regular activities of your day. People who regularly report breathing at rates of up to 30 full breaths per minute can reduce that number considerably with regular practice of deep abdominal breathing. The effects of correcting our breathing and practicing it regularly are profound and pleasant.

Breath Counting **Breath counting** is similar to the previous restful breathing relaxation exercise. When you practice breath counting, you simply focus directly on the breath as it comes in and goes back out. In this breathing exercise, you close your eyes, put your attention on your breath, and breathe normally. You inhale, and then as you exhale, you say, "one." The next inhale is followed by the exhale, and you say, "two." You continue through the number 4 and then repeat again from 1 to 4. You might include the silently spoken word "and" with each inhale. As you inhale, you say the word "and" followed by exhaling to the number.

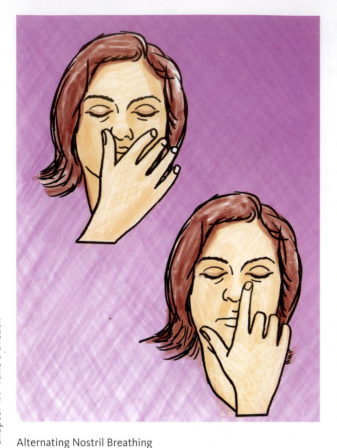

Alternating Nostril Breathing

Alternating Nostril Breathing Practitioners of meditation often include **alternating nostril breathing** (also known as balanced breathing) to relax the mind and body and to enhance their experience of meditation. Its purpose is to make the respiratory rhythm more regular, which in turn has a soothing effect on the entire nervous system. A few minutes of alternate nostril breathing is highly relaxing.[20]

This breathing exercise usually is done while seated or lying down. With the eyes open or closed, you bring one hand up to your face. In this technique, the thumb and forefinger are used to alternate pressing on either side of the nose. The focus is directly on the breath as you alternately exhale and inhale through one nostril, then exhale and inhale through the other nostril.

Beginning with the exhalation, push the thumb against one side of the nose to shut off that nostril as air passes freely through the other. During the following inhalation, continue to hold the nostril closed. On the next exhale, release the thumb and push against the nose with the forefinger on the opposite nostril closing this one off completely. Inhale while holding the same nostril closed. This pattern—switching back and forth from one nostril to the other—can be repeated as long as desired. Remember to place the focus on the breath.

Alternating nostril breathing can be adapted in several ways including single-sided nostril breathing techniques, which have been part of yoga tradition for generations. Although this is difficult to prove empirically, single-sided nostril breathing may either increase energy (right nostril) or calmness (left nostril).[21]

Right-Nostril Breathing (Energy)

1. Close off the left nostril with the index finger.
2. Inhale slowly and deeply through the right nostril until you feel a sense of fullness in the lungs.
3. Hold the breath for a count of 3 seconds.
4. Exhale slowly and completely through the right nostril.
5. Complete this cycle of breathing 7 to 10 times or until you obtain a sense of being energized.

Left-Nostril Breathing (Calmness)

1. Close off the right nostril with the index finger.
2. Follow the same procedure as for right-nostril breathing, except breathe through the left nostril for a sense of calmness.

If both calmness and energy are sought, an alternate nose-breathing technique is a quick, simple, and powerful breathing method that combines the left-nostril and right-nostril breathing techniques. It helps boost energy while maintaining a sense of calm.

1. Take a deep breath through the right nostril while closing the left nostril with the left index finger.
2. Hold your breath for a count of 3, then release the left nostril, close the right nostril, and exhale. Then inhale through the same nostril and hold your breath.
3. Releasing the right index finger, press against the left nostril with the left index finger again and exhale from the right nostril. This is considered one breath count.
4. Continue the above steps for 7 to 10 breaths or until you achieve a sense of calmed energy.

In his book *Conscious Breathing*, Gay Hendricks teaches this technique to help refresh and energize the body, clear and focus the mind, and improve overall mood. He advocates using this technique for easing a tired or scattered mood and for producing a clear, calm, focused state of mind.[22] Experiment with the various alternating nostril breathing techniques to determine what works best for you.

Full Breathing **Full breathing** involves breathing in first to the abdomen, then slowly filling up the rest of the lungs as you inhale. After holding your breath for a few moments, exhale by first releasing the air from the tops of the lungs, then slowly move down to the lower parts of the lungs so the abdomen moves back in at the end of the exhale.

Visualization Breathing While lying on your back, and with your eyes closed, place your hands over your stomach, just below your ribs. **Visualization breathing** combines full breathing with visualization. Practice full breathing for a few moments. As you inhale, visualize the inbreath moving down from your nose to the deepest parts of your lungs. If it helps to visualize it more clearly, imagine that your breath is colored, such as white. After a full inhale, hold the breath briefly and visualize it becoming energized in the lower parts of your lungs. As you begin slowly exhaling, visualize this energized air spreading to all parts of your body, bringing with it healing energy and purified oxygen. On the next inhalation, repeat this process. Continue breathing fully and imagine the energizing breaths spreading throughout your body for several minutes.

Command Breathing Tom Brown, an expert tracker and teacher of Native American spirituality, describes using what he calls the "command breath" to help bring the mind to a state of "sacred silence." The procedure for **command breathing** has some similarities to the other breathing exercises in this chapter. It can be done by oneself or with the help of a guide. Tom Brown suggests:

> This sequence begins with the guide telling the meditator to take a deep breath, hold it for a few moments, then at the command of the guide, releasing it completely. The guide tells the meditator that the next time the command breath is taken, he should focus all distraction, tension, and discomfort into that breath and let it all go with the exhalation. Let everything flow out with the air leaving the lungs. Now repeat the command breathing process about two to four times. Each time the meditator should imagine and believe that all distraction is passed out of the body and mind with each exhalation.[23]

Ujjayi Breathing One of the most important components of yoga is the focus on breathing throughout each pose. Breathing has been called the "bridge" that connects the mind and body. Baron Baptiste, a yoga instructor, describes one common form of breathing used in yoga called **ujjayi breathing.** This can be used in other types of activities, too. Baron gives the following instruction for ujjayi breathing:

> The breath we use for asana (yoga) practice is called *ujjayi breathing (oo-jeye-yee)*. The ujjayi breath is an audible breath that has a soothing, rhythmic, oceanic quality. It is done by contracting the whispering muscles in your throat to create a long, hairline thin breath. You do not breathe all the way down into your abdomen, but rather into your chest, lungs, and back.
>
> Here is a step-by-step breakdown of how to do it:
>
> 1. Bring your first or second finger to the soft spot between your collarbones.
> 2. With your mouth closed, breathe in through your nose, feeling the gentle retraction of those muscles beneath your finger. It should feel as though you are whispering in reverse. You are closing the airway a little, so it's kind of like breathing through a straw. Imagine the breath as a cleansing wind sweeping right in through that soft spot at the base of your throat.
> 3. For the exhalation, put your hand in front of your face as if it's a mirror. Gently retract your belly and, with your mouth closed and the muscles in your throat still contracted, exhale through your nose as if you were going to fog up that mirror. The exhalation is exaggerated and extended. It is important to keep your mouth closed or you will lose energy on the exhalation.
>
> This is the ujjayi breath. In, out, in, out … deep and free, rhythmic and steady. The volume of your breath both on the inhale and the exhale should be equal to each other. If you get dizzy, you're probably forcing it too much. Just relax and let it be effortless—not taking in too much or too little air. It's like a wood burning stove. Too much oxygen and you burn up the fuel too quickly, not enough and the fire goes out. A steady flow keeps the internal flame burning.[24]

Breathing While Stretching This breathing while stretching technique targets whole-body tension, diverting attention from anxiety-related physiological sensations toward feelings of relaxation and calmness through breathing.

1. Mentally scan your body for tension and rate yourself on a 1–100 scale for anxiety.
2. Stand or sit in a chair with your back straight.
3. Raise your arms parallel to your sides until they are directly overhead. Clasp your hands together and stretch toward the ceiling. While raising your hands upward, inhale slowly and deeply though the mouth, with lungs full when the hands reach their apex. Hold your breath for 3 to 5 seconds while stretching upward.
4. Slowly exhale through the nose while lowering the hands back to your sides.
5. Intertwine the fingers of both hands and with palms facing outward push away from the chest, arms parallel to the floor. While pushing away, take a deep breath through the mouth. When the arms reach maximum extension, push away from them, stretching the back and arms, holding the breath for 3 to 5 seconds.
6. Return the arms slowly to their resting position while exhaling slowly through the nose.
7. Repeat this exercise three to five times. Rate your body sensations and perceptions of anxiety on a 1–100 scale.
8. Repeat as necessary.

Individuals who are taught to identify their breathing patterns and body tension are surprised, and then excited, as they develop new body awareness. To become aware of our breathing patterns, we need merely to listen and focus on our breathing. Awareness empowers us to take steps to correct the pattern and to begin to breathe in a more natural and healthy way.[25]

Stress Relief Activities
Visit the Premium Website audio files to explore a variety of relaxation activities and techniques.

Conclusion

Conscious breathing is a component of nearly every relaxation technique. Used alone or in combination with other techniques, the beneficial results are immediately obvious. Above all else, the main focus in directing attention toward the breath is to consciously return breathing to its natural rhythm of deep, slow, and effortless inhaling and exhaling. As we do this, the stress response automatically turns off just as efficiently as it turns on when we sense any kind of danger or potential pain.

Of the many breathing techniques available, try them for several days and in various situations to determine the techniques that work best for you. Breathing—one of the most normal and natural processes—may turn out to be one of the most effective strategies for you in reducing stress and enhancing your sense of peace and well-being.

LAB

17.1   Restful Breathing

PURPOSE   To allow you to practice deep relaxation using relaxation breathing.

DIRECTIONS   Prepare your environment for relaxation. Follow along with the Restful Breathing instructions found in the Premium Website audio files. Practice this technique at least 2 times according to the instructions on the audio file. At least once, do it immediately before you sleep at night. Make sure it is the last thing you do before sleep. Do it at times when you will not be disturbed. Allow approximately 15 minutes to complete the exercise.
After completing Restful Breathing, respond to the questions below. Describe primarily how you were feeling in relation to your stress levels.

Afternoon:

1. How did you feel before the exercise?

2. What was your experience during the exercise?

3. How did you feel immediately after the exercise?

4. How did you feel several hours after completing the exercise?

Right before sleeping at night:

1. How did you feel before the exercise?

2. How quickly did you fall asleep?

3. How did you sleep, and how refreshed did you feel when you awakened the following morning?

4. How did this differ from a typical night's sleep?

Classroom experience (if applicable):

1. How did you feel before the exercise?

2. What was your experience during the exercise?

3. How did you feel immediately after the exercise?

4. How did you feel several hours after completing the exercise?

Summary After you have practiced the exercise and described your experiences, include a brief review of what you liked and/or did not like about this technique. Compare this technique to some of the others you have practiced. Would this be a relaxation technique you would consider using on a regular basis for stress management? Why or why not?

Key Points

- Breathing represents an important point of contact between mind and body because respiration links the voluntary and involuntary nervous systems.
- Shallow and irregular breathing reinforces stress and can have negative physical consequences, whereas deep breathing induces relaxation and promotes circulation.
- The two basic ways of breathing are: abdominal, or diaphragmatic, breathing; and chest, or thoracic, breathing.
- Thoracic breathing is frequently a signal that the fight-or-flight response is activated.
- Focused breathing is incorporated into most other relaxation techniques.
- Among the many breathing exercises to facilitate relaxation are simple diaphragmatic breathing, the reduce respiration technique, restful breathing, breath counting, alternating nostril breathing, full breathing, visualization breathing, command breathing, ujjayi breathing, and breathing while stretching.

Key Terms

abdominal breathing or diaphragmatic breathing

chest breathing or thoracic breathing

diaphragm

inbreath

pranayama

outbreath

simple diaphragmatic breathing

reduce respirations technique

restful breathing

breath counting

alternating nostril breathing

full breathing

visualization breathing

command breathing

ujjayi breathing

Notes

1. *The Best Alternative Medicine: What Works? What Does Not?*, by K. Pelletier (New York: Simon & Schuster, 2000).

2. *The Seven Mysteries of Life,* by G. Murchie (Boston: Houghton Mifflin, 1978).

3. *Full Catastrophe Living*, by J. Kabat-Zinn (New York: Dell Publishing, 1990).

4. *Your Maximum Mind*, by H. Benson (New York: Times Books/Random House, 1987).

5. *Minding the Body, Mending the Mind*, by J. Borysenko (New York: Bantam Books, 1988).

6. "Yoga-Based Therapy," by C. Patel. In P. M. Lehrer and R. L. Woolfolk (Eds.), *Principles and Practice of Stress Management* (2nd ed.) (New York: Guilford Press, 1993).

7. "Using Breathing Techniques to Ease Test Anxiety," by L. Wilkinson, W. Buboltz, and E. Seemann, *Guidance & Counseling 16*(3) (2001): 76–81.

8. *Spontaneous Healing,* by A. Weil (New York: Ballantine Publishing Group, 1995).

9. *Mind as Healer, Mind as Slayer*, by K. R. Pelletier (New York: Dell Publishing, 1992).

10. Pelletier, *Mind as Healer, Mind as Slayer.*

11. "Psychological Effects of Several Stress Management Techniques," by E. J. Forbes and R. J. Pekala, *Psychological Reports 72*(1) (1993): 19–27; "A Strategy to Enhance Humor Production Among Elderly Persons: Assisting in the Management of Stress," by F. J. Prerost, *Activities, Adaptation and Aging 17*(4) (1993): 17–24; "Effects of Visualization and Danjeon Breathing on Target Shooting with an Air Pistol," by J. Kim and L. K. Tennant, *Perceptual and Motor Skills 77*(3) (1993): 1083–1087; "Stress Management for Psychiatric Patients in a State Hospital Setting," by D. Starkey and H. Deleone, *American Journal of Orthopsychiatry 65*(3) (1995): 446–451.

12. "Impact of Regular Relaxation Training on the Cardiac Autonomic Nervous System of Hospital Cleaners and Bank Employees," by H. Toivanen, E. Lansimies, V. Jokela, and O. Hanninen, *Scandinavian Journal of Work, Environment and Health 19*(5) (1993): 319–325.

13. Wilkinson, et al., "Using Breathing Techniques to Ease Test Anxiety."

14. "Yoga, Pranayama, Thermal Biofeedback Techniques in the Management of Stress and High Blood Pressure," by A. U. Latha and K. V. Kaliappan, *Journal of Indian Psychology 9*(1) (1991): 36–46; "Efficacy of Relaxation Techniques in Hypertensive Patients. Fifth Joint USA-USSR Symposium on Arterial Hypertension," by T. A. Aivazyan, et al., *Health Psychology 7*(Suppl.) (1988): 193–200.

15. "Pain Control for Children," by S. Gerik, *Southern Medical Journal 98*(3) (2005): 399.

16. "Managing Menopause," by D. Schardt, *Nutrition Action Healthletter* (2004, July/August): 8–10.

17. Schardt, "Managing Menopause."

18. U.S Department of Health and Human Services, National Institute of Mental Health, Division of Communications and Education—*Plain Talk* series, Ruth Kay, Editor, retrieved December 7, 2008.

19. Wilkinson, et al., "Using Breathing Techniques to Ease Test Anxiety."

20. *Science of Breath*, by Y. Ramacharaka (Chicago: Yogi Publication Society, 1905).

21. *Perfect Health: The Complete Mind/Body Guide*, by D. Chopra (New York: Harmony Books, 1990).

22. *Conscious Breathing: Breathwork for Health, Stress Release and Personal Mastery*, by G. Hendricks (New York: Bantam Books, 1995).

23. *Awakening Spirits,* by T. Brown (New York: The Berkley Publishing Group, 1994).

24. *Journey Into Power*, by B. Baptiste (New York: Fireside, 2002).

25. Wilkinson, et al., "Using Breathing Techniques to Ease Test Anxiety."

18 Autogenics

■ I've never heard of autogenics. What is this, and how does it work? ■ Can people experience the benefits of relaxation from autogenics if they just try hard enough? ■ Why do my arms and legs feel warm and heavy when I do autogenics?

STUDENT OBJECTIVES

Study of this chapter will enable you to:

1. Describe how autogenics works for relaxation.
2. Explain the health-related benefits of autogenics.
3. Experience the benefits of autogenics.

Everything should be made as simple as possible, but not simpler.

—*Albert Einstein*

Students Experience Autogenics This first time I tried the autogenics exercise, I thought it was going to be a waste of time because of how I was feeling. I was totally awake and didn't think I'd be able to do it. But, to my surprise, this exercise gave me the deepest relaxation I think I've ever experienced, and I felt like going to sleep. My body was so heavy and relaxed. Just an hour later I felt completely rejuvenated.

—Jeff D.

* * *

Total relaxation is what I could call autogenics. I first did this at the end of the day with one of my roommates. Talk about melting into the floor! At first I had a hard time concentrating and feeling heavy. But it worked, and man did my body ever feel good after we were finished! The second time I did it right before bed and had an ever better experience. I was able to concentrate more and get more of the effect I think I was supposed to have. Once I was finished and in bed, my body didn't want to move. It still felt heavy but so relaxed that I probably stayed in the same position all night long. I really enjoyed this technique.

—Lindsay J.

* * *

This relaxation exercise has been my favorite so far. Before the autogenics exercise, I felt normal— not tired, hungry, or stressed. During the exercise, I relaxed easily and my body went limp. In fact I was so relaxed that I fell asleep. I woke up feeling like I was on top of the world. The second time I did the exercise, the same thing happened. I fell asleep again, but it was short and wonderful! I feel so good after I do that exercise. For the rest of the day it seemed like I could do anything. I had so much energy!

—Jennifer M.

Autogenics

The word *autogenic* comes from the Greek words *autos,* meaning self, and *genos,* meaning origin. Hence, **autogenics** is self-directed relaxation using suggestions to create feelings such as warmth and heaviness in the body.

The Power of Suggestion Autogenics is similar to hypnosis, in that both involve the use of suggestion. In hypnosis, a **suggestion** is any statement that the mind believes is true, accurate, or real. In autogenics this suggestion is self-directed. Hypnosis has been used as a means for changing how people think about things and as a way of helping them change their behaviors. Hypnosis will be explored more thoroughly in Chapter 20, on guided imagery. For now we want to address the power of suggestion, and how it relates to the effective method of relaxation called autogenics, or autogenic training (AT).

Background of Autogenic Training

Autogenic training is a method of reducing the stress response; the method was developed in Europe in the early years of the 20th century by the brain physiologist Oskar Vogt. Vogt was working with some of his most experienced hypnotic subjects when he noticed that as his subjects put themselves into a hypnotic state, their tension, fatigue, and headaches decreased.

Author Anecdote When I Say You Have Hot Shoes

At a high school assembly we were sitting in the gym bleachers. Down on the basketball court were 16 of our fellow classmates. They were peacefully sitting in chairs with their eyes closed. A man was walking around speaking into a microphone so everyone could hear what he was saying. He said in a firm voice, "When I say the words 'hot shoes,' you will have hot shoes and, boy, will you move! Your feet will feel like your shoes are on fire." After he said this, he told each of the hypnotized students to wake up and sit quietly in his or her chair.

The hypnotist then started speaking with them casually as if nothing at all had happened. As he was talking, he included the words "hot shoes" in one of his sentences. Immediately all of the students became uncomfortable. They looked down and started moving their feet. Soon they all had thrown their shoes (which in their minds had caught on fire) far away from where they were sitting.

From our point of view, the shoes had not changed in any way, but to the students sitting down there on the gym floor, those shoes had become unbearably hot and painful. We laughed, but those students sitting on the gym floor didn't. They were recuperating from the severe burns the "hot shoes" had inflicted on their feet. Of course, there were no hot shoes, nor were there burns on their feet. But in their minds, something painful had definitely happened.

—MO

In the 1930s, Johannes Schultz, a psychiatrist from Germany, continued the work of Professor Vogt and learned that those who were able to attain deep relaxation through hypnosis experienced two pleasant physical sensations. One was heaviness, and the other was warmth, primarily in their arms and legs. In addition, Shultz's subjects reported as an immediate benefit that their headaches went away.[1]

From these observations Schultz developed a system designed to activate the parasympathetic nervous system using suggestions focusing on warmth and heaviness. The simple suggestion to the mind caused the body to respond physically by increasing blood flow to the extremities and relaxing the muscles. Schultz found that those who practiced this simple method were able to attain deep levels of rest similar to the responses of people under hypnosis and meditation. Schultz's work, entitled *Autogenic Training*,[2] is the classic account of this autogenic training method.

One of Schultz's students, Wolfgang Luthe, immigrated to Canada from Germany and introduced the technique to North America. He also translated much of Shultz's work from German to English. Since then, autogenics has become a time-honored and effective means for reducing stress-related symptoms including insomnia, anxiety, and tension. Autogenics can be practiced anywhere. It is easy to learn and simple to practice and includes the positive aspects of hypnosis without requiring a trained hypnotist.

How Autogenics Works

The pleasant feeling of warmth in the extremities can be explained physiologically as the **vasodilation** (increase in the diameter) of blood vessels in response to parasympathetic nervous system activation. The parasympathetic nervous system is designed to bring the body to a state of homeostasis, or balance. In terms relating to the fight-or-flight response, vasodilation occurs when the impending threat has passed and there is no longer a need to run or fight. The pleasant feeling of heaviness is characteristic of muscles, formerly tensed to run or fight, becoming relaxed.

Benefits of Autogenics

Studies have demonstrated the effectiveness of autogenic training on a variety of stress-related problems and maladies. Autogenic training has been found to reduce heart rate, blood pressure, respiratory rate, and tension. Researchers have concluded that autogenic training is effective in dealing with anxiety, phobic disorders, and hysteria.[3]

Autogenics has been found to be a favorable cure for headaches, including tension headaches[4] and migraine headaches.[5] One such study showed a significant decrease in tension and also a decrease in migraine headaches, resulting in a significant decrease in consumption of migraine drugs and analgesics for subjects who practiced autogenics for an 8-month period. Subjects in this study showed immediate relief from headaches at the onset of the 8-month period, and the benefits continued throughout the course of the study.[6]

Findings from an interesting study with cancer patients who practiced autogenic training demonstrated a significant reduction in anxiety toward their cancer. They also showed an improvement in "fighting spirit" after practicing autogenics, compared to this attitude before learning the procedure.[7] "Fighting spirit" is defined as the open expression of emotions, either positive or negative. An improvement in fighting spirit has been shown to positively affect outcomes of cancer.[8] The subjects in this study showed an improved sense of coping. They also reported sleeping better as an apparent benefit of AT practice.

> **FYI**
>
> ### Case Study in Autogenics
>
> The effects of autogenics were demonstrated in a case study of a young woman (K.S.) who was suffering from severely disturbing nightmares almost every night as a result of a horrible automobile accident. After she began to practice autogenic training regularly, the frequency and severity of the post-traumatic nightmares dropped significantly, and they ceased altogether by the end of the treatment. The report stated:
>
> It is important to note that upon the completion of treatment, the patient began reporting positive changes in her anxiety levels, and she gradually became more socially active. Her sleep latency (the time it took for her to fall asleep) decreased from several hours to approximately 30 minutes. The patient estimated that the panic attacks diminished in intensity and ceased by the end of the treatment. Although it took K.S. some time to begin driving again, she actively began utilizing autogenic phrases in order to control and overcome her fear of "being behind the wheel." K.S. reported that the treatment helped her recover her sense of control over her anxieties via utilizing specific tools that she learned to master in a short period of time.
>
> **Source:** "The Treatment of Recalcitrant Post-Traumatic Nightmares with Autogenic Training and Autogenic Abreaction: A Case Study," by Micah R. Sadigh, *Applied Psychophysiology & Biofeedback* (1999) 24(3), 203.

RESEARCH HIGHLIGHT

Meta-analysis of Autogenic Training

Meta-analysis is the combining of data from several different research studies to gain a better overview of a topic than what was available in any single investigation.* In a meta-analysis** of autogenic training, AT was found to be positively beneficial for the following maladies:

Tension headache
Migraine headache
Mild-to-moderate essential hypertension
Coronary heart disease
Bronchial asthma
Somatoform pain disorder (unspecified type)
Raynaud's disease
Anxiety disorders
Mild-to-moderate depression
Functional sleep disorders

The same meta-analysis found AT to have a beneficial effect on mood, cognitive performance, quality of life, and physiological variables.

Sources:
Taber's Cyclopedic Medical Dictionary (19th ed.) (Philadelphia: F.A. Davis Co., 2001).
**"Autogenic Training: A Meta-analysis of Clinical Outcome Studies," by Friedhelm Stetter and Sirko Kupper, *Applied Psychophysiology & Biofeedback*, 27(1) (2002): 45.

Additional studies have shown that autogenics has been effective in dealing with insomnia[9] and muscle tension.[10] It also was found to help decrease the effects of post-traumatic stress disorder.[11] AT even seems to improve biathletes' shooting performance,[12] possibly because of its calming effect.

One study[13] examined the effect of autogenic training on pilots' flight performance. Compared to the control group, the group that received autogenic training showed a significant improvement in performance and a significant decrease in physiological arousal during emergency flying conditions. The pilots who practiced autogenics were able to remain calmer and more in control during stressful flying situations.

Other conditions that have shown favorable improvement with autogenic training include bladder problems, ulcerative colitis, irritable bowel syndrome, diabetes, thyroid disease, grief, eating disorders, PMS, asthma, circulation disorders, and peptic ulcers.[14]

Considering how the stress response is activated in the presence of a perceived threat and the illnesses that are attributed to this response, it becomes apparent why deep relaxation, such as what occurs while practicing autogenic training, can have such a powerful effect on improving the health of those who suffer from these disorders.

Experiencing Autogenics

Creating Favorable Conditions According to the authors of *Autogenic Training in Psychotherapy*, several factors are important for autogenic training to be successful.[15] Beneficial results are more likely with:

1. High motivation and cooperation
2. A reasonable degree of self-direction and self-control
3. Maintenance of a specific body posture conducive to success, including:
   a. Lying on a carpeted floor or on a bed (soft, flat surface)
   b. Hands resting comfortably to the sides, palms up, fingers loose and extended
   c. Feet forming a "V" with the heels not quite touching and the toes pointing outward
   d. The head and neck comfortably supported with a pillow
4. Reduction of external stimuli—turning off all possible sound-making devices including cell phones, telephones, television; reducing the possibility of being interrupted by others
5. Focus on internal processes to the exclusion of the external environment—focusing attention fully on what is happening internally
6. Presentation of the suggestions in a repetitive and monotonous manner, to avoid excitation and to create an environment conducive to passivity

For autogenics to work as intended, the person must have a passive attitude and not "try" to make anything happen. Those who practice it should make no conscious effort to force feelings of warmth, heaviness, or any other sensations that are suggested to the mind. Contrary to some of the other relaxation techniques that involve more willful mental activity, autogenics requires a passive alertness.

Tim Gallway described this attitude of passive alertness as **effortless effort,** signifying a lack of tension in allowing the sensations to happen. This is an attempt to be observant rather than to focus on how well or how badly relaxation is happening.[16] In taking this attitude, if nothing happens, that is okay. If sensations do happen, that is okay, too, but not to be overly celebrated. The individual should take what comes and continue passively.

Autogenics is best experienced lying on the floor or a bed. Autogenics also can be done sitting comfortably in a chair. In the seated position, sit comfortably in a high back chair with armrests for head and arms support. Feet should be flat on the floor with knees slightly apart. The individual can mentally repeat autogenic suggestions or someone else can read through a script of the suggestions. The latter is usually preferable when someone is learning autogenics. The Premium Website audio files contains the autogenics relaxation exercise to guide you through the process.

The autogenic suggestions usually follow this sequence:

1. Focus on heaviness in the arms and legs.
2. Focus on warmth in the arms and legs.
3. Focus on warmth and heaviness in the heart area.
4. Focus on breathing.
5. Focus on coolness in the forehead.

Stress Relief Activity
Practice the Autogenics Relaxation Technique found in the Premium Website audio files.

A Simple Autogenics Script

Make yourself as comfortable as possible. Gently close your eyes. Take in a nice, easy deep breath through your nose … and exhale. Again, a deep breath in … and exhale. Continue to breathe deeply in and out, keeping your eyes closed. (long pause)

Allow all thoughts of past and future to drift away. Bring yourself fully to this moment by focusing on your inner experience. (pause)

Now let your attention focus on your left arm and hand. Feel how they are gently supported by the surface below. Now, breathing slowly and evenly, focus passively on your left hand and arm while repeating to yourself, "My left hand and arm are heavy." Continue to repeat this silently to yourself for a few moments. (pause)

Now shift your attention to your right hand and arm, sensing how they are gently supported from below. Keeping your eyes closed and breathing evenly, repeat to yourself, "My right hand and arm are heavy." Continue saying this silently to yourself for a few moments. (pause)

Now let your mind focus on both hands and arms. Become deeply aware of how they feel. If you have trouble sensing both at the same time, shift your attention back and forth from one to the other. As you take deep, natural breaths, repeat silently to yourself, "My hands and arms are heavy." Continue saying this phrase to yourself for a few moments. (pause)

Now imagine that the feelings of heaviness and relaxation in your arms are spreading effortlessly throughout your body, flowing to every other part. Each time you breathe out, let yourself sink into deeper relaxation. (pause)

Now, keeping your eyes closed, let your attention focus on your left leg. Be aware of your left thigh, knee, lower leg, ankle, foot, and toes. Now, as you breathe evenly, repeat quietly to yourself, "My left leg is heavy." Continue saying this to yourself for a few moments. (pause)

Now let your attention move to your right leg, and as you breathe evenly and deeply, repeat to yourself, "My right leg is heavy." Silently repeat this phrase to yourself for a few moments. (pause) Notice the feelings of deepening relaxation in your right leg as you breathe evenly in and out. (pause)

Now focus easily on both legs. If you have trouble sensing both at the same time, simply shift from one to the other. Keeping your eyes gently closed and breathing evenly, repeat to yourself, "My legs are heavy." Repeat this phrase for a few moments to yourself. (pause)

Letting your attention move to your arms, say to yourself, "My arms are warm." Breathing slowly and evenly and letting the warmth spread in your arms, repeat this phrase for a few moments. (pause)

Now silently repeat to yourself, "My legs are warm." Continue saying this to yourself for a few moments as you breathe evenly, allowing sensations of warmth to flow throughout your legs. (pause)

Now let your mind scan your arms and legs. Notice how they feel. Silently describe these sensations to yourself. (pause)

Now, letting your attention easily move around your entire body, sense the spreading feelings of warmth and heaviness in your arms, neck, shoulders, chest, stomach, and legs. As you breathe evenly, say to yourself, "My entire body is warm and heavy." Continue for a few moments. (long pause)

Now mentally scan your body, being aware of any sensations of warmth, heaviness, and relaxation. Let these feelings spread for a few moments as you become more aware of these pleasant feelings. (pause)

Now, as you sink effortlessly into deeper relaxation, begin to sense the regular beat of your heart or the pulse in some other part of your body. Let yourself become very quiet, and very aware of your heartbeat and pulse. Breathing evenly and deeply, repeat to yourself, "My heart is calm and regular." (pause)

Move your attention to your breath as you say to yourself, "My breathing is slow and even." Continue this for the next few moments. (pause)

Move your awareness to your forehead and say to yourself, "My forehead is cool and relaxed." (pause)

Notice how comfortable, quiet, and still your body feels. Let yourself experience the slow, regular beating of your heart as you breathe easily and deeply. Feel the effortless spreading of relaxation throughout your body. Take a few moments to completely enjoy these pleasant sensations. (pause)

If you feel any areas of remaining tension, imagine feelings of wonderful warmth flowing easily to that place as you continue to breathe deeply. Passively let deep relaxation spread everywhere. (pause)

Completely enjoy this feeling of deep relaxation. Allow yourself to be still and rested. . . . (long pause)

As you prepare to end this session, take a deep breath in and out, filling your lungs fully and then easily releasing the breath. Gently begin to move your fingers, hands, arms, legs, and feet to revive the muscles. Keeping your eyes closed, turn your head from side to side while looking around the room. Gently stretch your whole body by extending your arms. As you bring your arms back down, turn to lie on your side, bringing your knees up toward your chest. Slowly open your eyes and slowly lift yourself up into a sitting position. Remain here for a few moments, enjoying the feelings of relaxation and stillness that you are feeling before retuning to normal activity levels.

You may want to modify this autogenics script to suit your own preferences. We're presenting this script to get you started and provide you with a format for introducing autogenics.

Author Anecdote So Relaxed She Feels Like She's Floating Autogenic training can be particularly powerful. Once, after leading a group through a good session of yoga, I had each of the participants lie on the floor and close their eyes. I led them through a relaxing autogenic sequence, which they seemed to enjoy.

Afterward, one of the members of the class came up and with some energy asked me, "What did you just do to me?!" Puzzled, I asked her what she meant. She told me that while she was doing the autogenic exercise, she became incredibly relaxed. After a few moments of deep relaxation, she said she felt like she was floating in the air, perfectly suspended about three feet off the ground. I asked her if this sensation was unpleasant. She said that it was one of the most wonderful, relaxing, peaceful feelings she had ever experienced. I assured her that she had stayed on the ground the whole time, but also congratulated her for reaching such deep levels of relaxation. She told me that she felt absolutely magnificent. I suggested to her that it sounded like her mind/body must really enjoy autogenics to have produced such a remarkably relaxing experience.

—MO

Stress Relief Activities
Visit the Premium Website audio files to explore a variety of relaxation activities and techniques.

Conclusion

Autogenics is self-directed relaxation using suggestion. The person experiences pleasant feelings of warmth and heaviness because of vasodilatation of blood vessels in response to activation of the parasympathetic nervous system. Meta-analysis showed autogenic training to be positively beneficial for a variety of stress-related conditions, including mood and quality of life.

18.1 Autogenics

PURPOSE To allow you to practice deep relaxation using autogenics.

DIRECTIONS Prepare your environment for relaxation. Follow along with the Autogenics instructions found in the Premium Website audio file. Practice this technique at least 2 times according to the instructions on the audio file. At least once, do it immediately before you sleep at night. Make sure it is the last thing you do before sleep. Do it at times when you will not be disturbed. Allow approximately 15 minutes to complete the exercise.

After completing Autogenics, respond to the questions below. Describe primarily how you were feeling in relation to your stress levels.

Afternoon:

1. How did you feel before the exercise?

2. What was your experience during the exercise?

3. How did you feel immediately after the exercise?

4. How did you feel several hours after completing the exercise?

Right before sleeping at night:

1. How did you feel before the exercise?

2. How quickly did you fall asleep?

3. How did you sleep, and how refreshed did you feel when you awakened the following morning?

4. How did this differ from a typical night's sleep?

Classroom experience (if applicable):

1. How did you feel before the exercise?

2. What was your experience during the exercise?

3. How did you feel immediately after the exercise?

4. How did you feel several hours after completing the exercise?

Summary After you have practiced the exercise and described your experiences, include a brief review of what you liked and/or did not like about this technique. Compare this technique to some of the others you have practiced. Would this be a relaxation technique you would consider using on a regular basis for stress management? Why or why not?

Key Points

- "Autogenic" comes from the Greek words *autos* meaning self, and *genos* meaning origin. Hence, autogenics is self-directed relaxation using suggestions.
- The pleasant feeling of warmth in the extremities can be explained physiologically as the vasodilatation of blood vessels in response to parasympathetic nervous system activation.

- Studies have demonstrated the effectiveness of autogenic training on a variety of stress-related conditions.
- Several factors outlined in this chapter are important for the practice of autogenic training to be successful.
- A simple autogenic script can be used to introduce you to autogenics.

Key Terms

autogenics

suggestion

autogenic training

vasodilation

meta-analysis

effortless effort

Discussion Time For Critical Thinking/Discussion Questions, please visit this book's Premium Website. www

Notes

1. *Mind as Healer, Mind as Slayer*, by K. R. Pelletier (New York: Dell Publishing, 1977).

2. *Das Autogene Training*, by J. Schultz (Stuttgart: Geerg-Thieme Verlag, 1953).

3. "Autogenic Biofeedback in Psychophysiological Therapy and Stress Management," by P. A. Norris and S. L. Farrion. In P. M. Lehrer and R. L. Woolfolk (Eds.), *Principles and Practice of Stress Management* (New York: The Guilford Press, 1984) pp. 220–254.

4. "Autogenic Training and Future Oriented Hypnotic Imagery in the Treatment of Tension Headache: Outcome and Process," by R. VanDyck, F. G. Zitman, A. C. Linssen, and P. Spinhoven, *International Journal of Clinical and Experimental Hypnosis 39*(1) (1991): 6–23.

5. "The Efficacy and Cost-Effectiveness of Minimal-Therapist-Contact, Non-Drug Treatments of Chronic Migraine and Tension Headache," by E. B. Blanchard, et al., *Headache 25* (1985): 214–220; "Temperature Biofeedback and Regulation Training in the Treatment of Migraine Headaches," by B. V. Silver, *Biofeedback and Self-Regulation 4* (1979): 359–366.

6. "Effect of Autogenic Training on Drug Consumption in Patients with Primary Headache: An 8-Month Follow-Up Study," by T. Zsombok, G. Juhasz, A. Budavari, et al., *Headache: The Journal of Head & Face Pain 43*(3) (2003): 251.

7. "A Quantitative and Qualitative Pilot Study of the Perceived Benefits of Autogenic Training for a Group of People with Cancer," by S. Wright, U. Courtney, and D. Crowther, *European Journal of Cancer Care 11*(2) (2002): 122.

8. *Mind/Body Health: The Effects of Attitudes, Emotions, and Relationships* (3rd ed.), by K. Karren, B. Hafen, N. Smith, and K. Frandsen (San Francisco: Benjamin Cummings, 2006).

9. "What to Use Instead of Sleeping Pills," by T. J. Coates and C. E. Thoreson, *Journal of the American Medical Association 240* (1978): 2311–2312.

10. "Biofeedback, Autogenic Training, and Progressive Muscular Relaxation in the Treatment of Raynaud's Disease: A Comparative Study," by J. F. Keefe, R. S. Surwit, and R. N. Pilon, *Journal of Applied Behavior Analysis 13* (1980): 3–11.

11. "Treatment of Posttraumatic Stress Disorder in Postwar Kosovo High School Students Using Mind–Body Skills Groups: A Pilot Study," by J. S. Gordon, J. K. Staples, A. Blyta, and M. Bytyqi, *Journal of Traumatic Stress 17*(2) (2004): 143–148.

12. "Effects of Autogenic and Imagery Training on the Shooting Performance in Biathlon," by A. Groslambert, R. Candau, F. Grappe, B. Dugué, and J. D. Rouillon, *Research Quarterly for Exercise & Sport 74*(3) (2003): 337.

13. "Autogenic Feedback Training Exercise and Pilot Performance: Enhanced Functioning Under Search-and-Rescue Flying Conditions," by P. S. Cowings, M. A. Kellar, R. A. Folen, W. B. Toscano, and J. D. Burge, *International Journal of Aviation Psychology 11*(3) (2001): 303.

14. http://stress.about.com/cs/relaxation/a/aa030501.htm

15. *Autogenic Training: A Psychophysiologic Approach in Psychotherapy*, by J. Schultz and W. Luthe (New York: Grune & Stratton, 1959).

16. *The Inner Game of Tennis*, by W. T. Gallway (New York: Random House, 1974).

19 Progressive Relaxation

- I don't understand how progressive muscle relaxation can work. How can tensing my muscles make me feel more relaxed? - What happens when a muscle contracts?

Study of this chapter will enable you to:

1. Describe contraction and relaxation of muscles.
2. Explain the benefits of progressive muscle relaxation.
3. Differentiate between active and passive relaxation methods.
4. Experience the difference between muscle relaxation and muscle tension.
5. Experience the benefits of progressive muscle relaxation (PMR) and passive progressive relaxation.

Tension is who you think you should be. Relaxation is who you are.

—*Chinese Proverb*

REAL PEOPLE, REAL STORIES

Students Share Their Experiences with PMR I really liked doing PMR. I asked my friend to do this with me, and afterward he couldn't quit saying to me how great he felt. I had to agree. I never thought that tensing your muscles and then releasing them would relax them so much. It was a normal day like any other when I decided to do this exercise, so I wasn't really tense, but I could always use a little relaxation. During the whole thing I was getting more and more relaxed. I really enjoyed this exercise and it put me in a good mood to just release that tension in my muscles. I think this is one of the relaxation techniques that could be used any time or any place. I felt good afterward and, believe it or not, this one didn't put me to sleep!

—Shantelle T.

* * *

The progressive exercise was different and really interesting. It was so helpful for me to see the differences between tension and relaxation. I know my body is tense a lot and my muscles are always sore from football. But I never really take the time to feel what it's doing to my body and to feel the immediate difference between tension and relaxation. When I would tense up my hands into a fist, my hands and arms were tight, and as soon as I breathed out and released all of the tension, I felt overwhelming relaxation. I noticed a big difference in my face and neck as well. My neck is always tense and my face, especially my eyes and jaw muscles, are constantly strained. When I allowed the relaxation to take over my body, I liked the feeling of heaviness in my muscles and the calm and peaceful feeling I had. This was a very good exercise.

—Tyler G.

* * *

My experience while doing the progressive relaxation was nice. I did it once after work and once before bed. I found it to be most relaxing after work because I get tense while I'm working. As I began the exercise, the first muscles we tensed were the hands and forearms. After I did that, it was like that part of my body was gone, sunk into the carpet. As I continued to do each muscle, they seemed to disappear, and after I had done every muscle, I felt like I'd sunk into a giant pillow. The comparison of contracting and releasing made my body seem so light. I felt totally relaxed, and my muscles had no tension whatsoever. The favorite muscle group to do was my thigh area. After it was completed, I felt entirely released of the tension I had gathered throughout the day. When I did PMR before bed, I fell asleep right away. Every time I've done any of these relaxation exercises, I've fallen asleep more easily. I usually have a hard time falling asleep because I have so much on my mind.

—Carli S.

Progressive Relaxation

Stiff neck, tension headache, tight shoulders, grinding teeth, low-back pain—all of these annoying symptoms can result from muscle tension. Although it is not life-threatening, muscle tension may be the most common and irritating symptom of stress. Muscles respond directly to thoughts of perceived danger by tensing in preparation for action. **Progressive muscle relaxation** (PMR) techniques are designed specifically to reduce muscle tension through focused attention.

Background

Edmund Jacobson, a doctor living in Chicago, first caught on to the idea of tension and relaxation in the muscles while he was working with patients who had a variety of maladies. He noticed one common characteristic in nearly all of his patients—muscle tension. Based on his previous research at Harvard and his current work with his patients, he recognized that the severity of many disorders could be diminished by reducing or relieving muscle tension.

Jacobson found that most of his patients had no idea that they had excess muscle tension in various places in their bodies. He noticed that as his patients were asked to consciously flex these tensed-up areas, and then consciously relieve that tension, the contracting muscles became relaxed. Jacobson understood that a muscle cannot contract and relax at the same time. By forcibly tensing a muscle and then consciously releasing the contraction, the muscles returned to their naturally relaxed position.

Thus was born the relaxation technique called progressive muscle relaxation. It also has been called **progressive neuromuscular relaxation,** which identifies the activation of the autonomic nervous system in initiating and turning off muscle tension. Although Jacobson's original technique has evolved and branched out into various adaptations, progressive relaxation remains a commonly used form of relaxation therapy in Western society today.

FYI

The Birth of PMR

Little did Edmund Jacobson know that a seemingly negative event during his days as a research assistant at Harvard in the early 1900s would provide an opportunity leading to the discovery of PMR, still a popular and effective stress management technique a century later.

Jacobson was a research assistant to Hugo Munsterberg, a professor who was considered one of the great minds of the day. When Jacobson's data supported theories in opposition to Munsterberg's own hypothesis, he fired Jacobson.

With time on his hands, Jacobson turned his attention to the study of the startle response, a sudden jerking or startle reaction that occurs naturally in response to unexpected loud noises. He discovered that deeply relaxed students demonstrated no obvious startle response to a sudden noise. This discovery proved to be the first systematic study of the effects of relaxation on the body and eventually led to the birth of PMR.

Source: *Mosby's Complementary and Alternative Medicine* (3rd ed.), by L. Freeman (St. Louis: Mosby, 2009).

Muscle Physiology

To understand how progressive relaxation works as an effective form of relaxation, it is helpful to have a basic understanding of how muscles work. The human body contains hundreds of voluntary skeletal muscles. Skeletal muscles are involved in several physiological functions, including generating force (strength and speed), generating heat, maintaining posture, and assisting in breathing.

Each skeletal muscle is composed of many muscle fibers (cells), each of which has the ability to contract or relax. A muscle fiber contracts when it receives a nerve impulse from the central nervous system (brain and spinal cord). After contracting, a muscle fiber relaxes until it receives another nerve impulse.

A **motor unit** consists of a single motor nerve and all the muscle fibers to which it sends impulses as demonstrated in Figure 19.1. When a motor unit receives a message from the nervous system, each of the muscle fibers responds with a burst of energy. When this happens, tiny filaments, which are the smallest parts of the muscle, pull on each other and cause a **muscle contraction** or shortening of the muscle fibers.[1]

All-or-None Principle

Muscle contraction is based on the **all-or-none principle.** A muscle fiber contracts completely or not at all. Skeletal muscles are naturally in a state of noncontraction, or relaxation. When a signal from the nervous system reaches a muscle motor unit anywhere in the body, all the muscle fibers in this motor unit contract completely. When the nerve impulse stops, the contraction stops and the muscle fiber relaxes, returning to its normally noncontracting state.

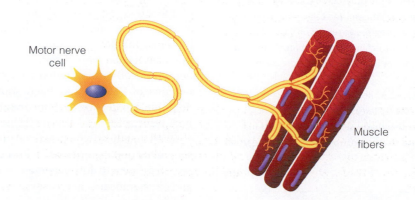

Motor nerve cell

Muscle fibers

FIGURE 19.1 Motor unit, composed of a motor nerve and muscle fibers

Muscles and Relaxation

What does muscle physiology have to do with stress management? Many muscles in the body remain in a chronically contracted state because they are continuously receiving the message from the nervous system that they should be contracting in preparation for fight-or-flight. But they don't receive the signal from the nervous system that the threat has passed and it is safe to relax. An example is often found in a person's shoulders, which might feel tight and sore because these muscles are continually tensed. Even while we sleep, thoughts in the unconscious mind can produce muscle tension. Common manifestations of muscle tension during sleep are jaw-clenching and teeth-grinding.

Recall from earlier chapters that one of the immediate actions of the fight-or-flight response is an increase in muscular tension to generate immediate power to either run or fight. This is an automatic response in the presence of a threat. As we also mentioned, most modern threats are those we create in our own mind. But because we still perceive threats in our environment, the autonomic nervous system responds to threats the same as it did in ages past—by gearing up to run or fight. As a result, our muscles become tense. The dilemma is that because our modern threats—daily work pressures, school requirements, or ongoing battles with a partner—do not come to an end immediately, the fight-or-flight response remains activated and, therefore, muscle contraction is continuous. The muscle tension doesn't turn off.

FYI

What Is Bruxism?

"Keep a stiff upper lip" or "get a grip!" That's often the advice we get—and give—on how to cope with stress. If you take it literally, the result could be grinding your teeth or clenching your jaws. Sometimes we grind our teeth—called bruxism—as we sleep. This is caused by stress and anxiety among other things. Symptoms include a dull headache, wearing down of the teeth, or a sore jaw. People who frequently grind their teeth are more likely to feel stressed out at work than those who don't clench their teeth, and women are more likely than men to say that they grind their teeth and that their jobs are stressful.[2] Your dentist can fit you with a mouth guard to protect your teeth while you sleep. If stress is causing you to clench or grind, you need to find a way to relax! Don't make your teeth the brunt of your stress.

How PMR Works

Progressive muscle relaxation activates the parasympathetic nervous system in a consciously directed way by first tensing a group of muscles and then consciously releasing the tension in that muscle group. This technique is called progressive muscle relaxation because you move progressively through the major areas of the body.

Of the many variations of the original PMR technique in use today, all have in common the objective of teaching a person to relax the muscles at will by first developing conscious awareness of what it feels like to be tense and then what it feels like to be relaxed. Once you learn to distinguish between tension and relaxation, you can control tension. The primary feature of this method is the ability to relax muscles selectively on command.

Author Anecdote
Progressive Relaxation and Yoga

We had just finished treating progressive relaxation in class, which included an exercise at the end of the session. One of the students approached me after class, eager to relate her experience. She clearly had gained much benefit from progressive relaxation, saying that she felt loaded with energy and at the same time peaceful and calm. Her comment to me—which I hadn't considered before—was that progressive relaxation seemed to her to be a lot like yoga. She explained that when she's stretching the body through the poses in yoga, the muscles contract. When the body releases from the stretch, the muscles naturally relax.

Each time she consciously contracted her muscles while doing PMR and then relaxed them afterward, she achieved the same feelings of deep release from tension as she did with yoga. This was a new idea to me, but one that makes sense as I think about it. Focusing on releasing muscle tension, using whatever method, works to release energy and relax the body. Relaxation is our natural state.

—MO

Benefits of Progressive Relaxation

Progressive relaxation effectively turns off the stress response and induces relaxation.[3] As a result, many of the adverse physical, mental, and emotional conditions associated with chronic stress have been reduced or eliminated with regular practice of PMR. It has been shown to be helpful in dealing with insomnia[4] and post-traumatic stress disorder.[5] One study showed that those who practiced progressive relaxation experienced a lower heart rate, less anxiety, lower perceived stress, and a significant decrease in salivary

PMR for Anxiety   Short-term feelings of anxiety may be an unavoidable part of life, but anxiety can be reduced through relaxation exercises such as PMR. In one study, high school students who received training in progressive muscle relaxation demonstrated significantly lower anxiety scores than those who had not received this training.* The researchers summarized their results by stating: "This should be exciting news for high school counselors and others who are looking for ways to help students who have high anxiety and the poor academic achievement that often is associated with it." If you want to relax before taking a difficult test, speaking in front of a group of people, or anything else about which you feel apprehensive, progressive muscle relaxation may be the tool that helps you get through it more easily.

Source: *"The Effects of Two Types of Relaxation Training on Students' Levels of Anxiety," by A. M. Rasid & T. S. Parish, *Adolescence, 33,* 99–102.

cortisol (indicating a physiological decrease in sympathetic nervous system activity) compared to control subjects. The subjects in this study also self-reported increased relaxation.[6]

Long and Haney found progressive relaxation to be as effective as aerobic activity in decreasing anxiety and increasing self-efficacy among working women.[7] In additional controlled studies, progressive relaxation has been effective in reducing the effects of other stress-related maladies, including reducing headaches,[8] depression,[9] aversion to chemotherapy,[10] low back pain,[11] postpartum depression,[12] and hypertension.[13]

How to Do Progressive Muscle Relaxation

Three forms of PMR are explained next—active progressive muscle relaxation; a variation called incremental muscle relaxation; and passive progressive relaxation.

Active Progressive Muscle Relaxation   In **active progressive muscle relaxation,** you tense a group of muscles fairly tightly—to about 70-80% of a maximum contraction. Once they are contracted sufficiently, you hold them in this state of tension for up to 8 seconds. Then you immediately release those flexed muscles for 15 to 30 seconds. During this relaxation phase, you consciously relax the muscles even more completely so you are as relaxed as possible.

As you exhale, imagine tightness and pain flowing out of your muscles. Feel the muscles become loose and limp, the tension flowing away like water out of a faucet. Notice the difference between tension and relaxation. By tensing your muscles first, you will find that you are able to relax your muscles more than you would if you were to try to relax your muscles directly. You focus awareness on the sensation of relaxation resulting from release of the tension and how this feeling differs from the feeling of tension. Careful examination of this change in tension is important.

While you are either seated or lying down, focus on a specific area of the body, such as your left arm and hand. Clench your fist, tightening your fist for several seconds and then relaxing your hand for 15 to 30 seconds.

Repeat this procedure at least once. If an area remains tense, repeat the tensing and relaxing up to five times. Progressively move through the body—such as the arms, the face, the torso, and the shoulders, tensing and releasing each muscle group as you go.

With some relaxation techniques the mind tends to wander to other thoughts because only the mind is involved. One of the biggest challenges of many relaxation techniques is a distracted mind. Because PMR involves both the mind and the body, it enables you to stay focused. Many individuals have great success with this technique because, by concentrating on tensing and relaxing muscle groups, they stay focused more easily.

Relaxation results from first tensing and then relaxing muscles.

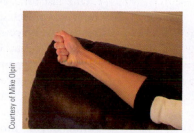
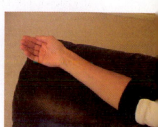

Courtesy of Mike Olpin

A More Western Way to Relax

Meditation, guided imagery, deep breathing, and several of the other stress management tools in this book have their roots in Eastern philosophy and practice. The function of these tools is to relax the mind or body in passive ways. By contrast, the roots of PMR are planted firmly in the West. Because it is an active form of relaxation, it seems to have broad appeal to our Western culture, where we often think that nothing happens unless we are actively engaged. If we are not "doing" something, nothing is happening. For individuals who struggle with the other types of relaxation exercises because their mind tends to wander too much or they get bored because they aren't sufficiently involved, PMR is an effective alternative.

Stress Relief Activity

Practice the Progressive Relaxation Technique found in the Premium Website files.

Incremental Muscle Relaxation   One effective variation of progressive muscle relaxation changes the process slightly. **Incremental muscle relaxation** is a method that sensitizes the individual to actual muscle tension levels. Working through each group of muscles, first tense the muscles maximally to what feels like 100% contraction. After 5 to 10 seconds of contracting maximally, relax that muscle group completely for 15 to 30 seconds. Contract the same muscles a second time, this time contracting to what feels like about 50% of maximal contraction. After 5 to 10 seconds of holding this contraction, relax the muscles completely for 15 to 30 seconds. On a third contraction of the same muscles, flex the muscles at no more than 10% of maximal contraction. At this point you are barely creating any tension. Hold this contraction for 5 to 10 seconds, and then relax the muscles completely for 15 to 30 seconds. Progress to the next set of muscles and follow the same procedure.

When learning PMR, a facilitator to guide you through the process will yield the best results. Included on the Premium Website audio files is a relaxation exercise titled Progressive Relaxation to guide your practice.

Active Progressive Relaxation Script   Make yourself as comfortable as possible. Gently close your eyes. Take a nice, easy deep breath in through your nose . . . and exhale. Again, a deep breath in . . . and exhale. Continue to breathe deeply in and out, keeping your eyes closed. (long pause) Allow all thoughts of your past and future to drift away.

When you tighten an area, do it only to a point at which you feel real tension but not pain. If a specific area or muscle is sore or uncomfortable, skip that area. As you tighten the various muscles during this session, you will inhale and hold your breath. As you exhale, you will release the tension.

Now make a fist with your hands, pressing the fingers against your palm, tightening the muscles in your wrists and forearms, until you feel moderate tension in that entire area. Feel the pulling tightness in your fingers, hands and forearms . . . hold it for a moment longer . . . and now, as you breathe out, let those muscles go limp like a rag doll. The tension drains naturally from your fingers, wrists, and forearms. Feel the pleasant relief of flowing relaxation. Notice how different this is from tension. (pause)

Again, tighten your fists and feel the tension build . . . hold it for a moment . . . and now, breathing out, let these muscles go limp, and say to yourself, "My arms and hands feel relaxed and calm." (pause)

Notice carefully how different this is from the tension. (pause)

One last time, make fists with your hands, while tensing your wrists, forearm, and upper arm muscles. Hold that tension and feel the stretching tightness . . . and now as you breathe out, let your hands and arms go limp, saying to yourself, "My hands and arms feel relaxed and calm." Let all remaining tension flow out through your fingertips, enjoying the sense of relief. (pause)

While letting your arms and hands remain deeply relaxed, now focus your attention on your face and head. Concentrating on how it feels, close your eyes tightly as if you were in a dust storm. Stretch your forehead muscles up as far as you can. Pull the corners of your mouth back and feel tension in every part of your face. Experience that sensation. . . . Now, breathing out, let all these muscles go completely limp and say to yourself, "My face and forehead feel relaxed and calm." Notice how different this is from the tension. Enjoy the sensation of relaxation. (pause)

Each time you exhale, feel your hands, arms, face, and forehead become even more deeply relaxed. (pause)

Now shift your attention to your neck muscles. These are usually the first ones to become tense when you encounter stress. Keeping your mouth closed, tighten your neck muscles by gradually moving your chin toward your chest and tightly forward until you feel tension around the base of your neck. Stretch those muscles and hold for a moment. . . . Now, breathing out, let these muscles go limp, allowing your head to return to a comfortable position. And as you breathe out again, say to yourself, "My neck feels relaxed and calm." Sense the flowing relief and notice how different it is from the tension. (pause)

Each time you exhale, feel any remaining tension flow out of your hands, arms, face, and neck. (pause)

Now, allowing your arms and neck to remain as relaxed as possible, focus attention on your shoulders. Move them up toward your ears as high as you can and feel tightness there. . . . Hold that tension for a moment . . . and now, breathing out, release the tension, letting your shoulders go limp as a rag doll. Say to yourself, "My shoulders are relaxed and calm." Notice how different this feels from the tension. (pause)

Now as you breathe comfortably, let all remaining tension flow out from your hands, arms, face, forehead, neck, and shoulders. Enjoy the calm feelings of spreading relaxation. (pause)

Now focus on your chest and stomach. Allowing your arms, shoulders, and neck to remain relaxed, take a deep breath, and hold it while you tighten the muscles in your stomach and around your chest . . . feel the tension build . . . and now let go completely, breathing out, and feeling relaxation flow through this whole area. Say to yourself, "My chest and stomach are relaxed and calm." Notice how different this feels from the tension. (pause)

Keeping your eyes gently closed, let your hands, arms, face, neck, shoulders, chest, and stomach become even more deeply relaxed. (pause)

Now think of the legs and feet. Tighten the muscles in your buttocks and thighs, and flex your feet by bending them up and toward your head. Feel the tension build . . . hold it for a moment . . . and now as you breathe out, let all these muscles go limp. Say to yourself, "My legs and feet feel relaxed and calm." Notice how different this feels from the tension. (pause)

Now each time you breathe out, feel all remaining tension flow out easily from your hands, arms, face, neck, shoulders, chest, stomach, legs, and feet. Repeat to yourself, "My entire body is relaxed and calm," as you easily and naturally breathe in and out. (pause)

Keeping your eyes closed, sense each part of your body. If you find any remaining areas of tension, tense them and then, breathing out, release the muscles until your entire body is comfortably, deeply relaxed. (long pause)

Passive Progressive Relaxation

Body Scan **Passive progressive relaxation** is a less active method of progressing through the various parts of the body using a technique called the **body scan.** This method does not involve active contraction of muscles but, rather, a passive scanning of the body. The body scan allows individuals to develop a focused, concentrated awareness of the body. Jon Kabat-Zinn, director of the Stress Reduction Clinic at the University of Massachusetts Medical Center, introduced this form of relaxation as the first method for patients to use to discover their bodies in a non-judgmental way and begin to find some relief from their stress-related symptoms.[14]

Often when an unpleasant sensation arises in the body, the immediate (and unconscious) reaction is to physically tense the muscles in that area. This tension can increase the physical discomfort. Focused attention allows individuals to learn subtle cues from the body that indicate an imbalance or the need for a specific intervention, such as a change in position or rest. The body becomes the teacher as individuals begin to identify subtle physical changes in the body that precede and accompany emotional responses.[15] This greater awareness of change, such as increased muscle tension, allows you to quickly do what is necessary to dissipate the tension.

While lying down, the person is guided to put his or her attention on a specific area of the body and simply tune in to what is happening in that part of the body. Kabat-Zinn then has the patient *progress* to another area of the body. Patients are instructed to remain as passive and non-judgmental as possible, while at the same time maintaining a detached thought process of careful observation of body parts, both deep inside and on the surface level.

Kabat-Zinn suggests that when practicing the body scan, a person also should become aware of thoughts that may arise spontaneously while focusing on a specific area of the body. As thoughts come to the surface, the person notes them, but does not add to them, and does not make judgments about those thoughts. For example, if a person were doing the body scan and her attention was on her knee, a thought might arise about how the knee was struck while snow skiing. These thoughts are simply observed but not added to or judged negatively. She would try to avoid adding thoughts about being depressed because she can't ski anymore or what other people think of her because she can't spend time with them on the slopes.

Detached observation may seem difficult at first, but according to Kabat-Zinn, passively progressing through the body in this way is profoundly beneficial. By allowing the breath and the awareness to move through the areas of the body, he believes the body is left in a state of balance and integrity. He refers to passive progressive relaxation as a form of meditation. It is an internal focus similar to methods of meditation described elsewhere in this book. Kabat-Zinn describes the ideal attitude that one should maintain while practicing this passive progressive internal focus. His words apply equally to any of the relaxation techniques found in this textbook:

> In its truest expression, meditation goes beyond notions of success and failure, and this is why it is such a powerful vehicle for growth and change and healing. This does not mean that you cannot progress in your meditation practice, nor does it mean that it is impossible to make mistakes that will reduce its value to you. A particular kind of effort is necessary in the practice of meditation, but it is not an effort of striving to achieve some special state, whether it be relaxation, freedom from pain, healing, or insight. These come naturally with practice because they are already inherent in the present moment and in every moment. Therefore, any moment is as good as any other for experiencing the presence within yourself. If you see things in this light, it makes perfect sense to take each moment as it comes and accept it as it is, seeing it clearly in its fullness, and letting it go. [16]

Observing, without judgment, directs healing energy to the area being observed. This concept does not immediately make sense to us because we think we aren't accomplishing anything by simply observing. But this is something you can test on your own. Kabat-Zinn explains, "Each time you scan your body in this way, you can think of it or visualize it as a purification or detoxification process, a process that is promoting healing by restoring a feeling of wholeness and integrity to your body." [17]

Included on the Premium Website audio files is a relaxation exercise titled Flowing Comfort, designed to help you receive guided practice for this type of passive progressive relaxation.

Passive Progressive Relaxation Script: The Body Scan [18]

1. Lie on your back in a comfortable place, such as on a foam pad on the floor or on your bed. This method is most effective for muscle relaxation, rather than to induce sleep. Muscles can stay in a contracted, tensed position, even during sleep, so the goal here is to first relax the muscles. A more peaceful sleep may follow. Make sure that you will be warm enough. You might want to cover yourself with a blanket.
2. Allow your eyes to close gently.
3. Feel the rising and falling of your belly with each inbreath and outbreath.
4. Take a few moments to feel your body as a "whole," from head to toe, the "envelope" of your skin, the sensations associated with touch in the places you are in contact with on the floor or the bed.
5. Bring your attention to the toes of the left foot. As you focus your attention to them, see if you can "direct," or channel, your breathing to them as well, so it feels as if you are breathing into your toes and out from your toes. It may take a while for you to get the hang of this. It may help to imagine your breath traveling down the body from your nose into the lungs and then continuing through the abdomen and down the left leg all the way to the toes and then back again and out through your nose.

Stress Relief Activity

Practice the Flowing Comfort Technique found in the Premium Website audio files.

6. Allow yourself to feel any and all sensations from your toes, perhaps distinguishing between them and watching the flux of sensations in this region. If you don't feel anything at the moment, that's fine, too. Just allow yourself to feel "not feeling anything."

7. When you are ready to leave the toes and move on, take in a deeper, more intentional breath all the way down to the toes, and on the outbreath allow them to "dissolve" in your "mind's eye." Stay with your breathing for a few breaths at least, and then move on to the sole of the foot, the heel, the top of the foot, and the ankle, continuing to breathe into and out from each region as you observe the sensation you are experiencing, and then letting go of it and moving on.

8. Each time you notice that your attention has wandered off, bring your mind back to the breath and to the region you are focusing on.

9. Continue to move slowly up your left leg and through the rest of your body as you maintain the focus on the breath and on the feeling of the particular regions as you come to them, breathe with them, and let go of them.

10. After you have completed scanning your body, focusing on each part with as little effort as possible, return to normal waking consciousness by slowly arousing various parts of your body. Gently begin to move your arms and hands, your legs and feet, your neck and shoulders, until you have revived yourself sufficiently to continue with your day.

Conclusion

Many muscles in the body remain in a chronically contracted state when they are continuously receiving the message from the nervous system that they should be contracting to enable them to fight or flee. These muscles do not receive the signal from the nervous system that the threat has passed and it is safe to relax. Active progressive muscle relaxation is a relaxation technique that reduces muscle tension and induces relaxation by first deliberately tensing muscles and then deliberately relaxing muscles. Through conscious awareness of how muscles feel in their relaxed state, an individual becomes more aware of muscle tension when it occurs. This is a trigger to actively relax the muscles.

Passive progressive relaxation is a more passive method of progressing through the various parts of the body, using a technique called the body scan. This method does not involve active contraction of muscles but, rather, a passive scanning of the body. Through detached awareness and observation, individuals discover their bodies in a non-judgmental way and begin to find some relief from their stress-related symptoms.

Both active and passive relaxation can be approached in many ways. Tailor your practice so it is fun and easy—and, most important, so it works for you.

Stress Relief Activities

Visit the Premium Website audio files to explore a variety of relaxation activities and techniques.

LAB

19.1 Progressive Relaxation and Flowing Comfort

PURPOSE To allow you to practice deep relaxation using active and/or passive progressive relaxation.

DIRECTIONS Prepare your environment for relaxation. Follow along with the Progressive Relaxation instructions to practice active progressive relaxation, or the Flowing Comfort instructions to practice passive progressive relaxation. These exercises are found in the Premium Website audio files. Practice the technique at least 2 times according to the instructions on the audio file. At least once, do it immediately before you sleep at night. Make sure it is the last thing you do before sleep. Do it at times when you will not be disturbed. Allow approximately 15 minutes to complete each exercise.

After completing Progressive Relaxation or Flowing Comfort, respond to the questions below. Describe primarily how you were feeling in relation to your stress levels.

Afternoon:

1. How did you feel before the exercise?

2. What was your experience during the exercise?

3. How did you feel immediately after the exercise?

4. How did you feel several hours after completing the exercise?

Right before bed:

1. How did you feel before the exercise?

2. How quickly did you fall asleep?

3. How did you sleep, and how refreshed did you feel when you awakened the following morning?

4. How did this differ from a typical night's sleep?

Classroom experience (if applicable):

1. How did you feel before the exercise?

2. What was your experience during the exercise?

3. How did you feel immediately after the exercise?

4. How did you feel several hours after completing the exercise?

Summary After you have practiced the exercise and described your experiences, include a brief review of what you liked and/or did not like about this technique. Compare this technique to some of the others you have practiced. Would this be a relaxation technique you would consider using on a regular basis for stress management? Why or why not?

Key Points

- Progressive muscle relaxation (PMR) is one of the most commonly used forms of relaxation therapy in Western society today.
- Many muscles in the body remain in a chronically contracted state because they are continuously receiving the message from the nervous system that they should be contracting in preparation for fight-or-flight.
- Progressive muscle relaxation involves consciously tensing and relaxing muscle groups progressively throughout the body. This reduces muscle tension.

- Adverse physical, mental, and emotional conditions associated with chronic stress have been found to be reduced or eliminated with regular practice of PMR.
- Passive progressive relaxation is a less active method of progressing through the various parts of the body using a technique called the body scan.
- The body scan focuses on detached observation and awareness of the body.

Key Terms

progressive muscle relaxation	muscle contraction	incremental muscle relaxation
progressive neuromuscular relaxation	all-or-none principle	passive progressive relaxation
motor unit	active progressive muscle relaxation	body scan

Discussion Time For Critical Thinking/Discussion Questions, please visit this book's Premium Website.

Notes

1. *Weight Training for Life* (9th ed.), by J. Hesson (Belmont, CA: Wadsworth/Cengage Learning, 2009).

2. "Grinding Down . . . Bruxism," by D. Blore, *Nursing Times* 91(26) (1995): 46–47.

3. "Effects of Progressive Relaxation and Classical Music on Measurements of Attention, Relaxation, and Stress Responses," by P. M. Scheufele, *Journal of Behavioral Medicine 23*(2) (2000): 207.

4. "Trait Anxiety and Sleep-Onset Insomnia: Evaluation of Treatment Using Anxiety Management Training," by M. Viens, J. De Koninck, P. Mercier, M. St-Onge, and D. Lorrain, *Journal of Psychosomatic Research 54*(1) (2003): 31–38; http://odp.od.nih.gov/consensus/ta/017/017_statement.htm

5. "Progressive Relaxation for Post-Traumatic Stress Disorder: A Case Study," by T. Charchuk, *Guidance & Counseling 15*(4) (2000): 23.

6. "The Impact of Abbreviated Progressive Muscle Relaxation on Salivary Cortisol," by L. A. Pawlow and G. E. Jones, *Biological Psychology 60*(1) (2002): 1.

7. "Coping Strategies for Working Women: Aerobic Exercise and Relaxation Interventions," by B. C. Long and C. J. Haney, *Behavior Therapy 19* (1988): 75–83.

8. "A Randomized Controlled Trial of an Internet-Based Treatment for Chronic Headache," by T. Devineni, and E. Blanchard, *Behaviour Research & Therapy 43*(3) (2005): 277–293; "Relaxation Therapy and Compliance in the Treatment of Adolescent Headache," by J. J. Wisniewski, J. L. Genshaft, J. A. Mulick, D. L Coury, and D. Hammer, *Headache 28* (1988): 612–617; "Two Studies of the Long-Term Follow-Up of Minimal Therapist Contact Treatments of Vascular and Tension Headache," by E. B. Blanchard, et al., *Journal of Consulting and Clinical Psychology 56* (1988): 427–432; "Cognitive Therapy and Relaxation Training in Muscle Contraction Headache: Efficacy and Cost-Effectiveness," by V. Attanasio, F. Andrasik, and E. B. Blanchard, *Headache 27* (1987): 254–260; "Relaxation Training for Tension Headache: Comparative Efficacy and Cost-Effectiveness of a Minimal Therapist Contact Versus a Therapist-Delivered Procedure," by S. J. Teders, et al., *Behavior Therapy 15* (1984): 59–70; "The Role of Regular Home Practice in the Relaxation Treatment of Tension Headache," by E. B. Blanchard, et al., *Journal of Consulting and Clinical Psychology 59* (1991): 467–470; "Placebo-Controlled Evaluation of Abbreviated Progressive Muscle Relaxation and of Relaxation Combined with Cognitive Therapy in the Treatment of Tension Headache," by E. B. Blanchard, et al., *Journal of Consulting and Clinical Psychology 58* (1990): 210–215.

9. "Efficacy of Two Relaxation Techniques in Depression," by A. Broota and R. Dhir, *Journal of Personality and Clinical Studies 6*(1) (1990): 83–90; "A Comparison of Cognitive-Behavioral Therapy and Relaxation Training for the Treatment of Depression in Adolescents," by W. M. Reynolds and K. I. Coats, *Journal of Consulting and Clinical Psychology 54* (1986): 653–660.

10. "Efficacy of Relaxation Training and Guided Imagery in Reducing the Adverseness of Cancer Chemotherapy," by J. N. Lyles, T. G. Burish, M. G. Krozely, and R. K. Oldham, *Journal of Consulting and Clinical Psychology 50* (1982): 509–529; "Providing Relaxation Training to Cancer Chemotherapy Patients: A Comparison of Three Delivery Techniques," by M. P. Carey and T. G. Burish, *Journal of Consulting and Clinical Psychology 55* (1987): 732–737; "Effectiveness of Relaxation Training in Reducing Adverse Reactions to Cancer Chemotherapy," by T. G. Burish and J. N. Lyles, *Journal of Behavioral Medicine 4* (1981): 65–78; "Conditioned Side Effects Induced by Cancer Chemotherapy: Prevention Through Behavioral Treatment," by T. G. Burish, M. P. Carey, M. G. Krozely, and F. A. Greco, *Journal of Consulting and Clinical Psychology 55* (1987): 42–48.

11. "Comparison of Group Progressive-Relaxation Training and Cognitive-Behavioral Group Therapy for Chronic Low Back Pain," by J. A. Turner, *Journal of Consulting and Clinical Psychology 50* (1982): 757–765.

12. "Relaxation Training and Expectation in the Treatment of Postpartum Distress," by J. S. Halonen and R. H. Passman, *Journal of Consulting and Clinical Psychology 53* (1985): 839–845.

13. "Relaxation Treatment of Hypertension: Do Home Relaxation Tapes Enhance Treatment Outcome?," by T. J. Hoelscher, K. L. Lichstein, S. Fischer, and T. B. Hegarty, *Behavioral Therapy 18* (1987): 33–37; "Relaxation Training for Essential Hypertension at the Worksite: I. The Untreated Mild Hypertensive," by M. A. Chesney, G. W. Black, G. E. Swan, and M. M. Ward, *Psychosomatic Medicine 49* (1987): 250–263; "Relaxation Treatment of Hypertension: Do Home Relaxation Tapes Enhance Treatment Outcome?," by T. J. Hoelscher, K. L. Lichstein, S. Fischer, and T. B. Hegarty, *Behavioral Therapy 18* (1987): 33–37; "Relaxation Training: Blood Pressure Lowering During the Working Day," by M. A. Southam, W. S. Agras, C. B. Taylor, and H. C. Kraemer, *Archives of General Psychiatry 39* (1982): 715–717; "Relaxation Training for Essential Hypertension at the Worksite: II. The Poorly Controlled Hypertensive," by W. S. Agras, C. B. Taylor, H. C. Kraemer, M. A. Southam, and J. A. Schneider, *Psychosomatic Medicine 49* (1987): 264–273.

14. *Full Catastrophe Living: Using the Wisdom of Your Body and Mind to Face Stress, Pain and Illness,* by J. Kabat-Zinn (New York: Dell Publishing, 1990).

15. "Mindfulness Meditation," by M. Ott, *Psychosocial Nursing and Mental Health Services 42*(7) (2004): 23–29.

16. Kabat-Zinn, *Full Catastrophe Living.*

17. Kabat-Zinn, *Full Catastrophe Living.*

18. Kabat-Zinn, *Full Catastrophe Living.*

20 Guided Imagery: Using Your Imagination

■ How does guided imagery work? ■ Can I still practice guided imagery if I'm not a "visual" person? ■ How are hypnosis and guided imagery related?

Study of this chapter will enable you to:

1. Summarize the relationship between the conscious mind and the subconscious mind.
2. Discuss how hypnosis relates to imagery.
3. Explain various uses for imagery.
4. Differentiate between guided imagery and visualization.
5. Experience relaxation guided imagery as a relaxation technique.

The image is more than an idea. It is a vortex or cluster of fused ideas and is endowed with energy.

—*Ezra Pound*

Students Experience Guided Imagery Before my first attempt at guided imagery, I was stressed! It was the end of the semester, and I felt like I had a million school things to take care of, not to mention all of my family/personal things that required my attention. During the guided imagery, it felt like a sanctuary! It was nice! I felt like I was on vacation. Immediately after the exercise, I had a complete stress level makeover; that is, until I remembered my economics assignment was still due! An hour after the guided imagery, I was focused and able to easily understand my Economics 101 reading and assignment. This is by far one of my favorite stress-relieving exercises.

Before my second experience with guided imagery I felt out of control. I swear my economics teacher is from another planet. I felt so overwhelmed and frustrated, almost to the point of tears. During the exercise, I felt relieved, although I was still anxious. As I was starting out, I felt my mind and body begin to relax. I felt more centered and comfortable. Immediately after this second attempt, I felt much better. I still felt frustrated, but I definitely felt more in control. An hour after the exercise, I felt better. I have the hardest time letting go of stress. I could still feel the anxiety lurking, but I felt calmer and better able to handle the day and any situations that may come up.

—Jamie S.

* * *

The first time I did guided imagery, I felt overwhelmed, stressed out, and impatient. As I tried the imagery, I became relaxed and calm. All the feelings I had before turned into peaceful, calm, relaxed feelings. I did this at night, and the next morning I woke up happy, ready for the day, and relaxed. The second time was in the morning, so I felt happy but a little nervous for the day ahead. During the exercise, I became aware of the beautiful scenery. It relaxed me and made everything full of serenity. I felt joyful afterward and energized to proceed with the day.

—Ashley H.

Guided Imagery: Using Your Imagination

In your imagination, visualize picking up a big, ripe, juicy lemon. Imagine yourself seeing the bright yellow lemon, feeling its texture, smelling its distinct lemony aroma. Next, see yourself taking a sharp kitchen knife, cutting the lemon into four quarters, taking one of those quarters, putting it into your mouth, and taking a huge, juicy bite. Imagine this clearly and notice that your mouth begins to salivate. Notice your mouth puckering up and watering.

Why would you salivate if there was no actual lemon? According to researchers at MIT,[1] there is no *real* difference between an imagined event and an event you perceive in your physical experience as far as how your mind interprets its meaning. You can either imagine eating the lemon or really eat the lemon and your brain will consider it as if the same thing is happening. This research has powerful implications for stress management.

Think for a minute about what this means. You can be sitting in your dorm studying for a test. If you can imagine yourself relaxing on a beautiful tropical beach in Bora Bora, your body will react as if you are actually there. Reversing the scenario, you actually can be on a beautiful beach in Bora Bora, and if your mind is imagining all the unpleasant things you have to do when you get home, your body will react by activating the stress response.

In this chapter you will learn how imagination relates to the conscious mind and the subconscious mind. You will learn how hypnosis works because of this connection. And you will learn to use the techniques of guided imagery and visualization to direct the imagination in a way that will subdue the sympathetic nervous system and elicit the relaxation response.

Background

Albert Einstein had some intriguing thoughts about imagination: "Imagination is more important than knowledge." We often hear that knowledge is power and the more knowledge you have, the more powerful you are. Why, then, would Einstein say that imagination is even more important?

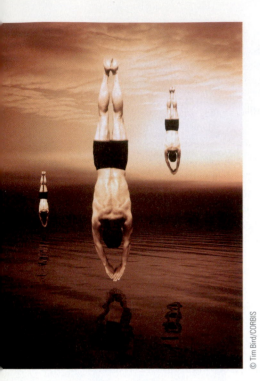

Imagining the perfect dive.

Golfer Jack Nicklaus, winner of 73 PGA tour victories, commented, "I never hit a shot, even in practice, without this color movie: First I 'see' the ball where I want it to finish, nice and white and sitting up high on the bright green grass. Then the scene quickly changes and I 'see' the ball going there—its path, trajectory, and shape, even its behavior on landing. Then there's a sort of fade-out, and the next scene shows me making the kind of swing that will turn the previous images into reality."[2]

Stephen Covey said, "All things are created twice."[3] He explained that first we have a mental creation, the picture in mind of what we want to create. The second creation occurs when we do the things necessary to bring into the physical dimension the picture that was first created in the mind.

The case could be made that virtually nothing exists in our experiences that we do not imagine in some way beforehand. A simple example demonstrates how this works: A person may begin to feel hungry. In his mind he thinks to himself that a bowl of cereal would satisfy that hunger. This is the first, or mental, creation. Very soon he finds himself filling a bowl with cereal and sitting down to eat. This is the second, or physical, creation. This occurs in nearly every action we pursue. First we see it in our mind, then we act on that image.

When we fear something, our worry and fear produce images that we create about future events. We see the potentially painful outcomes happening in our imagination. These painful images are what initiate the stress response. The imagined event is as real to the mind as the event that actually is happening in our physical experience.

Sports psychology is built on the premise that the body/mind does not know the difference between an actual event and an imagined one.[4] So, whether you are eating a lemon, improving your golf game, or learning to relax, what you first experience in your mind affects your physical experience. You can learn to consciously use your imagination to influence your experience in a positive manner.

298

Visualization. It has been called "going to the movies" and it may be the most important part of your mental package.

—*Ray Floyd, winner of the PGA, Master's, and U.S. Open golf tournaments*

The Mind and How It Works

Understanding the theory behind how hypnosis works and the connection between hypnosis and the conscious and subconscious mind will help you understand how relaxation techniques such as guided imagery work and why they are so effective in reducing stress. Hypnosis is not a relaxation technique you will be practicing; however, understanding some of the underlying theory can help you think about how guided imagery works.

Hypnosis **Hypnosis** can be defined as a state of attentive, focused concentration with suspension of some peripheral awareness. It is characterized by extreme suggestibility, relaxation, and heightened imagination. When you are under hypnosis:[5]

- Your attention is more focused.
- You are more responsive to suggestions.
- You are more open and less critical and disbelieving.

Hypnotherapists say that hypnosis creates a state of deep relaxation and quiets the mind. When you are hypnotized, you can concentrate intensely on a specific thought, memory, feeling, or sensation while you are blocking out distractions. You are more open than usual to suggestions, and you can use this to improve your health and well-being.[6]

Although how hypnosis works is not entirely clear, it seems to affect how your brain communicates with your body through nerve impulses, hormones, and body chemicals. The predominant

FYI

Mesmerizing Idea
The father of modern hypnotism is Franz Mesmer, an Austrian physician. He believed hypnosis to be a mystical force flowing from the hypnotist into the subject and called it "animal magnetism." Although critics quickly dismissed the magical element of his theory, Mesmer's assumption that the power behind hypnosis came from the hypnotist and was in some way inflicted upon the subject took hold for some time. Hypnosis was originally known as mesmerism, after Mesmer, and we still use its derivative, "mesmerize," today.[7]

school of thought on hypnosis is that it is a way to access a person's subconscious mind. Normally, you are aware only of the thought processes in your conscious mind. Scientists think that the deep relaxation and focusing exercises of hypnotism work to calm and subdue the conscious mind so it takes a less active role in your thinking process.

The Conscious and Subconscious Mind
Consider the mind as having two parts: the conscious and the subconscious. We can liken these two parts of our mind to the two people who run a coal-powered steam engine. The conscious mind is like the engineer who is sitting in the front of the train. His job is to guide the train wherever it has to go. If he sees that a hill is coming up, he decides that the train will require more power. If he sees a sharp curve ahead, he determines the need to slow down so the train can negotiate the turn safely. The conscious mind (engineer) understands things such as right or wrong, good and bad, yes and no, and so on, and makes decisions accordingly. This is the choice-making part of our mind.

The subconscious mind is like the person in the back of the engine who is shoveling coal into the fire—the stoker. He receives directions from the engineer and does exactly as he is told. When the engineer says, "We need more power!" the stoker says, "Okay, I'll put more coal into the fire, as you wish." He doesn't give the command any more thought about how appropriate or inappropriate this command is. He doesn't try to second-guess the engineer. He doesn't think of possible consequences of his actions. He just dumps some more coal into the fire. He only knows to respond exactly as he is told without question, without doubt.

Such is the subconscious mind and its relationship to the conscious mind.

Author Anecdote Hypnosis Day at School! The school was always buzzing for several days after the stage hypnotist performed at our high school. One year I was taking a class from a man, Mr. Ward, who claimed he knew how to hypnotize people just like the stage hypnotist. We were skeptically curious. Mr. Ward told us that when people are hypnotized, they are able to do things they wouldn't normally be able to when their disbelieving mind gets in the way.

One day in class we asked Mr. Ward to give us a demonstration. Somewhat reluctantly, he agreed. In the past he had hypnotized a couple of the girls who happened to be in the class. He informed us that they could "go under" simply when he called their name, counted to three, and then snapped his fingers. We didn't believe this for a moment, but we played along.

Before doing this, Mr. Ward asked for one of the strongest boys in the class to demonstrate his muscle strength. We all chose Rick, who was a football player, and clearly the strongest person in the class. Mr. Ward set up two chairs facing each other about 4 feet apart. He then asked Rick to suspend himself between the chairs with his head and neck on one of the chairs and his ankles and feet on the other. Mr. Ward asked Rick to place himself on the chairs as if he were lying on the floor facing the ceiling. His body, from his neck down to his calves, was to remain suspended. Mr. Ward asked Rick to remain in that position for as long as he could without buckling or bending his body.

We watched with eagerness. Within a few seconds, Rick's body started to shake, especially his stomach muscles. He lasted about 15 seconds in that position until he could hold it no longer. To Rick, 15 seconds seemed like a long time to hold himself in that suspended position.

Mr. Ward then went up to one of the girls and said to her, "Paulina, one, two, three," and then snapped his fingers. Immediately Paulina collapsed to the floor like a rag doll. Mr. Ward asked Paulina if she could hear him and if she felt fine (her eyes were closed as if she were asleep). She responded affirmatively. Interested, we watched, but we were pretty sure she was faking it. Then he gave her a command or suggestion. He told Paulina that when he counted to three and snapped his fingers, her body would immediately become stiff like a steel beam like the ones used in construction. He suggested to her that it would be impossible for her body to bend regardless of what would happen. He said this to her a few more times, then asked her if she understood.

Still with her eyes closed, she said she did. Mr. Ward then counted to three and snapped his fingers. We watched with anticipation as we saw Paulina begin to straighten her body on the floor. Mr. Ward asked a couple of guys in the class to carefully pick her up and place her in the same suspended position between the chairs, supported only by her feet at one end and her neck and head on the other. Paulina was probably the smallest girl in the class. She had never lifted any weights, nor had she ever considered doing sit-ups to strengthen her abdominal muscles.

We watched in dumbfounded amazement as Paulina remained in this suspended position for nearly a minute without bending. I couldn't believe my eyes. What she was doing was superhuman. There was no way she could fake this. Something powerful was happening here. (I probably should add that Paulina was very sore the next few days!)

—MO

The subconscious mind is depicted as being much larger than the conscious mind because it contains all the thoughts, images, and memories that we have had throughout our entire life. Figure 20.1 shows how this might look.

Whatever the conscious mind focuses on, believes, thinks, and directs is what the subconscious mind responds to; it follows through without question. Whereas the conscious mind has doubts, fears, reservations, and considerations about what it thinks can or can't be done, the subconscious mind simply does as it is told. When we repeatedly or with conviction say to ourself that we can't learn math, or that we are shy, or that we have any other limitation such as a belief that we can't quit smoking, our subconscious mind simply follows the direction given to it and says: "Oh, okay, I'll act shy" … "I'll be bad at math" … "I'll make it really hard to give up this smoking addiction."

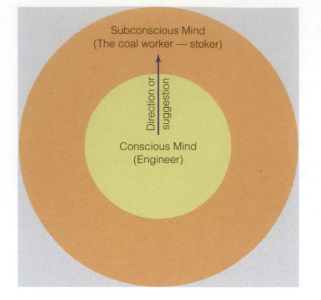

FIGURE 20.1 The engineer represents the conscious mind; the stoker represents the subconscious mind. Directions move from the conscious to the subconscious mind.

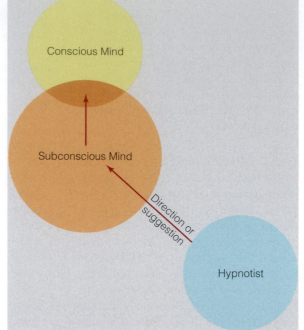

FIGURE 20.2 During hypnosis, the conscious mind takes a back seat. Suggestions are given from the hypnotist directly to the subconscious mind which follows through on the suggestion with exactness.

When a person is hypnotized, an interesting thing happens with the conscious mind. The hypnotized person goes into an altered state where the conscious mind, which is more critical and more analytical, moves off to the side for a while and the person doing the suggesting (making the commands, such as the hypnotist or hypnotherapist) talks directly to the subconscious mind. Figure 20.2 shows how this looks.

When the subconscious mind is spoken to directly, without the filtering of the conscious mind, the subconscious simply does as it is told. It doesn't know limitations, so whatever it is told to do, it simply says, "Oh, okay, I'll put in some more coal" (or whatever it is told to carry out). The conscious mind is still aware during hypnosis, but it doesn't become involved in the action of analyzing and critiquing the suggestions given to the subconscious mind. It is important to note that while suggestibility is a major component of hypnosis, the therapist or hypnotist does not have *control* of the person. Individual motivation is required for successful hypnosis, and the individual will not submit to suggestions that are in opposition to his or her values.

Imagery and Visualization

Imagery is a flow of thoughts that includes sensory qualities from one or more of the senses. It is the thought process that invokes the senses. Imagination has a powerful impact on the body and mind. **Visualization** relates more specifically to using the imagination to picture or see a place or thing. The focus in visualization is on the sense of sight.

Even though the terms *imagery* and *visualization* often are used interchangeably, they have a subtle difference in that visualization focuses on visualizing or seeing a place or thing while imagery can include smell, touch, hearing, taste, position, and motion as well as visual images.[8] Imagery is a broader term. The more clearly you can imagine the scene and the more senses you involve, the more real it becomes to your mind.

It's All in Your Mind

Researchers have studied patterns in the brain's cerebral cortex that occur during hypnosis. Hypnotic subjects showed reduced activity in the left hemisphere of the cerebral cortex, while activity in the right hemisphere often increased. Neurologists believe that the left hemisphere is the logical control center of the brain, operating on deduction, reasoning, and convention. The right hemisphere, in contrast, controls imagination and creativity. A decrease in left-hemisphere activity fits with the hypothesis that hypnosis subdues the inhibitory influence of the conscious mind. Conversely, an increase in right-brain activity supports the idea that the creative, impulsive, subconscious mind takes the reins. This theory lends credence to the idea that hypnotism opens up the subconscious mind.[*]

Guided imagery works in a manner similar to hypnosis. Research has found a correlation between the ability to use imagery and the ability to be hypnotized.[**] Although imagery shares some similarities with hypnosis, it differs in several important ways. Imagery is not characterized by a lessening of the person's own will, nor does it emphasize responding to a hypnotist's suggestions. Imagery does not attempt to access unconscious materials, rather imagery is vividly remembered.[†]

Sources:
[*]http://science.howstuffworks.com/hypnosis
[**]*The best alternative medicine: What works? What does not?* by K. Pelletier. (New York: Simon & Schuster, 2000).
[†]*Complementary & Alternative Medicine: A Research-Based Approach* by Lyn Freeman. St. Louis: Mosby, 2009.

Uses of Imagery

The authors of the book *The Mental Game Plan*[9] describe several different uses of mental imagery, including the following:

1. *Improvement of performance skills.* Imagery is used to mentally rehearse a skill in preparation for the real event. This could be something like seeing yourself doing well on a test or performing in an athletic event. You might view yourself performing to perfection immediately prior to participating in an activity, much like Jack Nicklaus did prior to each golf shot. One study showed that students who prepared for a test and used visualization remained calmer and more at ease during the exam. They were better able to remember the information and material they studied.[10]

2. *Improvement of confidence and positive thinking.* You can do this by replaying in your mind previous times when you performed at a high and satisfying level. For example, if you were preparing to give a speech in front of a large group of people, you could review earlier times when you gave talks successfully and let the images of those successful presentations help you build confidence for the upcoming speech.

3. *Tactical rehearsal and problem solving.* You can use this method to visualize possible outcomes that may arise in a given situation and decide on possible alternatives for handling the outcomes. For example, imagine different scenarios for how your boss will respond to your request for a raise. Picture yourself in the situation and imagine how you would respond to questions from your boss.

4. *Performance review and analysis.* Soon after completing or participating in an event, you can use your imagination to review your performance and assess yourself for strengths to build on and weaknesses to improve upon.

5. *Control arousal and anxiety.* Guided imagery is effective in helping to reduce the stress response by imagining relaxing scenes and even including yourself in those images. Commonly, these images occur in nature and in other peaceful places. The simple act of imagining these peaceful places can have a profound effect on reducing stress levels.

Stress Management and Peak Performance in Sports

Applying guided imagery and other mental strategies can help you relax and perform better in many settings. The goal of most athletes, as well as performers in a variety of other settings including dancing, business, and theater, is to operate at their peak during as much of the performance as possible. In terms of physical talent, collegiate athletes often stack up fairly evenly. So, what is it that separates those who wish they were winners from the peak performers? Most coaches and sports psychologists agree, the difference is what is taking place in the mind of the performer, both prior to and during the performance.

(Continued)

The mental activities that set apart the peak performers from the rest are easy to learn and within everyone's capabilities. All the psychological tools that you need to perform at your peak are found in this book. Combining them into a systematic practice can help any performer learn to think the way winners do. If you want to improve your performance, these five mental tools will help:

1. *Relax*—This first tool happens to be the essence of this book. The performer must learn how to relax. This doesn't mean chillin' in front of the television or hangin' out with some friends. It means regular practice of those relaxation techniques that are specifically designed to turn off the stress response.

    Consider the golfer who is lining up a putt. By thinking that there may be some bad outcome if he or she misses, the body interprets this as a threat, and the stress response activates automatically. When this happens, the running and fighting muscles, rather than the putting muscles, are activated. The shot is more likely to go awry and performance will suffer.

    Learning how to relax the mind and body through repeated practice helps prevent the onset of the stress response. The more frequently the performer practices relaxation techniques, the more that relaxed state becomes one's natural state during wakeful parts of the day, including during performance. So learning to relax is the first, and possibly most important, tool to help the athlete perform optimally. Chapters 16–22 of this book give you the best techniques for relaxation.

2. *Be mindful*—Stay in the moment. A successful track coach shared the advice he gives his runners to help them stay focused, "Keep your brain in your lane." Keeping your mind steadily focused on what you are doing, while keeping the mental chatter to a minimum, allows you to concentrate more fully. The chapter on mindfulness gives you a very thorough analysis of how to do this.

3. *Monitor your self-talk*—Take the time to listen to what you consistently say to yourself during performance. Negative messages, self-doubt, and criticism will hinder performance and turn on the stress response. Replace this negative self-talk with positive affirmations like, "I have trained well and will perform at my best. I can do this!" Control of self-talk, as well as the best ways to manage how you consistently think, is outlined in Chapter 6.

4. *Imagine your success*—The fourth tool, guided imagery, is the focus of this chapter. Clearly imagining your perfect performance is a strong skill that prepares you to perform more closely to perfection in the actual event. Each time you imagine the perfect performance in your mind, you gain more confidence in your abilities. The subconscious part of your mind doesn't easily distinguish between an imagined event and a real one. As a result, when you visualize your performance, it is almost as if you are actually doing it. This instills greater confidence and reduces stress.

    Use imagery to involve as many of your senses as possible. See yourself performing perfectly, but also include how it would feel kinesthetically. Sense how it feels to shoot the foul shot that goes through the hoop. Imagine what you might hear, smell, or taste, such as the sweat mixing with your saliva or the aroma of the event. Put yourself, mentally, into the actual scene and then observe yourself performing flawlessly. Imagine you are watching yourself on a television, or you could view the scene as if looking out from your own eyes. Run the mental movie over and over and watch your confidence grow each time you succeed.

5. *Let go and get out of your own way*—The ability to perform physically is already a part of the advanced athlete. So, most successful athletes will tell you that once the physical training has been done, their top performances came by letting go and allowing the process of playing to happen through them, rather than thinking about and deliberating about how it should happen. This higher level of functioning is described as "being in the zone or in the flow" of the game. It can not be forced or coerced. You can't "try" to make it happen. Curiously, it seems to happen when we are least trying to make it happen. At this stage, the athlete doesn't need to think about the "how" of doing the sport. The physical tools are already in place. Letting go involves letting those skills go to work on their own without letting thoughts about how it's done get in the way.

By applying these mental skills to your pre-performance time as well as during the action, the likelihood of experiencing these peak performance moments increases dramatically. Those are the times when playing and performing are the most enjoyable.

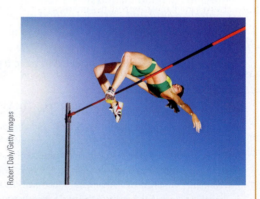

Robert Daly/Getty Images

Athletes use principles of stress management to help them perform at their peak.

Seeing Sacred Symbols
Visualizing sacred symbols is a spiritual ritual used in many cultures. Hindus and Buddhists use a *mandala,* a graphic representation depicting the universe. Sacred symbols can help individuals connect with their deep subconscious awareness and create a meditative state.

Source: *Spirituality, Health, and Healing,* by C. Young and C. Koopsen (Thorofare, NJ: Slack Inc., 2005).

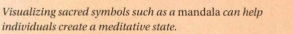

Ian Woodcock/Getty Images

Visualizing sacred symbols such as a mandala *can help individuals create a meditative state.*

So, even though imagery has several applications, the remainder of this chapter will focus primarily on using the imagination to control arousal and anxiety. The technique for doing this is called relaxation guided imagery (RGI).

Relaxation Guided Imagery: What Is It?

Relaxation guided imagery is the technique used to connect with the subconscious mind in a way that will activate the relaxation response. Guided imagery implies using the imagination in a directed way toward a specific image, scene, or sensation. By imagining a relaxing scene, for example, your mind and body respond as if you were actually in this relaxing spot. This relaxing imagery decreases the arousal of the stimulating, or sympathetic, branch of the autonomic nervous system, which helps reduce anxiety and perception of pain.

Guided imagery is similar to hypnosis in that what we imagine can be translated into changes in our physiology, biochemistry, and, as a result, in health outcomes. Because the subconscious mind doesn't know the difference between something experienced and something clearly imagined, it can be used to help a person deeply relax. Images of relaxing scenes can be imagined in our minds. As our mind thinks of something or somewhere relaxing, the subconscious mind automatically responds physiologically as if we were really in that place. Part of this response includes a complete lack of a threat. Because there is no threat, the parasympathetic nervous system is activated, and the body relaxes and returns to a state of homeostasis.

Benefits of Guided Imagery Athletes, performers, businesspeople, inventors,[11] and even people who are trying to overcome various illnesses[12] have used the imagination to help them produce desired outcomes. Guided imagery also has been helpful in treating many stress-related symptoms, including headaches, muscle spasms, chronic pain, and general or situation-specific anxiety.[13]

Research has demonstrated that RGI is effective in improving health outcomes for a myriad of medical conditions, including cancer, HIV, migraine headaches, hypertension, and post-surgical healing.[14]

O. Carl Simonton and Stephanie Simonton pioneered the application of imagery in cancer patients. Their patients were encouraged to imagine their immune system cells engulfing and devouring vulnerable cancer cells. Although a definitive study that demonstrates whether this works has not been undertaken, many patients found it helpful, even if they were not cured, and reported relief of anxiety and pain, better toleration of chemotherapy and radiation, and an increased sense of control.[15]

Research on guided imagery has found it to be effective for improving many stress-related maladies. It also has been used successfully in areas such as sports performance and recovery from chemical dependencies. It is especially effective in producing deep relaxation in those who practice it regularly. This is another powerful way to produce quick and noticeable relaxation. Don't take it lightly because of its simplicity!

Guided Imagery for Youngsters with Asthma

Asthma is a common disease of the respiratory system, especially among younger people in our culture. People who have asthma have difficulty breathing because the bronchial airways are temporarily blocked, caused by constriction of the muscles surrounding the airways. A person with asthma doesn't struggle with inhaling but, instead, has a difficult time exhaling. Asthma often is triggered by emotional distress.

A study reported in the journal *Psychology in Schools* examined the effectiveness of guided imagery as a means for reducing stress and the severity of an asthma attack in young people with asthma. Junior high students who had been diagnosed with asthma were selected for the study. Each of the subjects experienced mild to severe levels of asthma when emotionally upset.

In the study, which lasted 8 weeks, the students were taught relaxation guided imagery (RGI), which involved a specific script incorporating (a) general relaxation exercises (i.e., letting the tension go in each part of the body and imagining being in a pleasant, peaceful place); (b) guided imagery in which the participant imagines specific biological healing mechanisms in the bronchial tubes and lungs; (c) instructions to imagine doing a favorite activity during which the participant has no problems with his or her asthma; and (d) guided imagery in which the participant visualizes breathing in special colored air that completely clears the airways and lungs.

Students engaged in the RGI exercises for 20 minutes for an average of four times per week. At the end of the study, each of the subjects reported a noticeable decrease in feelings of anxiety, which tend to trigger asthma attacks. The RGI exercises led to improvements in lung function over time, but the greatest increases were immediately following the RGI exercises. The overall results suggest that RGI is a promising intervention in treating children with asthma as an adjunct to medical intervention.

Source: "Relaxation and Guided Imagery: A School-based Intervention for Children with Asthma," by H. L. Peck, M. A. Bray, & T. J. Kehle, *Psychology in the Schools*, 2003, *40*(6).

Guided Imagery as a Technique for Relaxation

When guided imagery is used as a method for relaxing, it usually is best done lying on a couch or bed or sitting up in a chair. Other environmental conditions that maximize the effects of guided imagery are similar to the other relaxation techniques: It should be done in a place where you won't be disturbed and where the lights can be turned down. Sometimes using relaxing music is helpful. It is important to monitor yourself for how warm or cool you might feel. Have a blanket ready to cover you in case of a chill. Once situated, your eyes are closed and the process of guided imagery begins.

Because the imagination is unlimited, there is virtually no end to the things you can imagine in order to develop a relaxed state. A typical RGI session begins with some brief and simple relaxation exercises, such as meditation, deep, restful breathing, a body scan, or progressive relaxation. No more than 2 or 3 minutes will go by until you begin to relax the mind and body before going into the imagery.

Next, begin to use your imagination. Some common and simple images that can help you turn off the stress response include walking along the beach with gentle ocean waves caressing your legs and feet, walking peacefully through a forest, being in the mountains or by a still lake, or sitting by a running river. You can picture yourself drifting slowly down a lazy stream, sitting atop a silent peak overlooking a majestic view, or resting in the stillness of a quiet field. Something is highly relaxing about seeing ourselves in nature. You can experiment until you find the most peaceful, relaxing place you can possibly imagine.

Although some people clearly see a relaxing setting when using RGI, for others it will be more elusive and more like a general impression of relaxation. Shakti Gawain, author of the book *Creative Visualization*, suggests:

> Don't get stuck on the term "visualize." It is not at all necessary to mentally see an image. Some people say they see very clear, sharp images when they close their eyes and imagine something. Others feel that they don't really "see" anything, they just sort of "think about" it or imagine that they are looking at it, or become aware of a feeling impression. That's perfectly fine. We all use our imaginations constantly; it's impossible not to, so whatever process you find yourself doing when you imagine is fine.[16]

To enhance your relaxation experience even more, increase the amount of sensory information you put into your imagination. For example, as you are walking along the beach, add the colors of the blue sky with puffy white clouds overhead. You might add the sounds of gulls, the feel and sound of a gentle breeze, and the feel of soft, grainy sand under your feet as you walk. The more senses you involve in the imagery, the more powerful the effect—the more you will feel like you are really there. By fully and clearly using your senses in your imagination and imagining scenes that are pleasant and relaxing, you quickly bring feelings of deep relaxation into your mind and body.

Guided imagery typically is done by having someone read a script or by using a recording that directs your imagination through a relaxing situation or scene. You will find some examples of guided imagery at the Premium Website audio file. You may want to simply use your imagination freely on your own to create the imagined scene.

Suggestions for Improving Guided Imagery Practice

The ability of each individual to access all of the senses for imagery practice will vary, depending on his or her preferred and most easily used sensory expression and motivation. It will also depend, to some extent, on each person's natural and innate ability to *imagine.* If you are one of those individuals who lack a vivid imagination, don't be dismayed. Research has identified one key factor to imagery success in persons with less vivid imaginations. Strong motivation to engage in imagery can produce some benefits even in individuals with limited abilities to imagine.[17]

Here are some tips to facilitate a positive outcome with guided imagery:

- Think in terms of the unlimited—no limits, no barriers in your imagination. If you want to fly in your imagination, you are free to fly. If you can imagine it … anything is possible.
- Release all thoughts of what others might think. There are no "others" in your imagination so don't be shy. Act boldly and freely.
- Include relaxing music in the background, such as classical or New Age music without lyrics.
- Be playful. Don't be too serious when you are working in your imagination. The harder you try, the harder it will be to "view" your imageries well.

A Simple Guided Imagery Script

Here is a simple guided imagery script for you to practice. Ask someone to read the script while you relax and experience guided imagery.

Lie down with your arms resting comfortably at your sides. Separate your feet and turn them slightly out. Make yourself as comfortable as possible. Gently close your eyes. Take in a nice, easy, deep breath through your nose … and exhale. Again, a deep breath in … and exhale. Continue to breathe deeply in and out. (long pause)

Allow all thoughts of your past and future to drift away. Bring yourself fully to this moment. Be patient with yourself as you visualize. Don't try too hard. If the scenes don't appear immediately in your imagination, try to sense the image, but don't force it.

Now, with your eyes closed, picture in your imagination a beautiful mountain scene. Imagine that you are in the mountain scene and that you are enjoying the beauty and peace of this beautiful place. It is one of the most beautiful places you have ever seen. Picture the large majestic mountains reaching up to the blue sky. Notice a few puffy, white clouds overhead and some clouds at the peaks of the highest mountains in view. (pause)

At the base of these mountains is a large forest of trees. This forest is rich with deep greens and browns. You notice the trees sway gently in the breeze. Feel the warm sun as it lands on your arms and face. This place is so peaceful and serene. Experience this place fully in your imagination. (pause)

Shortly, you notice a path that moves toward this forest. Step on the path and begin walking toward this grove of trees. Smell the fragrances of this forest as you reach the trees along this path. Breathe deeply and fill your lungs with the forest smells. (pause)

As you walk along this path, you notice, through the trees, a clearing up ahead. This clearing opens up to a majestic view of a large, sandy beach and the ocean extending as far in the distance as your eyes can see. Look around and notice the variety of colors you see all around you … the color of the sand, the sky, the ocean. (pause)

See yourself moving toward this sandy beach. Soon you begin walking barefoot in the sand and you notice that the sand is warm and soft. With each step, your feet feel more comfortable. Everything is perfect here. You feel safe and secure. The only sound you can hear is the gentle surf as it moves toward you and then away again like the ocean breathing

Stress Relief Activities
Visit the Premium Website audio files for examples of guided imagery.

in and out. Stop and gaze out at this majestic ocean. Notice how completely relaxing this ocean appears. It is so peaceful and strong. Enjoy this perfect place for a few moments. Take in the warmth of the sun and the serenity of this magnificent ocean. You are completely at peace, warm and calm. Nothing can disturb this peaceful feeling. (pause)

Imagine sitting down at a perfect place in the sand, closing your eyes and just listening ... feeling the peacefulness ... the restfulness of this place. Imagine yourself lying down in a comfortable position ... and letting go of your worries and tensions ... and relaxing. ... Imagine the warmth of the sun ... and the cool breeze playing on your face ... as you relax ... and breathe quietly in ... and out. ... (pause)

Listen to the quiet sounds around you ... feel the sun on your skin, warming you, soothing away all tensions and cares ... feel the breeze playing on your skin. ... This place is so restful, so full of peace. ... Let the faint smells and silence of this marvelous place gently relax you. (pause)

Breathe in gently and deeply and relax. Your body is rested and at peace. ... You are drawing strength and energy from the sunlight. ... As you breathe in, the energy fills you. ... Your lungs are filled with oxygen that spreads nourishing and healing energy to every part of your body. As you inhale this pure fresh ocean air, visualize this healing energy spread through your entire body. You feel completely at peace, rested and content. Enjoy these feelings as you relax in the wonder of your place by the ocean. (pause)

Now, with a deep breath, remind yourself that you can easily return to this relaxing place to bathe in the stillness. Completely enjoy this feeling of deep relaxation. Allow yourself to be still and rested. ... (long pause)

Now prepare to end this session. When you return to normal waking consciousness, you will feel relaxed, alert, refreshed, wide awake, and energized. (return slowly)

Conclusion

The imagination has a powerful impact on body and mind. Guided imagery works in a manner similar to hypnosis to connect directly with the subconscious mind in such a way that your body responds directly to what you are imagining. Relaxation guided imagery is a technique that you can use to calm your body and mind by suppressing the sympathetic nervous system and creating homeostasis.

If you can imagine yourself relaxing on the beach in Hawaii with a refreshing breeze blowing in from the ocean, you can activate the relaxation response just as if you actually were on the beach relaxing. It can work both ways: If you actually are on the beach in Hawaii and your mind is imagining all the problems and work you left at home, your body will respond as if you are home dealing with the stresses. The stress response will be activated.

Truly relaxing and taking time away from work and school responsibilities is valuable to restore us mentally and physically. Maybe you can't take a trip to Hawaii, but you can take 20 minutes to imagine you are there! Your body and mind will appreciate the break.

LAB

20.1 Guided Imagery

PURPOSE To allow you to practice deep relaxation using guided imagery.

DIRECTIONS Prepare your environment for relaxation. Follow along with the guided imagery instructions found in the Premium Website audio file. You can select the Guided Imagery—Mountain Lake or the Guided Imagery—Floating Through Colors exercise. You may want to try them both. Practice the technique at least 2 times according to the instructions on the audio file. This exercise is probably best done sitting in a comfortable position rather than lying down. It is not one that is used to help you fall asleep so much as it is used to deeply relax you while remaining conscious. Allow approximately 15 minutes to complete the exercise.

After completing guided imagery, respond to the questions below. Describe primarily how you were feeling in relation to your stress levels.

First Practice:

1. How did you feel before the exercise?

2. What was your experience during the exercise?

3. How did you feel immediately after the exercise?

4. How did you feel several hours after completing the exercise?

Second Practice:

1. How did you feel before the exercise?

2. What was your experience during the exercise?

3. How did you feel immediately after the exercise?

4. How did you feel several hours after completing the exercise?

Classroom experience (if applicable):

1. How did you feel before the exercise?

2. What was your experience during the exercise?

3. How did you feel immediately after the exercise?

4. How did you feel several hours after completing the exercise?

Summary After you have practiced the exercise and described your experiences, include a brief review of what you liked and/or did not like about this technique. Compare this technique to some of the others you have practiced. Would this be a relaxation technique you would consider using on a regular basis for stress management? Why or why not?

Key Points

- Imagery is a flow of thoughts that encompasses sensory qualities from one or more of the senses. It is the thought process that invokes the senses.
- Visualization relates more specifically to using the imagination to picture or see a place or thing.

- Guided imagery works in a manner similar to hypnosis to connect directly with the subconscious mind in such a way that the body responds directly to what you are imagining.
- Relaxation guided imagery is a technique that can activate the relaxation response.

Key Terms

hypnosis
imagery

visualization

relaxation guided imagery

Discussion Time For Critical Thinking/Discussion Questions, please visit this book's Premium Website.

Notes

1. "Mental Imagery of Faces and Placed Activates Corresponding Stimulus-Specific Brain Regions," by N. Kanwisher and K. O'Craven, *Journal of Cognitive Neuroscience 12*(6) (2000): 1023–1034.
2. *Golf My Way,* by J. Nicklaus (New York: Fireside, 1974).
3. *Seven Habits of Highly Effective People,* by S. Covey (New York: Fireside, 1989).
4. *Imagery for Getting Well: Clinical Applications of Behavioral Medicine,* by D. Brigham (New York: Norton, 1994).
5. http://www.mayoclinic.com
6. http://www.mayoclinic.com
7. http://science.howstuffworks.com/hypnosis
8. *The Best Alternative Medicine: What Works? What Does Not?,"* by K. Pelletier (New York: Simon & Schuster, 2000).
9. *The Mental Game Plan: Getting Psyched for Sport,* by S. J. Bull, J. G. Albinson, and C. J. Shambrok (Cheltenham, UK: Sports Dynamics, 1996).
10. "Test Anxiety and Hypnosis: A Different Approach to an Important Problem," by H. E. Stanton, *Australian Journal of Education 21* (1977): 179–186.
11. *Superlearning,* by S. Ostrander and L. Schroeder (New York: Dell Publishing Corp., 1979).
12. *Love, Medicine & Miracles,* by B. Siegel (New York: Harper & Row Publishers, 1986).
13. *The Relaxation & Stress Reduction Workbook,* by M. Davis, E. R. Eshelman, and M. McKay (Oakland, CA: New Harbinger Publications, 1988).
14. "Guided Imagery: A Psychoneuroimmunological Intervention in Holistic Nursing Practice," by J. F. Giedt, *Journal of Holistic Nursing 15* (1997): 112–127.
15. Pelletier, *The Best Alternative Medicine.*
16. *Creative Visualization,* by S. Gawain (New York: Bantam Books, 1985).
17. *Complementary & Alternative Medicine: A Research-Based Approach* (3rd ed.) by Lyn Freeman. St. Louis: Mosby, 2009.

21 Meditation

STUDENT OBJECTIVES

After studying the material in this chapter, you should be able to:

1. Explain the four factors necessary for mantra meditation.
2. Distinguish between the various types of meditation.
3. List the benefits of meditation.
4. Participate in, and experience the relaxing benefits of, meditation.

Buero Monaco/Getty Images

Meditation is not a way of making your mind quiet. It's a way of entering into the quiet that's already there—buried under the 50,000 thoughts the average person thinks every day.

—*Deepak Chopra*

Student Meditation The first time I did meditation, I had a tension headache. As I began to focus on my mantra, I could feel the tension releasing out of my head and neck. I don't know how long I sat there, but the longer I was there, the better I felt. I finished feeling like I'd never had a headache to begin with, and that's a rare occasion.

—*Emily A.*

* * *

When we were first given the assignment to meditate, I was skeptical about doing it. I thought it was going to be some weird hippie thing that you see in movies, but I soon found out that I was wrong. The first time I tried the exercise, I was surprised at how easy it was. I thought for sure that it was going to be hard for me to get into, but my mind eased right into the mantra and I found myself relaxing with no trouble. The word that I chose to use was "love." I found that the more I repeated the word, the easier it was to keep it in place in my mind. Other thoughts came into my mind during my meditation, but they quickly left.

By the end of the exercise, my mind felt lighter (for lack of better description). It was almost like I was somewhere else looking at myself on the outside. At first I wasn't completely aware of all of my surroundings, but the more I came out of meditation, the more aware I became of everything. I also was very aware of how much my breathing had slowed down compared to when I started. I was so excited about trying meditation again that I did it every day this week.

The best result I've had so far was a few days ago. I had a really bad headache and didn't feel like meditating, but I had committed myself to do it anyway. I stayed in my meditation about ten minutes longer than I had the other days, and as I concentrated on my word (love), I found that I wasn't thinking of my headache anymore. By the end of my meditation, my headache was completely gone. I am still amazed that it was something that simple that got rid of the headache, especially since medication usually doesn't even make a dent in the pain. So now I'm hooked. I've put time in my planner to meditate at least three days a week to start, and I hope I can do more. I've developed some relaxing exercises over the course of the semester, but this is the easiest and the best I've experienced. So I guess you can say that I'm hooked on the "weird hippie stuff" that I had always been skeptical of!

—*Brandy B.*

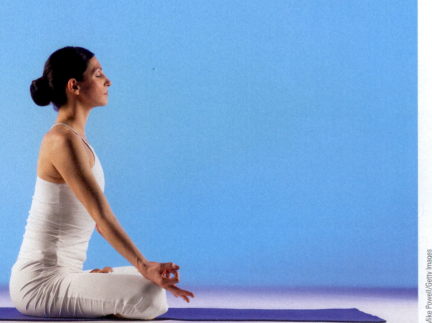

The lotus position is often associated with meditation.

© Mike Powell/Getty Images

Meditation: It's Not What You Think

What images come to your mind when you think of the word *meditation*? Perhaps you think of a Tibetan monk or an Indian guru sitting in the **lotus position** (cross-legged with each foot resting on the alternate thigh) with hands resting on knees, forefingers touching thumbs, eyes closed, repeating what sounds like the word "hum" again and again.

You probably have heard some people say that meditation is simply focusing the mind on a certain image. Others say it is like daydreaming or like doing a guided imagery. Meditation has even been equated with prayer. Many people are leery of meditation because they don't quite know what it is. One thing we do know is that meditation has blossomed into numerous forms that are practiced by many cultures throughout the centuries. People around the world incorporate some variation of this powerful relaxation technique into their daily routine. This ancient spiritual practice is finding new uses as both a stress-management technique and in the treatment of mental and physical disorders.

Meditation: What Is It?

So what is meditation? **Meditation** is a conscious mental method of systematically allowing the mind to focus gently on a single item. In the process, the mind tends to think more clearly as the mental chatter quiets. The result is a mental state of alert relaxation. When you clear the clutter from your mind, your mind and body settle naturally into a state of balance, or homeostasis. Through focus and concentration, your mind opens to new perspectives and self-awareness. The calming mental exercises of meditation are a proven antidote to stress and tension.

Of the many ways to meditate, nearly all have some requirements in common:

- A quiet environment where you will not be disturbed
- A comfortable, relaxed position, usually sitting
- A point of mental focus

Meditation means different things to different people. Meditation may simply mean prayer or contemplation while focusing your mind on a single thought or idea, on an object such as a flower, on a simple shape, on a sound, or on an image. People have been known to meditate with their eyes wide open while continuously looking at and focusing on the flame of a candle or at one point on a wall or ceiling. People can meditate with their eyes half open, with eyes barely open to let in just a sliver of light, or they may meditate with their eyes completely shut. In this chapter you will have the opportunity to try different meditation techniques. As you experiment with them, you will discover which ways work best for you.

Many books, articles, and Websites describe meditation as a means for creating enlightenment, for developing one's inner energies, and for reaching transcendental awakening. These and other uses of meditation may be interesting and useful, and you may want to explore these more fully on your own. The scope of meditation as it is discussed in this text is limited to its uses as a powerful and effective method for preventing and reducing stress and the disorders associated with chronic stress.

What Meditation Is Not

Thoughts about meditation might conjure up images of a person who is capable of making the mind become completely still to a point at which no thoughts are happening. Let's consider the possibility that meditation is the process of deleting all thoughts and creating a perfectly still mind.

Author Anecdote   My Introduction to Meditation   Many years ago I worked in a city public library. One of the joys of working in this library was that I had the opportunity to see the many books that had been written on almost any topic. I noticed one section of books having to do with meditation. Not knowing anything about meditation at the time, I was intrigued as I read some of the claims about meditation that were noted in the books. Among the results of regular meditation, these books mentioned a decrease in blood pressure, slower brainwave activity, lower resting heart rate, reversing the aging process, feeling more alive and more alert all day long, and many other claims.

I was eager to learn this method of relaxation called transcendental meditation (TM), but one challenge seemed too big for me as a young, poor, working college student. I discovered that if I was going to learn how to meditate, it would cost me $500 to be personally taught how to do it. That seemed pricey, but I badly wanted to learn this technique, so I went to the introductory presentation, scraped together the necessary cash, and signed up to learn how to meditate.

A week later I found myself in a room with the same man who had given the presentation the previous week. I was eager to get started. In this room incense was burning, rose petals were strewn everywhere, and pictures of men I had never before seen were displayed around the room. Music that sounded like it came from the movie *Gandhi* was playing lightly in the background.

The man asked me to sit down, we talked for a few moments, and he asked me to remain quiet while he began speaking in another language that sounded like a prayer of some kind. I didn't recognize it, and I thought this whole thing was a little bit strange. My thoughts were that I came to learn how to meditate, not to be converted to some Far Eastern religion. Toward the end of this prayer, he began saying a word again and again. I didn't recognize the word, nor did I have any idea what it meant. He told me to start repeating it with him quietly aloud to myself. His voice grew quieter, and he prompted me to continue saying the word again and again. Thinking that I needed to get my money's worth, I did just what he said to do. He prompted me to begin saying the word more quietly to myself, until at some point he directed me to simply repeat the word silently to myself again and again and again. He told me to close my eyes and simply continue whispering the word to myself without vocalizing. I did this for about 15 minutes, when he instructed me to stop repeating the word and slowly open my eyes.

When I was through, I was astonished at how different I felt. I felt so dramatically peaceful and content—like I had never felt before. I felt like I had slept for 16 hours. This was incredible! I had gotten my money's worth and more! I didn't understand it in the least, but I felt absolutely terrific!

For more than two decades I have continued to meditate the exact same way I did that first time (without all of the mystical aspects of that first evening), and the effects are always dramatic. I have more energy. I feel more alive, more alert, and more easily able to focus on everything I do. Few things have had a greater impact on my sense of well-being than meditation.

—MO

Take a moment to try this little experiment: Close your eyes, and for about 30 to 60 seconds try to create a still mind. Try to eliminate every thought in your mind for about 30 to 60 seconds. Use as much effort as possible, and use any method that you can think of to make your mind go completely blank. Do this now.

What did you discover? Did you find this an easy thing to do? Most people who try this report that it was even harder to create a still mind by thinking about making it happen. As you were trying to still your mind, you probably noticed thoughts popping in and out of your head at lightning speed, coming from nowhere into your consciousness, leading to other thoughts, which led to still other thoughts, and so on, seemingly out of your control. As hard as you try, you notice that it is virtually impossible to force your mind to become blank.

A favorite example is the impossible demand, "Don't think about a white bear." The harder we try not to think of something, the more it stays in our mind. The harder we try to empty our mind, the more it fills with thoughts. Trying to empty your mind in any determined way is not meditation. The result of this thinking process can hardly be considered peaceful.

Meditation Put into Practice

We are told that meditation is good for us, that it relaxes us, that it is healing, that it stills the mind, and that it brings enlightenment. So how can you learn and practice meditation in your daily life? Meditation does not take years of practice, nor does it involve venturing off to some spiritually enlightened sage who lives in the Himalayas. It also does not involve forceful attempts to still the mind. To help get you started, try these two simple, easy-to-learn techniques—mantra meditation and breathing meditation.

Mantra Meditation

Of the many ways to meditate, no clear evidence indicates that one type of meditation is far better than the rest. Based on years of research on the physiology of meditation, Herbert Benson of Harvard Medical School found that any meditation practice could produce the relaxing physiological changes known as the relaxation response as long as four factors were present:[1]

1. A mental device (constant and repetitive focus of attention)
2. A passive attitude
3. Decreased muscle tone facilitated by a comfortable position
4. A quiet environment

Mantra meditation is a technique that combines these four factors. Let's look at each of these in more depth to help you put this information into action.

Mental Device Meditation involves focusing the mind on a single item. One of the most common mental devices that allows this to happen is a **mantra,** which is simply a repeated word, a sound, or a phrase used as a point of focus during meditation. "Mantra" comes from the Sanskrit words for mind (*man*) and sound (*tra*). Mentally repeating a word or phrase can quiet the mental chatter that fills your mind.

Mantra meditation is easy to learn and simple to put into practice. Begin by choosing your mantra—one that is easy to remember and has associations that are relaxing. Some people prefer one- or two-syllable words such as *one, peace, still, love, now, serene, peaceful, success, soothe, happy, calm,* or *relax.* Others prefer a phrase such as, "I feel calm" or "I am peaceful."

Once you have selected your mantra, find a quiet place where you will not be disturbed, turn down the lights, sit in a comfortable chair, close your eyes, focus inwardly on your breath and bodily sensations for about 30 seconds, and then begin saying your mantra again and again silently to yourself: for example, "One…one…one…one…one…one…one…one…one…one…one…one…one…one…one…one…one…one…one…one…one…one…one…one…." Repeat the mantra slowly and passively. That's all there is to it. The only effort you make is the intention of silently repeating the mantra. As other thoughts come and go, simply allow the gentle repetition of your mantra to be the focus.

Magical Mantra?

Does each individual have a certain "right" mantra? Herbert Benson and others at Harvard did some interesting studies on **transcendental meditation** (TM). TM is unique in that it involves going into a meditative state by repeating a special, individualized mantra—a Sanskrit sound without meaning. The researchers wanted to know if the study participants could realize the same effects by using words other than those the trainers of TM gave them. They wanted to know if there is something special and unique about the individualized mantra that is necessary for meditation to be successful.

The researchers concluded that it makes no difference what word or phrase you repeat. They found that the process of focusing on, and repeating, a sound was the crucial component. It seems that the positive benefits of meditation could be achieved without any of the Eastern mystical features commonly found with TM.

Source: The *Relaxation Response*, by Herbert Benson (New York: Morrow Books, 1975).

Passive Attitude When you meditate, you should exert as little effort as possible. Working at meditation does not work. You should not try to make anything happen. Relax, focus, and let it happen. This may seem contrary to the way you have done most things in your life. Most of us have been taught that we need to work hard to accomplish anything significant. Meditation is different. When you meditate, you should have only one intention: the simple act of repeating the mantra, when it occurs to you to do so, with as little effort as possible. Do not try to do anything else or try to make anything else happen. The attitude that works best for meditation, and most of the relaxation exercises discussed in this book, is called "effortless effort."

Comfortable Position Meditation begins by sitting in a comfortable position. You may choose to sit on the floor, in a chair with a straight back, in the lotus position, or any other seated position that is comfortable to you. Try to sit up comfortably straight. Jon Kabat-Zinn suggests that sitting for meditation is different from simply sitting down casually. He describes this as "sitting with dignity."[3]

To avoid falling asleep while meditating, you probably should not meditate lying down. When you meditate, you commonly go into levels of deep rest with altered brainwave activity, yet you usually remain awake and aware. It is as if you are resting deeply but not sleeping. Meditation is not sleeping, and the benefits are different. You do not want to associate meditation with sleeping, which is what you are apt to do when you lie down.

Quiet Environment Finding a place where you will not be disturbed is beneficial. Set your chair in a closet, or go to a room where you know the phone will not ring and no one will interrupt you. Many people find it beneficial to select a special spot for their daily meditation routine. Though not a requirement, it is recommended that the lights be turned down or off. To avoid visual distractions and enhance concentration, best results are achieved by meditating with the eyes closed.

These are the ideal conditions, but with time, people have been known to practice this type of meditation almost anywhere, including in airports, cars, boring classes, or at the tops of mountains. The effects are still the same. Environmental noises should not be considered a hindrance to meditation but should be treated the same as your internal thoughts. Simply let them happen and gently focus on your mantra.

Ending Meditation To achieve the greatest benefit, you should end your meditation correctly. Have you ever been asleep and in the middle of a dream when suddenly the phone rang and you were awakened abruptly? When this happens, you may feel out of balance and irritated. While meditating, you will achieve a level of restfulness similar to that during deep sleep. You *do not* want to come out of meditation quickly. End meditation by returning slowly to normal consciousness. Give yourself 2 or 3 full minutes to quietly

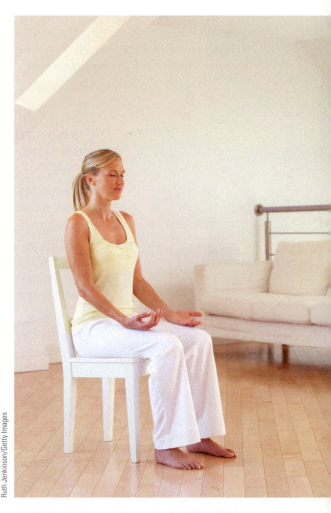

Ruth Jenkinson/Getty Images

Meditation is commonly practiced while sitting in a chair.

Brainwave Activity

A classic meditation study involved an analysis of brainwave activity of people who meditate. The researchers connected people who were meditating to an electroencephalogram during meditation. They wanted to see if brainwave activity changed in any unique way while meditating.

Brainwave activity is measured in cycles or rhythms. Brainwave activity occurs in four basic patterns. The first and highest level is called *beta*. People who exhibit beta brainwave levels are usually awake, alert, and fully aware of what is happening. Higher beta brainwave levels correspond with higher stress levels. The next level of brainwave activity is called *alpha*. Alpha brainwave activity usually occurs during daydreaming, in the early periods of sleep, in light hypnosis, and during most relaxation techniques. The next two, slower, levels of brainwave activity are *theta* and *delta*. These slow levels of brainwave activity occur almost exclusively during deeper sleep, while we dream, and during deep hypnosis. During these slower brainwave rhythms, our body undergoes its most restorative rest. As we sleep at these deeper brainwave rhythms, our body repairs itself from cuts and bruises, the immune system works more powerfully to fight off diseases, and we get critical rest and inner repair work.

During a typical night of sleep, our mind usually takes an hour or two to settle down to these deeper levels of brainwave activity and allow the deep healing to occur. The researchers found that during meditation people were able to reach these deep levels of brainwave activity and enjoy deep rest in as few as 5 minutes. These meditators were aware and conscious, rather than asleep, as they meditated. The researchers called this level of deep rest while meditating a *hypometabolic state*. Along with the slowing of brainwave activity, other calming events were taking place in the body. The meditators' heart rates decreased dramatically and breathing rates slowed dramatically. Both of these measures indicate a decrease in the stress response.

Source: "The Physiology of Meditation," by R. K. Wallace and H. Benson. *Scientific American*, 1972, 226(2), 84–90.

sit in your chair, enjoying the peacefulness of the experience. This may sound trivial, but it is important. Take your time when you are returning. *Don't be in a rush to end your meditation sessions!*

Mantra Meditation: Putting It All Together You are ready to put it all together. Follow these simple steps:

1. Sit with dignity and close your eyes.
2. Repeat your mantra.
3. When your mind wanders, return your focus to passively repeating your mantra.
4. Do not be in a hurry to end your meditation, regardless of its duration.
5. Enjoy the benefits of profound relaxation.

Breathing Meditation

Mantra meditation is one type of meditation. A second type of meditation for you to try is **breathing meditation.** This form of meditation is traced back to Buddha, from *Buddha's Little Instruction Book.*[4]

To begin meditation, select a quiet time and place. Be seated on a cushion or chair, taking an erect, yet relaxed posture. Let yourself sit upright with the quiet dignity of a king or queen. Close your eyes gently and begin by bringing your full, present attention to whatever you feel within you and around you. Let your mind be spacious and your heart be kind and soft.

As you sit, feel the sensations of your body. Then notice what sounds and feelings, thoughts and expectations are present. Allow them all to come and go, to rise and fall like the waves of the ocean. Be aware of the waves, and rest seated in the midst of them. Allow yourself to become more and more still.

In the center of all these waves, feel your breathing, your life-breath. Let your attention feel the in-and-out breathing wherever you notice it, as coolness or tingling in the nose or throat, as a rising and falling of your chest or abdomen. Relax and softly rest your attention on each breath, feeling the movement in a steady,

Author Anecdote Meditation Feels Good Few things have as dramatic and immediate an effect on how a person feels as mantra meditation. After having learned and practiced this simple technique in stress-management class, Brandon slowly opened his eyes and sat quietly in the back of the room. He appeared to be in a daze of sorts. Class members started talking about their experience. Brandon raised his hand and remarked to the class, "I have never felt this good in my entire life." It is not unusual to have students remain in the room after class is over and just sit there, in their chairs, enjoying the stillness and serenity they feel after meditation.

—MO

easy way. Allow the breaths to follow any rhythm, long or short, soft or deep. As you feel each breath, concentrate and settle into its movement. Let all other sounds and sensations, thoughts and feelings continue to come and go like waves in the background.

After a few breaths, your attention may be carried away by one of the waves of thoughts or memories, by body sensations or sounds. Whenever you notice you have been carried away for a time, acknowledge the wave that has done so by softly giving it a name such as "planning," "remembering," "itching," "restless." Then let it pass and gently return to the breath. Some waves will take a long time to pass, and others will be short. Certain thoughts or feelings will be painful, and others will be pleasurable. Whatever they are, let them be.

At some sittings you will be able to return to your breath easily. At other times in your meditation, you will be aware mostly of body sensations or of plans or thoughts. Either way is fine. No matter what you experience, be aware of it, let it come and go, and rest at ease in the midst of it all. After you have been sitting for 20 or 30 minutes in this way, open your eyes and look around you before you get up. Then, as you move, try to allow the same spirit of awareness to go with you into the activities of your day. In this type of meditation, the focus is primarily on the breathing rather than a mantra. The mind is trying neither to forcibly think a certain way nor to inhibit thoughts from coming and going. There is simply a calm and passive mental return to focusing on the in-and-out movement of the breath. Most meditation treats rambling thoughts gently and forgivingly. If thoughts ramble and stray from the intended focal point, there is no criticizing or belittling oneself for not meditating correctly. The goal is to return and continue putting attention on the breath. When this happens, the mind tends to become more still, more calm and peaceful.

Try both mantra meditation and breathing meditation for several days and see what works best for you. Of the many versions and variations of meditation, let's look at some additional forms that are particularly effective for relaxation.

Types of Meditation

The most important component of meditation is the process of bringing the mind to focus on a single object, word, or idea to the exclusion of all others and to remain focused for a period of time. You have learned two forms, mantra meditation and breathing meditation. Following is a brief description of some additional ways of meditating that strive to allow the mind to focus more fully. Several of the following meditation exercises come from Lawrence LeShan's book, *How to Meditate: A Guide to Self-Discovery.*[5]

Contemplation

In the **contemplation** form of meditation, begin by selecting an item such as a natural object—a rock, a twig, a leaf, a seashell. Or you could choose something like a piece of cloth, a small ball, a piece of jewelry, or even a shoelace. You should choose an object that you can hold comfortably in your hands. Hold the object at a comfortable visual distance and be flexible about this distance.

In contemplation, the goal is to simply look at the object. You are to make no attempt to judge the object, or to try to analyze or understand the object. You simply place your attention on it and observe it passively. Let yourself connect with the object through touch as well as by sight. Just pay attention to the object, nothing more. As your attention wanders, gently bring it back to the object. This is a form of mindfulness, which was treated more fully in Chapter 7.

Breath Counting

This type of meditation is somewhat similar to the restful breathing relaxation exercise you learned in Chapter 17, as well as the breathing exercise earlier in this chapter. When you practice breath counting, you simply focus directly on the breath as it comes in and goes back out.

Do this **breath counting meditation** by closing your eyes, putting your attention on your breath, and breathing normally. You inhale, and then when you exhale, you say the number "one." The next inhale is followed by the exhale and saying the number "two." You continue through the number "four" and then repeat again from "one" to "four." You also might include the silently spoken word "and" with each inhale. As you inhale, say the word "and" followed by exhaling to the number.

Thought-Watching

You practice **thought-watching** by picturing yourself sitting peacefully at the bottom of a clear lake. Begin with the understanding that large bubbles tend to rise from the bottom of the lake to the top in an easy and effortless fashion. With this idea in mind, tune your attention to your thoughts as they pass into your mind. As a thought comes in, picture the thought as a bubble rising slowly and easily to the surface above you and then out of your attention. Follow this by the next thought that gently rises to the surface. LeShan suggests that each bubble rises from the bottom to the top in about 5 to 8 seconds. As each thought comes in, do not try to analyze or judge the thought. Simply approach each thought or sensation with the attitude of "Oh, that's what I'm thinking. How interesting." Then, as it passes out of visual space, you move to the next one.

If sitting at the bottom of a clear lake is an uncomfortable image for you, you may use the image of watching puffs of smoke rise from a large campfire on a windless day. You also may use the image of your thoughts as logs floating down the river, first coming into view and then passing across and soon fading out of your view.

Chakra Meditation

Chakras are the energy centers in the body through which spiritual and emotional energies flow. The word *chakra*, taken from Hindi, means "wheel of energy." Proponents of Hindu philosophy believe that the free, unblocked flow of energy through the chakras is vital for the health and well-being of the whole person. The belief is that when the flow of **prana,** or energy, is blocked, disease results.

Although chakras have not been established as measurable physiological centers in Western science, many individuals have experienced the benefits of chakra meditation. In **chakra meditation,** each of the seven chakras within the body corresponds to a specific color. These chakras are the point of focus. Each chakra has certain characteristics and influences a different aspect of the personality.

The base chakra (red): controls the basic human survival instincts and provides an essential "grounding." Our most basic human instincts originate from this chakra.

The sacral chakra (orange): is linked to sexuality and reproductive capacity.

The solar plexus chakra (yellow): is said to direct our awareness of self within the world. This is the seat of our emotional life and existence.

The heart chakra (green): is connected to love and compassion. This chakra is the center of feelings of love, harmony, and peace.

The throat chakra (blue): is linked to individual creativity and communication.

The brow chakra (indigo): forms the seat of both intuition and awareness. It is seen as the seat of perception, often perception beyond our physical senses.

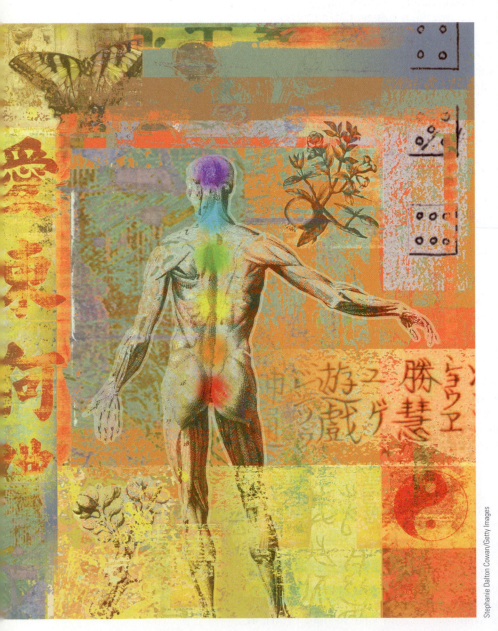

Stephanie Dalton Cowan/Getty Images

The main chakras within the body each correspond to a specific color. In chakra meditation, the point of focus is on each of these chakras.

The crown chakra (violet or white): links our spiritual connection to the universe around us, the link with the divine. This chakra also balances the interior and exterior energies of our existence, connecting us to the world around us.

When you practice chakra meditation, you focus inwardly, creating these chakras in your imagination. You may visualize the chakras as circles, balls, or wheels of colors that correspond to each chakra at each location. You may visualize each chakra spinning, pulsating, or radiating the colors. Focus directly on each one and allow your imagination to freely create this inner experience.

Walking Meditation

Another type of meditation that has great appeal for some people incorporates the principles of mindfulness you learned in Chapter 7. **Walking meditation** involves the use of movement rather than a mantra or the breath as one's focus.

The focus should be on the movement of each foot, broken up into three stages: lifting, moving, and placing. The simple objective is to be aware, noting each sensation as it occurs. Of course, as in sitting meditation, the mind will wander and has to be brought gently back to the object of meditation—in this case the movement of each step. Through practice and simple awareness, the mind increasingly concerns itself only with what *is*.[6] Psychotherapist Nancy J. Napier describes how to practice walking meditation:[7]

1. Begin by deciding where you're going to walk—someplace where you won't be disturbed. Be sure you are wearing comfortable clothing and shoes and that you have set aside whatever time you need to do this meditation.
2. Take a few moments to direct your attention to the bottoms of your feet. Feel how your feet make contact with the surface under you.
3. Remind yourself that your feet support your body and the surface under you supports your feet. There's no effort here. Just be aware of the support available to you.
4. Now slowly take a step forward. As you do, notice how you lift one foot and, as you move forward, the foot still on the ground begins to roll forward as well, and you naturally shift your weight. Do this slowly enough so you can feel the various elements of taking a step.
5. Pay attention to how your other foot touches the ground as you move into the step. Very slowly, simply allow the step to unfold and notice the movement of your body. Do this in whatever way allows you to keep your balance comfortably. The point here is not to get anywhere. It's to be aware of each element of your steps, to bring awareness to the process of walking mindfully.
6. As you walk, also notice your surroundings, the colors, shapes, textures, smells. Allow into your awareness whatever arises, and invite yourself to refocus on the bottoms of your feet and the steps you're taking if you find that your mind has drifted away from the meditation.
7. Also notice your breathing. Notice how it feels to settle your awareness in your belly, as well as in the bottoms of your feet. Your goal is to be present in your body as you notice your experience of walking slowly in this moment.
8. If you notice any feelings or thoughts arise, whether you experience them as comfortable or uncomfortable, name them—"thought," "feeling"—and then let them just keep moving through. Notice that if you will allow it, every thought, feeling, and sensation that arises naturally moves through and moves on.
9. When you have walked for the time you allowed, stop and take a moment to notice how you feel, physically and psychologically.
10. As you come back to everyday activities and awareness, notice what happens if you continue to inhabit yourself the way you did during your walking meditation.

The important component of walking meditation is continual awareness of movement as it is happening. As your mind wanders, gently bring it back to the process.

Benefits of Meditation

By relaxing the body and calming the mind, meditation can reduce the harmful effects of tension and stress—factors associated with many medical conditions. Although meditation has its roots in Eastern religious practice, the health benefits seem to be independent of the spiritual and philosophical components of meditation. You can bring your own beliefs and worldview to the meditative experience.

Members of many Eastern religions have long realized the benefits of meditation, but most Westerners have approached the practice with a skeptical eye. New imaging technology, however, is providing scientific information supporting the benefits of meditation. Functional magnetic resonance imaging (fMRI) has been used to identify and characterize the brain regions that are active during meditation. This research suggests that various parts of the brain known to be involved in attention and in the control of the autonomic nervous system are activated, providing a neurochemical and anatomical basis for the effects of meditation on various physiological activities.[8] For example, meditation has been shown in one study to produce significant increases in left-sided anterior brain activity, which is associated with positive emotional states. Moreover, in this same study, meditation was associated with increases in antibody titers to the influenza vaccine, suggesting potential linkages among meditation, positive emotional states, localized brain responses, and improved immune function.[9] Recent studies such as these involving imaging are advancing the understanding of meditation and other mind/body mechanisms. [10]

Herbert Benson and his colleagues at Harvard conducted research on volunteer practitioners of TM to determine if meditation could counter the physiological effects of stress. Their research showed that during meditation:

heartbeat and breathing rates slow,

oxygen consumption falls by 20%,

blood lactate levels, which are known to rise with stress and fatigue, drop, and

electroencephalograms (EEGs) show an increase of alpha brain wave patterns, another sign of relaxation.

Many stress-related illnesses have responded favorably to meditation. Meditation has been correlated with[11]

improvement in the breathing patterns of patients with bronchial asthma,

lower blood pressure in both pharmacologically treated and untreated hypertensive patients,

reduced premature ventricular contractions in patients with ischemic heart disease,

fewer symptoms of angina pectoris,

lower serum cholesterol levels in hypercholesterolemic patients,

relief of sleep-onset insomnia,

amelioration of stuttering,

lower blood sugar levels in diabetic patients, and

reduction in the symptoms of psychiatric illness including depression.

Meditation has been found helpful in alleviating fibromyalgia,[12] headache pain,[13] and stress in caregivers of dementia patients.[14] One report suggested that practicing meditation can positively influence chronic illness and can serve as a primary, secondary, and/or tertiary prevention strategy.[15] In research on meditation and its effects on anxiety, results have shown reduced anxiety levels in individuals after they begin to practice meditation regularly.[16]

In addition to the many physiological benefits of meditation, research[17] has shown that meditation has many psychological benefits including:

improved job performance and satisfaction,

improved academic performance in high school and college,

better long-term and short-term recall,

sounder sleep,

less anxiety,

less fear,

fewer phobias,

more positive mental health, and

increased empathy.

Mellow, Empathic Meditators

In a 2005 study, researchers measured brain electrical activity before, immediately after, and 4 months after a 2-month course in meditation. They found persistent increased activity on the left side of the prefrontal cortex, which is the area of the brain associated with joyful and serene emotions.*

And that's not all: researchers at the University of Wisconsin have used advanced brain images to show that certain types of meditation may increase the human capacity for empathy, defined as the ability to understand and share another person's experience. In the study, researchers compared brain activity in meditation experts with that of subjects just learning the technique. They measured brain activity, during meditation and at rest, in response to sounds—a woman in distress, a baby laughing, and a busy restaurant—designed to evoke a negative, positive, or neutral emotional response.

The researchers found that both the novice and the expert meditators showed an increased empathy reaction when in a meditative state. However, the expert meditators showed a much greater reaction, especially to the negative sound, which may indicate a greater capacity for empathy as a result of their extensive meditation training.

An increased capacity for empathy, the authors say, may have clinical and social importance. The next step, they add, is to investigate whether compassion meditation results in more altruistic behavior or other changes in social interaction.**

Sources:
*"Meditation in Psychotherapy," *Harvard Mental Health Letter*, 2005, *21*(10), 1–4.
**Lutz A, Brefczynski-Lewis J, Johnstone T, et al. Regulation of the neural circuitry of emotion by compassion meditation: effects of meditative expertise. *PLoS ONE* [online journal], March 2008. Accessed on May 28, 2008.

Meditation can be seen as a useful and effective intervention in reducing stress and in dealing with a wide variety of stress-related illnesses. Over the years, many carefully designed studies have investigated the benefits of meditation and deep relaxation. These comprehensive studies support the physiological and psychological benefits.

Frequently Asked Questions about Meditation

Following are some questions and answers to topics that frequently arise when you are learning meditation. Use these hints and suggestions to enhance your experience of meditation.

How do I stay focused when I meditate? Regardless of the type of meditation you choose, a question that warrants special consideration is, "What do I do when my mind begins to wander?" We will use mantra meditation as an example.

Three things can happen as you begin repeating your mantra. Not all of these will happen every time, but each time that you practice, you will experience one or more of them. First, you will continue repeating the word for most of the time your eyes are closed. You'll keep saying, "one … one … one … one … " for most of or the entire time you have set aside to meditate. In the typical experience, you will not remain focused on the word the entire time, but occasionally you will.

Another typical occurrence during meditation is that soon after you begin repeating your mantra, your mind begins to wander. Thoughts of what is going on in your life will come and go, and you will stop thinking of repeating the mantra. This is not rare, *nor is it a bad thing*, nor do you have to be concerned about it. When this happens—and it most certainly will—you simply intend to bring your awareness back to the mantra.

Your thoughts might sound something like this, "one … one … one … one … one … one … one … one … one … one … I wonder what I'm going to wear tonight when I go to that party … I hope Rick comes to the party … he's such a nice guy … I should have gone shopping yesterday when those sales were on. … those cool things probably won't be on sale again soon … but I did study for that test that's tomorrow. … I wish I had more time to study. … " At some point in this thought process, you will catch yourself thinking about all these other things; you will become aware of your chain of thoughts. When this happens, you will gently bring yourself back to repeating your mantra. "Oh, yeah, one … one … one … one … " Each time this happens, you do the same thing.

The third thing that may happen is that you may fall asleep. If so, you may well experience one of the deepest sleeps you have had in a long time! If this happens (and it will from time to time), gently, as you awaken from your deep sleep, repeat the mantra for a few more minutes before you end your meditation. Do not reprimand yourself for falling asleep. Take advantage of this opportunity to get some deep rest. If you fall asleep regularly when you meditate, this is a good indication that you need more sleep.

Always be gentle with yourself during meditation. Never think that you are a bad meditator, or that you cannot meditate because your mind wanders so much. People who have practiced meditation for many years still notice that their mind wanders as they are intending to repeat the mantra. This is normal. Whatever happens during meditation is appropriate as long as you have the single intention of repeating the mantra and returning to it when you wander off. Whenever it occurs to you to do so, simply insert the mantra in under all of your other thoughts that come and go. This is your only intention.

When is the best time to meditate? Only you can answer this question as you practice meditating on your own, but here are some general guidelines:

- Many people get optimal results when they meditate at least once a day, and twice is ideal. Typically, there are two times of the day that work best: immediately after waking up in the morning, and in the early afternoon, sometime between 4 o'clock and 6 o'clock p.m. This is a wonderful way to rejuvenate yourself for your evening activities. Your meditation schedule will depend on what works for you.
- Meditating before eating rather than afterward is better. When you meditate after eating, energy is diverted to digesting food. You will be more likely to fall asleep from fatigue if you meditate immediately after a meal.
- You should avoid using meditation as a means to help you fall asleep, because you don't want to associate meditation with sleep. Many individuals find that they are more alert and refreshed after meditation. Other techniques in this book are effective for helping you fall asleep immediately.

How long should I meditate? With any of the methods of meditation, begin with sessions that last about 10 minutes. With practice, and if it feels good to you and is producing good results, you may want to increase your meditation periods to 15 to 20 minutes or more. But only you can answer the question, "How long should I meditate?" With practice, you will become aware of what your body needs. If you have only 5 minutes to meditate before an important meeting, a test, or an eventful evening, take those 5 minutes and enjoy meditating. Any amount of time meditating is time well spent.

Will meditation get easier with practice? Some people practice meditation for years and still have days when their mind wanders and the calmness of meditation escapes them. A distracted mind is one of the great challenges to the practice of meditation. Even the great meditation masters often refer to their daily meditation as "practice" because it is not a finished product. Your motivation and the attention you bring to your practice have a great deal to do with the benefits you receive.

A person does not necessarily get better at meditation with regular practice any more than a person gets better at eating breakfast every day. The way it is done doesn't change. What we find, however, is that the physiological and psychological effects of meditation tend to expand with practice. For example, the resting heart rate during meditation may decrease to as low as 30 beats per minute in those who have practiced meditation for years. Some report that their breathing rate—the number of breaths they take per minute— becomes as low as one inhalation and exhalation during an entire minute. These are definite signs that we are decreasing our demand for energy during meditation, that we are slowing down our systems, and in the process are restoring, balancing, healing, and turning off the stress response.

Another typical occurrence in regular meditation is that as practice becomes regular, the effects of meditation remain throughout the day. You feel calm and peaceful and enjoy all the benefits of feeling relaxed during the entire day.

Does it matter if I lie down, rather than sit, during meditation? Earlier in the chapter we discussed sitting with dignity during meditation. What is so special about sitting? Here is what Jon Kabat-Zinn says about the importance of sitting during meditation:

> Sitting down to meditate, our posture talks to us. It makes its own statement. You might say the posture itself is the meditation. If we slump, it reflects low energy, passivity, a lack of clarity. If we

sit ramrod-straight, we are tense, making too much of an effort, trying too hard. When I use the word "dignity," everybody immediately adjusts his or her posture to sit up straighter. But they don't stiffen. Faces relax, shoulders drop, head, neck, and back come into easy alignment. The spine rises out of the pelvis with energy. Everybody seems to instantly know that inner feeling of dignity and how to embody it.[18]

So, when you practice meditation, sit in a way that affirms an attitude of presence, openness, calmness, and dignity.

How will I know if I'm getting the best results from meditation? Contrary to what you might think, the quality of a good meditation is not what happens during meditation but, instead, how you feel afterward. This is why it makes little difference what happens while you are meditating as long as you intend to return to your point of focus. How you feel afterward is the crucial determinant in whether the meditation is having positive effects for you. Do you feel more alert, more alive, calmer, more energized? If you do, this feedback tells you that the meditation is having positive effects and you should continue with your regular practice of meditation.

Conclusion

Meditation is simple and powerful. Although we may not entirely understand why or how it works, we know that it works to enhance our health and well-being. Of the several types of meditation and unlimited variations, you can adapt your meditation practice to work for you. Mantra meditation and breathing meditation are excellent techniques to get you on your way to experiencing the benefits of meditation. For students who have learned meditation, few methods are as warmly embraced for regaining balance, restoring energy, and bringing peace and tranquility.

21.1 Mantra Meditation

PURPOSE To allow you to practice deep relaxation using mantra meditation.

DIRECTIONS Prepare your environment for relaxation. Practice doing mantra meditation at least two times according to the instructions in this chapter. This exercise is best done sitting in a comfortable position rather than lying down. It is not one that is used to help you fall asleep so much as it is used to deeply relax you while remaining conscious. Allow approximately 15 minutes to complete the exercise.

After completing mantra meditation, respond to the questions below. Describe primarily how you were feeling in relation to your stress levels.

First Meditation:

1. How did you feel before meditating?

2. What things did you notice happening while you meditated (mental, emotional, physical)?

3. How did you feel while you meditated?

4. How did you feel after meditating (both immediately and several hours after meditating)?

5. Any other thoughts, concerns, or insights you had regarding your experience meditating?

Second Meditation:

1. How did you feel before meditating?

2. What things did you notice happening while you meditated (mental, emotional, physical)?

(Continued)

3. How did you feel while you meditated?

4. How did you feel after meditating (both immediately and several hours after meditating)?

5. Any other thoughts, concerns, or insights you had regarding your experience meditating?

Classroom experience (if applicable):

1. How did you feel before meditating?

2. What things did you notice happening while you meditated (mental, emotional, physical)?

3. How did you feel while you meditated?

4. How did you feel after meditating (both immediately and several hours after meditating)?

5. Any other thoughts, concerns, or insights you had regarding your experience meditating?

Summary After you have practiced the exercise and described your experiences, include a brief review of what you liked and/or did not like about this technique. Compare this technique to some of the others you have practiced. Would this be a relaxation technique you would consider using on a regular basis for stress management? Why or why not?

Key Points

- The most important component of meditation is the process of bringing the mind to focus on a single object, word, or idea to the exclusion of all others, and to dwell on it for a period of time.
- Herbert Benson's research found four key factors that result in the relaxation response: a mental device, a passive attitude, a quiet environment, and a comfortable position.
- A mantra is a repeated word, a sound, or a phrase used as a point of focus during meditation.
- Regular meditation has extensive physiological and psychological benefits.
- Many forms and variations of meditation allow you to determine the practice that produces optimal results for you.

Key Terms

lotus position
meditation
transcendental meditation
mantra meditation
mantra

faith factor
breathing meditation
contemplation
breath counting meditation
thought-watching

chakras
prana
chakra meditation
walking meditation

Discussion Time For Critical Thinking/Discussion Questions, please visit this book's Premium Website.

Notes

1. *The Relaxation Response*, by H. Benson (New York: Morrow Books, 1975).

2. *Stress Management for Wellness* (4th ed.), by W. Schafer (Belmont, CA: Wadsworth/Thomson Learning, 2000).

3. *Wherever You Go, There You Are*, by J. Kabat-Zinn (New York: Hyperion, 1994).

4. *Buddha's Little Instruction Book*, by J. Kornfield (New York: Bantam Doubleday Del Pub. Group, 1994).

5. *How to Meditate: A Guide to Self-Discovery*, by L. LeShan (Boston: Little, Brown and Company, 1974).

6. http://buddhism.about.com/od/meditation/a/walking.htm

7. http://www.nancyjnapier.com

8. Lazar, S. W., Bush, G., Gollub, R. L., et al. Functional brain mapping of the relaxation response and meditation. *Neuroreport.* 2000;11(7):1581-1585.

9. Davidson, R. J., Kabat-Zinn, J., Schumacher, J., et al. Alterations in brain and immune function produced by mindfulness meditation. *Psychosomatic Medicine.* 2003; 65(4): 564–570.

10. Mind/Body Medicine: An Overview. NCCAM Publication No. D239, December 1, 2008.

11. "Modern Forms of Meditation," by P. Carrington. In P. M. Lehrer and R. L. Woodfolk (Eds.), *Principles and Practice of Stress Management* (2nd ed.). (New York: Guilford Press, 1998) pp. 139–168.

12. "The Impact of a Meditation-Based Stress Reduction Program on Fibromyalgia," by K. H. Kaplan, D. L. Goldenberg, and M. Galvin-Nadeau, *General Hospital Psychiatry 15*(5) (1993): 284–289.

13. "Mind-Body Therapies for the Management of Pain," by J. A. Astin, *Clinical Journal of Pain 20*(1) (2004): 27–33.

14. "A Pilot Study of a Yoga and Meditation Intervention for Dementia Caregiver Stress," by L. C. Waelde, L. Thompson, and D. Gallagher-Thompson, *Journal of Clinical Psychology 60*(6) (2004): 677–688.

15. "Meditation's Impact on Chronic Illness," by R. Bonadonna, *Holistic Nursing Practice 17*(6) (2003): 309–319.

16. "Modern Forms of Meditation," by P. Carrington. In P. M. Lehrer and R. L. Woolfolk (Eds.), *Principles and Practice of Stress Management* (2nd ed.). (New York: The Guilford Press, 1993) pp. 139–168.

17. *The TM Book: How to Enjoy the Rest of Your Life*, by D. Denniston and P. McWilliams (Allen Park, MI: Versemonger Press, 1975).

18. Kabat-Zinn, *Wherever You Go, There You Are.*

22 Yoga

> ■ Do I have to twist myself into the shape of a pretzel to enjoy the benefits of yoga? ■ Is yoga the same thing as meditation? ■ What can I do to prepare myself for practicing yoga to get the most out of it? ■ Is yoga a New Age cult or a religion? ■ How many times a week should I do yoga, and for how long?

Study of this chapter will enable you to:

1. Explain the meaning, purpose, and benefits of yoga.
2. Differentiate between types of yoga.
3. Learn how to prepare for yoga practice.
4. Practice various yoga poses designed to promote well-being and relaxation.

Before you learn to stand on your head, you need to learn to stand on your own two feet.

—*Swami Satchidananda*

Students Experience Yoga While I was doing the yoga, I noticed myself gradually begin to relax. My muscles loosened up, and I could feel my body, as well as my mind, begin to relax. I felt calmer, and my body felt much better after doing all of that stretching. I felt like I had fully stretched my body, and it felt good. Before I had actually tried yoga, I thought of it as all of these weird stretching poses that weren't extremely helpful. After doing some of the yoga poses, I can testify that they are helpful and relaxing. I also was impressed by how good I felt after practicing the poses and how relaxing it actually can be. Now I'm a believer in the power that yoga can have on the body.

—*Kathryn R.*

* * *

I thought yoga was easy, but after doing it, I realized that it's a lot harder than it looks. I realized that I'm not as flexible as I used to be and that yoga would help me to be more flexible. Before I tried yoga, especially being a guy, I thought it was just for flexible women. I didn't think I could benefit from yoga, and I thought it looked easy. Now I know that yoga is for everyone, whether they are flexible or not, and I know that it isn't as easy as it looks, but it also is very relaxing and refreshing.

—*Brett M.*

* * *

I went to the yoga class last Friday and, to be honest, I was a little skeptical. I thought it would be great to do and help my body with flexibility, but I didn't think it would have the effects on my body that it did. After the session my body felt great, I had a high energy level for the rest of the night. I didn't have a problem going to sleep, and when I woke up in the morning, I had the best night's sleep! After yoga, mentally, I had the same feeling I get when I'm done jogging, and it was less painful on my knees. I definitely enjoyed the session and will make yoga a regular in my exercise routine.

—*Amy H.*

* * *

Yoga

When you think of yoga, what images come to mind? You may think of slender people from India putting their bodies into contorted, pretzel-like positions and making humming sounds. This is a familiar image because of the origins of yoga. But behind this inaccurate stereotype lies a rich, practical method of achieving peak physical health, psychological well-being, and deep inner peace.

Yoga is a course of exercises and postures intended to promote control of the body and mind and to attain physical and spiritual well-being.[1] The term *yoga* comes from the Sanskrit root *yuj*, which means "to join" or "to yoke together." It literally signifies union of the body, mind, emotions, and spirit into one harmonious, integrated whole. Swami Rama[2] described yoga as an attempt to take into account all three sides of human life—the body, the mind, and the soul—or, to put it differently, the physical, the mental, the emotional, and the spiritual. The idea is that a healthy body is necessary to house the inner soul.

Unfortunately, a physically healthy person may lack spiritual awareness, and even those who are both physically fit and spiritually aware may not have a proper relationship with others. Yoga philosophy teaches ways of establishing harmony between and among the various sides of life. Once the mind and body have established harmony, once they have become integrated and still, healing takes place at all levels.

This chapter introduces you to the effective stress-management strategy known as yoga. You will discover that yoga is not designed to make you withdraw from the world and accept a reclusive lifestyle, as some people think. To the contrary, yoga is about learning how to live life more fully, to accomplish more, with more joy and less stress.

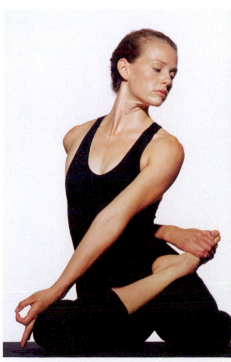
© Ronnen Eshel/CORBIS

When you think of yoga, what images come to mind?

Being myself includes taking risks with myself, taking risks on new behavior, trying new ways of being myself, so that I can see how it is I want to be.

—*Hugh Prather*

Background

Yoga is said to have originated in India nearly 5,000 years ago. The exact dates of its inception are not known, but stone carvings found in archeological sites depicting figures in yoga positions have been found in the Indus Valley dating back 5,000 years or more.[3] In general, the tradition has been passed down from generation to generation by word of mouth, and from teacher to student.

The Indian sage Patanjali is believed to have assembled a collection of yoga theories and practices known as the **yoga sutras** (aphorisms or thoughts). The system he wrote about has eight limbs or eight branches of yoga, consisting of:[4]

1. **yama,** meaning "restraint"—refraining from violence, lying, stealing, casual sex, and hoarding
2. **niyama,** meaning "observance"—purity, contentment, tolerance, study, and remembrance
3. **asana**—physical exercises
4. **pranayama**—breathing techniques
5. **pratyahara**—preparation for meditation, described as withdrawal of the mind from the senses
6. **dharana,** concentration—being able to hold the mind on one object for a specified time
7. **dhyana,** meditation—the ability to focus on one thing (or nothing) indefinitely
8. **samadhi,** absorption—realization of the essential nature of the self

Most yoga classes, books, and videos today focus on the third, fourth, and fifth branches of yoga—namely, asanas (postures or poses), pranayamas (breathing techniques), and pratyahara (meditation). Collectively, these three make up what is commonly known as **hatha yoga.** They are designed specifically to, among other things, reduce stress and restore balance.

Other ways of practicing yoga[5] include the yoga of wisdom (jnâna yoga), the yoga of service (karma yoga), and the yoga of devotion (bhakti yoga). One can spend many hours studying the yoga disciplines, such as fasting, vegetarianism, disciplined thinking, and many other yoga philosophies. A wide range of information is available through classes, books, videos, and yoga Websites if you are interested in exploring yoga in more depth.

Yoga has no political or religious boundaries. Anyone can practice yoga, regardless of age, sex, or physical condition. Those who are interested in beginning regular yoga practice would do well to seek a class with a qualified teacher who can provide guidance and instruction so the initial experience with yoga will be positive. You will find tips for selecting a qualified, effective instructor later in this chapter.

Overview of Yoga Styles[6]

Classical hatha yoga is the traditional approach to hatha yoga. It is called "classical" because it has not been adapted in any way. This form of yoga involves simple poses that flow from one to the other at a comfortable pace. Participants are encouraged to proceed at their own pace, taking time to concentrate on breathing and meditation in their practice. This yoga style is ideal for winding down at the end of a tough day.

Iyengar yoga is a classical style of yoga that is softer on the body and is well-suited for beginners and those who haven't exercised in a while. It uses props such as chairs, straps, blocks, pillows, and sandbags to compensate for a lack of flexibility, which is helpful for those who have back or joint problems.

The key to any style of yoga is to learn the proper fundamentals and form. Iyengar yoga emphasizes symmetry and alignment, and also meditation. The person holds each pose longer than in most other yoga styles, developing a state of focused calm.

Benefits of iyengar yoga include toning muscles, eliminating tension, and easing chronic pain. When weak areas of the body are strengthened and stretched, the body returns to its correct alignment.

Ashtanga yoga (power yoga) is the preferred choice for athletes, because ashtanga yoga is light on meditation but heavy on developing strength and stamina. The poses are more difficult than those performed in other styles, and students move quickly from one pose to another in an effort to build strength, stamina, and flexibility.

This style is suitable for anyone in reasonable physical condition, but those who are new to exercise should avoid this style of yoga. Even "beginner" routines can be physically demanding workouts. Ashtanga yoga takes students through a warming up of the body to "activate" the muscles. Students then move from one pose to another in a continual flow, and combine the inhale and exhale of the breath with movements.

The cornerstone of power yoga is the sun salutation, a 12-pose flowing series that is modified in various ways known as the primary and secondary series. This form pays attention particularly to linking the breath to each of the movements.

Kundalini yoga incorporates mantras (chanting), meditations, visualizations, and guided relaxation. It focuses on healing and "purifying" the mind, body, and emotions. Kundalini yoga is designed to activate the kundalini energy in the spine.

This energy activation is achieved with poses, breath control, chanting, and meditation. Kundalini yoga is beneficial in dealing with addictions, and many people find it to be a natural way of releasing endorphins through breathing and doing the poses.

Bikram yoga is done in a hot room, 90 to 105 degrees Fahrenheit, replicating the temperature of the birthplace of yoga in India. This style of yoga moves sequentially through 26 postures that are performed in a precise order. The Bikram series warms and stretches muscles, ligaments, and tendons in the order in which they should be stretched according to Bikram Choudhury, developer of this style of yoga.

When combined with the heat, Bikram yoga makes for a tough workout. The exercises are more physical than most, with high intensity. This style is recommended for yoga veterans and extremely fit individuals.

Kripalu yoga is more spontaneous, flowing, and meditation-orientated. The first stage of Kripalu yoga involves primarily postural alignment while intertwining the breath and movement. The individual holds the poses only a short time.

The student progresses to the second stage, which includes meditation, and holds the poses longer. Finally, the practice of poses becomes a spontaneous dynamic movement. The individual experiences the essence of Kripalu yoga through a continuous flow of postures while meditating, for gentle, yet dynamic yoga.

Sivananda yoga has a series of 12 poses, with a foundation of the sun salutation, breathing exercises, relaxation, and mantra chanting.

You may want to experiment with various styles of yoga to determine which best suits your needs. For relaxation, hatha yoga is often a preferred choice.

What Is Hatha Yoga?

Hatha yoga, which is especially effective for inducing a state of energized relaxation, will be the focus of the rest of this chapter. Hatha yoga consists of regulating the mind and body through 14 breathing exercises (pranayamas) and more than 200 balanced physical postures or poses (asanas) that exercise and lengthen all the muscles in the body.[7] The physical postures require one to control, regulate, and become aware of one's physical existence. The emphasis is on giving complete mental attention to each movement to the exclusion of everything else. With practice, different body functions become more integrated with one another, with all parts functioning together harmoniously. Energy from within is awakened, and the person practicing yoga feels radiant with vitality and energy.[8]

The practice of yoga postures (asanas) differs significantly from conventional exercise such as aerobics, weight training, and jogging. The goal of asana practice is to restore the mind/body to its natural condition of well-being, alertness, and potentially peak performance. Developing muscle strength and cardiovascular fitness and achieving other health benefits are possible in the process but usually are considered secondary objectives.

Benefits of Yoga

The regular practice of yoga produces general health benefits as well as specific relaxation benefits. These benefits come together for overall well-being of body, mind, and spirit. Yoga specialist John C. Kimbrough describes the benefits of regular yoga relaxation practice:[9]

- Results in better overall physical and mental health.
- Relieves and delays the onset of fatigue and makes up for lost sleep.

- Helps access and cultivate the skillful and healthy elements of the unconscious mind. This brings about a spiritual unfolding and leads to better mind/body integration and harmony and effortless living.
- Minimizes and alleviates illusions, fatigue, confusion, and nonessential burdens, and develops a living that is more skillful, which allows us to let go of disturbing thoughts and feelings. It helps us deal with our life stresses and brings about greater freedom from negative conditioning and repressed memories.
- Prepares the mind, body, and breath for sitting concentration/meditation practice.

Every unhealthy condition that results from chronic activation of the stress response can be improved through regular practice of yoga. During yoga practice, most feel a decrease in the stress response through the duration of a yoga session. As a result, the body functions that are altered when we perceive a need to run or fight return to homeostasis. This balanced physiological state allows the body to correct problems that have arisen from chronic stress for lasting results long after the yoga session has ended.

An early study with Indian yogis, most of whom practiced hatha yoga, reported that the following characteristic pattern of physiological alterations occurred during regular yoga practice:

1. An extreme slowing of respiration to 4 to 6 breaths per minute
2. More than a 70% increase in electrical resistance based on galvanic skin response (GSR), indicating a state of deep relaxation
3. A predominance of alpha brainwave activity
4. Slowing of the heart rate to 24 beats per minute from the normal rate of 72 beats per minute[10]

Each of these alterations in physiology indicates deep levels of relaxation.

Asanas are gentle stretching movements designed to rejuvenate and bring balance to the entire body. This happens in several ways.

First, yoga postures increase blood supply to specific areas of the body and stimulate them with a squeezing action that gently massages the internal organs. The asanas make use of gravity to further increase blood flow to targeted areas. For example, an inverted pose such as the headstand increases blood flow and oxygen to the brain, enhancing its ability to function optimally. The shoulder stand produces an increase in blood flow to the thyroid gland. With an emphasis on long, deep breathing, oxygen-rich blood flows throughout the body.

Second, yoga poses increase flexibility in the spine. This ensures a nervous-system connection to all parts of the body because the nerves from the spine extend to all body tissues, organs, and glands. The yoga postures are designed to stretch and relax muscles, increase flexibility in the joints, and stretch ligaments and tendons. Most asanas work on more than one area of the body at the same time. For example, the twisting asanas bring benefits to the spine, adrenal glands, liver, pancreas, and kidneys.

The asanas are a discipline for the body, which in turn positively affects the mind. Asanas balance the nervous system. They increase flexibility, improve circulation, strengthen muscles, aid in digestion, improve the immune system, and increase breathing capacity and elasticity of the lungs.

Yoga postures work on all dimensions of the mind/body:

1. *Physically,* the body experiences healing, muscle strengthening, stretching, and relaxation. All tissues and organs in the body get a workout, and even the nervous system returns to a more balanced state. Yoga makes the physical body healthy, fit, flexible, and more immune to disease, which helps to alleviate those physical disorders that have a connection to psychological or system imbalance.
2. *Mentally,* the mind cultivates peacefulness, alertness, and a heightened ability to focus and concentrate. Because of this, one can relax, study, and understand oneself better to develop a more balanced state of mind.
3. *Emotionally,* yoga frees the mind from anxiety, worry, and tension, and transforms negative emotions and behaviors into positive and higher states. Yoga also may help people overcome being at the mercy of their emotions and unhealthy conditioned responses. It can lead an individual to become more sensitive and compassionate to the needs of others.

For those wounded
by civilization,
yoga is the most
healing salve.
—Terri Guillemets

Yoga Helps Reverse Heart Disease

Dean Ornish, author of *Dr. Dean Ornish's Program for Reversing Heart Disease,* uses a yoga-based therapy scientifically with his patients. In one of his studies, he and his colleagues randomly assigned 48 middle-aged male and female outpatients with coronary artery disease to experimental and usual-care control groups. Patients in the experimental group were prescribed an extremely low-fat vegetarian diet and moderate exercise, were trained in stress management including enhancement of social support among the group members to increase compliance, and were advised to stop smoking.

The stress-management training included yoga-based stretching exercises, breathing techniques, meditation, relaxation, and visual imagery. The patients were asked to practice these exercises at least 1 hour per day, and were given 1-hour audiocassette tapes to help them practice. The patients in the control group were not asked to make any similar lifestyle changes but were free to do so.

The experimental group, compared to the control group, realized:

- a significantly greater drop in total cholesterol levels (24.3%) and low-density lipoprotein cholesterol levels (37.4%)
- significant reduction in the frequency, duration, and severity of angina pain
- a decrease in constriction of coronary arteries

The authors of the study commented that coronary artery disease is progressive, and that results from the control group demonstrated that the usual advice to change lifestyle and medications were not sufficient to halt its progression. Results of the experimental group gave early indications that, for heart disease, changes in lifestyle including yoga-based therapy may be a potent alternative.

Sources:
Dr. Dean Ornish's Program for Reversing Heart Disease, by D. Ornish (New York: Ballantine Books, 1990); "Can Lifestyle Changes Reverse Coronary Heart Disease?," by D. Ornish and S. E. Brown, *Lancet 336* (1990): 129–133; "Yoga-Based Therapy," by C. Patel. In P. M. Lehrer and R. L. Woolfolk (Eds.), *Principles and Practice of Stress Management* (2nd ed.). (New York: Guilford Press, 1993); "The Use of Hatha Yoga as a Strategy for Coping with Stress in Management Development," by F. S. Heilbronn, *Management Education & Development* 23(2) (1992): 131–139.

4. *Spiritually,* yoga prepares one for meditation as it develops inner strength. Yoga experts claim that yoga helps an individual evolve spiritually as it enables him or her to understand and accept life's situations and experiences from a broader perspective, thereby increasing faith in a more elevated purpose for life and faith in a higher power and the goodness of life.

5. *Behaviorally,* yoga redirects wasted energy away from behaviors that could be detrimental to well-being. It leads to a more balanced and harmonious interaction with others and an inner peace of mind. Yoga brings about a deeper state of relaxation that makes an individual more fruitful and more able to enjoy life.

> **Author Anecdote** Yoga Makes the Headache Go Away For two years I was a yoga instructor at a fitness center. Each week we would go through a routine of poses that seemed to be helpful to the participants because they kept coming back for more. One older woman came nearly every single week like clockwork. She never said a word but seemed to enjoy herself while she was in class. One day I bumped into her as we were leaving, and I took a moment to ask her about her experience with the class. She said that she enjoyed the class tremendously. But what struck me as being most interesting was when she said that she always came to class with a headache from the stress of her day—and she always left without it.
>
> —MO

In a study conducted in Japan with female college students, hatha yoga was compared to progressive relaxation and its effects on heart rate, blood pressure, physical self-efficacy, and self-esteem. Both treatments were found to be effective in lowering heart rate and blood pressure and in improving self-esteem.[11]

The American Yoga Association provides details on how yoga alleviates the symptoms of the following conditions:[12]

Addiction	Depression
AIDS/HIV	Diabetes
Anxiety and stress	Fibromyalgia
Arthritis	Headaches
Asthma	Heart health
Back and neck pain	Hypertension
Chronic fatigue	Incontinence

Infertility	Pain management
Insomnia	PMS/menopause
Multiple sclerosis	Weight management

Directly related to stress management, yoga activates parasympathetic nervous system activity, which, as mentioned in earlier chapters, unleashes energy, restores the immune system, and fixes many problems that stem from a chronically activated fight-or-flight response. Yoga relaxes us deeply.

In addition, yoga helps us develop and grow. When individuals are in a given pose, they move in the direction of their physical limits of flexibility. Once they have found that limit, they ease back a little and then, with each exhalation, move through that limitation, slowly, gently, and easily. This process of moving through the limitations is translated into other areas of life in which they have set up perceived barriers. As they meet challenges that seem difficult, they step back a bit, breathe, and do what is necessary to easily move through that barrier. Little by little, they expand and grow in all areas of life with confidence because they have practiced doing it every time they practice yoga.

How to Practice Yoga

Yoga asanas are designed to develop the body with three primary facets of fitness: power, flexibility, and balance. Every pose combines one or more of each of these fitness factors. Some poses may develop balance more than flexibility. Other poses are designed to develop strength and power. Working on a wide variety of poses develops each of these aspects of fitness throughout the entire body.

Each pose has a specific Sanskrit name and a corresponding English equivalent. For example, the standing forward bend is called *uttanasana* (OOT-tan-AHS-ahna). Many of the asanas have animal names, such as the camel posture and the eagle posture. This is because yogis created their asanas in part by observing animal behavior. They noticed how animals instinctively stretch and contract their bodies. For example, after a cat is finished with a nap, it instinctively stretches, arching the spine in both directions. You do not have to know the names of the various poses to do them correctly, but you should try to perform them correctly. With time and practice, the names become a natural part of your yoga practice.

Asana practice for beginners and experienced yogis is essentially the same, the difference being the intensity of the poses and the student's flexibility. A typical yoga session proceeds through a series of poses, being mindful of what is happening in the body, entering and ending each pose slowly, breathing fully and deeply in and out through the nose, and enjoying the process.

Yoga poses are done in a variety of positions including standing, sitting, kneeling, lying on the back, lying on the stomach, on the hands and knees, and in inverted positions. Each asana might have a number of variations. Depending on one's skill level, the poses may be modified to any of the variations. This is why yoga is appropriate for individuals of all levels of fitness and flexibility.

If you have not done yoga before, you might find that many of the poses resemble the stretching exercises you did when you were in physical education classes in junior high and high school or when you stretched in preparation for a sporting event. Many of the poses are the same, with more emphasis on fluid movement between postures and increased awareness of breathing.

As you move into and out of each pose, keep a part of the mind's focus on the flow of breathing. In general, inhalation takes place during expansion phases of a pose and exhalations occur during the contracting phases of a pose. As you hold a pose, allow the breath to flow like a circle, going in through the nose, down into the lowest parts of the lungs, turning around and coming back out through the nose. Visualize the flowing breath like a Ferris wheel slowly moving around in a smooth, circular pattern. The breath should not be jerky, nor should there be long pauses in the flowing breath between an inhale and exhale or between an exhale and inhale.

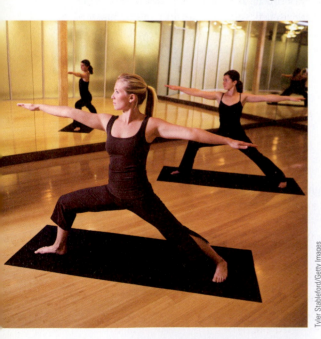

Nearly every yoga pose has an English name and a Sanskrit name. This one is called Warrior II Pose or Virabhadrasana II.

Tyler Stableford/Getty Images

Move slowly into each pose and back out of the pose. Never jerk through a range of motion. Take your time and allow your body to move smoothly from beginning to end of a pose. Hold each pose for at least 20 seconds; longer is better. The muscles, tendons, and ligaments require about 20 seconds to release and move into a stretching mode. Some poses involve movement rather than static stretching. Move through these slowly and easily.

Stretch to an almost maximal range of motion, and then ease back a little from there. This is where you start. As you are holding the pose, allow yourself to move ever so slightly more into the stretch each time you exhale. Let the exhale assist you in expanding. With practice, you will find your body responding by easing you gently through your physical limits.

Keep your attention focused directly on what is happening in your body. Do not let your mind wander. As you maintain your focus, gently move through your limits and extend yourself while at the same time making sure that you are not overextending and causing unnecessary damage to tissues. *Never push yourself through the range of a stretch to a point where you feel pain.* A feeling of slight muscle pulling is okay, but pain is never a good thing when doing yoga. If you feel pain, the tissue is sending a message that it is being pulled or pushed too far. That leads to injuries and also fear connected to that pose in the future.

Staying focused on what is happening inside, paying attention to the sensations, and easing back when you feel pain will prevent any damage and lead to a positive yoga experience. If you are someone who is not very flexible, yoga is an ideal exercise for you. Your flexibility will increase gradually with regular practice, and you will realize that everyone has a different level of flexibility. Where you are now is just fine. Yoga is not limited to the most limber among us. Everyone experiences the healing effect, no matter how far he or she can stretch into the poses.

Yoga usually is done barefoot, wearing comfortable athletic attire or loose clothing that breathes easily. The same attire that you wear to the gym is appropriate for practicing yoga. You might find it helpful to bring a towel with you, and a yoga mat is especially useful on hard floors. You can practice yoga nearly anywhere—at home, at school, in the office, at the beach, in a park, or anywhere you have some open space, peace and quiet, and some fresh air.

Taking Precautions Before Starting Yoga

Yoga, overall, is generally considered very safe. But there are some situations in which yoga can pose a risk. Check with your doctor or other health care provider before starting a new yoga program. This is especially important if you have certain health conditions, such as joint problems or a history of low back or neck pain. You may need to avoid certain yoga positions depending on your condition because of the undue strain it may cause.

Also see your health care provider before you begin yoga if you have any of the following conditions or situations, since complications can arise:

- High blood pressure that's difficult to control
- A risk of blood clots
- Eye conditions, including glaucoma
- Osteoporosis
- Pregnancy
- Artificial joints[13]

You may be able to practice yoga in these situations if you take certain precautions. For instance, if you're pregnant, avoid any poses that put pressure on your uterus, such as those that require you to twist at the waist.

Tips for Enhancing Your Yoga Experience

- Do yoga on an empty stomach. A full stomach inhibits your range of motion for many poses. A full stomach also drains your energy while your body diverts energy to digestion. Refrain from eating 2 to 3 hours before a yoga session. If you become extremely hungry before beginning yoga, experiment with a light snack such as a few nuts, yogurt, or some juice. Be sure to drink plenty of water before, during, and, most important, after a yoga session.

- Experience the benefits of yoga by practicing as little as 1 hour per week. Certainly, the more you do it, the more you will experience its positive effects. Most yoga classes last approximately 1 hour to 1½ hours. The recommendation for beginners is to try to practice about two or three times per week. One positive aspect of yoga is that if you have only 15 or 20 minutes to practice, you can select a few poses and do them fully in that amount of time. You might find that after continued practice, your desire to do yoga will increase just as those who exercise regularly come to enjoy working out regularly.

- When possible, practice at the same time every day. Morning is a great time to work out stiffness from the previous night's sleep and create energy and balance for the day. In the afternoon and evening, the muscles are warmer and looser, allowing greater stretching. Be careful during these times that you don't overdo and push yourself too far.

- Go at your own pace. Don't compare your progress or your flexibility to anyone else. Where you are is fine, and how fast you are progressing is fine.

- Take responsibility for your progress. If you are going to a class or following a video, listen to the feedback your body is giving to you. If you feel refreshed and energized an hour after practicing *and* the following day, you are on the right track. If you have noticeable discomfort or pain at either of these times, lower the intensity of your yoga practice.

- Be patient with yourself. Don't look for immediate results. Release any and all expectations of how you *should* be progressing, and simply let the experience of regular practice be sufficient. Yoga develops the body and mind at many levels, some of which may not be observable immediately. Trust the process, and simply concentrate on regular practice.

- Enjoy the experience. Associate pleasure with the joy of stretching, breathing, and smooth body movement. Your body will tell you that this is a healthy and useful thing to do. You will experience a flood of positive feelings both during and after yoga.

Finding a Yoga Class

If you've decided to try yoga for stress management or relaxation, look around for classes in your area to see what's offered. You can also learn yoga from books and videos. But beginners usually find it helpful to learn with an instructor. Classes offer camaraderie and friendship, which are important to overall well-being.

When you find a class that sounds interesting, contact the instructor and get all of your questions answered so that you know what to expect. Questions to ask can include:

- What are the instructor's qualifications? Where did he or she learn yoga, and how long has he or she been teaching?

- Does the instructor have experience working with students with your needs or health concerns? If you have a sore knee or an aching shoulder, can the instructor help you find poses that won't aggravate your condition?

- Is the class suitable for beginners? Will it be easy enough to follow along if it's your first time? Can you observe a class before signing up?

- What is the focus of the class? Is it aimed at your needs, such as stress management or relaxation, or is it geared for people who want to reap other benefits?

- What do you need to take along to class? Some classes require you to bring a mat or towel to sit or stand on while doing poses. Other classes will provide a mat.

At the end of a yoga class, you should feel invigorated, yet relaxed and calm. If this isn't the case, talk to your instructor. He or she might have suggestions for you. Otherwise there may be another yoga class better suited to your needs for stress management and relaxation.[14]

Sample Poses

Table 22.1 is a demonstration of common yoga poses. There are many more poses than these represented here, and in addition, variations for each. This table contains asanas that you would see at yoga classes or in yoga productions (videos/DVDs/books) available at most major bookstores. Figure 22.1, Salutation to the Sun, combines several poses into a flowing sequence.

As you practice these poses, try to put yourself in the same position as you see in the illustrations. The pictures demonstrate the poses being done one way. For example, Side Angle Pose below shows him with his left foot forward and right foot back. Be sure to do the opposite by switching so the right foot is forward and the left foot is back. Do the poses both ways in every case where this can happen. At first you probably will find that you aren't able to match the examples as presented here. With regular practice, however, your body will develop sufficient flexibility, strength, and balance to do them. To enhance your experience with the poses, keep in mind the suggestions and tips outlined in this chapter.

TABLE 22.1 Common Yoga Poses

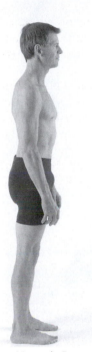

Mountain Pose

Standing Forward Bend

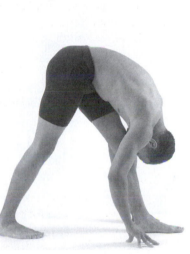

Side Angle Pose

Dancing Pose

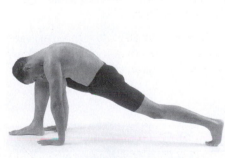

Warrior I

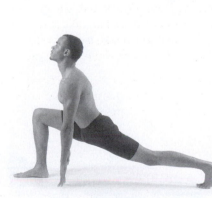

Warrior I (continued)

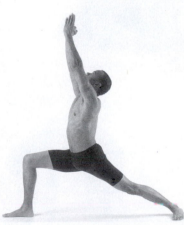

Warrior I (continued)

(Continued)

TABLE 22.1 (Continued)

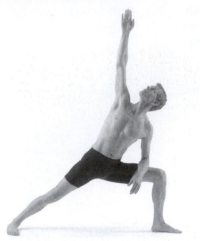

Side Angle Pose

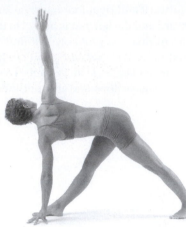

Twisted Triangle Pose

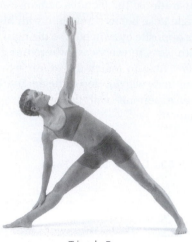

Triangle Pose

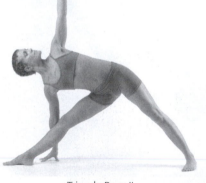

Triangle Pose II

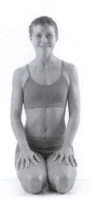

Thunderbolt

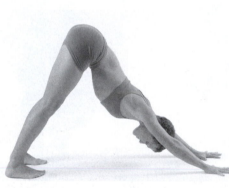

Downward Dog

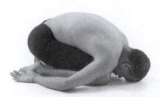

Child's Pose

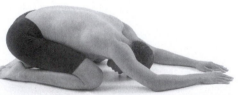

Stretched Child's Pose

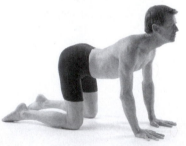

Tiger Breathing (inhale)

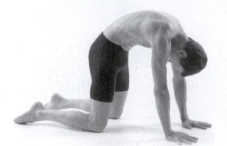

Tiger Breathing (exhale)

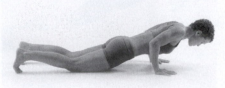

Half Boat

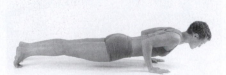

Half Boat (continued)

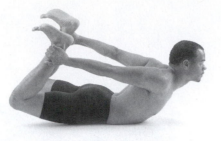

Bow

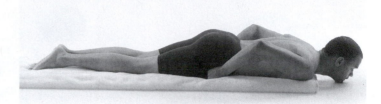

Full Locust

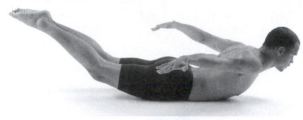

Full Locust (continued)

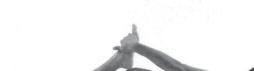

Half Bow

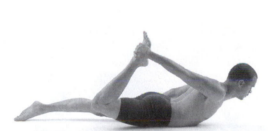

Half Bow (continued)

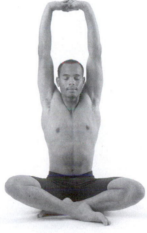

Sitting Side Bend

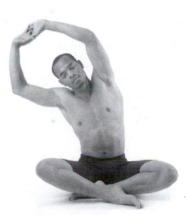

Sitting Side Bend (continued to both sides)

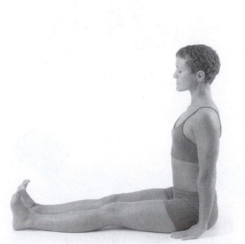

Staff Pose

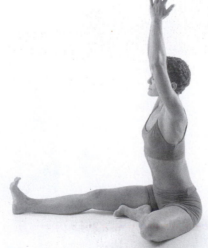

Head to the Knee

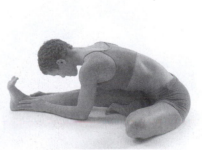

Head to the Knee (continued)

(Continued)

TABLE 22.1 (Continued)

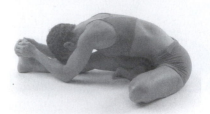

Head to the Knee (continued)

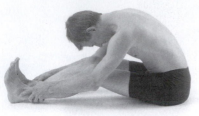

Back Stretch

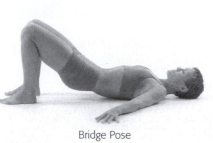

Back Stretch (continued)

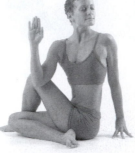

Spiral Twist (both sides)

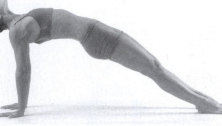

Front Body Stretch

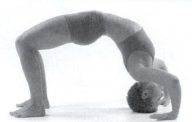

Bridge Pose

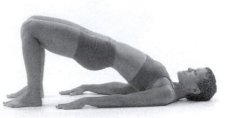

Bridge Pose (continued)

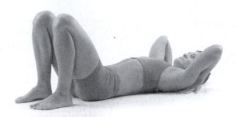

Upward Bow

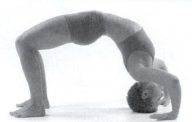

Upward Bow (continued)

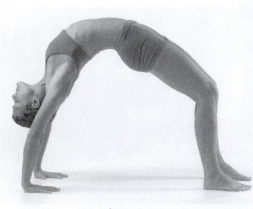

Upward Bow (continued)

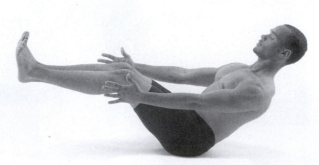

Boat Pose

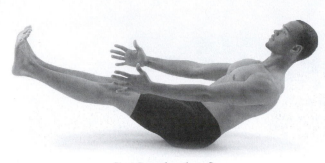

Boat Pose (continued)

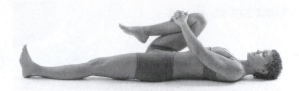

Single Knee to Chest (do each knee)

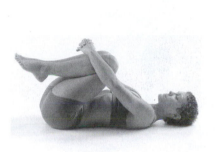

Knees to Chest

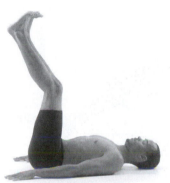

Upward Straight Legs

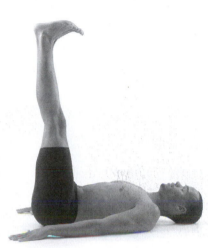

Upward Straight Legs (continued)

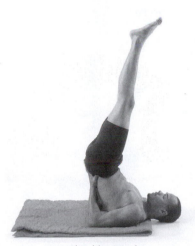

Shoulder Stand

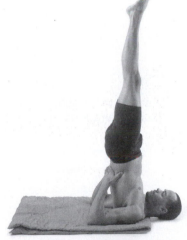

Shoulder Stand (continued)

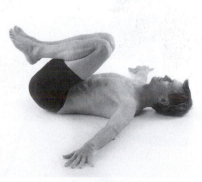

Belly Turning Pose

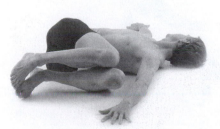

Belly Turning Pose (left side)

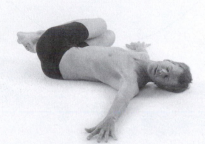

Belly Turning Pose (right side)

(Continued)

TABLE 22.1 (Continued)

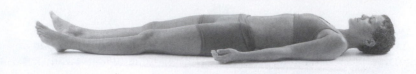

Corpse Pose

Source: *Yoga for Fitness and Wellness*, by R. Dykema (Belmont, CA: Wadsworth/Thomson Learning, 2006).

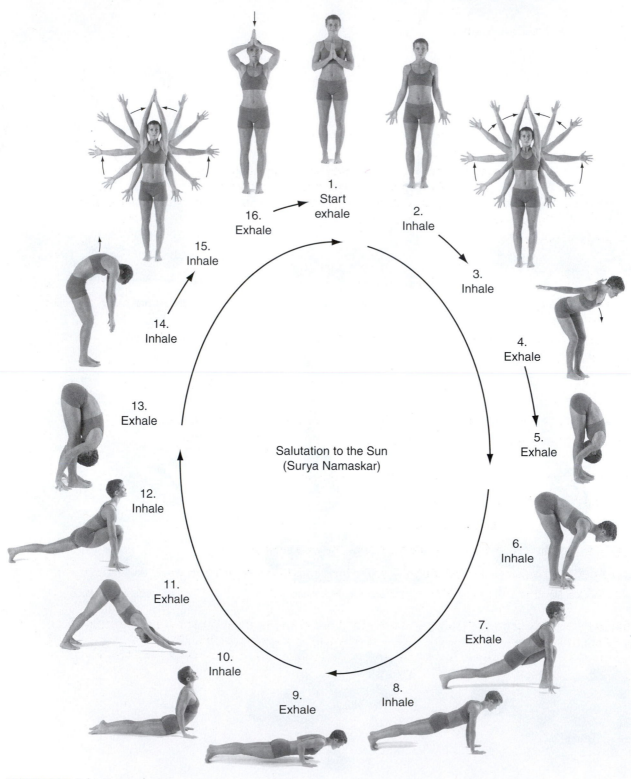

Salutation to the Sun
(Surya Namaskar)

1.
Start
exhale

16.
Exhale

2.
Inhale

3.
Inhale

15.
Inhale

14.
Inhale

4.
Exhale

13.
Exhale

5.
Exhale

12.
Inhale

6.
Inhale

11.
Exhale

7.
Exhale

10.
Inhale

8.
Inhale

9.
Exhale

FIGURE 22.1 Salutation to the Sun

Conclusion

Yoga signifies union of the body, mind, emotions, and spirit into one harmonious and integrated whole. Yoga has many styles and variations. Hatha yoga focuses on simple, flowing poses, along with breathing and meditation, making it especially effective for relaxation. Yoga postures work on all dimensions of the mind/body to activate the parasympathetic nervous system and initiate the relaxation response.

22.1 Yoga Practice

PURPOSE To allow you to experience relaxation through the practice of yoga.

DIRECTIONS On two separate occasions, experiment with a variety of poses according to the instructions and pictures in the text. Follow the guidelines, tips, and pointers for proper yoga as they have been explained to you. There are many poses, but select at least 10 per session and do them exactly as they appear in this chapter. Among the poses that you try, include the following simple poses:

- Standing forward bend
- Triangle pose I
- Thunderbolt
- Downward Dog
- Child's pose I
- Head to the Knee
- Spinal Twist
- Bridge
- Belly Turning pose
- Salutation to the Sun (Be sure to follow this carefully as it is a series of sequential poses.)
- Corpse pose (Always end with this one.)

Report After you have practiced yoga, respond to the following:

1. Which poses did you choose each time?

2. Which did you find difficult, easy, or impossible?

3. How did you feel before, during and after doing the yoga sessions?

4. After actually doing yoga, describe how your perceptions have changed from what you perceived yoga to be before you did your sessions.

Summary Include a brief review of what you liked and/or did not like about yoga as a relaxation technique. Compare yoga to some of the other relaxation techniques you have practiced. Would this be a relaxation technique you would consider using on a regular basis for stress management? Why or why not?

Key Points

- Yoga is a course of exercises and postures intended to promote control of the body and mind and to attain physical and spiritual well-being.
- Yoga is said to have originated in India nearly 5,000 years ago.
- Many styles of yoga exist.
- Hatha yoga consists of regulating the mind and body through 14 different breathing exercises (pranayamas)

and more than 200 balanced physical postures or poses (asanas) to exercise and lengthen all the muscles in the body.
- Hatha yoga is especially effective in reducing stress and restoring balance.
- Studies find a variety of physiological and psychological health benefits from regular practice of yoga.

Key Terms

yoga	pratyahara	ashtanga yoga
yoga sutras	dharana	kundalini yoga
yama	dhyana	Bikram yoga
niyama	samadhi	Kripalu yoga
asana	hatha yoga	Sivananda yoga
pranayama	iyengar yoga	

Discussion Time For Critical Thinking/Discussion Questions, please visit this book's Premium Website. www

Notes

1. http://www.websters-online-dictionary.org
2. *Book of Wisdom—Ishopanishad,* by R. Swami (Honsdale, PA: Himalayan International Institute, 1972).
3. http://www.americanyogaassociation.org
4. http://www.americanyogaassociation.org
5. http://www.americanyogaassociation.org
6. http://www.yoga.org.nz; http://www.ytoc.org
7. "Yoga-Based Therapy," by C. Patel. In P. M. Lehrer and R. L. Woolfolk (Eds.), *Principles and Practice of Stress Management* (2nd ed.). (New York: Guilford Press, 1993).
8. Patel, "Yoga-Based Therapy."
9. http://stress.about.com
10. "Electrophysical Correlates of Some Yogi Exercises," by B. K. Bagchi and M. A. Wenger. In L. van Bagaert

and J. Radermecker (Eds.), *Electroencephalography, Clinical Neurophysiology and Epilepsy* (Vol. 3). (London: Pergamon, 1959).
11. "The Short-Term Psychophysiological Effects of Hatha Yoga and Progressive Relaxation on Female Japanese Students," by J. A. Cusumano and S. E. Robinson, *Applied Psychology: An International Review* 42(1) (1993): 77–90.
12. http://www.americanyogaassociation.org; http://www.santosha.com
13. http://www.mayoclinic.com/health/yoga/cm00004
14. http://www.mayoclinic.com/health/yoga/cm00004

23 Complementary and Alternative Health

> ■ A friend said that acupuncture helped her feel much better by balancing the flow of energy in her body. I haven't heard of this. Does energy really flow through our bodies—and what does it have to do with feeling good? ■ What is reiki? ■ I've become friends with an exchange student from China. He was explaining that, when his mother was sick, she was treated with herbs, massage, and acupuncture. What's that all about, and if it works, why don't we do it in the United States?

Study of this chapter will enable you to:

1. Explain the five categories of complementary and alternative medicine.
2. Describe complementary and alternative healthcare practices that relate to stress management within each of the five categories.
3. Discuss the stress-related health benefits of complementary and alternative healthcare.
4. Differentiate between the various types and techniques of massage.
5. Contrast the typical Western medicine approach to health with alternative medical approaches to health and healing.

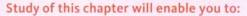

We doctors do nothing. We only help and encourage the doctor within.

—*Albert Schweitzer*

© Karen Su/Getty Images

The Magic of Massage For her birthday, Jackie received from her best friend a gift certificate for a massage. As she walked into the room for her first-ever massage, she felt both excited and nervous. Her massage therapist, Diane, explained that there are several types of massage and asked Jackie what she hoped to gain from her massage. They decided that the Swedish relaxation massage best fit Jackie's needs. Diane explained that they would have complete privacy and Jackie could either remove all her clothes or leave on her underclothes if that would be more comfortable for her. Diane explained that Jackie would be covered with a soft sheet throughout the massage.

As Diane began to massage the warm oil over Jackie's back, Jackie felt a powerful sense of relaxation—an emotionally soothing experience accompanied by the sound of a bubbling fountain and the scent of relaxing lavender filling the warm, cozy room. Jackie could feel herself relaxing as she took a couple of deep breaths. She could hardly believe how quickly the hour passed. She couldn't remember when she had so totally allowed herself to be in the moment and surrender to the relaxation. Jackie decided immediately that massage would be a regular part of her self-care program.

Complementary and Alternative Health

The interest in complementary and alternative health has exploded as individuals seek more balanced approaches to health and healing. A wide variety of techniques fall under the broad heading of *alternative healthcare.* An estimated 60 to 90% of visits to healthcare professionals are for stress-related disorders,[1] yet many people have found that our current healthcare system is not especially effective in helping them deal with stress. People are turning to alternatives to replace or complement the "take a pill" approach for stress and stress-related problems.

A growing body of research and the swell of public interest have raised awareness of techniques and practices such as acupuncture and acupressure, biofeedback, massage, tai chi, and herbals. Many of these practices have been used successfully throughout history and in cultures around the world to promote balance and well-being. Several of these strategies, including meditation, guided imagery, yoga, music therapy, and prayer, are described in other chapters. In this chapter we will learn about additional alternative health strategies that can help you prevent and manage stress.

Understanding Complementary and Alternative Health

The National Center for Complementary and Alternative Medicine (NCCAM) is the official government agency of the National Institutes of Health that is responsible for research on complementary and alternative health. This Center defines **complementary and alternative medicine** (CAM) as a group of diverse medical and healthcare systems, practices, and products that are not presently considered to be part of conventional medicine. CAM covers a spectrum of ancient to new-age approaches that purport to prevent or treat disease. The list of what is considered to be CAM is revised continually, as therapies that are proven to be safe and effective are adopted into conventional healthcare and as new approaches to healthcare emerge.[2]

Complementary medicine, as its name suggests, is used *together with* conventional medicine. An example is using aromatherapy to lessen a patient's discomfort following surgery. By contrast, **alternative medicine** is used *in place of* conventional medicine. An example is to use meditation instead of medication to treat stress. The preferred terminology, as defined by NCCAM, is **integrative medicine,** which combines mainstream medical therapies and CAM therapies.

Regardless of what you call it, the number of people using complementary and alternative health (CAH) practices is growing. Several of these practices and techniques have special relevance for managing stress. A common aspect of nearly every CAH practice is the component of balance.

The art of healing comes from nature and not from the physician. Therefore, the physician must start from nature with an open mind.

—*Paracelsus*

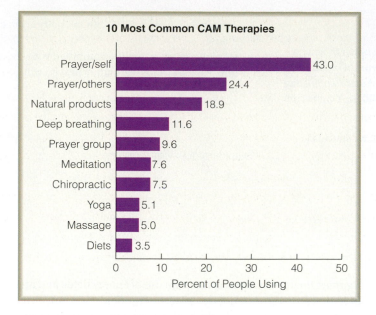

FIGURE 23.1 10 Most Common CAM Therapies

Source: Centers for Disease Control 2002 National Health Interview Survey, conducted by National Center for Complementary and Alternative Medicine (NCCAM)

10 Most Common CAM Therapies

- Prayer/self — 43.0
- Prayer/others — 24.4
- Natural products — 18.9
- Deep breathing — 11.6
- Prayer group — 9.6
- Meditation — 7.6
- Chiropractic — 7.5
- Yoga — 5.1
- Massage — 5.0
- Diets — 3.5

Percent of People Using

Most Common CAM Therapies

According to the Centers for Disease Control 2007 National Health Interview Survey, almost 4 out of 10 adults had used CAM therapy in the past 12 months, with the most commonly used therapies being nonvitamin, nonmineral, natural products; deep breathing exercises; meditation; chiropractic or osteopathic manipulation; massage; and yoga. Between 2002 and 2007, increased use was also seen for acupuncture, massage therapy, and naturopathy.

FYI

The Guru of Alternative Medicine Andrew Weil,

Harvard-educated physician and botanist, is frequently described as the guru of alternative medicine. He has written a number of best selling books, including *The Healthy Kitchen* and *Eight Weeks to Optimum Health*, *Spontaneous Healing*, and *Natural Health*, *Natural Medicine*.

Dr. Weil, an internationally recognized expert on medicinal herbs, mind/body interactions, and integrative medicine, places great importance on diet, exercise, deep breathing, and peace of mind as the primary components of healing and living a healthy life. Dr. Weil is director of the Program in Integrative Medicine at the University of Arizona. He founded the Polaris Foundation, with the mission of advancing integrative medicine and optimum health around the world.

When prayer specifically for health reasons is included in the definition of CAM, the number of U.S. adults using some form of CAM in the past year rises to 62 percent.[3] As shown in Figure 23.1, many of these practices relate to relaxation and stress management. The survey found that CAM approaches were used most often to treat back, neck, and joint pain or problems; colds; and anxiety and depression.

Categories of Complementary and Alternative Medicine

NCCAM classifies CAM therapies into the following five categories, or domains:

1. *Alternative medical systems.* Alternative medical systems are built upon complete systems of theory and practice. Often, these systems have evolved apart from and earlier than the conventional medical approach used in the United States. Examples include homeopathic medicine, naturopathic medicine, traditional Chinese medicine, and ayurveda.

2. *Mind/body interventions.* Mind/body medicine uses a variety of techniques designed to enhance the mind's capacity to affect the body. Some techniques that were considered CAM in the past have become mainstream—for example, cognitive–behavioral therapy, which you learned about in Chapter 6. Other mind/body techniques still considered CAM include meditation, prayer, mental healing, biofeedback, and therapies that use creative outlets such as art, music, and dance.

3. *Biologically based therapies.* Biologically based therapies in CAM are substances found in nature, such as herbs, foods, and vitamins. Examples include dietary supplements and herbal products.

Culturally Based Healing Arts

Traditional Oriental medicine (such as acupuncture, shiatsu, and reiki), Indian systems of healthcare (such as ayurveda and yoga), and Native American healing practices (such as the Sweat Lodge and Talking Circles) all incorporate the beliefs that:

- Wellness is a state of balance between the spiritual, physical, mental, and emotional "selves."

- An imbalance of forces within the body is the cause of illness.
- Herbal/natural remedies, combined with sound nutrition, exercise, and meditation/prayer, will correct this imbalance.

Source: http://www.mentalhealth.org

4. *Energy therapies.* Energy therapies involve the use of energy fields and are of two types:
   a. **Biofield therapies** are intended to affect energy fields that purportedly surround and penetrate the human body. Some forms of energy therapy manipulate biofields by applying pressure or manipulating the body by placing the hands in, or through, these fields. Examples include qi gong, reiki, and therapeutic touch.
   b. **Bioelectromagnetic-based therapies** involve the unconventional use of electromagnetic fields.
5. *Manipulative and body-based methods.* These methods in CAM are based on manipulation or movement of one or more body parts. Examples include chiropractic and osteopathic manipulation and massage.[4]

Applications of the Five Categories of CAM to Stress Management

Examples of some of the stress-management practices that relate to each of the five CAM categories will communicate the importance of integrative stress-management practices you can incorporate into your life.

Alternative Medical Systems Worldwide, most medical systems differ significantly from the Western healthcare approach. It can be argued that the Western approach is more of a disease management system than a true healthcare system.

Although it is beyond the scope of this book to discuss in detail each of the alternative medical systems, a brief description of a few of these will help you compare and contrast the Western healthcare approach to other therapeutic approaches. As you read about the various medical systems, reflect on how the approach would impact the treatment of stress-related conditions.

Traditional Chinese Medicine (TCM) **Traditional Chinese medicine (TCM)** is the contemporary version of the 3,000-year-old medical practice of China. TCM includes a variety of carefully formulated techniques, such as acupuncture, herbal medicine, massage, qi gong, and nutrition.

Ayurvedic Medicine **Ayurveda,** India's traditional system of natural medicine, is claimed to be the oldest system of natural healing on Earth. Ayurvedic medicine is described as "knowledge of how to live." Asians have practiced this holistic form of medicine continuously for approximately 5,500 years, and it now is gaining interest and support in Western countries including the United States.

An integral component of ayurvedic medicine is teaching people how to release stress and tension through meditation and yoga, which you read about in Chapters 21 and 22. Taking a holistic approach to the individual, ayurveda believes that all facets of life contribute to health—including nutrition, hygiene, sleep, weather, and lifestyle, as well as

Traditional Chinese Medicine around the World

Approximately one-fourth of the world's population uses TCM, including some 12 million people who go to TCM practitioners in the United States.

Source: *The Best Alternative Medicine: What Works? What Does Not?*, by K. Pelletier (New York: Simon & Schuster, 2000).

The art of medicine consists of amusing the patient while Nature cures the disease.

—*Voltaire*

Patient Care Deepak Chopra explains that ayurvedic physicians are more interested in the patients they see than in their diseases. He recognizes that what makes up the person is experience—sorrows, joys, fleeting seconds of trauma, long hours of nothing special at all. The minutes of life silently accumulate and, like grains of sand deposited by a river, the minutes eventually can pile up into a hidden formation that comes into view above the surface as a disease. In ayurveda, understanding what is causing stress in a person's life is integral to health and healing.

Take a few minutes to reflect on the typical approach to health and disease in the U.S. health/medical system. Does your healthcare provider seem more interested in you or in your disease? Reflect on cultural differences in how ayurveda approaches health and disease compared to the approach in traditional Western medicine. As you reflect, consider the words of Hippocrates: "It is more important to know what sort of person has a disease than to know what sort of disease a person has."

Source: *Quantum Healing: Exploring the Frontiers of Mind/Body Medicine,* by D. Chopra (New York: Bantam Books, 1989).

physical, mental, and sexual activities. It also takes emotional factors into consideration, as anger, fear, anxiety, and unhealthy relationships are believed to contribute to illness. A healthy emotional state is considered to be the very foundation of physical health.[5]

Naturopathic Medicine **Naturopathy** encompasses the diagnosis, treatment, and prevention of disease, as well as the promotion of health. One of the oldest forms of medicine, naturopathy weaves the healing traditions of China, India, Greece, and Native American cultures together with modern scientific principles and technology. Treatment is individualized, with significant time and attention devoted to lifestyle counseling. Naturopathic medicine makes recommendations on diet, exercise, and stress management. Modern naturopathy is founded on six basic principles:[6]

1. *Nature has the power to heal.* The physician's role is to support the self-healing process by removing obstacles to health.
2. *Treat the whole person.* Disease rarely has a single cause, so every aspect of the patient must be brought into harmonious balance.
3. *First, do no harm.* A physician should use methods and substances that are as nontoxic and noninvasive as possible.
4. *Identify and treat the cause.* Rather than suppress symptoms, the physician should treat the underlying causes of disease.
5. *Prevention is as important as cure.* A physician should help create health, as well as cure disease.
6. *Doctors should be teachers.* Part of the physician's task is to educate the patient and encourage self-responsibility.

Clearly, most of these alternative medical systems emphasize the wholeness of body, mind, and spirit, and the unity of the individual with the natural environment. This is in sharp contrast to Western medicine's mechanistic approach, in which the body is seen as a machine with parts to be fixed when they are broken. The main focus of Western medicine is on the treatment of disease, often with drugs and surgery, rather than on the holistic promotion of health.

Mind/Body Interventions

A clear connection exists between mind/body interventions and stress management. Considerable research supports mind/body interventions, such as meditation, and the impact on stress management and health. Increasingly, meditation is no longer considered a CAH practice but, rather, a mainstream practice. Interventions such as prayer, cognitive techniques, and music therapy have been discussed in other chapters.

A mind/body intervention that has not been discussed previously is biofeedback. **Biofeedback** is a method that uses electronic devices to help a person learn how to consciously regulate bodily functions, such as breathing, heart rate, muscle tension, skin temperature, and blood pressure, in order to improve overall health. The electronic instruments accurately measure, process, and "feed back" information about autonomic activity, permitting development of voluntary control over physiologic processes.[7]

> The natural healing force within each one of us is the greatest force in getting well.
>
> *—Hippocrates*

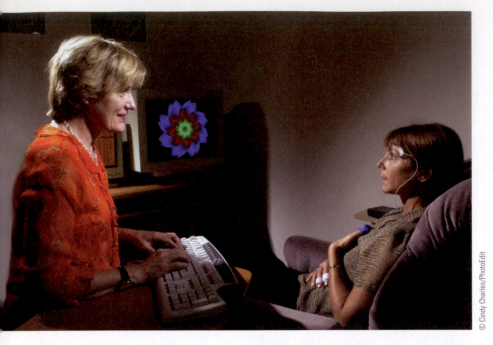

Biofeedback machines can help you learn to control autonomic functions.

Since the 1970s, research has demonstrated that humans can gain control over several autonomic nervous system functions. This discovery—that people can control internal physiologic events—has had profound implications for health. The application of biofeedback to the treatment and prevention of stress conditions is logical, based on decades of stress research demonstrating that chronic arousal of the autonomic nervous system is what contributes to many stress-related disorders.

Biofeedback is used to reduce stress, eliminate headaches, recondition injured muscles, control asthmatic attacks, and relieve pain. It is also proving to be an effective treatment for a variety of stress-related problems including hypertension, irritable bowel syndrome, and fibromyalgia.[8] It has been found to be helpful for other stress-related maladies like hot flashes, Raynaud's disease, nausea and vomiting associated with chemotherapy, irregular heartbeats (cardiac arrhythmias), chronic low back pain, chronic constipation, incontinence, and epilepsy.[9]

Different types of biofeedback can be used for a variety of purposes. Common types of biofeedback include:

Electromyogram (EMG) EMG is the most common form of biofeedback. It uses electrodes or other types of sensors, commonly connected to the forehead, jaw, or shoulder muscles, to measure muscle tension. When the electrodes sense tension, the biofeedback machine produces a signal, such as a sound or a colored light. As you are alerted to muscle tension, you begin to sense how it feels and immediately take steps to relax the tension. EMG is commonly used to promote relaxation of the muscles involved in backaches, headaches, neck pain, and grinding teeth (bruxism).

Temperature biofeedback A common symptom of the stress response is a decrease in skin temperature in the hands and feet. Sensors attached to your fingers indicate skin temperature levels and can alert you when the stress response has been activated with lower skin temperatures. When you're under stress, a low temperature reading can give you immediate feedback that it is time to relax.

Galvanic skin response (GSR) Somewhat like a lie detector machine, GSR sensors measure the activity of your sweat glands and detectable amounts of perspiration on the skin. The GSR biofeedback device senses the increase in this physiology and gives immediate feedback to the user.

Electroencephalogram (EEG) An EEG uses sensors placed on the scalp and linked to a computer with an EEG-biofeedback instrument to monitor the brainwave activity associated with different mental states, such as heightened stressful alertness, normal wakefulness, relaxation, calmness, light sleep and deep sleep (the brainwaves have been labeled beta, alpha, theta, and delta). If there is an increase in the strength of particular frequencies of this signal, it means a person is functioning at a particular mental state. If, for example, you read slow-wave patterns or theta waves, it means the person being monitored is inattentive or drowsy.

There are many products and devices from which you can select to help you explore the amazing world of biofeedback. These devices not only can help you relax, but they are enjoyable to use. They frequently come with games or activities that turn the process of relaxing into an interesting adventure or a fun challenge. A couple of examples of these products are FreezeFramer and Journey to the Wild Divine. As you connect to the computer, you are guided through the activities that help you learn to focus your thinking in more relaxing ways. As technology continues to advance, we will continue to see more ways to enhance the communication between the mind and body.

Here is an example of how biofeedback might look if you were to try it. Imagine that you are sitting in front of a computer and you have one or more of your fingers comfortably connected to a "sensor" that is attached to your computer.

You see on your computer screen an animated person juggling some colorful balls. You are instructed to think happy, peaceful thoughts. As you do, the person juggling the balls begins to toss them higher into the air. As you practice, you see the connection between the way you think and the height of the juggled balls.

To experiment, you decide to think of a recent argument in which you got really angry. As you dwell on the argument and try to relive it in your mind, you notice that as you get angrier, the man juggling the balls tosses them lower and lower in the air until he is just holding the balls in his hands.

Realizing how your thoughts have made this happen, and also not feeling so good because you've just relived an unpleasant event, you decide to apply relaxation imagery to imagine one of the most pleasurable, delightful experiences you've ever had. Perhaps it happened on a recent vacation. It was a time when you felt incredibly relaxed, happy, and peaceful. As you dwell on this new picture in your mind, the man juggling the balls begins to toss the balls high into the air again. You have just witnessed the clear connection between the mind and body.

Biofeedback devices often are used in conjunction with deep breathing, meditation, or guided imagery, to monitor the ability of these techniques to reduce the stress response. Again, biofeedback is merely a means of providing information concerning the body and relaxation. It does not take the place of relaxation techniques. Once individuals learn to relax using biofeedback, they can eliminate the special instrument by relying upon breathing, visualization, or one of the many forms of meditation.[10]

Biologically Based Therapies Ongoing research is exploring the connection between natural substances (such as herbs, dietary supplements, and vitamins) and stress and anxiety relief. Among American consumers, herbs are popular as a means to help the body adapt to physical and emotional stressors. Ginseng, for example, is frequently used to induce relaxation. Valerian is an herb often consumed as a tea to enhance sleep,[11] and melatonin is a pineal hormone touted for the same purpose.[12]

The herb kava may reduce anxiety and induce sleep. Although kava has been found to be effective for treating stress, the Food and Drug Administration has issued a consumer advisory warning of a possible association between kava products and liver problems. This effect is still under investigation but serves as a reminder that biologically based products can have powerful effects, both positive and negative.

People must use caution when taking herbals or other biologically based therapies. Although compelling evidence indicates that some of these products are effective for inducing relaxation, adequate studies often have not been conducted to determine potential side effects or contraindications with other drugs.

Energy Therapies

Energy therapies involve the use of energy fields including **meridians**—invisible channels of energy that flow in the body—or energy fields outside the body. In Chinese healing theory, each person has flowing through the body a vital energy called *chi* (also called *qi*), which sustains life and from which all other activities flow. The chi flows through the body by way of meridians. When a person has a sickness or diseases, the underlying cause of the problem is thought to be a blockage of this energy flowing through the meridians. The therapy creates a release of the blockage and restores the energy flow to normal, high functioning levels. Some techniques, such as reflexology, acupressure, acupuncture, and shiatsu, combine energy balance with massage.

Reflexology is based on the Oriental theory that meridian lines or pathways carry energy throughout the body, with points in the hands and feet that correspond to all areas of the body. Because each zone or part of the body has a corresponding reflex point on the feet, stimulating that reflex point causes the natural energy of the related organ to be restored. If a certain area feels tender when pressure is applied, this may indicate a

Meridians are energy pathways that flow throughout the body. In Chinese healing theory, when a person has a sickness the underlying cause of the problem is thought to be a blockage of energy flowing through the meridians.

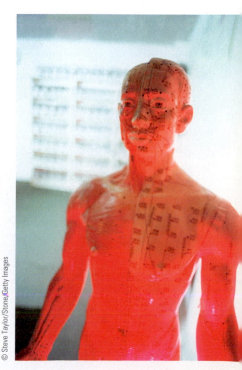

© Steve Taylor/Stone/Getty Images

Calming Kava

Kava is a slow-growing plant that is a member of the pepper family. The root of this plant is used for medicinal purposes. Historically, kava has been grown in islands in the Pacific, where it is valued as a ceremonial drink. Kava drinkers describe a sense of tranquility, relaxation, sociability, well-being, and contentment after drinking the liquid. They say it lessens fatigue and anxiety.

Kava is recommended for treating nervous anxiety, stress, and restlessness. In a scientific study, 101 outpatients experiencing anxiety participated in a 25-week trial using an extract of kava. From week 8, the treatment group demonstrated significantly superior outcomes compared to a placebo, as assessed by a variety of tools and measures.

The researchers concluded that kava may be beneficial as a treatment alternative to prescription medications in anxiety disorders. Kava had none of the tolerance problems or potential addictive qualities associated with the other medications. Although kava is an effective herb for reducing anxiety, ongoing research is necessary to determine the safety of long-term use, as explained below.

Sources: *Mosby's Complementary and Alternative Medicine: A Research-Based Approach,* by L. Freeman, (St. Louis: Mosby, 2004); *The Complete German Commission E Monographs: Therapeutic Guide to Herbal Medicines,* by M. Blumenthal (Boston: Integrative Medicine, 1998); "Kava-Kava Extract WS 1490 versus Placebo in Anxiety Disorders—A Randomized Placebo-Controlled 25-week Outpatient Trial" by H. Volz and M. Kieser. *Pharmacopsychiatry 30*(1) (1997): 1–5.

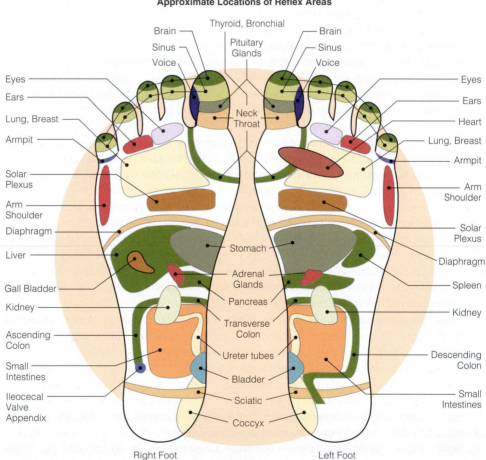

Approximate Locations of Reflex Areas

Brain · Sinus · Voice · Thyroid, Bronchial · Pituitary Glands · Brain · Sinus · Voice · Eyes · Ears · Heart · Lung, Breast · Armpit · Arm Shoulder · Eyes · Ears · Lung, Breast · Armpit · Solar Plexus · Arm Shoulder · Diaphragm · Liver · Gall Bladder · Kidney · Ascending Colon · Small Intestines · Ileocecal Valve Appendix · Neck Throat · Stomach · Adrenal Glands · Pancreas · Transverse Colon · Ureter tubes · Bladder · Sciatic · Coccyx · Solar Plexus · Diaphragm · Spleen · Kidney · Descending Colon · Small Intestines

Right Foot · Left Foot

FIGURE 23.2 Reflexology: Approximate Locations of Reflex Areas

dysfunction in the corresponding part of the body. Continued gentle pressure is applied to these locations (see Figure 23.2) on the feet and hands to restore normal functioning and health.

Four related energy therapies are acupuncture, acupressure, emotional freedom technique (EFT), and shiatsu. These therapies are intended to open the flow of chi, restore balance, and support the natural healing of the body. Feelings of deep relaxation and increased vitality are common benefits of these treatments.

1. **Acupuncture** involves inserting hair-thin, sterile needles into the body at specific points (acupoints) to manipulate the body's flow of energy to balance the body's systems. This manipulation is believed to regulate functions such as heart rate, body temperature, and respiration, as well as sleep patterns and emotional changes such as the relief of stress and anxiety.[13]

Although researchers are not certain how acupuncture works, theories suggest that it corrects the balance of chi, the vital energy or life force flowing through the meridians. These meridians are linked to specific organs and organ systems. Although needles are the common method of application, practitioners also may apply heat, pressure, friction, suction, or impulses of electromagnetic stimulation to the needle points.

2. **Acupressure** often is described as "acupuncture without the needles." Pressure is applied to pressure points thought to be areas of chi concentration.

3. **EFT (emotional freedom technique)** is an alternative medicine tool based on the theory that negative emotions are caused by disturbances in the body's energy field. Tapping on the meridian endpoints on the face and body while thinking of a negative emotion alters the energy field, restoring it to balance. The theory behind EFT is that it provides a bridge between energy-based therapies such as acupuncture and acupressure and mind/body therapies wherein achieving proper mental and emotional states contributes to enhanced health. EFT is newer form of energy therapy, but the healing effects of this modality are showing positive results with a variety of physical and emotional problems. Exploratory studies specifically for EFT are now underway.

4. **Shiatsu** means "finger pressure" in Japanese. It originated as a synthesis of acupuncture and traditional Japanese massage. This system of finger pressure is applied to specific points along acupuncture meridians.

Four additional energy therapies are the following:

1. **Qi gong** (pronounced chee gong or chee gung), a Chinese exercise involving physical movement and breathing exercises designed to circulate the internal vital energy.

2. **Tai chi,** the most popular form of exercise in China, consisting of a precise sequence of slow, graceful movements, accompanied by deep breathing and mental attention, to achieve balance between body and mind and to focus vital energy.

3. **Therapeutic touch,** based on the premise that the human body is surrounded by, and permeated with, an energy field that is connected with the universal life energy. Therapeutic touch may or may not involve physical contact, but contact is always made with the client's energy field. For the practitioner, intentionality (compassionate, focused attention on the recipient) is the most important factor in healing.

4. **Reiki,** a healing technique that channels the universal life energy to recipients by the laying on of hands. A complete treatment involves placing the hands on the head and shoulder area, and then the stomach area, ending with the feet. The underlying belief is that healing energy can be transferred from a practitioner to a recipient.

Manipulative and Body-Based Methods

Several practices that are used to reduce stress fall under the category of manipulative and body-based methods. Massage, an important body-based method with stress management implications, will be discussed in detail. Some of the benefits of these methods relate to something as seemingly simple as touch. We will begin by exploring the benefits of touch and massage.

Muscle Tension Take your thumb and push in on your thigh with moderate force. Notice if you feel any pain. Now, with your thumb or forefinger, push with equal force somewhere between your neck and shoulder on one of those "rope-like" muscles that

---

Author Anecdote   Acupuncture and Cluster Headaches   While I was in graduate school, I lived next door to another graduate student who had incredibly painful cluster headaches (he said a cluster headache feels like a migraine headache multiplied by 10). He told me that sometimes he wanted to shoot himself and end it all because the pain was so intense. Nothing seemed to work to make the headaches go away. No doctor in Illinois had any answers for him, and no drug seemed to work.

A woman in the department where he was working on campus happened to mention to him that she was an acupuncturist and would be happy to do what she could to help him. He told me he was so desperate that he was willing to try anything. I asked if I could watch when she came to his house, as I had never seen acupuncture done and was curious.

The student lay on the couch in his living room while I watched the woman put needles into various places in his body—his feet, his ears, his eyebrows—all places that to me had nothing to do with an aching head. When it was over, he told me that the pain he had felt in his head was mostly gone. She returned for a follow-up session.

In the following weeks and months, I asked my neighbor if he was still getting the cluster headaches. He said he hadn't felt any pain since the acupuncture treatments. In the time that we lived next to him, he never mentioned cluster headaches again.

—MO

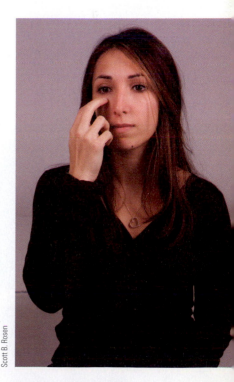

Scott B. Rosen

EFT (Emotional Freedom Technique) is a new type of energy therapy based on acupuncture and acupressure.

The Touch Factor

Investigators at Ohio State University studied the effects of a diet high in fat and cholesterol in rabbits, specifically as it affected the process of atherosclerosis. In humans, this process of cholesterol deposition results in vascular diseases of various types, such as heart attacks and stroke.

Results of this study should have been rather predictable, because previous studies supported that a diet high in fat and cholesterol led to atherosclerotic changes in the arterial systems of rabbits. Surprisingly, a certain group of the test rabbits demonstrated atherosclerotic changes that were 60% less than that of the overall group.

The investigators were astonished and could come up with no obvious explanation for this unexpected result. Finally they discovered an unplanned and unexpected variable in the experiment: The rabbits that were affected less severely were those that were fed and cared for by one of the investigators who, during the course of the experiment, regularly took them from their cages and petted, stroked, and talked to them.

Was this mere coincidence? Many scientists would have considered laughable the possibility that rabbit–human interchanges could play a role in atherosclerotic vascular disease. After all, atherosclerotic vascular disease is an objective affair rooted in molecular processes and the battle against it should be fought on the battleground of the cell, not the psyche—or so the theory of molecular medicine goes.

To test this "coincidence," systematic, controlled studies were designed in which two groups of rabbits again were fed the same diet and were treated identically except that the rabbits in one group were removed from their cages several times a day for petting and were talked to each time by the same person. The result? The rabbits that received affection once again demonstrated a 60% lower incidence of atherosclerosis.

Not content with the possibility of two coincidences, the Ohio State investigators repeated the study. The results were the same. In an unexplained way, the "human factor" emerged. Touching, petting, handling, and gentle talking were the crucial determinants in the disease process that will affect many of us—atherosclerosis.

Source: "Social Environment as a Factor in Diet-Induced Atherosclerosis," by R. M. Nerem, M. J. Levesque, and J. F. Cornhill, *Science 208* (1980): 1475–1476, as quoted in L. Dossey, *Space, Time and Medicine* (Boston: Shambhala Publications, 1982).

feels noticeably hard. If you are like many of us, you will feel more discomfort when you press on your neck and shoulder muscles. This is because stress-related tension can become chronic and often settles into the muscles of the upper back and shoulders. Again, muscles become tense with activation of the fight-or-flight response. Because these muscles maintain a constant state of activation, they are chronically contracting. When this happens, the muscles contact pain receptor nerves and we feel muscle pain.

Another outcome of chronically tensed muscles is fatigue. To understand this, try to hold your arm outstretched for a long time. Soon the tightened muscles that are holding up your arm become tired and painful. This is the case with many muscles in our body. Muscles remaining in a constant state of contraction become painful and fatigued. As a result, you feel tired and exhausted.

The purpose of massage is to work on these tension-packed muscles, to relax the muscles directly by pressure and rubbing. As massage is applied to muscles, they relax and the pain receptor nerves no longer are being stimulated by the tensed, contracting muscles. The result is at least two healthy outcomes:

1. Pain is relieved.
2. The energy being expended in the muscles is freed and can be used elsewhere in the body.

Touch and Massage Touch has both physical and emotional benefits, making it important for managing stress and

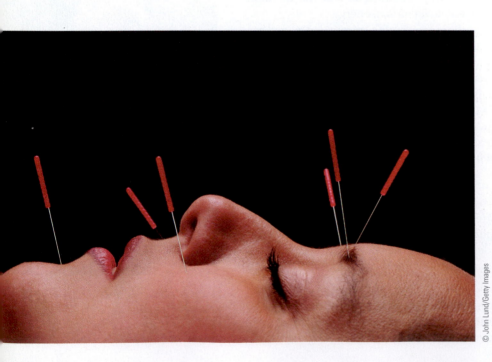

© John Lund/Getty Images

Acupuncture involves inserting hair-thin, sterile needles into the body at specific points to manipulate the body's flow of energy and restore the balance of chi, the vital energy or life force flowing through the meridians.

improving health. Touch has been found to improve heart irregularities. People with a certain type of irregular heartbeat attained a more normal rhythm in the minute after they were touched as their pulse was being taken. Touch has also been found to relieve depression. Children and adolescents who were hospitalized for depression scored better on depression and anxiety measures after receiving daily massage.[14]

What is true for rabbits (see Research Highlight) seems to be true for humans as well. Researchers from the University of Miami Medical Center found that massage helps babies handle the increased stimulation after leaving the womb, and it helps the babies relax when they are experiencing stress.[15] In the study, the premature infants were massaged for 15 minutes three times a day over 10 consecutive days. The babies who were touched:[16]

- averaged 47% greater weight gain per day than the premature infants who were not massaged.
- were more active and alert and demonstrated more neurological development than the premature infants who were not massaged.
- required 6 fewer days in the hospital than the control group.

Whether the benefits come from touch or from massage is difficult to determine. Massage techniques have been used for years to induce relaxation and are effective in part because of the touch factor, but additional factors also determine the effectiveness of massage for relaxation.

Therapeutic touch is based on the premise that the human body is surrounded by, and permeated with, an energy field that is connected with the universal life energy. For the practitioner, compassionate, focused attention on the recipient is the most important factor in healing.

Typical Benefits of Therapeutic Massage

Therapeutic massage typically leads to physical, mental, emotional, and other benefits. These are explained briefly.

1. *Physical benefits.* Massage therapy is intended to stretch and loosen tight muscles. Among the resulting benefits are that it can:
   - loosen joints and improve range of motion
   - relieve cramps and muscle spasms
   - lessen muscle fatigue
   - improve blood flow and the movement of lymph throughout the body
   - facilitate the removal of metabolic waste resulting from exercise or inactivity
     - increase the flow of oxygen and nutrients to cells and tissues, which speeds healing from injury or disease
     - relieve symptoms of disorders such as headache, chronic and acute pain, asthma, arthritis, carpal tunnel syndrome, temporomandibular joint (TMJ) dysfunction, and athletic injuries

   In addition, massage stimulates the release of endorphins, the body's natural painkiller.

2. *Mental benefits.* Massage therapy provides a relaxed state of alertness, reduces mental stress, and enhances the capacity for calm thinking and creativity. Massage also can improve the duration and quality of sleep and increase the ability to concentrate.
3. *Emotional benefits.* Massage therapy satisfies some of the need for caring and nurturing touch. It can improve feelings of well-being, and it reduces anxiety.
4. *Additional benefits.* Massage can help combat the negative effects of aging by enhancing tissue elasticity, improving immune system functioning, and relieving muscle aches and stiffness. Athletes and other performers commonly use massage to help them relax, prepare for performances, and hasten repair from injury. After receiving a massage, people frequently report feeling lighter, more energized, and more peaceful.

Author Anecdote **Healing Touch** Years ago, when I was a student nurse at Lutheran Deaconess Hospital in Minneapolis, I learned an important lesson about touch. Part of the routine A.M. and P.M. care for every patient was a backrub. Our nursing instructors were clear that this nursing intervention was as important as any. I wanted to get on with the "real" work of nurses—starting IVs, administering medications, conducting assessments—but soon came to realize the almost magical power of the backrub. For 10 minutes, these patients each had my undivided attention and often related important information that was vital to their health and recovery.

My caring touch somehow relaxed the body and opened the mind in a way that allowed healing to happen. Now, research on touch and massage supports what my teachers knew many years ago: Touch heals.

—MH

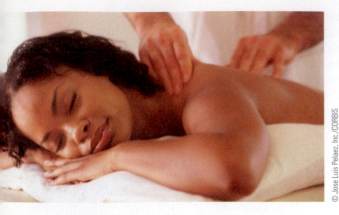

Swedish massage includes long, gliding strokes, kneading, friction, tapping, and shaking motions on the upper or more superficial layers of the muscles.

Types of Massage

The most common type of basic relaxation massage is Swedish massage. Additional bodywork modalities are briefly described as well.

Swedish Massage Dr. Pehr Henrik Ling, a Swedish doctor, developed this first modern method of massage in the 1820s through his study of physiology, gymnastics, and massage techniques borrowed from China, Egypt, Greece, and Rome. **Swedish massage** usually is done with lotions or oils and includes long, gliding strokes, kneading, friction, tapping, and shaking motions on the upper or more superficial layers of the muscles. Swedish massage affects nerves, muscles, glands, and circulation and promotes health and well-being.

Other Types of Massage and Bodywork Along with Swedish massage, other types of bodywork modalities used to help the body and mind relax and promote healing include the following:

1. **Deep tissue massage:** used to release the chronic patterns of tension in the body through deep muscle compression with the heel of the hand, the pads of the thumb, and even the elbow pressing deliberately along the grain of the muscle. With continuous pressure, deeply held patterns of tension, as well as toxins, can be released.

2. **Myotherapy:** also known as trigger-point therapy, designed to reduce pain, relax muscle spasms, and improve circulation. Trigger points are intense knots of muscle tension that often cause pain in other areas of the body. When a trigger point is under excessive emotional or physical stress, it can result in painful muscle spasms. Spasms, in turn, cause pain. Trigger points are diffused or erased by concentrated pressure applied to the trigger points for a short time (several seconds to 2 or 3 minutes) by the fingers, knuckles, and elbows.

3. **Craniosacral therapy** (CST): a gentle, hands-on method of evaluating and enhancing the function of a physiological body system called the craniosacral system. The craniosacral system is made up of the membranes and cerebrospinal fluid that surround and protect the brain and spinal cord and sustains the environment in which the nervous system functions. The system extends from the bones of the skull, face, and mouth (collectively known as the cranium) all the way down to the tailbone area (sacrum). Problems or imbalance in this system can result in sensory, motor, and neurological disabilities.

   Just as the cardiovascular system has a pulse, the craniosacral system has a rhythmic pulse. This delicate rhythm is generated by spinal fluid as it is pumped

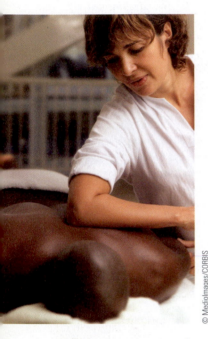

Deep tissue massage is used to release the chronic patterns of tension in the body through deep muscle compression by pressing deliberately along the grain of the muscle.

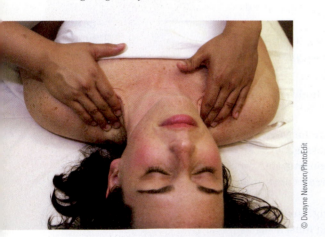

Myotherapy is designed to ease trigger points, intense knots of muscle tension that often cause pain. Trigger points are diffused or erased by concentrated pressure applied to the trigger points.

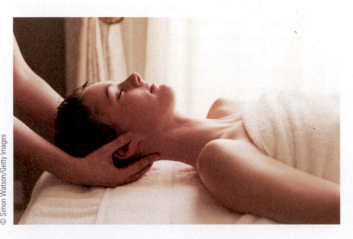

Craniosacral therapy is a gentle, hands-on method of evaluating and enhancing the function of the craniosacral system.

through the brain and spinal cord. A skilled therapist can monitor the quality, strength, and amplitude of this rhythm at specific locations on the body to pinpoint the source of problems and imbalances. Once the problem has been determined, using a touch usually no heavier than the weight of a nickel, the practitioner can assist the natural movement of the fluid and related soft tissue to restore balance and allow the body to heal itself of many associated problems.

Craniosacral therapy has been helpful in reducing stress, as well as improving spinal cord and brain functions. It typically is used to treat conditions such as chronic fatigue, migraine and other headaches, chronic neck and back pain, sinusitis, central nervous system disorders, temporomandibular joint syndrome (TMJ), post-traumatic stress disorder, and orthopedic problems.

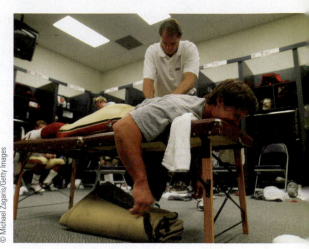
© Michael Zagaris/Getty Images

4. **Sports massage:** a special type of massage focusing on muscle systems specific to the performance of athletes, to help them perform optimally without injuries. The athletes receive massages before, during, and after competition to drain away fatigue, relieve swelling, reduce muscle tension, and improve flexibility. Massage is often combined with practices such as icing and compression. Sports massage can enhance the body's recovery process after performance and reduce the risk of injury during performance.

5. **Chair massage:** also known as on-site massage or corporate massage, is administered while the person receiving the massage is fully clothed and seated in a specially designed chair. A massage chair usually slopes forward, allowing better access to the large muscles of the back. This type of massage typically lasts between 10 and 20 minutes. It frequently is available at airports, in health clubs, in malls, or when a massage therapist visits business offices.

6. **Hot stone massage:** typically used by health spas, where stones are heated and positioned on specific locations on the body. The stones are gently moved to other locations on the body and light pressure is applied directly to the stones.

Self-Massage Many of us would like the idea of a daily massage, but giving over our bodies to the trained hands of a professional massage therapist is not always possible. Still, according to the ancient Indian medicinal tradition of ayurveda, massage is as vital to our routine as washing our hair or brushing our teeth. Rather than relying on someone else, self-massage is a nurturing, stress reducing addition to our daily ritual.

The practice of self-massage in ayurveda is mentioned in written texts that are more than 3,000 years old. Beginning in infancy, parents massage babies to increase their suppleness and flexibility, improve digestion, soften the skin, soothe the nervous system, and enhance bonding. Later, children are taught self-massage, which they continue throughout their lives.

Self-massage initially can seem overwhelming. After all, who has time to squeeze one more thing into the day? But these few minutes can set the tone for the rest of the day and also can provide an amazing array of benefits. Massage currently is a hot topic for medical research, and studies have shown an array of benefits, including reduced anxiety and cravings, increased energy, lowered pain, fewer headaches, better lymphatic drainage, and quicker recovery time after athletic activity.

Felicia Tomasko[17] offers these suggestions for a relaxing self-massage routine:

1. **Using Oils** According to ayurveda, oil is the most effective medium for massage. It nourishes both the skin and the deeper tissues. Cooling oils such as coconut or sunflower oil are soothing in the summertime, and warming oils such as sesame oil increase circulation in the cold of winter. Neutral oils—shea butter, almond, sunflower, and jojoba—can be used year-round.

2. **Optimal Time of Day** Morning is the recommended time for massage, before bathing or showering. Warm water helps oil penetrate into the skin, cleansing the lymphatic system and relieving muscular tension. Morning massage stimulates the nervous system, softens stiff muscles, and can even substitute for a strong cup of coffee!

Sports massage is a special type of massage focusing on muscles specific to the performance of athletes. Sports massage can enhance the body's recovery process after performance and reduce the risk of injury during performance.

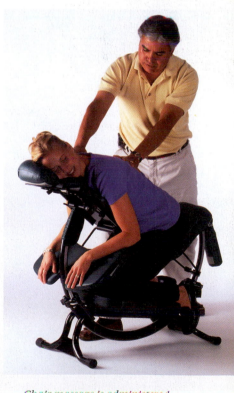
© SW Productions PhotoDisc/Getty Images

Chair massage is administered while the person receiving the massage is fully clothed and seated in a specially designed chair.

3. **How to Do Self-Massage** In ayurveda, massage is administered from the head to the feet. You can either apply oil to your scalp, or massage with dry hands. Vigorously rub your fingertips on your scalp to stimulate pressure points, increase circulation, and calm the mind. Then use your fingertips to massage around your face and forehead. Continue the treatment down the sides of your nose and along your jaw, cheeks, and ears. Face massage prevents sinus congestion and relieves stress and muscular tension. Working the earlobes and the area around the ears especially soothes the nervous system by stimulating pressure points.

Moving down your neck, chest, abdomen, and back, use your whole hand, giving particular attention to stiff areas such as your shoulders, neck, or lower back. To relieve stress, press the points halfway between your neck and the edge of your shoulder (the center of the trapezius muscle). Massage under your arms and along the sides of your chest and ribs to encourage lymphatic drainage by stimulating the high concentration of lymph nodes there.

Vigorous massage around the hips and low back relieves tension that collects from too much sitting. Circular motions around the abdomen encourage healthy digestion and elimination of wastes. When massaging your arms and legs, use long strokes on the large bones to increase circulation, release muscular tension, and move *prana* or chi (life force), but use circular motions around the joints to increase flexibility and stimulate the release of synovial fluid, the joint's lubrication.

An ayurvedic ritual for foot massage is to massage the feet with oil before going to sleep. This practice can calm the entire body by stimulating pressure points on the soles of the feet.

Just a few minutes of massage can encourage relaxation and well-being.[18]

As you have learned—and hopefully experienced—massage has therapeutic effects for a range of conditions and often is accompanied by pleasurable feelings of relaxation and well-being. Massage promotes relaxation through increased blood flow and the release of neurochemicals, such as endorphins, that are the body's "natural opiates." The tactile and neurochemical effects of massage interrupt patterns of stress held in the body. Massage induces a state of deep rest from which the recipient can emerge feeling more balanced, relaxed, and energized.[19]

Conclusion

All five categories of CAM therapies clearly relate to stress management. As the research continues and as the public increasingly uses these techniques, CAM therapies will have an expanded role in stress management and health promotion.

Groucho Marx once said, "Be open-minded, but not so open-minded that your brains fall out." The effectiveness of some of the alternative approaches to health and healing has not been proven through rigorous scientific study. This by no means indicates that the techniques aren't effective. It often means that we simply have no scientifically acceptable way to measure the effects. Research indicates that many forms of CAM are highly effective, especially for preventing stress-related conditions and for promoting balance and well-being.

The bottom line is that you must take responsibility to investigate what is acceptable, safe, and effective for you. Experiment with the therapies that seem interesting and feasible, and discover some options for stress management and health that may seem new and unusual. For generations, people around the world have found that they work.

23.1 Contrasting Health Systems

PURPOSE   Contrast the traditional Western medicine health system approach to stress management to the naturopathic medicine approach.

DIRECTIONS   You know that stress is epidemic and a contributor to many of the diseases and health problems that plague our society. A consistent theme throughout this book is that much of this stress we experience can be prevented. Promoting health and preventing disease is an integral aspect of many of the complementary/alternative strategies presented in this chapter. For this assignment, you will need to do some research using references in addition to your textbook.

Respond to the statements below:

1. Explain how stress management and prevention is typically approached in the traditional Western medicine health system.

2. Based on the six basic principles of naturopathic medicine found in this chapter, explain how stress management and prevention would be approached in naturopathic medicine.

3. Discuss your perception of the strengths and weaknesses of how stress would be addressed from both the Western medicine and naturopathic medicine perspectives.

4. Cite your sources.

Key Points

- An estimated 60 to 90% of visits to healthcare professionals are for stress-related disorders, yet many people have found that the current U.S. healthcare system is not especially effective in dealing with stress.
- Integrative medicine combines mainstream medical therapies and CAM therapies.
- Many complementary and alternative therapies are effective in stress management.
- The National Center for Complementary and Alternative Medicine (NCCAM) has identified five categories of CAM medicine: alternative medical systems, mind/body interventions, biologically based therapies, energy therapies, and body-based methods.
- Alternative medical systems such as traditional Chinese medicine, ayurveda, and naturopathic medicine focus on the holistic promotion of health.

- Biofeedback is a mind/body intervention that facilitates conscious control of autonomic body functions.
- Biologically based therapies, such as herbal remedies, are well-accepted in many countries. Herbals are a popular choice for relaxation and sleep.
- Energy therapies such as reflexology, acupuncture, acupressure, emotional freedom technique, shiatsu, qi gong, tai chi, therapeutic touch, and reiki restore the flow of chi and support the body's natural healing.
- Massage is especially effective for relaxation because it reduces muscle tension, fatigue, and pain.

Key Terms

complementary and alternative
   medicine
complementary medicine
alternative medicine
integrative medicine
biofield therapies
bioelectromagnetic therapies
traditional Chinese medicine (TCM)
ayurveda
naturopathic medicine

biofeedback
meridians
reflexology
acupuncture
acupressure
emotional freedom technique
shiatsu
qi gong
tai chi

therapeutic touch
reiki
Swedish massage
deep tissue massage
myotherapy
craniosacral therapy
sports massage
chair massage
hot stone massage

Notes

1. *Health Promotion in Nursing Practice* (5th ed.), by N. Pender, C. Murdaugh, and M. Parsons (Upper Saddle River, NJ: Pearson Education, Inc., 2005).

2. http://nccam.nih.gov

3. http://www.cdc.gov/nchs/nhis.htm

4. http://nccam.nih.gov

5. *The Best Alternative Medicine: What Works? What Does Not?*, by K. Pelletier (New York: Simon & Schuster, 2000).

6. Pelletier, *The Best Alternative Medicine.*

7. "Using Biofeedback to Make Childhood Headaches Less of a Pain," by K. Allen, *Pediatric Annals 33*(4) (2004): 241–245.

8. Allen, "Using Biofeedback to Make Headaches Less of a Pain."

9. http://www.mayoclinic.com/

10. Pelletier, *The Best Alternative Medicine.*

11. "Critical Evaluation of the Effect of Valerian Extract on Sleep Structure and Sleep Quality," by F. Donath, S. Quispe, K. Diefenbach, et al., *Pharmacopsychiatry 33*(2) (2000): 47–53.

12. "Melatonin in Patients with Reduced REM Sleep Duration: Two Randomized Controlled Trials," by D. Kunz, R. Mahlberg, C. Muller, et al., *Journal of Clinical Endocrinology and Metabolism 89* (1) (2004): 128–134.

13. http://www.mentalhealth.org

14. Mayo Clinic Health Letter, June 1994, 7.

15. *Infant Massage: A Handbook for Loving Parents*, by V. S. McClure (New York: Bantam, 1989).

16. "Tactile/Kinesthetic Stimulation Effects on Preterm Neonates," by T. Field, S. Schanberg, F. Scafidi, C. Bauer, N. Vega-Lahr, R. Garcia, J. Nystrom, and C. Kuhn, *Pediatrics 77*(5) (1986): 654–659.

17. http://www.healinglifestyles.com

18. http://www.healinglifestyles.com

19. *Holistic Health and Healing,* by M. Bright (Philadelphia: F.A. Davis Company, 2002).

24 More Stress-Reduction Strategies

■ Why do I feel so good after watching a funny movie or TV show? ■ What kind of music is best for relaxation? ■ Even if my favorite types of music are not necessarily relaxing, is it bad or harmful to listen to them? ■ I feel better after a good cry. Besides crying, are there other ways to relieve upset feelings? ■ I feel better when I write down my thoughts in my journal, but I'm concerned that other people will read my private thoughts. Should I tear up the pages I've written, or is it better to keep my written thoughts and refer to them later to see where I've been and how far I've come?

Study of this chapter will enable you to:

1. Describe the impact of humor on stress and health.
2. Describe the positive effects of music.
3. List the most effective types of music for stress management.
4. Become aware of additional ways to reduce stress.
5. Avoid ineffective options for reducing stress.

Rule number one: Don't sweat the small stuff.
Rule number two: It is all small stuff.

—*Robert Elliott*

Amy's Story I got married when I was 18. My husband was 20. We made plans like so many newly married couples do . . . careers, buying a house, starting a family. Two short years into our marriage, our dreams were shattered. I was three months pregnant when we learned that my husband had brain cancer. His prognosis was extremely poor, and I was told that he probably wouldn't live to see our baby born.

This was not acceptable to my husband. He told me that he was going to live—not only long enough to see the birth but long enough so his child would get to know him and remember him. Thus our battle began. This was more than a battle with the cancer. It was with the medical professionals who told us that he had only six months to live.

I started reading books to him in his hospital bed, often not knowing if he could even hear me. I found compilations of funny stories and jokes. I laughed—most of the time so I wouldn't cry. Then came the day when he laughed with me. He became alert and oriented and ready to take on each day with a smile. He became the talk of the hospital unit. The staff members were amazed at his progress and commented that he always had a smile on his face. He was always good for a joke.

Our daughter was born in March. My husband was by my side. He was there on her first day of preschool, kindergarten, first grade, and second grade.

Almost four years have gone by since my husband passed away. Not until he died could I fully see his strength and lust for life. The stress I felt in knowing that I was going to lose my husband surely must have been outmatched by the stress he felt, knowing that he was the one who was going to die. He never showed it—which is what helped me cope throughout his illness. His strength and sense of humor carried us both. I thank him for that. I thank him for not giving up and for having the courage to laugh at his six-month prognosis. I thank him for showing me that life is not just black and white. I thank him for helping me put things into perspective. I thank him for teaching me that laughter is good medicine. I thank him for laughing his way into our daughter's life.

If you ask our daughter, she will say, "My daddy was a funny man."

More Stress-Reduction Strategies

Chapters 16 through 23 presented methods that work to turn off the stress response. Those techniques were designed to bring about relaxation and restore balance. This chapter looks at a smorgasbord of additional ways to reduce stress, though they may not initially be considered to serve that purpose. They are things we typically include in our lives that, by their nature, can make us feel better. First we will discuss humor and laughter for relaxation. Then we will explore music as an important strategy for relieving stress. The chapter will conclude with a list of other methods that people commonly use to help them feel better, as well as a brief look at those things we should avoid in trying to reduce stress.

Although some of these stress-reduction methods have not been as thoroughly examined scientifically, strong anecdotal evidence supports their effectiveness. The best attitude for the approaches described in this chapter is that of discovery. Experiment with the strategies and see which ones work for you. If you are like most people, you will find positive results as you incorporate several into your lifestyle and daily activities.

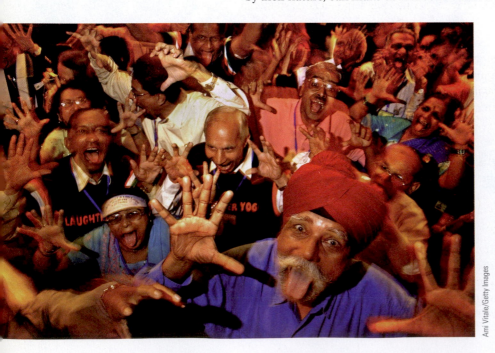

Ami Vitale/Getty Images

In India the 'lion laugh' proves to be a great stress reliever. Try it!

Laughter and Humor

Life can seem serious at times, but we can do much to bring balance to our lives through humor. An Apache myth tells how the Creator endowed human beings with the ability to do everything—talk, run, see, and hear. But he was not satisfied until they could do just one thing more: laugh. And so men and women laughed and laughed and laughed! Then the Creator said, "Now you are fit to live."[1]

Healthy children laugh as many as 400 times a day, and adults only about 15 times a day.[2] Maybe we learn to repress our emotions, or maybe our lives become so filled with responsibility and stress that we simply don't feel like laughing. Whatever the reason, the adage that "laughter is good medicine" has proven to be true. Laughter can help prevent stress and it has positive health benefits.

Even though the terms **humor** and **laughter** may seem to be interchangeable, they involve different processes. You do not need a sense of humor to laugh. If you have ever watched a 6-month-old baby burst into laughter spontaneously at the funny faces dad is making, you come to understand that laughter is innate and a sense of humor is learned. A sense of humor is an intellectual process, while laughter spontaneously engages every major system in the body.[3] So people with a terrific sense of humor may or may not laugh, and people may laugh without a sense of humor. The bottom line is that both laughter and humor can be beneficial to prevent and reduce stress.

A darker side of humor is **sarcasm.** In contrast to humor, which has the power to heal and uplift, sarcasm can be a form of aggression used to put people down. Saying "I was just kidding" is often the back door out of a put-down and is not usually humorous.

Benefits of Laughter

The late Dr. Norman Cousins brought attention to laughter as a legitimate tool for relieving stress and pain. He found that 10 minutes of laughter allowed him 2 hours of pain-free sleep while dealing with a painful, chronic illness called ankylosing spondylytis. After this personal experience, he spent the rest of his life investigating the positive emotions and their relationship to health.

The harmful effects of stress upon an individual's health are well known. You have learned that stress and negative emotions have been associated with immunosuppression and increased epinephrine and cortisol blood levels. The pleasant feelings associated with mirthful laughter may modify some of the neuroendocrine components of the stress response. In addition, stress hormones that constrict blood vessels and suppress immune activity decrease after being exposed to humor.[4] Laughter has been shown consistently to improve mood and reduce stress.

How Laughter Works

Laughter creates predictable physiological changes in the body in a manner similar to exercise. Laughter exercises the diaphragm and the cardiovascular system and has even been referred to as "internal jogging." The body responds to laughter like it does to exercise, in two stages:[5]

1. The *arousal phase*, with an increase in physiological measures including pulse, respirations, and blood pressure.
2. The *resolution phase*, during which physiological measures return to resting values or lower values, creating a relaxation response.

Researchers hypothesize that although laughter invokes a form of stress, it is different in effect from the stress that results in an increase in stress hormones and in a compromised immune system. Laughter seems to create the positive stress known as *eustress.* Laughter is associated with a release of tension and an increase in the natural mood-lifters known as **endorphins**—mood-elevating, pain-relieving chemicals produced naturally by the brain.

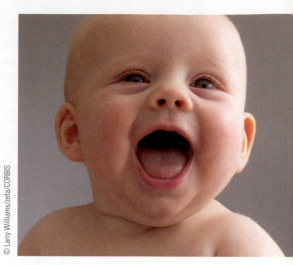

© Larry Williams/zefa/CORBIS

If you have ever watched a 6-month-old baby burst into laughter at the funny faces Dad is making, you come to understand that laughter is innate.

A cheerful heart is good medicine, but a downcast spirit dries up the bones.
—*Proverbs*

The arrival of a good clown exercises a more beneficial influence upon the health of a town than of twenty asses laden with drugs.
—*Thomas Sydenham, M.D., 17th-century physician*

The Power of Laughter

Michael Miller, director of preventive cardiology at the University of Maryland Medical Center, theorized that laughter might promote healthier arteries by reducing mental stress, which has been shown to constrict blood vessels and reduce blood flow. He tested his theory on 20 volunteers, monitoring their blood pressure, cholesterol, blood-sugar levels, and how their blood vessels reacted to stress. Then he asked them to watch scenes from two movies. The first scene, chosen to provoke stress, was the opening scene from the realistic 1998 war movie *Saving Private Ryan.* The second scene was from the 1996 comedy *Kingpin.*

A total of 160 blood vessel measurements were taken before and after the laughter and mental-stress phases of the study. The study found that the lighthearted movie reliably relaxed the blood vessels and increased blood flow in 19 of the 20 volunteers. The reactions probably were prompted by the release of nitric oxide, which relaxes blood vessels much like the endorphins released during exercise.

Miller said, "A good belly laugh a day would be a big step toward heart health."*

In a similar study, Lee Berk and colleagues at Loma Linda University conducted a study to assess the effects of laughter on stress hormones. They hypothesized that laughter would elicit neuroendocrine responses different from those invoked by the stress response. Blood hormone levels were compared when the experimental participants were shown a humorous video and the control participants sat quietly for the same length of time.

The findings showed significant reductions in stress hormones, including cortisol, in the video watchers, compared with the resting control group. The authors described the effects of laughter as eustress, a healthy, positive form of stress.**

Sources:
*"For a Hardy Heart, Have a Hardy-har-har," by S. Sternberg, *USA Today*, March 8, 2005, 18A.
**"Neuroendocrine and Stress Hormone Changes during Mirthful Laughter," by L. Berk et al., *American Journal of Medical Science* 298(6) (1989): 390.

Humor also can empower people by giving them a different perspective on life's problems. When individuals can learn to see humor in stressful situations, the response to the perceived threat often changes.[6] Amy's story in the opening vignette illustrates this idea. Her husband made a decision to take control of what he could during a situation in which much was out of his control. Through humor and laughter, he had a positive impact on his health and even the well-being of those around him.

Subjective Nature of Humor

Laughter and humor vary widely between genders, ages, and cultures. Humor may affect men and women differently, as a study of 131 undergraduate students indicated. Although humor reduced stress-related physical symptoms in men and women alike, it reduced stress-linked anxiety more significantly in men. The researchers theorized that men may prefer humor as a more appropriate way of expressing emotions such as anxiety, whereas women are more likely to use self-disclosure—confiding in a friend, for example.[7] Women might note that the next time a male friend or relative cracks a joke at a most inappropriate time, he might be dealing with his anxiety in the way more typical of his gender.

Humor Strategies for Stress Prevention

- Keep a "funnies file" with your favorite cartoons and jokes.
- Choose a comedy rather than a violent movie.
- When the news is depressing, turn it off.
- When something makes you laugh out loud, share it with a friend and multiply the mirth.
- Keep a "humor journal" in which you write things that make you laugh, such as funny things children say or humorous errors in the newspaper. By being more aware, you will notice the fun and funny things happening around you every day.
- Plan a weekly 'funny movie night' with family or friends. Take turns picking the movie.
- Read your favorite newspaper cartoons every day.
- Spend time with fun, lighthearted people who find the joy in life.

What makes us laugh is different for different individuals. What is important is to find ways to laugh every day. Find ways to spend time with people who add joy and laughter to your life. Laughter is not just fun. It is healthy.

Music

Music and Mood Music creates the mood for many settings. Those who select music for various environments and events recognize that it sets the tone for sporting events, parades, restaurants, shopping centers, television shows, advertisements, and dances. The music selection is usually precise and purposeful to create an atmosphere appropriate for that setting.

When you are shopping at a major department store, you may not be aware of the music that is playing, but the music has been selected to encourage shoppers to spend more time enjoying their shopping experience. Happy shoppers stay longer and buy more. Music at an all-you-can-eat buffet will be different than an expensive, top-quality restaurant. In the all-you-can-eat restaurant, the music usually is louder and peppier because the owner wants you to hurry up, eat, and leave. In the expensive restaurant, the music is likely soft and peaceful, encouraging you to stay and order more food.

> I think I should have no other mortal wants, if I could always have plenty of music. It seems to infuse strength into my limbs and ideas into my brain. Life seems to go on without effort, when I am filled with music.
>
> —*George Eliot*

Think about any scary movie you have seen. Now think about the most frightening part of that movie and everything about the terrifying scene. What would happen if you were to remove the music during the chilling sequence? Suddenly it becomes far less frightening. The dramatic music creates the mood of fear. Music has long been used to affect our mood and influence how we feel.

History of Music Music has been used throughout history to calm the body, mind, and spirit. The term **music therapy** is fairly new, yet the practice of using music to heal can be traced back to antiquity. The healing power of music therapy is even recorded in the Bible: "And whenever the evil spirit from God was upon Saul, David took the lyre and played it with his hand; so Saul was refreshed, and was well, and the evil spirit departed from him." (1 Samuel, 16:23)

FYI

The Gift of Music
How ironic—one of the supreme masterworks of music, which has enthralled listeners through the ages, was meant to put its first audience to sleep! Russian Envoy Count Kayserling suffered from miserable insomnia. To deal with the problem, he hired one of Johann Sebastian Bach's finest pupils, the fourteen-year old Johann Gottlieb Goldberg, to play music for him during his restless nights. The Count installed Goldberg in a room nearby, ready to play at the Count's command. To soothe the Count, Bach wrote a special piece, formally entitled *Aria With Diverse Variations for Harpsichord with Two Manuals*, in 1741. In gratitude, the Count sent Bach 100 louis d'or, an extraordinary sum far exceeding his annual salary. We know this composition today as the "Goldberg Variations."

Source: *Superlearning*, S. Ostrander and L. Ostrander (New York: Dell Publishing, 1979).

People who were imprisoned in Auschwitz, a Nazi concentration camp during World War II, used music to help them cope with some of the most difficult situations imaginable. People were separated from family and friends and forced into slave labor. They watched as people around them were executed and knew their turn to die was coming. The people in these camps seemed to have little to live for, yet many remained strong and endured the trial. Some turned to music as a source of strength.

In one story, prisoners about to enter the gas chamber joined together in their final moments to sing with feeling and passion the Czechoslovakian national anthem, and then a Hebrew song, "Hatikvah," as a way to give each other strength for what was ahead of them. Music was a way for them to find peace, even in death.[8]

The Effects of Music on the Body and Mind Musicologist David Tame says this in his book, *The Secret Power of Music:*

> To the question, "Does music affect man's physical body?" modern research replies in the clear affirmative. There is scarcely a single function of the body that cannot be affected by musical tones. The roots of the auditory nerves are more widely distributed and possess more extensive connections than those of any other nerves in the body. Investigation has shown that music affects digestion, internal secretions, circulation, nutrition, and respiration. Even the neural networks of the brain have been found to be sensitive to harmonic principles.[9]

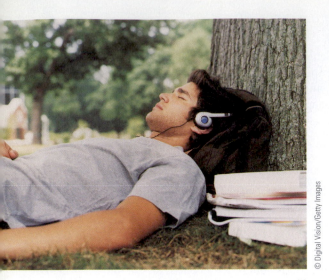

Music has the power to touch us deeply and can help tune out the stresses of daily life.

According to Sari Harrar, health news editor for *Prevention* magazine, "Music has the power to soothe the savage, stressed out beast." After reviewing clinical studies and anecdotal evidence from music therapists, Harrar concludes that music helps to:[10]

- Manage pain
- Improve mood and mobility
- Reduce the need for pain relievers and sedatives accompanying surgery
- Relieve anxiety
- Lower blood pressure
- Ease depression
- Enhance concentration and creativity

Further studies show that music has measurable physical effects on the body. Certain kinds of music have been found to lower heart rates, respiratory rates, and blood pressure, increase tranquil mood states,[11] and increase oxygen levels in the blood.[12] For individuals with hypertension and related conditions, music can be combined with other therapies to promote health. Here are findings from other studies:

- Surgical patients exposed to music reported significantly lower pain intensity and required less morphine compared to a control group.[13]
- Subjects with osteoarthritis reported less arthritic pain when music was played, compared to a control group of subjects who simply sat quietly.[14]
- People undergoing surgery have been shown to require less anesthesia, awaken from anesthesia more quickly and with fewer side effects, and heal more rapidly when healing music is played before, during, and after the surgical procedure.[15]
- Individuals suffering from depression need less medication and have more success in psychotherapy when music is added to their course of treatment.[16]
- Grief, loneliness, and anger are all managed better when appropriate music is added to therapy.[17]
- Autistic children and children diagnosed with brain damage all react positively to music therapy.[18]

Ronald Kotulak wrote in the *Chicago Tribune:*

What is it that touches us so deeply when we listen to the music we love? It could be that we are listening to an inner voice attached to one of humankind's earliest languages. Whatever the solution to the mystery, this Chicago musician and songwriter finds nothing calms a screaming infant better than the songs he and his wife present to their child.

Almost everybody enjoys a beautiful melody. It takes root into the brain, priming the imagination, arousing passions, sedating anxieties and inspiring the body to move in rhythm. A person who is born deaf and never has heard a note can still learn to dance by feeling the vibrations music makes.[19]

Whether easing pain, relieving loneliness, or even calming the cries of a screaming baby, music affects us profoundly.

How Music Works Music can affect the body and mind in two distinct ways:

1. Directly, as the effect of sound upon the cells and organs
2. Indirectly, by affecting the emotions, which in turn influence numerous bodily processes

Following are examples of each of the two ways music can affect the body.

Medical Resonance Therapy Music One development in the use of music therapy is **medical resonance therapy music** (MRT-Music). This music, composed by German musicologist Peter Huebner, is based on the principle of resonance. **Resonance** means that the precise harmony contained in a given musical structure resonates inside the human body, from the ears to the brain and from the brain to various organs. In this way, it also becomes an important tool for preventing disease.[20]

Soothing Music Affects Stress Hormones

In a Japanese study, levels of the stress hormones ACTH and cortisol were measured in surgical patients just before anesthesia was administered. Patients who listened to soothing music immediately before anesthesia showed a drop in stress hormones by more than 50%. The opposite happened to those who did not listen to music. Their hormone levels showed a rise of more than 50%. The researchers concluded that any music a patient finds pleasurable will reduce levels of stress.

Source: "Sound & Healing," by J. Klotter, *Townsend Letter for Doctors and Parents* (Feb/March 2003) p. 28.

The effects of MRT-Music have been studied for years in people with various conditions, including individuals with cancer, skin diseases, high-risk pregnancies, in crisis situations, and surgery patients.[21] One study investigated the effect of MRT-Music on women with high-risk pregnancies. In the course of 5 years, 140 women with high-risk pregnancy were individually studied at stages throughout their pregnancy. The women listened to MRT-Music for 8 sessions that lasted about 40 to 60 minutes each.

These researchers found that with continued use of MRT-Music, the anxiety levels of each woman decreased. The women also had an increased threshold of pain sensitivity in labor, meaning they were able to handle higher levels of pain, and a reduced labor time. The heart activity of the developing fetus increased, indicating a strongly developing heart. The number of interrupted pregnancies was reduced by about half, and no harmful side effects were observed in the study.[22]

The underlying principle of MRT-Music is that music actually can influence our body directly at the cellular and organ levels.

Perception of Music

If you have ever been brought to tears by a song, you know that music also affects us at an emotional level. The individual meaning attached to music influences our reaction to the music. This subjective emotional response to music activates a physiological response. Different types of music affect us differently.

To ease stress, you have to enjoy the music you are listening to. Individual perception and preference may be the most important factor in determining which music provides you with optimal benefits.

Which Music Is Best for Stress Management?

What type of music is best for reducing stress or for helping to create a relaxing environment? As we have discussed, individual choice and preference are important factors. Two genres of music—classical and New Age—have been found to be relaxing for many.

Classical Music

Classical music is one of the best types of music for relaxation and meditation. One type of early classical music that seems to be the most effective in reducing the stress response is music from the baroque musical period.[23] Composers representative of the baroque period include Bach, Handel, and Vivaldi, among others.

Researchers who studied the effects of classical music found that when people are connected to an electroencephalogram (EEG) machine that records brainwave activity while listening to classical music, they had brainwave activity similar to that commonly found in meditators. The researchers looked specifically at the **adagio movements** of the baroque and early classical compositions, with a tempo of about 60 beats per minute. These

---

FYI

Music Affects Plants

Dr. T. C. Singh, head of the Botany Department at Annamalai University, India, has conducted research into the effects of music on plants. He discovered that constant exposure to classical music caused plants to grow at twice their normal speed. In his experiments, the violin was found to be one of the most life-enhancing instruments of all. Perhaps the most significant of all of Dr. Singh's findings was that later generations of the seeds of musically stimulated plants carried on the improved traits of larger size, more leaves, and other characteristics. Music had changed the plants' chromosomes!

Source: *The Secret Power of Music*, D. Tame (Northamptonshire, England: Turnstone Press, Ltd., 1984).

movements seemed to be the most relaxing and produced heightened alpha brainwave activity similar to what occurs during deep relaxation, hypnosis, and meditation. The music of Mozart has become so popular as a healing tool that the treatment now is known as the **Mozart effect.**

A well-known example of an adagio composition of baroque music is Pachelbel's "Canon in D." Whether it is Pachelbel's Canon, Mozart's classical compositions, or any of the other varieties of classical music, this genre of music lends itself well to relaxation.

New Age Music Another genre that has become well-accepted and effective for relaxation is **New Age music.** Sub-classifications of New Age music include New Instrumental, Space Music, Music for Meditation, and Acoustic Guitar, among others. One of the earliest New Age music composers, Steven Halpern, described New Age music as music that does not build mainly on the principle of tension and release (like most music in general) but, rather, functions like wallpaper (meaning that it rests quietly and almost unnoticed in the background), which can create a positive, even healing atmosphere. New Age music is available to suit every type of relaxing activity, from yoga and deep meditation to increasing energy after a draining day.

Don Campbell, teacher and researcher in the fields of music, sound, health, and learning, believes that to get in touch with music that allows access to the unconscious and inner depths, one must listen to the masterpieces of baroque, classical, romantic, and impressionist composers, who have, in his opinion, encoded many of their works with messages of divine inspiration and unity. He believes that great compositions offer keys to personal transformation and the understanding of wholeness to those who listen.[24]

In summary, certain genres of music may affect us directly at a cellular level. Classical and New Age music seem to be especially effective in calming the body. Still, individual perception and preference may be the most important factor in determining what music works best for you. In any case, music affects us profoundly. In the words of Nietzsche, "Without music, life would be a mistake." Music that is appealing and relaxing can be a powerful part of any personal stress-management program.

What Else Can I Do?

This chapter has introduced you to two effective ways of affecting stress levels—laughter and music. You can do a variety of other "little things" to help reduce stress each day. Following are some of these ways.

- *Listen to your body.* When you are under stress, your body will send signals indicating that it is on overload. Typical signs of overload, discussed in earlier chapters, include fatigue, headache, muscle pain, irritability, and inability to concentrate. Tune in to these signals and become familiar with those that occur most frequently. If you notice a headache coming on each time you feel overwhelmed, this is a signal that your stress response is up and running in high gear. Pay attention to the other signals that your body sends during tense times. At the onset of these symptoms, do something immediately to reduce the stress you are feeling so you can deal with the situation appropriately, without the additional false sense of alarm.

- *Deal directly with the cause.* Identify your stressors specifically and determine if you can do something to eliminate or modify the most stressful of these. If stress comes from your relationship with a person, take the time to iron out your differences. If tension comes from an unfinished task, restructure your priorities so you can fulfill that responsibility. Examine your routines at home, at work, and at school, and eliminate unnecessary activities.

- *Distance yourself.* Parents sometimes use "time-out" for misbehaving kids. Most adults also can benefit from time-outs. A time-out can be an effective tool to help someone step out of a stressful situation, cool down, and refocus on what is really important. When you find yourself in an emotionally charged situation, step back and ask yourself, "Is this working?" If not, take a few moments to separate yourself from the situation. Remove yourself from the battle zone and let your emotions subside. From an emotional distance, you sometimes can see the situation more clearly.

- *Talk yourself through a situation.* We readily feel anxious and worried when we are surrounded by negative feedback, especially from ourselves. Instead of saying, "I'll never get this done in time," say, "I've been in similar situations before and managed it all right!" Be your own cheerleader; give yourself pep talks instead of self-scoldings.

- *Pat yourself on the back.* A little bit of self-congratulation can go a long way toward feeling a lot of self-worth. Mentally pat yourself on the back when you have accomplished something, no matter how small. When you are successful at something, take a moment to allow yourself to feel good about a job well done. Curiously, we are quick to judge our actions negatively when we think we haven't measured up. Why not choose the opposite route when we have made the grade successfully?

- *Be creative.* When you are in a stressful situation, take a few minutes to write down every possible solution to the problem, regardless of how impossible or crazy it might seem. Writing your list of options reminds you that you do have the freedom to select your course of action, that you do have some control. This thought alone can reduce stress, and you probably will come up with a brilliant solution to the problem.

- *Change your attitude.* Anytime you catch yourself thinking or saying that something is a problem, change how you think and speak of it by calling it a challenge. Challenges are viewed differently than problems. On the one hand, problems are viewed as annoying and difficult and often involve discomfort. Challenges, on the other hand, usually are viewed as opportunities. They allow you to rise to the occasion and grow as you meet the challenge head on.

- *Keep agreements.* An agreement is a verbal or nonverbal commitment that we intend to complete a certain action. If we say we will do something, and then we do it, we have kept an agreement. When we keep agreements, things work out; the systems in which we live run smoothly. When we keep agreements, we also maintain our integrity. When we don't keep agreements, things do not run as smoothly and integrity is lost. Lying, cheating, and stealing are examples of not keeping agreements.

  We make agreements every day. We tell others that we will meet them at a certain place at a certain time, or we agree to do a certain amount of work on a job. We even make agreements with ourselves. We say to ourselves that we will get up on time, clean the house, forgive someone, or not drink any more caffeinated beverages. Keeping agreements is one of the greatest demonstrations that you are choosing to be responsible for your life and the outcomes you create. Whenever you say that you intend for something to happen, be responsible for making it happen.

- *Take short naps.* Naps are short periods of rest that recharge the body for the remainder of the day. People take naps that last anywhere from 30 minutes to 2 hours. Often, when people awaken after longer naps, they don't feel any better than they did prior to napping and may even feel a decline in alertness and performance. Researchers believe this is so because when a person sleeps for longer periods during the day, the mind begins to do the same thing it normally would do at night: Brainwave activity goes into deeper sleeping patterns, just as it would during a typical night's sleep. Upon awakening, the sleeping

It's the Little Things That Add Up

Each individual stressor that we experience can work together with the others to produce a large mountain of stress. Viewed on the positive side, immersing ourselves in many small, positive things can also add up to a large contribution toward a more relaxing lifestyle. Here are some examples of small things that add up to a more contented life:

- Simplify mealtimes.
- Play with children at a playground, and do all the fun things they do.
- Look for the positive aspects of situations.
- Say something nice to somebody.
- Fly a kite.
- Walk in the rain.
- Go dancing and let loose for a while.
- Say hello to a stranger.
- Read a good book while you're curled up in a warm bed.
- Go to a museum or a place where art is presented.
- Hum or whistle your favorite tunes.
- Plant a tree.
- Feed the birds.
- Work in the garden.
- Make a paper airplane and throw it from a high place.
- Learn a new song.
- Go on a picnic.
- Take a different route to work.
- Watch your favorite movie.
- Make and eat popcorn.
- Write a letter to an old friend.
- Cook a meal and eat it by candlelight.
- Talk less and listen more.
- Freely praise other people.

You could add many simple, yet relaxing things to this list of "little things." We can view most things that we do as pleasant when we apply the proper attitude.

FYI | Short Naps Are Best

Researchers have found that a brief afternoon nap of only 10 minutes was more recuperative than a 30-minute nap in terms of improved alertness and performance in the hour following napping.

Sources: "The Recuperative Value of Brief and Ultra-Brief Naps on Alertness and Cognitive Performance," by A. J. Tietzel and L. C. Lack. *Journal of Sleep Research 11*(3) (2002): 213–220.

rhythms are still in a deeper nighttime sleeping mode. As a result, the person takes substantially longer to return to the usual levels of activity compared to the immediate improvement following shorter naps. Additional research on napping indicates that a quick afternoon nap does not seem to hinder the ability to enjoy a good night's sleep.[25]

- *Change your physiology; change your feelings.* We can change how we are feeling by changing how our body is positioned. An energized, happy person holds herself in a certain way. Her face looks a certain way—happy and confident. She holds her body in a certain way—upright and secure. Her shoulders are up and back, her chest held high, and she's breathing a certain way—fully and deeply.

  Conversely, a depressed person positions herself in a very different way. She may move more slowly, her shoulders may sag, and even her voice may become shallow and hard to hear. You can trick your emotions into feeling better by putting your body into the position that it usually feels when you are happy, energized, and alive. Curiously, emotions will follow the body's physiology.

  Try this: Begin by smiling. Next, push your shoulders back, and sit up or stand up straight. Take a full, deep breath to completely fill your lungs with air. Raise your head and look up. Raise your eyebrows and clap your hands several times above your head. As you do this—as unusual as it sounds—you will notice yourself immediately feeling better. A smart way to change your physiology, and thereby change how you feel, is by exercising. Doing something active requires more oxygen, which requires deep breathing, alertness, and a positive, energetic body posture.

- *Write about it.* Keeping a diary, or **journaling,** is a proven way to release emotions. In a study published in the *Journal of the American Medical Association,*[26] researchers found a psychological improvement from emotional problems among subjects after they wrote about their stress. Keeping a "stress diary" can help you identify stressors in your life. Once you identify them, you can manage these stressors more easily.

  Giving yourself a few minutes to put your thoughts into words may be effective in helping you deal with the problem at hand. Many people find stress relief through the simple act of writing down thoughts that are racing around in the mind. Once you move those thoughts from your mind to paper, you may want to throw them away, or you may choose to reflect on the thoughts. The stress-relieving value often comes from the simple act of getting the thoughts out of your head and down on paper, where you can see them.

  You can practice journaling in a variety of ways: You can unload all of your thoughts and feelings about something, or you might write a single note or two about an event that you can deal with later at a more appropriate time. Some people like to get their thoughts on paper immediately after something painful has happened. Some prefer to wait until they have quiet time before going to sleep. Others do their journaling in the morning after a refreshing night's sleep because "sleeping on it" helps them gain perspective on the situation and brings to the surface new ideas or solutions previously unseen. Sometimes, if a person doesn't write down ideas immediately, they slip back into the subconscious mind waiting for another ideal time to resurface.

  Mindful writing—writing whatever happens to be on the mind at the moment—is a powerful way to allow the insights and inspiration from one's intuition to bubble to the surface.

  Brenda Ueland, author of the book *If You Want to Write,* said:

  Writing, the creative effort, the use of the imagination, should come first—at least some part of every day of your life. It is a wonderful blessing if you will use it. You will become happier, more enlightened, alive, impassioned, light-hearted and generous to everybody else.[27]

  She explains how you can bring your best ideas to the surface.

  You sit down to write, to think. . . . No logical thought comes in the first minute or two that you try it. A sort of paralysis follows, a conviction of your mental limitations, and you disconsolately go downstairs to do something menial and easy like washing the dishes, while doing so (though not knowing it) having some wonderful, fascinating, extraordinary, original, illuminating thought. Not knowing that they are thoughts at all, or "thinking," you have no respect for them and do not put them down on paper—which you are to do from now on! That is, you are always to act and express what goes through you.[28]

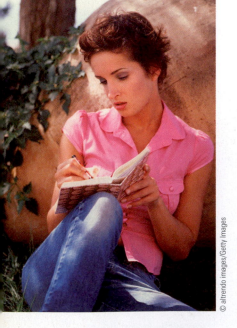

Many people find stress relief through the simple act of writing down thoughts that are racing around in the mind.

Spend 10 to 15 minutes at a time putting down your feelings on paper. Don't worry about grammar, syntax, or spelling. You are the only one who will read your written work. Unload on paper the events of the day and, *more important,* how you feel about the events, especially the events in which you found yourself getting upset, angry, or stressed.

Above all, don't let journaling or diary writing become a stressor in itself. You should write, as a method of emotional release, when you feel the urge. Don't force writing to happen, but when you do feel the urge to write, follow the urge.

- *Talk it out.* Don't bottle up anger, worries, or frustrations. Sometimes, discussing problems with a trusted friend can help clear your mind so you can concentrate on solving problems. Learning to talk things over with someone you trust can release the pressure, make you feel better, and help you come to a new understanding of the problem.

- *Cry it out.* We can find relief from stress by physically releasing these emotions. Sometimes crying is the best way to do this. Some people believe that one of the reasons that women tend to live longer than men in our society may be their willingness to release emotional distress by crying. As a result, they release potentially damaging stress. Many people report feeling relieved after releasing pent-up emotions by crying it out.

- *Scream it out.* Similar to crying, the act of releasing pent-up energy by loud verbal emissions or screaming has been found to be useful in releasing emotional energy for many people. Do this by turning up the radio in your car and singing your favorite song at the top of your lungs, or putting your face into your pillow and blasting away with all your might.

We should note that screaming directly at other people probably has the opposite effect and usually leads to further problems. When you decide to use scream therapy, be sure you are not using it to attack another person but, instead, to simply release the energy you are feeling.

- *Sing it out.* Music can be a powerful way to release tension and stress, as has been discussed. Many people relax by playing their favorite instrument. Singing can be a relaxing way to relieve stress, too. People sing in the shower, while driving, or while doing chores. Many people add music to make work less stressful. This might be at the office or while studying at home. Whatever songs you prefer, you can have a lot of fun enjoying yourself and releasing your stress by singing.

- *Dance it out.* The combined benefits of exercise and music can come together in a fun and relaxing way when we dance to relieve stress. In his book *Tuesdays with Morrie,* Mitch Albom describes how his old professor, Morrie Schwartz, experienced the moment through dance:

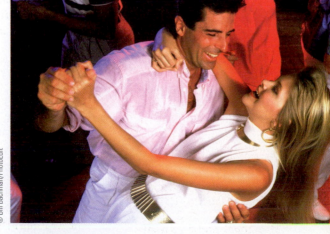

Dance your cares away. The combined benefits of exercise and music can come together in a fun and relaxing way when we dance to relieve stress.

© Bill Bachman/PhotoEdit

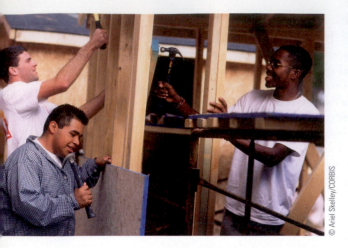

Doing something to help others takes our mind off our own problems—and it feels good too!

© Ariel Skelley/CORBIS

He had always been a dancer, my old professor. The music didn't matter. Rock and roll, big band, the blues. He loved them all. He would close his eyes and with a blissful smile begin to move to his own sense of rhythm. It wasn't always pretty. But then, he didn't worry about a partner. Morrie danced by himself.

He used to go to this church in Harvard Square every Wednesday night for something called "Dance Free." They had flashing lights and booming speakers, and Morrie would wander in among the mostly student crowd wearing a white T-shirt and black sweatpants and a towel around his neck, and whatever music was playing, that's the music to which he danced. He'd do the lindy to Jimi Hendrix. He twisted and twirled, he waved his arms like a conductor on amphetamines, until sweat was dripping down the middle of his back. No one there knew he was a prominent doctor of sociology, with years of experience as a college professor and several well-respected books. They just thought he was some old nut.

Once he brought a tango tape and got them to play it over the speakers. Then he commandeered the floor, shooting back and forth like some hot Latin lover. When he finished, everyone applauded. He could have stayed in that moment forever.[29]

It is easy to imagine the fun and relaxation that Morrie must have experienced. Why not make exercise fun through dancing?

- *Focus on the needs of others.* Taking attention from our own problems and shifting it to the needs of someone else tends to help us forget about the rough times we are going through. As people see the challenges others are facing, they often gain a new perspective on their own challenges. They develop an attitude of gratitude instead of self-pity. They also feel fulfillment from helping others in need.
- *Have sex.* The sexual response involves a sequence of events that involve the body and mind. The physiological experience of the sexual response typically has a relaxing effect on both. During the orgasm phase of the sexual response, many muscles throughout the body tense. Following orgasm, those tensed muscles automatically relax. This leaves the body feeling deeply relaxed. Consensual sex can be a great way to relieve stress and tension.
- *Soak in the tub.* The warmth of the water is relaxing to the muscles. Being by yourself without anything else to do except enjoy the water is relaxing as well. As a pleasant way to unwind after a rough day, place lit aromatic candles around the bathtub. Soak in warm water while playing relaxing music, and let the peaceful environment and soothing warm water completely relax the body and mind.
- *Gaze at the sky.* Sit back and observe the heavens. Simply enjoy the view. Pondering the vastness of the universe can make many problems seem insignificant. If it is daytime, watch the blue sky and the clouds. Realize that the sky is perfect in every way, yet it is always changing. Consider this as a good metaphor for your own life.

"Solutions" to Avoid

In Chapter 15 we discussed some of the unhealthy lifestyle habits, such as drinking and drugs, that some people use as a means of coping with stress. Following are some additional coping strategies that are best avoided.

Don't:

- *Gossip.* When people don't feel so good about themselves, they sometimes resort to talking about other people. The psychological reasoning for this is if they can bring someone else down, it will elevate them, in some way, above the other person. By talking about someone else, they can have the feeling that they are in control, more in the know, and that they have more value and worth. Unfortunately for them, this is not possible, as no one has any more value or worth than anyone else.

Remember—we are what we think. Spreading negative thoughts creates and intensifies negative feelings and emotions. It may bring a short-term pleasurable feeling, but in the long run, gossip creates negative social and emotional problems as well as guilt. People who frequently gossip often entertain mistaken paranoid thoughts that others are talking unfavorably about them as well.

- *Whine and complain.* Like gossiping, thinking and speaking in a complaining, poor-me way may seem like a solution, but it does nothing to solve problems and is a possible cause of stress. Whining doesn't deal with the problem directly but, instead, makes the problem seem bigger than it really is by expanding it in the mind. Nobody enjoys being around someone who is constantly telling everyone how bad things are by vying for sympathy or pity for their problems.

- *Blame others.* A surefire way to release yourself from responsibility and convince yourself that you don't have to deal with a problem is to blame others. But this solution is short-lived. On the surface, this way of dealing with problems makes people feel more in control of the situation, but blaming someone else for the consequences of your actions merely shows an unwillingness to accept responsibility. If you don't accept responsibility, you deny yourself the opportunity to effectively problem-solve. Blaming also damages relationships and leads to feelings of anger, frustration, and helplessness.

- *Self-inflict pain.* When a person is stressed, the fight-or-flight response is hard at work gearing up to avoid a potential pain. Sometimes we already feel severe emotional pain because of emotional traumas such as abuse or neglect. One way that some people choose to try to deal with that emotional distress is to create a physical pain to replace it. Typical examples of self-inflicted pain are deliberately cutting oneself, pinching, pulling out hair, or hitting oneself. Experiencing a physical pain to try to drown the emotional distress may result in temporary relief, but as an alternate method of managing stress, it is ineffective because it adds emotional stresses including guilt, shame, and embarrassment. If this is used as a method to cope with emotional distress, the best solution may be to get help from a counselor or a licensed therapist.

- *Overdo it.* Any activity that is healthy in moderation becomes unhealthy and leads to more stress when it is overdone. Eating food, for example, is a healthy and positive part of effective living. But overeating can lead to an unhealthy existence with the added risk of disease and a compromised lifestyle. Sufficient and satisfactory sleep is a key component in reducing stress levels, but oversleeping to avoid important activities or to waste time can be detrimental. Frequently, when people oversleep, they don't feel any better. The body and mind need only a certain amount of sleep for optimum functioning. More sleep than this can be counterproductive. Natural sleep patterns are interrupted and a person may feel groggy and sluggish throughout the day.

  No harm comes from watching a moderate amount of television as a diversion or distraction from the stressors of the day, but spending many hours in front of the television can prevent people from doing the important things in life. Other common activities that can become problematic when they are overdone include working, talking on the phone, surfing the Net, playing video games, or spending time with friends. Even leisure activities such as exercising, which normally would be stress-reducing, can become troublesome. Almost anything can be unhealthy if it is done in excess.

  How can we tell if we are overdoing something? As mentioned in an earlier chapter, our body and mind will give us feedback that indicates we are overdoing it. If we don't feel well after we are finished, if we are not living according to our highest values, if we are ignoring important things in life, if we feel uneasy or apathetic, we should see these signals as feedback that we are overdoing something. We need to look again at how much time or energy we should spend on that activity.

- *Attempt suicide.* The worst option for managing stress is suicide. Attempting suicide indicates that a person believes he or she has run out of options. Suicide eliminates the possibility for all other possibilities and devastates family members and friends. Something else always can be done even if it isn't immediately apparent.

  If you are considering suicide as a way to deal with your stress, get help. Even if you don't think anyone else could possibly assist you, every problem has an answer. Sometimes it requires the assistance of someone else to discover alternatives. Asking for help is not a sign of weakness. It is a sign of love—love of yourself. Even if you don't feel worthy of love, you are worth it. Don't permit suicide to be an option!

  There are many positive, healthy options for preventing and managing stress. Take control of your life so you don't let these unhealthy options take control of you. You deserve better.

Stress Management for LIFE—Planning for the Future

Now that you have completed the final chapter in your book, take the opportunity to focus on synthesizing your learning, reflecting on your growth, and planning how to implement what you have learned for a lifetime of better stress management and an improved quality of life. Your textbook is called *Stress Management for **Life*** with the intention that you can incorporate what you have learned for a lifetime of better stress management.

Throughout this book, you have learned a plethora of tools and techniques for stress management. You will each have your favorites. Some of you found prevention techniques, like applying the POPP formula or Living Above the Line, to be most helpful. Others of you found great meaning in prioritizing your values, keeping a gratitude journal, or committing Random Acts of Kindness. Few students miss the importance of understanding the power of how perceptions determine reality. Many students report that the time management and money management chapters help them take control and literally change their life. From the relaxation techniques, the favorites run the gamut from meditation to PMR to autogenics to guided imagery to yoga. The Power Nap and Restful Breathing are always popular choices.

You now have the knowledge, tools, skills, and abilities to take control of your life through the prevention and management of stress. The Stress Management Lab for this chapter will help you continue on the path to an improved quality of life. Enjoy the journey!

Conclusion

This chapter has presented many additional ways to reduce stress, including laughter, music, and many "little" things you can incorporate into your daily routine. The methods you choose are up to you, but feel confident that you now have a toolbox full of stress-relieving tools. Your personality and the situations in which you find yourself will determine which tools will work most effectively for you. With practice, the tools become sharper and more proficient at handling the stressors with which you are dealing. Reflecting on your learning and planning for your future stress management is the next important step.

LAB

24.1 Synthesis

PURPOSE This lab provides you with an opportunity to reflect on your learning and plan for your future. This assignment is the synthesis and analysis of what you have learned throughout the semester and your plan for incorporating your learning into your life.

Review:

Start by taking some time to review your work throughout the semester. Review the assignments you have completed, the relaxation exercises you have practiced, your journals, and the reading from your textbook. When you have completed this, write your response to the following questions:

1. What are the three most important things you have learned from this course and why? Give this some careful thought and include your rationale for the relevance of this learning to your life.

2. You practiced a variety of stress-reduction techniques throughout the semester. List the two that worked best for you and why you think each of these were effective for you. Are there specific reasons for which you would use each of these? If so, explain.

Planning:

Complete the Stress Management for Life Contract found at the Premium Website in Chapter 24 of your Student Activities Manual. You do not need to submit your contract, but when you have completed it, answer the following:

1. List your two stress management goals. Be specific about what you will do and write your goals in the SMART format (see Chapter 12 in your text for a review on writing SMART goals).

2. Explain what you will do to facilitate the accomplishment of your goals. What specific things will you do that will help you be successful?

3. What payoffs will you realize by fulfilling your goals?

Sharing:

Select one person whom you trust and whose input you value. Choose someone who will listen to you with an open mind and who will be honest in providing feedback. Share with that person the three most important things you learned this semester. Include what you have been working on in the course, including your major stressors, why you think your quality of life could improve if you managed stress better, some of the techniques you have used to prevent and manage stress and your plan for the future. Ask for their perspective on both your stressors and your plan. After you have talked with this person, write your response to the following questions:

1. Who did you talk to and why?

2. What input, advice, and observations did this person offer? What, if any, of this person's feedback was useful to you?

3. What did you learn from this sharing?

Key Points

- Laughter is stress-relieving and has a positive impact on health.
- Music can have a powerful stress-reducing effect.
- Music affects both the mind and body by its direct effect on cells and organs, and indirectly by affecting the emotions.
- Certain types of music, particularly classical and New Age, are especially effective for relaxation.

- A variety of simple strategies help release pent-up emotional and physical tension.
- Some ineffective options for dealing with stress should be avoided and can be dangerous.

Key Terms

humor
laughter
sarcasm
endorphins
music therapy

medical resonance therapy music
resonance
classical music
adagio movements
Mozart effect

New Age music
journaling
mindful writing

Discussion Time For Critical Thinking/Discussion Questions, please visit this book's Premium Website.

Notes

1. *Healing Beyond the Body: Medicine and the Infinite Reach of the Mind,* by L. Dossey (Boston: Shambhala, 2001).

2. *Mosby's Complementary & Alternative Medicine: A Research-Based Approach* (3rd. ed.), by L. Freeman (St. Louis: Mosby, 2009).

3. *Fundamentals of Complementary and Alternative Medicine,* by M. Micozzi (New York: Churchill Livingstone, 2001).

4. "The Laughter-Immune Connection: New Discoveries," by L. Berk, *Humor and Health Journal* 5(5) (1996): 1–7.

5. "Humor, Laughter, and Play: Maintaining Balance in a Serious World," by P. Wooten. In B. Dossey, C. Guzetta, and L. Keegan, (Eds.), *Holistic Nursing: A Handbook for Practice* (3rd ed.) (Gaithersburg, MD: Aspen Publishing, 2000).

6. "Jest 'n' Joy," by M. Baim and L. LaRoche. In H. Benson and E. Stuart, (Eds.), *The Wellness Book: A Comprehensive Guide to Maintaining Health and Treating Stress-Related Illness* (New York: Fireside, Simon & Schuster, 1993).

7. "Interaction of Humor and Gender in Moderating Relationships Between Stress and Outcomes," by M. Abel, *Journal of Psychology* 132(3) (1998).

8. "Transcending Circumstance: Seeking Holism at Auschwitz," by L. H. Freeman, *Holistic Nursing Practice* 16(5) (2002): 32.

9. *The Secret Power of Music,* by D. Tame (Northamptonshire, England: Turnstone Press, Ltd., 1984).

10. "Got Pain? Got the Blues? Try the MUSIC CURE," by S. Harrar, *Prevention* 51(8) (1999): 100.

11. "Effects of Music Listening on Depressed Women in Taiwan," by Y. Lai, *Issues in Mental Health Nursing* 20(3) (1999): 229.

12. "Plugged-in Preemies," by M. Munson and R. Iconis, *Prevention* 47(7) (1995): 42.

13. "A Comparison of Intra-Operative or Postoperative Exposure to Music—a Controlled Trial of the Effects on Postoperative Pain," by U. Nilsson, N. Rawal, and M. Unosson, *Anaesthesia* 58(7) (2003): 699.

14. "Issues and Innovations in Nursing Practice: Effect of Music on Chronic Osteoarthritis Pain in Older People," by R. McCaffrey and E. Freeman, *Journal of Advanced Nursing* 44(5) (2003): 517.

15. "Music for Surgery," by L. Rogers, *Advances: The Journal of Mind-Body Health* 11(3) (1995): 49.

16. "Using Music Techniques to Treat Adolescent Depression," by C. Hendricks, B. Robinson, L. Bradley, and K. Davis, *Journal of Humanistic Counseling, Education & Development* 38(1) (1999): 39.

17. "Music Therapy in Grief Resolution," by R. Bright, *Bulletin of the Menninger Clinic* 63(4) (Fall 1999).

18. "In the Key of Therapy," by T. O'Neill, *Report/Newsmagazine* (BC Edition), *28,* Issue 22 (11/19/2001).

19. O'Neill, "In the Key of Therapy."

20. http://www.mrtmusic.org

21. "Effects of ME Therapy Music on Patients with Psoriasis and Neurodermatitis—A Pilot Study," by I. Lazaroff and R. Shimshoni, *Integrative Physiological & Behavioral Science* 35(3) (2000): 189–198.

22. "Clinical Application of Medical Resonance Therapy Music in High-Risk Pregnancies, by V. N. Sidorenko, *Integrative Physiological & Behavioral Science* 35(3) (2000): 199–208.

23. *Superlearning,* by S. Ostrander, L. Schroeder, and N. Ostrander (New York: Dell Books, 1994).

24. *Music and Miracles,* by D. Campbell (Wheaton, IL: Theosophical Publishing House, 1992).

25. "The Prevalence of Daytime Napping and Its Relationship to Nighttime Sleep," by J. J. Pilcher, K. R. Michalowski, and R. D. Carrigan, *Behavioral Medicine* 27(2) (2001): 71.

26. "Effects of Writing About Stressful Experiences on Symptom Reduction in Patients with Asthma or Rheumatoid Arthritis: A Randomized Trial," by J. M. Smyth, A. A. Stone, A. Hurewitz, and A. Kaell, *Journal of the American Medical Association* 281(14) (1999): 1304–2309.

27. *If You Want to Write,* by B. Ueland (St. Paul, MN: Graywolf Press, 1987).

28. Ueland, *If You Want to Write,* p. 59.

29. *Tuesdays with Morrie,* by M. Albom (New York: Doubleday, 1997).

Glossary

A

ABCDE technique   Cognitive method that involves examining irrational beliefs that make us anxious, changing those beliefs, and envisioning more positive consequences of our actions.

ABC123 prioritized planning   Time management method designed to move from crisis management and "putting out fires" toward doing those things that are most important on a daily basis.

Abdominal breathing or diaphragmatic breathing   Inhaling in a way that causes the **diaphragm** to contract and move down, drawing air into the lungs.

Active progressive muscle relaxation   Dynamic form of progressive relaxation characterized by tightly tensing muscle groups and then relaxing them.

Acupressure   Therapy in which finger pressure is applied to points on the body thought to be areas of chi concentration; described as **acupuncture** without the needles.

Acupuncture   Therapy in which hair-thin, sterile needles are inserted into the body at specific points (acupoints) to manipulate the body's flow of energy and thereby create balance, relieve pain, or produce regional anesthesia.

Acute stress   Stress that results from short-term **stressors**.

Adagio movements   Baroque and early classical compositions with a tempo of about 60 beats per minute; suggested to aid in relaxation.

Adrenal cortex   Outer portion of **adrenal glands**.

Adrenal glands   Two triangle-shaped glands, one positioned on top of each kidney, from which stress hormones are secreted during the stress response.

Adrenal medulla   Inner portion of **adrenal glands**, where **epinephrine** and **norepinephrine** are secreted.

Affirmation   A statement written in the present tense as a positive "I" statement and applied to the clarifying paragraph that describes one's values.

Affluenza   Disease-like epidemic causing people in society to seek more and more material possessions, resulting in growing debt.

Agape   Unselfish love that gives of itself and expects nothing in return.

All-or-none principle   A muscle fiber contracts completely or not at all.

Alternating nostril breathing   Also known as balanced breathing, a technique that uses gentle occlusion of a nostril through a full breath, then switches to the other nostril, and continues back and forth.

Alternative medicine   Therapies that are used in place of conventional medicine.

Altruism   Helping or giving to others without thought of self-benefit.

Anger   A transient emotional response based on the way one chooses to think about events, usually triggered by perceived provocation or mistreatment.

Anorexia   Eating disorder characterized by self-starvation and excessive weight loss.

ANS   *See* Autonomic nervous system.

Antiplanning   Setting goals and being firm about where one wants to go, but at the same time being flexible on how to get there.

Anxiety   A heightened emotional state that is a psychological and physiological response to worry.

Appraisal support   Type of help that provides affirmation, feedback, and information for self-evaluation.

Aromatherapy   Therapeutic use of essential oils.

Asana   Postures or physical exercises of **yoga**.

Ashtanga yoga   Also known as power yoga; has more difficult poses than those in other yoga styles and requires moving from one pose to another in an effort to build strength, stamina, and flexibility.

Assertiveness   Standing up for one's personal rights and expressing thoughts, feelings, and beliefs in direct, honest, and appropriate ways that do not violate another person's rights.

Autobiographical listening   Listening from the perspective of one's own experience.

Autogenics   Self-directed relaxation technique using suggestions that focus on warmth and heaviness in the body.

Autogenic training   Method of reducing the stress response that uses suggestions focusing on warmth and heaviness; originated in Europe in the early years of the 20th century by the brain physiologist Oskar Vogt.

Autonomic nervous system (ANS)   Branch of the nervous system responsible for many functions in the body that occur involuntarily, such as digestion, heart rate, blood pressure, and body temperature.

Awfulizing   Mentally turning inconveniences or difficult situations into something awful, horrible, or terrible.

Ayurveda   India's traditional system of natural medicine holding that all aspects of life contribute to health, including nutrition, hygiene, sleep, weather, and lifestyle, as well as physical, mental, and sexual activities.

Bikram yoga   A style of yoga that is done in a room 90 to 105 degrees Fahrenheit; moves sequentially through 26 postures performed in a precise order.

Binge eating disorder   An eating disorder characterized primarily by periods of uncontrolled, impulsive, or continuous eating beyond the point of feeling comfortably full.

Bioelectromagnetic therapies   Treatments that involve the unconventional use of electromagnetic fields.

Biofeedback   A method that uses electronic devices to help a person develop voluntary control and consciously regulate autonomic activity, such as breathing, heart rate, muscle tension, skin temperature, and blood pressure, in order to improve overall health.

Biofield therapies   Treatments intended to affect energy fields that purportedly surround and penetrate the human body.

Body composition   Makeup of the body in terms of fat tissue in relation to lean body tissue (muscle, bone, organs).

Body scan   A form of **passive progressive relaxation** involving focused, concentrated, non-judgmental observation of the body.

Breath counting meditation   A type of meditation where one focuses directly on the breath as it comes in and goes back out while counting from 1 to 4.

Breathing meditation   A type of **meditation** that uses the breath as the primary focus.

Bruxism   Grinding, gnashing, or clenching the teeth during sleep or during situations that make one feel anxious or tense.

Budget   A plan to manage money in which the budgeter prioritizes spending to accomplish financial goals.

Bulimia   Eating disorder characterized by a secretive cycle of binge eating followed by purging.

CAM   *See* Complementary and alternative medicine.

Cardiorespiratory fitness   Ability of the heart, lungs, and blood vessels to process and transport oxygen required by muscle cells to meet the demands of prolonged physical activity.

Carotid pulse   Heart rate measured at the carotid artery on the neck just under the jaw.

Chair massage   A form of massage administered while the person receiving the massage is fully clothed and seated in a specially designed chair.

Chakra meditation   A form of **meditation** that uses the **chakras** as the primary focus.

Chakras   Energy centers in the body through which spiritual and emotional energies flow.

Chest breathing or thoracic breathing   Breathing that is relatively shallow, in which the chest expands and the shoulders rise as the lungs take in air.

Chi   Internal energy flow.

Chromotherapy   A discipline that uses colors to treat individuals who have certain specific disorders.

Chronic stress   Continuing stress provoked by unrelenting demands and pressures that go on for an extended time.

Classical music   Traditional genre of music that seems to be highly effective in reducing the stress response.

Cognition   Mental process that encompasses thinking and reasoning skills.

Cognitive appraisal   One's interpretation of a **stressor**.

Cognitive dissonance   A disparity or contradiction between one's behavior and beliefs, values, or self-image.

Cognitive distortion   Magnifying thoughts out of proportion to their seriousness, resulting in excess stress.

Cognitive restructuring   Changing the meaning or interpretation of **stressors**.

Cognitive therapy   Helping a person think in new ways by focusing on cognitive distortions and then relearning thought processes as a way to alter negative emotions.

Comfort zone   Any place, situation, relationship, or experience in which one does not feel any threat.

Command breathing   Technique designed to release distractions, tensions, and discomforts with each exhalation.

Complementary and alternative medicine (CAM)   A group of diverse medical and healthcare systems, practices, and products that presently are not considered to be part of conventional medicine.

Complementary medicine   Therapies that are used together with conventional medicine.

Conditioned response theory   Theory proposing that when things happen in our environment, we are conditioned to respond in certain ways.

Conflict   Expressed struggle between at least two independent parties who perceive incompatible goals, scarce rewards, and interference from the other party, in achieving their goals.

Connectedness   Feeling of relatedness or regard to others, a sense of relationship to all of life, a feeling of harmony with self and others, and a feeling of oneness with the universe and/or a universal element or Universal Being.

Contemplation   A form of **meditation** that uses a physical object as the primary focus.

Control   Deeply held belief that one can directly influence a situation.

Cortisol   One of the key stress hormones released from a portion of the **adrenal glands** called the **adrenal cortex**.

Craniosacral therapy   A gentle, hands-on method of enhancing the function of a physiological body system called the craniosacral system.

Culture   A pattern of learned behaviors based on values, beliefs, and perceptions of the world.

Decibels (dB)   A unit for measuring the intensity of sounds.

Deep tissue massage   Muscle compression with the heel of the hand, pads of the thumb, and even the elbow pressing deliberately along the grain of the muscle to release chronic tension in the body.

Detached observation   Observing without judgment or expectations.

Dharana   Concentration; being able to hold the mind on one object for a specified time.

Dharma   A Hindu principle that holds that finding one's place in the puzzle of life results in satisfaction and in feeling fulfilled, happy, and worthwhile in life.

Dhyana   The ability to concentrate on one thing (or nothing) indefinitely; **meditation**.

Diaphragm   Large, umbrella-shaped sheet of muscle that is attached to the rib cage and is integral to breathing.

Diencephalon   Central portion of the brain, responsible for regulating emotions, among other things.

Dietary Guidelines for Americans   Science-based advice to promote health and reduce risk for major chronic diseases through diet and physical activity.

Discomfort zone   A place where we do not naturally gravitate and usually try to avoid.

Distress   The negative effects of **stress** that drain us of energy and surpass our capacity to cope.

Distributed study   Spacing learning periods with rest periods between sessions.

Doodads   Expenses, often unnecessary or unexpected, that negatively affect a budget more than a person might think.

Dopamine   A chemical naturally produced by the body that makes us feel good and can help offset pain.

E

Ecospirituality   The personal relationship between an individual and the environment.

Effortless effort   Allowing directed action to happen without tension, based on an attitude of passive alertness.

Emotional freedom technique   An alternative medicine tool based on the theory that negative emotions are caused by disturbances in the body's energy field and that tapping on the meridian endpoints on the face and body while thinking of a negative emotion alters the energy field, restoring it to balance.

Emotional health   One of the five dimensions of health; involves the ability to understand feelings, accept limitations, and achieve emotional stability.

Emotional problems   In **rational emotive behavior therapy**, disturbances over which one has total control.

Emotional support   Help in building esteem and in providing comfort, love, trust, concern, and listening.

Empathic listening   Active listening, seeking to truly understand the other person before seeking to be understood.

Endorphins   Mood-elevating, pain-relieving chemicals produced naturally by the brain.

Environment   Everything both internal and external to an individual.

Environmental stressor   Some aspect of the environment that is perceived as annoying, distracting, uncomfortable, or stressful.

Epinephrine   Also known as adrenaline, a hormone secreted by the medulla (inner) portion of the **adrenal gland**, which (together with **norepinephrine**) brings about changes in the body known as the **fight-or-flight response**.

Episodic acute stress   Frequent bouts of **acute stress**.

Ergonomics   The study of individual workers and the tasks they perform, for the purpose of designing appropriate and safe living and working environments.

Eustress   Positive, desirable **stress** that keeps life interesting and helps to motivate and inspire.

External locus of control   A belief that whatever happens to one is unrelated to one's own behavior; what happens to a person is beyond his or her control.

F

Faith   Belief in, or commitment to, something or someone that helps a person realize a purpose. Faith is belief without proof.

Faith factor   The concept that explains that power is added when one combines the quieting effect of **meditation** with the power of one's beliefs.

Fear   Anxious or agitated feeling based on the perception of impending danger or threat.

Feng shui   Ancient Chinese study of the natural environment based on the belief that physical and emotional well-being is strongly influenced by the immediate environment.

Fight-or-flight   The body's automatic physiological response that prepares the individual to take action upon facing a perceived threat or danger.

Flexibility   Ability of the joints to move freely through a full range of motion.

Forgiveness   Psychological peace that comes when psychologically injured people release their grievances against others.

Full breathing   Technique that involves breathing in first to the abdomen and then slowly filling up the rest of the lungs while inhaling.

G

General adaptation syndrome   Process in which the body tries to adapt to chronic stress; consists of three stages—alarm, resistance, and exhaustion.

Glycemic index   A measure of foods, and how quickly they convert into blood sugar.

Going with the flow   Accepting situations one can't control.

Guilt   Conscious preoccupation with undesirable past thoughts and behaviors.

H

Hardiness   The term used to describe a combination of personality characteristics including the traits of commitment, challenge, and control.

Hassles   The irritating, frustrating, or distressing incidents that accompany everyday existence.

Hatha yoga   Collectively, **asanas** (postures or poses), **pranayamas** (breathing techniques), and **pratyahara** (meditation); designed to reduce stress and restore balance.

Healing environment   Surroundings in which one is supported and nurtured, in which one feels calm, and in which health and well-being are promoted.

Heat effect   The observed higher rates of aggression by people in hot environments compared to cooler environments.

Heat hypothesis   Theory holding that hot temperatures can promote aggressive motives and behaviors.

Holistic health   A view of health that encompasses physical, intellectual, emotional, spiritual, and social dimensions.

Homeostasis   The body's natural state of balance or stability.

Hostility   An attitude motivated by hatefulness and animosity.

Hot stone massage   Form of massage using stones that are heated and positioned on specific areas of the body.

Humor   An intellectual expression intended to induce **laughter**.

Hypnosis   A state of attentive, focused concentration with suspension of some peripheral awareness characterized by extreme suggestibility, relaxation, and heightened imagination.

Hypothalamus   Chief region of the brain for integrating **sympathetic** and **parasympathetic** activities from higher-order thinking.

I

Imagery   Flow of thoughts that incorporates sensory qualities from one or more of the senses.

Important   In time management terms, refers to those things that would make a long-term difference.

Inbreath   Physiological process of bringing air into the lungs.

Incremental muscle relaxation   Progressive relaxation exercise done by tensing muscle groups first maximally, then 50% of maximal, then 10% of maximal, holding each tense for 15 to 30 seconds followed by resting periods of 15 to 30 seconds between each tensing.

Informational support   A form of help consisting of intangible things such as giving advice, suggestions, and directives.

Instrumental support   A type of assistance that provides tangible things such as money, use of a car, or a place to stay.

Instrumental values   Values that consist primarily of personal characteristics and character traits that tend to lead toward **terminal values**.

Integrative medicine   Therapies that combine mainstream medical therapies and **complementary and alternative medicine** (CAM) therapies.

Integrity   The ability to carry out a worthy decision.

Intellectual health   One of the five dimensions of health, refers to the ability to think and learn from experiences, assess and question new information, and be open to new learning; also termed **mental health**.

Interleukins   Chemical messengers that enable **lymphocytes** to communicate with each other.

Internal locus of control   The belief that your own actions result in specific outcomes, that what you experience is based on your actions and efforts.

Iyashi   Japanese word denoting a combination of healing, calming, and getting close to nature.

Iyengar yoga   A classical style of **yoga** that is softer on the body than other forms; well-suited for beginners and those who haven't exercised in a while.

J

Journaling   A way of releasing emotions by writing down one's thoughts about them.

K

Karoshi   Japanese word meaning death by overwork.

Koyaanisqatsi   A Hopi Indian word meaning crazy life, life in turmoil, or life out of balance.

Kripalu yoga   A form of **yoga** that is more spontaneous, flowing, and meditation-orientated than other forms.

Kundalini yoga   A form of **yoga** that incorporates mantras (chanting), meditations, visualizations, and guided relaxation.

L

Latte factor   A metaphor referring to spending money on things, like daily lattes, that if cut back on or eliminated would make a significant difference in a budget but would not involve a significant lifestyle change.

Laughter   A vocal expression of amusement or good **humor**.

Learned optimism   The outcome of positive **self-talk** and **thought stopping**.

Learned response theory   Theory stating that when one associates a specific environment with something painful in that environment, the two get linked together.

Levels of responding   Ways by which people commonly react to situations, and the accompanying emotional consequences.

Lifebalance   A healthy time-management method that promotes purposeful planning combined with going with the flow.

Locus of control   The way we ascribe our chances of success or failure in a future venture to either internal or external causes.

Lo-pan   A special compass, used by practitioners of *feng shui*, designed to determine the energy characteristics of a building or room.

Lotus position   Sitting on the floor or a mat cross-legged with each foot resting on the opposite thigh.

Lymphocytes   White blood cells with the function of killing infectious agents.

M

Management   The art or manner of controlling.

Mantra   A repeated word, sound, or phrase as a point of focus during **meditation**.

Mantra meditation   A type of **meditation** that combines the four factors common to most meditation: (1) a mental device, (2) a passive attitude, (3) decreased muscle tone, and (4) a quiet environment.

Massed study   Time spent learning in concentrated, unbroken intervals.

Medical resonance therapy music   Music originally composed by German musicologist Peter Huebner, used as therapy and based on the principle of **resonance**.

Meditation   A conscious mental method of systematically allowing the mind to focus gently on a single item.

Melatonin   A sleep-related hormone that is secreted in increased levels in the dark.

Mental health   A dimension of health in which the mind is engaged in lively, healthy interaction both internally and with the surrounding world; also termed **intellectual health**.

Meridians   Invisible channels of energy that flow in the body.

Meta-analysis   A system of combining data from several different research studies to gain an overview of a topic that is more significant than a single investigation.

Mindful writing   Writing whatever comes to mind at the moment, to allow insights and inspiration from the intuition to bubble to the surface.

Mindfulness   The state of being attentive to, and aware of, what is taking place in the present.

Mindfulness-based stress reduction   A participatory wellness program based on mindfulness meditation, wherein participants are taught how to work with aspects of awareness.

Mindfulness self-efficacy   The level of confidence a person must have to maintain non-judgmental awareness.

Mindlessness   A state of mind in which one's thoughts are not in the present moment and when one tunes out what is happening here and now.

Monochromic time   Time seen as linear, things occur one at a time.

Motor unit   A single motor nerve and all the muscle fibers to which it sends impulses.

Mozart effect   Using the music of Mozart as a healing tool in therapeutic treatment.

Muscle contraction   Shortening of the muscle fibers.

Muscle endurance   Ability of muscles to function over time with support from the respiratory and circulatory systems.

Muscle fitness   A combination of muscle strength and endurance.

Muscle strength   The ability of skeletal muscles to engage in work; relates to the force a muscle can exert.

Music therapy   The practice of using music to heal.

Myocardial stunning   A unique medical condition in which severe emotional stress causes heart abnormalities, including heart failure.

Myotherapy   A form of massage characterized by concentrated pressure applied to the trigger points for a short time (several seconds to 2 or 3 minutes) by the fingers, knuckles, and elbows to reduce pain, relax muscle spasms, and improve circulation.

MyPyramid   The newest food guide pyramid that has replaced the original version.

N

Namaste   Translated, it says, "I honor the place in you where the entire universe resides. I honor the place in you, where lies your love, your light, your truth, and your beauty. I honor the place in you, where ... if you are in that place in you ... and I am in that place in me ... then there is only one of us."

Natural killer cells   Specialized cells that seek out and destroy foreign invaders in the body.

Naturopathic medicine   One of the oldest forms of medicine; combines the healing traditions of many cultures with modern principles to encompass the diagnosis, treatment, and prevention of disease, as well as the promotion of health.

New Age music   A genre of modern music characterized by a relaxing or peaceful quality based on quiet harmonies.

Niagara syndrome   The feeling, comparable to a mid-life crisis, that occurs when people don't take a good look at who they are and where they are going.

Niyama Yoga   Term for "observance," relating to purity, contentment, tolerance, study, and remembrance.

Nocebo effect   Sickness and death resulting from expectations of negative outcomes and from the associated emotional states.

Norepinephrine   Also known as noradrenalin, a hormone secreted by the medulla (inner) portion of the **adrenal gland**, which (together with **epinephrine**) brings about changes in the body known as the fight-or-flight response.

O

Optimists   Those who tend to see what is right and good about situations.

Outbreath   The physiological process of expelling air from the lungs.

P

Parasympathetic nervous system   Branch of the **autonomic nervous system** that returns the physiology to a state of **homeostasis**, or balance, after the threat, danger, or potential pain is no longer perceived to be imminent.

Pareto's law   A principle suggesting that in many activities, 80% of the potential value can be achieved from just 20% of the effort and the remaining 80% of effort results in relatively little return.

Passive progressive relaxation   A method of progressing through the various parts of the body that promotes relaxation using a focused observation technique called the **body scan**.

Perceived noisiness   Subjective assessment of noise that combines the decibel level and the context in which a noise occurs.

Perception   A person's cognitive (mental) interpretation of events.

Pessimism   A general attitude of assuming the worst.

Pessimists   Those who tend to see what is wrong and bad about situations.

Physical health   One of the five dimensions of health; involves the cells, tissues, organs, and systems functioning together in good working order.

Pineal gland   Gland in the brain that produces **melatonin**.

Placebo   A drug or treatment used as an inactive control in a test; although a placebo is believed to lack a specific effect, it often elicits a positive response because of the patient's expectation of benefits.

Placebo effect   A result created by the belief that one will benefit from an intervention.

Planning   The act of bringing future events into the present so appropriate control can be applied.

Polychromic time   Time seen as a natural rhythm in which several things can happen at once, and not controlled by human beings.

Power language   Speaking that boosts a feeling of control simply by changing the words used.

Power Nap   A means of relaxation that combines deep breathing, **mindfulness**, and **yoga** to relax and rejuvenate body and mind.

Practical problems   According to **rational emotive behavior therapy**, experiences over which the individual has little, if any, control.

***Prana* Yoga**   Term for energy that flows through the body.

Pranayama   Sanskrit term referring to control of breath: *prana* (life energy), and *ayam* (control); in yoga, breathing techniques.

Pratyahara   In preparation for **meditation**, withdrawal of the mind from the senses.

Premature cognitive commitments   Efforts to bring about results that coincide with one's self-limiting beliefs.

Procrastination   Avoidance of doing a needed task that needs to be accomplished.

Progressive muscle relaxation (PMR)   Muscle relaxation in which each muscle is forcibly contracted, then released in sequence. Another term for **progressive neuromuscular relaxation**.

Progressive neuromuscular relaxation (PNR)   Muscle relaxation in which each muscle is forcibly contracted, then released in sequence. Another term for **progressive muscle relaxation**.

Progressive relaxation   Another term for **progressive neuromuscular relaxation**.

Psychoneuroimmunology   Interactions among the nervous system, the psyche, and the immune system, and their implications for health.

Psychophysiological   Synonym for **psychosomatic**.

Psychosomatic   A descriptive term originating from the core words *psyche*, meaning the mind, and *soma*, meaning the body, and usually referring to conditions that have both a mind and body component.

Q

Qi gong   A Chinese therapy involving physical movement and breathing exercises designed to circulate the internal vital energy.

Quadrant Planning   Time management method focusing on activities with reference to importance and urgency, and putting "first things first."

R

Radial pulse   Heart rate measured at the radial artery on the thumb side of the wrist.

Rapid eye movement (REM) sleep   Sleep phase when dreaming occurs.

Rational emotive behavior therapy   Treatment based on the premise that stress-related behaviors are initiated by self-defeating perceptions that can be changed.

Reality   What is; what is happening.

Recommended Dietary Allowances (RDA)   The daily amount of a nutrient considered adequate to meet the known nutrient needs of almost 98% of all healthy people in the United States.

Reduce respirations technique   Breathing method designed to lower the breathing rate to between 10 and 12 breaths per minute and even slower.

Reference anxiety   State of mind that stems from people judging their possessions in comparison with others, not based on what they need.

Reflexology   Therapy based on a system of points in the hands and feet that are believed to correspond to areas of the body.

Reframing   Another term for **cognitive restructuring**.

Reiki   A healing technique that channels the universal life energy to recipients by the laying on of hands.

Relaxation   The process of effectively moving the mind/body from the stress response to the relaxation response.

Relaxation guided imagery   Technique designed to connect with the subconscious mind in a way that will activate the relaxation response by using the imagination in a directed way toward a specific image, scene, or sensation.

Religiosity   Extent of participation in, or adherence to, the beliefs and practices of an organized religion.

Resonance   Precise harmony contained in a musical structure that resonates inside the human body, from the ears to the brain and from the brain to various organs.

Respiration rate   Number of breaths taken in 1 minute.

Restful breathing   Technique designed to allow the breath to go as deep as possible into the lowest parts of the lungs.

Road rage   Aggressive and dangerous driving behaviors directed at other motorists.

Runaway eating   The consistent use of food and food-related behaviors—such as purging or exercising excessively—to deal with unpleasant feelings and the sense that these feelings are out of control.

S

Samadhi   Absorption; realization of the essential nature of the self.

Sarcasm   An element of **humor** that can be used as a form of aggression to put people down.

Seasonal affective disorder (SAD)   A condition characterized by depression related to lack of light in seasons with short days.

Self-efficacy   Belief in one's ability to accomplish a goal or change a behavior.

Self-limiting beliefs   Faulty notion that one does not have the ability to carry out specific tasks.

Self-talk   The messages one sends to oneself; internal dialogue.

Sensory overload   A cluttered mind that results from accumulating thoughts that compete for attention.

Serendipity   Quality that, through good fortune and sagacity, allows a person to discover something good while seeking something else.

Serotonin   A mood-enhancing chemical that the body produces naturally.

Shalom   A Hebrew term that means more than wellness or wholeness and can best be translated as "peace."

Shiatsu   Japanese-based therapy system that uses finger pressure applied to specific points along acupuncture meridians.

Simple diaphragmatic breathing   Technique that focuses on the in and out movement of the abdomen during inhalation and exhalation.

Sivananda yoga   A form of **yoga** that has a series of 12 poses and, as its foundation, the sun salutation, breathing exercises, relaxation, and mantra chanting.

SMART goals   Goals that are **S**pecific, **M**easurable, **A**ction-oriented, **R**ealistic, and **T**ime-based.

Social health   One of the five dimensions of health; refers to involvement with others and expressing care and concern for others.

Social support   An individual's knowledge or belief that he or she is cared for and loved, belongs to a network of communication, and has a mutual obligation with others in the network.

Spiritual   Refers to a belief in, and devotion to, a higher power beyond the physical realm.

Spiritual dimension   One of the five dimensions of health, an inner quality that goes beyond religious affiliation and strives for inspiration, reverence, awe, meaning, and purpose.

Spiritual health   The result of discovering a basic purpose in life and learning how to experience love, joy, peace, and fulfillment.

Spirituality   A means of giving meaning to existence, a sense of purpose in life, and a relationship or sense of connection with a higher power.

Sports massage   A special type of massage involving muscle systems specific to athletic participation.

Stream of consciousness   The constant flow of thoughts through the mind.

Stress   The physiological response that is activated when the mind perceives a threat.

Stressor   Any event or situation that an individual perceives as a threat; precipitates either adaptation or the stress response.

Suggestion   Statement that the mind believes is true, accurate, or real.

Sutoresu   Japanese word for stress.

Swedish massage   Massage, usually done with lotions or oils, consisting of long, gliding strokes, kneading, friction, tapping, and shaking motions on the upper or more superficial layers of the muscles; the most common type of basic relaxation massage.

Sympathetic nervous system   Branch of the **autonomic nervous system** (ANS) responsible for initiating the fight-or-flight response each time one perceives potential danger or pain.

T

Tai chi   A popular form of exercise in China that consists of a precise sequence of slow, graceful movements, accompanied by deep breathing and mental attention, to achieve balance between body and mind and to focus vital energy.

Technosis   A state of being so immersed in technology that one risks losing identity.

Technostress   Feelings of dependence, incompetence, anxiety, and frustration associated with technology.

Tend-and-befriend response   Theory proposing that females are more likely than males to respond to stressful circumstances by nurturing offspring to protect them from harm (tending), and befriending (creating and joining social groups to exchange resources and provide protection).

Terminal values   Outcomes that one works toward or believes are most important and desirable; end-states of feeling.

Therapeutic touch   Therapy based on the premise that the human body is surrounded by, and permeated with, an energy field that is connected with the universal life energy.

Thought stopping   Ceasing negative thoughts when they enter the **stream of consciousness**.

Thought-watching   Inner mindfulness **meditation** that uses one's random thoughts as the primary focus.

Time   The occurrence of events in sequence, one after another.

Time management   The art or manner of controlling the sequence of events in life.

Time zapper   Something that takes away time from what is more important.

Traditional Chinese medicine (TCM)   Therapies that involve a variety of carefully formulated techniques, such as **acupuncture**, herbal medicine, **massage**, **qi gong**, and nutrition.

Transcendental meditation (TM)   A type of **meditation** in which one goes into a meditative state by repeating a special, individualized **mantra**.

U

Ujjayi breathing   Method of breathing that has a soothing, rhythmic, oceanic quality and is commonly done while practicing yoga.

Unreality   What is not; what is not happening.

Urgent   Describes things that demand our immediate attention.

V

Value   A belief upon which one acts by preference.

Values acquisition   The conscious assumption of a new **value**.

Values clarification   The process of defining and applying what one truly values.

Vasodilation   Increase in the diameter of blood vessels in response to activation of the **parasympathetic nervous system**.

Vipassana   Literally, "seeing clearly."

Visualization   Using the imagination to picture or see a place or thing.

Visualization breathing   Breathing technique that combines **full breathing** with visualization.

W

Walking meditation   A form of meditation in which physical movement is the primary focus.

White noise   The soft sounds of nature, such as running water or rainfall, or soft music that is used to help drown out other sounds that may be distracting and stressful.

Worry   Conscious preoccupation with events yet to come.

Y

Yama   Yoga term for "restraint," relating to refraining from violence, lying, stealing, casual sex, and hoarding.

Yerkes–Dodson principle   A tenet holding that a certain amount of stress is healthy, useful, and even beneficial, but when stress exceeds one's ability to cope, the overload contributes to diminished performance, inefficiency, and even health problems.

Yoga   A course of exercises and postures intended to promote control of the body and mind and to attain physical and spiritual well-being.

Yoga sutras   A collection of yoga theories and practices assembled by the Indian sage Patanjali.

Index